Study Guide

for

Pharmacology and the Nursing Process

Fifth Edition

Linda Lane Lilley, RN, PhD
Scott Harrington, PharmD
Julie S. Snyder, MSN, RN, BC

Study Guide prepared by
Julie S. Snyder, MSN, RN, BC
Adjunct Faculty
School of Nursing
Old Dominion University
Norfolk, Virginia

With special thanks to
Linda K. Wendling
for her contribution to the first edition

Study Skills by
Diane Savoca
Coordinator of Student Transition
St. Louis Community College at Florissant Valley
St. Louis, Missouri

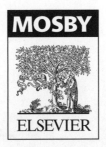

MOSBY

ELSEVIER

11830 Westline Industrial Drive
St. Louis, MO 63146

STUDY GUIDE FOR PHARMACOLOGY AND THE NURSING
PROCESS, FIFTH EDITION

ISBN: 978-0-323-04489-9

Notice

Knowledge and best practice in this field are constantly changing. As new research and experience broaden our knowledge, changes in practice, treatment and drug therapy may become necessary or appropriate. Readers are advised to check the most current information provided (i) on procedures featured or (ii) by the manufacturer of each product to be administered, to verify the recommended dose or formula, the method and duration of administration, and contraindications. It is the responsibility of the practitioner, relying on their own experience and knowledge of the patient, to make diagnoses, to determine dosages and the best treatment for each individual patient, and to take all appropriate safety precautions. To the fullest extent of the law, neither the Publisher nor the Authors assumes any liability for any injury and/or damage to persons or property arising out or related to any use of the material contained in this book.

The Publisher

Previous editions copyrighted 2004, 2002, 1999, and 1996.

ISBN: 978-0-323-04489-9

Acquisitions Editor: Kristin Geen
Developmental Editor: Jamie Horn
Publishing Services Manager: Jeff Patterson
Senior Project Manager: Clay S. Broeker
Cover Design Direction: Paula Ruckenbrod

Printed in the United States of America

Last digit is the print number: 9 8 7 6 5 4 3 2

Contents

Student Study Tips

CHOOSE TO MANAGE YOUR TIME

Time and money have much in common. They can be spent, saved, invested, given away, stolen, and wasted. The big difference between these two commodities is that you can earn more money. Your time is limited. Learn to mange your time now and the quality of your life will increase because you will have more time to do what you enjoy.

You may not enjoy studying. What you want is to be a nurse, and studying is one choice that will get you what you want. Being a nurse will bring you the satisfaction that you need. I, for one, am very thankful that you have made this decision. The world needs dedicated skilled nurses. To meet this need you must make the decision to manage your time effectively.

Establish Goals and Create Action Plans

One key to time management is having clear goals and an action plan to accomplish these goals. This is more than saying, "I want to be a nurse" or "I want to ace my pharmacology midterm." It is a decision to spend time now to get clarity and direction so that you will have more time later to relax. The following guidelines can help you get what you want.

Guidelines for Setting Goals

There are some basic guidelines to follow when setting goals:
- **Be realistic.** The goal must be something that you can reasonably expect to accomplish. A goal of scoring 100% on each and every unit test is not realistic, but a goal of scoring 85% or better is.
- **Be specific.** Goals must set out exactly what needs to be done. Do not simply state, "I will study for the exam." Specify how many hours, what days, and what times you will study. The more specific the goal statement, the easier it is to establish a plan, complete that plan, and thus achieve the goal set.
- **Establish a time limit.** Specify a time limit for completing each step in the plan and an overall deadline for accomplishing the goal.
- **Make the goal and actions measurable.** State the goal and each step in the plan for achieving it in a way that will enable you to measure your progress toward completion.

The following is an example of how this goal and action process works: You have a chapter test a week from today. The test will cover approximately 45 pages of text material, and there are 40 specific pharmacologic terms you must know. In addition, you have been given about 20 pages of supplementary handouts in class. What will you do in the next 7 days to prepare for this test?

Goal Statement:
I will study to make a good grade on this exam.
This is a poor goal statement because it is not specific, sets no time limits, and offers no real way to measure progress. The intent is good, but the implementation of such a vague goal is usually poor.

Revision 1:
I will spend 2 hours a day studying for the next chapter test in order to get at least an 80% score.
This is a better goal statement. If one assumes that 2 hours per day is realistic, then the goal is more specific, the grade goal is measurable, and there is a time limit of sorts. This goal statement might be good enough, but it could still be improved.

Final Version:
I will spend 2 hours per day, from 2:30 to 4:30 PM, for the next 7 days studying for the chapter test in order to score at least 80%.
This is what is needed. This version states how much time, when, how many days, and for what purpose. Setting clear goals helps you get started and serves as a motivator to keep you working.

Guidelines for Action Statements

A goal, no matter how well stated, is not enough. There must be action statements to help you make day-to-day progress toward meeting the goal. The guidelines that apply to defining your goal also apply to establishing the action statements—they should be realistic, specific, measurable, and time limited. They spell out what is going to be done day to day. Here are three examples of good action statements for the sample goal:

- I will master six pharmacology terms each day.
- I will spend from 2:30 to 3:00 PM each day reviewing class handouts.
- I will review 10 pages of text material from 3:00 to 4:00 PM each day.

These examples should give you a good idea of how to go about developing a clear goal and a set of actions to carry out to achieve that goal.

Organize Tasks and Create Schedules

It takes time to make time. It is your choice. Either you set your schedule or others will do it for you. It is 2:30 PM. The phone rings and friends want you to go out or your boss wants you to work overtime or your sister wants you to watch the kids. When you have an action plan and a schedule, your choices are clear. This is the time you scheduled to review class handouts. Can you reschedule this review or do you want to keep this promise you have made to yourself to accomplish your goal? No matter what you decide, you have maintained control over your time.

Your goals and action plans are the foundation for your time management. The next key is to organize tasks and create schedules.

Guidelines for Organizing Tasks

1. Divide tasks into three categories:
   a. Jobs that **have to be done,** such as going to class, going to work, eating, and getting adequate rest. These jobs are the easiest to accomplish because the consequences of not doing them are serious. If you do not go to class, failure is almost a sure thing. If you do not go to work, soon there will be no paycheck. The consequences of not eating or sleeping are obvious.
   b. Jobs that **should be done,** such as studying, paying bills, cleaning the house, and all of those other necessary but unpleasant tasks that are part of life. The "should-be-done" jobs are the most difficult to accomplish because they are the jobs that are all too easy to put off doing. These are also the jobs for which time management skills are most essential.
   c. Things that you **want to do.** These include all of the fun things that provide pleasure and escape from the routines of class, study, and work. Most of us are very successful at finding time to do what we want to do, even when there is a sizable backlog of "should-be-done" chores waiting. This choice can lead to procrastination and stress. The important things are maintaining balance and staying focused on your goals.

2. Prioritize items in your **"have-to-be-done" category** based on your physical and mental health needs. Examine the consequences of not doing these activities. If you can live without doing an activity, then it is not a need.

3. Prioritize your **"should-be-done" category** based on your physical and mental health needs. Examine the consequences of not doing these activities. Can you accomplish your established goals without doing a given activity? If so, then it is not a need.

4. Prioritize your **"want-to-do" category.** Some recreational time is absolutely essential in any effective time management system. "Want-to-do" activities can often be used as incentives for completing what should be done.

5. Use incentives to accomplish what you should do. For each person the rewards will be different. Spend a little time determining what will work for you. It might be watching your favorite reality show, prime time drama, or comedy show; going to the movie theater to see a new release; reading a book for pleasure; or just spending some time with family or friends.

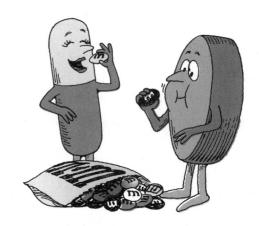

Guidelines for Creating Workable Schedules

You will need three types of schedule: **master, weekly, and daily.**

Start by developing a **master schedule** table on your computer that has seven columns and 15 to 17 rows. The columns are the days in the week and the rows are the hours in the day. The left-hand column will represent Sunday and the far right will be Saturday. Start at the top of each column with the time you usually get up in the morning and end each column with the time you usually go to bed. A typical master schedule might begin at 6 AM and end at 11 PM.

Once the blank schedule sheet is prepared, the next step is to fill in those hours that correspond to the activities

	SUN	MON	TUES	WED	THUR	FRI	SAT
7:00		GET UP		GET UP		GET UP	
8:00		TRAVEL		TRAVEL		TRAVEL	
9:00	GET UP	CLASS		CLASS		CLASS	
10:00	CHURCH	CLASS	TRAVEL	CLASS	TRAVEL	CLASS	
11:00	CHURCH		PRACTICUM		PRACTICUM		
12:00		CLASS	PRACTICUM	CLASS	PRACTICUM		
1:00			PRACTICUM		PRACTICUM		
2:00		PERSONAL	PRACTICUM		PRACTICUM		
3:00		PERSONAL					
4:00		AEROBICS		AEROBICS		AEROBICS	
5:00							
6:00		DINNER	DINNER	DINNER	DINNER	DINNER	
7:00							FUN
8:00							FUN
9:00							FUN
10:00							FUN
11:00	BEDTIME	BEDTIME	BEDTIME	BEDTIME	BEDTIME	BEDTIME	FUN

▼ **FIGURE 1-1.** The master schedule. This is an essential first step in managing time effectively.

you have to do. These are the hours others control, and the activities are those that occur at the same hour, on the same day or days, and for several weeks or longer. For example, the semester's schedule of classes is the first set of activities to enter into the master schedule. Other activities such as work, travel, worship services, and any other regular activities also belong in the master schedule.

The master schedule should contain only those recurring activities that cannot be done at any other time. Activities such as doing the laundry, watching television, and shopping should not be included, because the time when you do them is more flexible. The idea behind compiling the master schedule is to establish those times of the day that are "spent" and therefore cannot be used for any other activities. The empty blocks that remain represent the time you have to do everything else. Figure 1-1 shows a sample master schedule.

Creating a master schedule takes no more than a half-hour, and it will generally serve you for an entire semester. The only reason to compile a new master schedule is that a significant schedule change has occurred. You may get a new work assignment or your nursing practicum site may change and require an additional 15 or 20 minutes of travel time. Then a new master schedule should be drawn up to accommodate the increase in time that is now necessary. Once the master schedule is completed, make four or five copies of it. These copies will be used to prepare the detailed weekly schedule.

Next, move on to developing your **weekly schedule.** The master schedule helps you identify the time you have available to complete the **"should-be-done"** and **"want-to-do"** task lists. The weekly schedule is more complex. It is intended to help you plan for study, recreation, family time, and all those other activities that you want to fit into a typical week. To prepare the detailed weekly schedule, take one of the copies you made of the master schedule and begin to fill in activities in the open blocks of time. The first blocks of time you should assign are the most important ones for any student—study time. This is what time management is all about—scheduling the needed hours of study (Figure 1-2).

When filling in study hours, consider these important factors:

■ **Amount of planned study time.** There is an old rule pertaining to study time, and even though it is an old rule, it is still a very good guideline. The rule is to plan 2 hours of study time for each 1 hour spent in class. For example, a three-credit-hour course meets 3 hours per week, so you need to plan 6 hours of study time per week for this course. Remember, this is a general rule. Some courses will not actually require as much time as you allot, whereas others will require more. The reason for beginning a semester with this approach is simple. It is easy to find things to do with time you do not need for study, but once a semester is under way it can be very difficult to find additional study time. If you do not plan enough study time at the beginning, you will soon find yourself in a constant battle to keep up. The result is frustration, anxiety, and a sense of impending doom—feelings

	SUN	MON	TUES	WED	THUR	FRI	SAT
7:00		GET UP		GET UP		GET UP	
8:00		TRAVEL		TRAVEL		TRAVEL	
9:00	GET UP	CLASS	*STUDY*	CLASS	*STUDY*	CLASS	
10:00	CHURCH	CLASS	TRAVEL	CLASS	TRAVEL	CLASS	*STUDY*
11:00	CHURCH	*LUNCH*	PRACTICUM	*LUNCH*	PRACTICUM	*LUNCH*	STUDY
12:00		CLASS	PRACTICUM	CLASS	PRACTICUM		PERSONAL
1:00		*STUDY*	PRACTICUM	*STUDY*	PRACTICUM	*STUDY*	PERSONAL
2:00	*FREE*	*STUDY*	PRACTICUM	*STUDY*	PRACTICUM	*STUDY*	PERSONAL
3:00			*TRAVEL*		*TRAVEL*		.
4:00		AEROBICS		AEROBICS		AEROBICS	
5:00							
6:00		DINNER	DINNER	DINNER	DINNER	DINNER	
7:00	*STUDY*	STUDY	*STUDY*	STUDY	*STUDY*	STUDY	FUN
8:00	*STUDY*		*STUDY*		*STUDY*		FUN
9:00	*STUDY*	*REVIEW*	*REVIEW*	*REVIEW*	*REVIEW*		FUN
10:00							FUN
11:00	BEDTIME	BEDTIME	BEDTIME	BEDTIME	BEDTIME	BEDTIME	FUN

▼ **FIGURE 1-2.** The detailed weekly schedule. Study times should be filled in first.

you do not need when you want to perform at your very best.

- **Personal prime time.** Do you wake up early, ready to charge forward, but find it difficult to be productive after 10 PM? Do you do your best work in the afternoon and early evening and prefer to sleep until 10 AM? Are you a night owl? Answers to these questions will reveal your prime time, those times of the day when your ability to concentrate is at its best and you can accomplish the most. These are the times you want to use for study. It is not always possible, because of class and work schedules, to schedule all study time in your prime hours, but it is essential that those hours be used for study as much as possible. It would be foolish to plan to study your toughest material between 9 and 11 PM when you know that is a time when just reading the daily paper is a challenge.
- **Study hours for specific courses and general study hours.** The reason for scheduling both general and specific study times is that the study demands of different courses vary from day to day and week to week. For instance, you will need some hours of study every week to master new material, terms, and concepts in pharmacology, but the study time demands will increase in the days just before exams, midterms, and project due dates. The hours set aside for specific courses are for accomplishing

the day-to-day study demands; the unassigned study hours are for meeting the changing demands posed by these special circumstances. These unassigned study hours also let you meet unexpected demands. No matter how carefully you plan your time, something will happen to prevent you from using the time block you had set aside for learning.

Be patient and evaluate what works for you. It usually takes two or three attempts over a period of 3 weeks to arrive at a detailed schedule that works well for you. There is a tendency on the first attempt to try to schedule some important activity for every waking hour. Ultimately such a schedule will make you feel as though there is no time for fun. Determine what is not working for you and make appropriate adjustments. Each week your schedule will come closer to being realistic and effective. The need to evaluate and revise is the reason for making several copies of the master schedule. Or you may want to use an electronic calendar. It saves time in the revision process, and saving time is, after all, what time management is all about.

Your last scheduling activity is to create **daily schedules and lists.** No matter how carefully and thoughtfully you prepare the detailed weekly schedule, it cannot include all the tasks you will face. You will have small tasks, infrequent tasks, and unexpected tasks that will need to be added to your schedule. Each day as you think of things you want or need to do the next day, write them down. Carry a small notebook that will fit into a pocket or purse. Many cell phones have a list and/or calendar feature. Once a day, review the list and set priorities for the next day.

Consider the following when setting priorities:

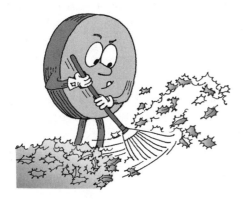

- **There are only 24 hours in each day.** Be realistic about what you are able to accomplish. Do not plan to review three chapters of text material on a day when you know there will not be enough time to cover more than half of one chapter.
- **Everything is not important.** Rank your tasks as A, B, or C, with A being the most important and C being the least important. Then go about completing your As. Procrastinating about your B and C lists is not a sin. For example, going to the dry cleaners is critical if the outfit you must wear tomorrow is there, but if you do not absolutely have to have that outfit tomorrow, then the trip to the cleaners is a low priority and can be postponed to another day. Then it will be on your A list.
- **Rewriting to-do lists can steal your time.** You may want to make one weekly list and mark the tasks as A, B, or C. Put only A tasks on your daily to-do list. If you have extra time you can look at your weekly list. Or you can keep your tasks on note cards and then each day stack them in priority order.
- **Planning your route can save you time.** Look at the small tasks listed, such as picking up milk and dog food, dropping off dry cleaning, and going to the bank. Not only plan to do those errands but also think about the order in which they should be done. Planning your route so that it completes a circle from home to the cleaners to the grocery store to home will be much more time efficient than going from home to the grocery store, back home, then to the cleaners, and finally back home again.
- **As you complete a job on the daily list, cross it off.** Crossing it off tells you that you are making progress and motivates you to move to the next item on the list. If not every item is crossed off, remember that tomorrow is another day. Celebrate what you did get done and create a plan for tomorrow that will help you accomplish your goals.

- **Remember your goals and planned action steps.** When unexpected daily tasks push them onto the B list, be sure to revise your plan to get back onto your time line. Put planning on your A list.
- **Waiting time can be a gift.** Small blocks of time are often lost or wasted because it does not seem as though anything significant could be accomplished during them. If you learn to use these small blocks effectively, you can free up larger blocks for more time-consuming or fun tasks. If a class ends 10 minutes early or if you are waiting for your ride, use the time for study. Take advantage of such "found" time to review five vocabulary terms, rework a set of class notes, or preview the next five pages of assigned reading. Using the odd minutes in the day to your advantage can really help you achieve your goals as a student.

Your time is a valuable resource for you to manage or to waste. The choice is yours. Stop for a few minutes and think over the previous strategies on how to manage your time: establishing goals and creating action plans, organizing tasks, and creating schedules. Which of these strategies will you choose to apply?

CHOOSE TO USE YOUR RESOURCES

This Study Guide is one of the resources that will help you be successful in this course. When you choose to apply these study tips, they will help you to be successful in all of your course work. Three other resources are your textbook, your instructor, and your classmates.

Your Textbook

The authors of your textbook have taken great care in organizing the information provided in a manner that will assist your learning. Each part starts with study skills tips that build on the tips that are presented in the Study Guide. At the beginning of each chapter, you will find specific objectives describing what you are expected to know and be able to do as a result of studying each chapter. Each chapter also contains learning activities and a glossary of terms. Take 10 minutes right now to perform a survey of your textbook so that you know what to expect over the term of this course. Look for chapter titles and Points to Remember. Later in this Study Guide you will find tips for mastering your textbook.

Your Instructor

Some students look at their instructor in awe. She or he is so smart and has so much experience. This is true, but he or she is also a teacher who cares about pharmacology and your learning. Your instructor wants to hear your questions because this demonstrates that you are interested in learning and you are actively engaged with the material in your textbook and lectures. The instructor is an expert on the content and the type of tests that will be given in the class. Ask questions about what will be covered on a test and the type of questions you can expect. Office hours are designed to make your instructor available to you. Choose to get your money's worth and use them!

Your Classmates

We all have different learning styles, strengths, and perspectives on the course material. Participating in a study group can be a valuable addition to your nursing school experience. These groups can be a fun way to learn. Teaching others helps us to learn and aids in organizing the course material. A study group is made up of students who are in the same class and who want to learn by discussing the course material. There are guidelines for organizing successful study groups.

1. Carefully **select members** for your group.
   - Choose students who have **abilities and motivation** similar to your own. Socializing and gossiping can eat up valuable study time. Noncommitted and underprepared classmates can be a drain.
   - Look for students who have a **common time to meet.**
   - Select classmates who have **different learning styles** from yours. They might understand the reading material or lecture material better than you. They may be able to draw a diagram that will help your learning.
   - Find students who have good communication skills—people who know how to listen, ask good questions, and explain concepts.

2. Clarify the **group's purpose and expectations.**
   - Where and when will you meet?
   - How often will you meet? How long will the meetings be?
   - How much individual preparation between meetings is expected?
   - Can family members, children, or other students come to the meetings?

3. **Exchange names, phone numbers, addresses, and E-mail addresses.** Have a plan in case of emergencies.

4. **Plan an agenda** for each meeting.
   - Put the date and goal for the session on the top.
   - List the activities that will help you accomplish the goal.
   - At the end of the study session, list the results of your efforts and set the date and time for your next session.
   - Make assignments for the next session.

There are also some useful strategies to follow:

1. Exchange lecture notes and discuss content for clarity and completeness.

2. Divide up difficult reading material and develop a lesson to teach the information to each other.

3. Quiz each other by turning objectives at the beginning of each chapter into questions.

4. Use the Critical Thinking and Application and Case Study sections in this Study Guide as a basis for discussions.

5. Create and take your own practice tests. Discuss the results.

6. Develop flash cards that review key vocabulary terms.
   This list could go on and on. Work with your group to design the strategy that works for you. Each study group you work with will be different.

Often in career programs like those in nursing, medical, and law schools, the course study group will turn into a learning group. **Learning groups may meet over several semesters even when the members are not taking the same classes.** Learning groups help you to prepare for licensing examinations, laboratory work, clinics, or practicum experiences. They focus on understanding and application in the field.

CHOOSE TO DEVELOP YOUR VOCABULARY

Participating in study groups and learning groups is an asset when you are working to develop a new vocabulary. Every specialty or discipline has its own language that must be learned for full mastery to occur. When you learn vocabulary with a group, you can hear others using the terms and they start to become real to you. Courses such as this one on pharmacology contain extremely complex material, and terminology is a major component of that complexity. As you learn to integrate this vocabulary into your discussions of the discipline, it will seem less like a foreign language. In technologic, scientific, and medical areas, mastering the vocabulary can make the difference between being successful and struggling constantly to understand the ideas and concepts being presented. It is therefore helpful to adopt some strategies that can make the process of vocabulary development easier and more effective. Working with a study group is one strategy, but there are several more.

Use Dictionaries

You must have a good current desk reference dictionary. *Current* means the most recent edition of whatever dictionary you choose. A dictionary published 10 or 15 years ago may contain most of what you need, but unless there have been periodic revisions, as shown on the copyright page, it is almost certain to lack some information, and this may cause you problems. A desk reference dictionary is a hard-bound dictionary and not a condensed or paperback version. Paperbacks are convenient to carry around, but to get the dictionary to this convenient size, some words have been omitted and some definitions have been shortened. This is not what you want. You need the most complete and current edition you can find and afford.

You may or may not need a medical dictionary. You will probably have access to one or more at your college or departmental library. The best way to decide whether you need to invest in such a specialized dictionary is to ask your instructor for his or her advice.

Reference the Text Glossary

As soon as you look at any of the chapters in this text, you will discover the glossary. A glossary is nothing more than a text-specific dictionary. It contains the terms and definitions the authors consider essential for a full understanding of the material. The glossary will not necessarily contain every term that is unfamiliar to you. (This is why you need a good dictionary.) You can begin the process of mastering vocabulary by paying particular attention to the glossary and key terms.

Create Flash Cards

Obtain a supply of note cards. Pick the size that best accommodates your handwriting style and size. If 5″ × 7″ cards do not fit into your notebook, pocketbook, or book bag and this discourages you from carrying them around with you, then use 3″ × 5″ cards. Remember, the flash cards these become are one of the best things you can study on the run.

Use What You Know

When you encounter an unfamiliar word, do not automatically assume that you have no idea what it means. Use the knowledge you have already acquired in other nursing courses and throughout your life.

For instance, *psychotherapeutic* appears in the chapter title for Chapter 15. Your first reaction may be that you do not know what this term means. By using what you know, however, you may be able to make an educated guess as to the meaning of the word without consulting either the text glossary or a dictionary.

This is how you make that educated guess. Consider that the first part of the word is *psycho*. By this point in your career as a student, you know that *psycho* refers to the mind. This is a good start. Now consider the next part of the word. The meaning of *therapeutic* may or may not be evident to you, but it should remind

you of a simpler word, *therapy,* which is the treatment used to cure or alleviate an illness or condition. Put *mind* and *treatment* together, and it would seem that *psychotherapeutic* must refer to the treatment of mental problems.

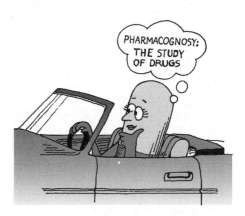

Note that this is an educated guess. It may not be a perfect definition, but it will give you a basis for acquiring a fuller understanding when the term is defined in the glossary or introduced and defined in the text of the chapter. The first sentence in Chapter 15 confirms that this educated guess is very close to the actual meaning: "The treatment of emotional and mental disorders is called *psychotherapeutics.*" Using this approach to analyzing the meaning of a word not only confirms that you have a basic understanding of the word but also cultivates a mental link between what you know and the more specific definition provided in the text. Words and their meanings learned in this way are usually easier to grasp and easier to retain. Unfortunately, this technique will not work with some of the terms used in pharmacology because they are so specialized and specific to the field. This calls for the use of other techniques.

Learn the Standard Abbreviations

Make sure as you read that you pay attention to the "shorthand" used. For example, in Chapter 12, the abbreviation *CNS* is used repeatedly. The first time it is presented, the author identifies it as standing for *central nervous system* by putting the abbreviation in parentheses after the term. Thereafter, the abbreviation is used in lieu of the long term. The same thing is done for *REM* in this chapter. It is essential that you learn these abbreviations and recall each, not as a set of meaningless letters but as a key term that must be mastered.

Establish Relationships

REM is an abbreviation for *rapid eye movements,* and this term refers to a particular stage of sleep. Chapter 12 deals with CNS depressants. Relating REM to the focus of this chapter will help you remember that

CNS depressants are used to influence sleep. The idea is to establish a clear relationship between the terms used and the ideas presented. Words should not be learned in isolation from the material; otherwise, you may know a lot of words and their meanings but not be able to relate them to ideas and content. *On tests, you are not likely to be asked just to repeat memorized definitions.* Instead, you will be asked to integrate these meanings into your answers to questions about nursing practices and applications.

Another important way of relating words to meanings is to link the meanings of closely related terms. The words *hypnotic* and *sedative* are good examples of this. In looking at the meanings in the glossary, you will find that each refers to a certain class of drugs. Both classes of drugs influence the CNS, but the drugs in each have a somewhat different effect. It is useful to start with the understanding that both affect the CNS but then to appreciate how the terms relate to each other. Sedatives inhibit the CNS but do not cause sleep; hypnotics at low dosages have the same effect, but at higher dosages they may induce sleep. In this learning method, you learn meanings by looking at the general similarities and then at the specific differences between terms. In doing this, you have learned both words and should never have any problems relating the words to their meanings.

CHOOSE TO TAKE EFFECTIVE LECTURE NOTES

Why Take Notes?

The primary reason for taking notes is to help your memory. It is impossible to remember everything that is said during a 1- to 2-hour lecture. The very act of writing something down helps strengthen learning and memory. In addition, note taking helps to focus attention on the lecture. It is very easy to take mental vacations during a lecture; note taking helps keep you involved.

Note-Taking Problems

1. **Selectivity** is the biggest challenge. How do you know what is really important?

2. **Unfamiliar vocabulary** causes confusion. This is particularly true in a course heavy in technical, medical, and pharmaceutical terminology such as this one.

3. Hard-to-read or even **illegible handwriting** is frustrating.

4. It is **difficult to listen and write at the same time.** It splits one's focus and often gets in the way of understanding.

Note-Taking Solutions

1. Realize that note takers are made, not born. You can learn to be more effective as both a note taker and note user, but **this requires some practice** and a willingness to adopt new techniques.

2. **Use the vocabulary development** strategies previously discussed so that you will have a better understanding of the lecture material.

3. **Note taking is a five-stage process** that is spread out over the days and weeks between lectures and the time when you are reviewing your notes in preparation for a test.

Stage 1: Be Prepared

Note taking begins before the lecture. Read assigned material before class. This provides you with the background needed to listen intelligently to the lecture and to be selective when taking notes. You will have less unfamiliar vocabulary. The lecture will bring the textbook content to life for you.

Go to class a few minutes early and review your notes from the previous lecture. This will help warm up your brain so it will be ready to receive new information.

Stage 2: Active Listening

Taking quality class notes requires active listening. This is one of the most challenging aspects of being a good note taker. It requires an awareness of both the lecturer's language and his or her nonverbal style. You have to pay attention not only to what is said, the verbal aspect, but also to the visual, nonverbal, aspect of the presentation.

Active listening requires selectivity. If you spend the lecture time trying to write down every word, you will not be able to listen to and therefore grasp the ideas. Focus on the most important ideas, terms, and facts to be recorded for later review. Writing less and listening more is a good rule to follow for note taking.

Learn to listen for key words and phrases. These vary with the subject content and with the individual lecturer, so there is no way to provide a single, definitive list of them. However, there are some verbal signals (words) that will give you clues that the lecturer is about to give important information:

- Sequence words—*first, second, next, then, last, finally*
- Contrast words—*but, however, on the other hand*
- Importance words—*significant, key, main, main point, most important*

The use of words and phrases such as these is the lecturer's way of signaling the relative importance and progression of certain facts and ideas. As important as these words are, however, it is also necessary to be aware of the volume, tone, and pace of delivery. Some instructors will slow down or repeat ideas that are important. Other instructors may speak louder and point into the air to emphasize a point. Get to know your instructor's style and you will be able to anticipate what will be on the test. Of course, if the instructor says, "One of the most important drugs in the treatment of …," then you should immediately know that what follows is an important point for your notes. The instructor has even told you it is important. As you practice active listening and observing in the lecture environment, you will find that your ability to discern the important ideas will improve.

Stages 1 and 2 are preparation for the real work that goes on in the last three stages.

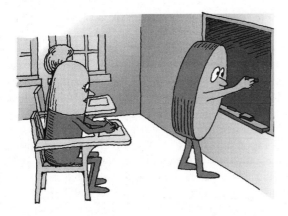

Stage 3: In-Class Note Taking

The split-page note format requires a change in the way you set up your note paper. In this method, each sheet is divided into two parts by drawing a line down the full length of the page to create a left-hand column that is 2½ to 3 inches in width and a right-hand column that is 5½ to 6 inches in width. The right-hand column should be used for taking class notes. (The function of the left-hand column will be explained in the description of Stages 4 and 5.)

There is no magic formula for note taking. Simply take the best notes you can. Remember, notes are personal. Do not judge your notes against those of other classmates. Some will take a lot of notes, and others with a different background and expectations will take far fewer notes. The key point is to do what works for you. When what you are doing stops working, then try another strategy.

Here are some tips for taking effective lecture notes that may make the process easier and more effective for you:

- **Write in your own words** most of the time. Writing ideas in your own style will make them easier to learn and remember.
- **Leave space** between main points. When you sense that the lecturer has moved to a new idea, leave a couple of lines blank on your note paper. That way,

if the lecturer returns to this point later, you will have room to add further notes. Even if there is no need for additional notes, the blank lines will help you see the organization of the ideas and the relationship between them. This space can also be used to add information that is from the textbook.

- Indicate **direct cues** from the lecturer, such as "This will be on the test," "This is a difficult concept," or even "Know this." Put a star or a check in your notes so you will remember to study this information when preparing for the test.
- Be especially aware of the **visual presentation.** This consists of information written on the chalkboard or presented using an overhead projector, slide projector, Power Point display, or other electronic display. Many lecturers outline key points on the chalkboard as a means of staying focused on the points they want to cover. Use this information to help you stay equally focused. Electronic displays are often chosen because the ideas can best be understood when they are presented visually.
- The **repetition** of certain points is the single most useful tip that they are really important. When an idea, term, or fact is important, the lecturer will almost certainly repeat it. For instance, the lecturer will introduce a new term, define it, give a couple of examples to clarify the definition, and finally redefine the term. This repetition is a signal that it is very important for you to learn the information.
- Be alert for **questions directed to the class.** These questions are another way the speaker stresses important information and are also a way for him or her to find out how well the students have understood what has been said. Such questions are thus also cues that certain information is important.
- Be **actively involved** in what is going on in class. This means being willing to respond to a question directed to the class. It also means asking questions when things are not clear. Do not feel that because no one else is asking questions you are the only person who does not understand something. It is highly probable that there are others who are just as confused. Your objective in class is to understand the lecture and record key ideas in your notes so that you can study effectively. Questions are not dumb if they relate to the material being presented.

Stage 4: Out-of-Class Reworking

The notes you take in class are only one part of the effective study of lecture material. Out-of-class reworking of these notes is critical, and this is where the left-hand column of your note paper comes into use. Ideally, this reworking should be done immediately after the class ends, but this is not always possible. It must be done within 24 hours, however, to get full benefit from this strategy.

Reworking class notes will not take more than 10 to 15 minutes to complete, but it will save you hours of study time later on.

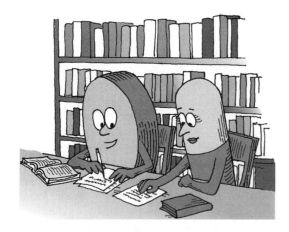

The following is the recommended method for reworking your class notes:

- **Read over the class notes.** Look for major topics, key ideas, terms, and the organization pattern. At this point you are not trying to remember everything you got from the lecture. You are looking for places where your notes are incomplete or confusing. If you read your notes soon after the lecture, you will be able to clarify points or add missing material because most of what was said will still be fresh in your mind. If you wait until the next day (or worse, the next week), what is now only confusing will by then be a complete mystery. Taking the time to read your notes over soon after you take them will save much time and frustration later on.
- **Write topic heads for lecture segments** in the empty left-hand column of your notes. As you read your notes, identify the major topics that were discussed. For example, look at Chapter 11 in the text. The chapter title tells you that it is about general and local anesthetics, but the information does not stop there. Further topics are discussed and divided into subgroups. Headings are necessary to break down very complex material into understandable blocks. You should be doing the same thing with your notes. Limit your labels to three to five words. You are not trying to rewrite class notes but to make the organization of the ideas crystal clear. Sometimes the notes on the chalkboard or Power Point slide will provide the labels for you. Sometimes the labels will be included in a lesson outline furnished by the instructor. Often, however, you will have to compose your own labels. With practice you will develop this skill. Keep at it. These labels are an essential aspect of the final stage of this note-taking method.
- **List vocabulary.** The left-hand column is also a great place to put content-specific vocabulary. Look again

at Chapter 11. Notice that there is a glossary of terms for that chapter. This is provided so that you can immediately begin to focus on the content-specific vocabulary you will have to master for that chapter. You can create your own personal glossary of the terms used in the lecture. As you read over your notes, each time you encounter terms from the text or new terms introduced in the lecture, note the word in the left-hand column. Doing this will help you learn the needed vocabulary.

- **Expand.** Often during a lecture, you will only have time to write fragments of information. These may be meaningful at the time you write them but can be confusing later. Therefore, as you read your notes, fill in those places where there may be such gaps; otherwise, what was a small problem will become a big one later on. It will not take long, and it will pay off. You may use the left-hand column or the lines that you left blank for adding such information.

Remember: The reworking must be done the same day as the lecture for it to be efficient and productive. The longer the interval between the lecture and this reworking, the greater the likelihood of forgetting. When you read notes the same day as the lecture, you will be able to recall almost everything said. The reworking process will only take 10 minutes or so to complete, but it will pay off in a significantly improved set of class notes. Of equal importance is the fact that the reworking process is preparation for the final, critical stage in the note-taking process.

Stage 5: Frequent, Active Review

Notes, no matter how good, need to be **studied early and often.** Learning and memory depend on rehearsal, or review, and this must be an active process. Rereading notes will improve your understanding and memory somewhat, but there is a technique you can use that will accomplish much more. This technique will help you to be an active learner and encourage frequent rehearsal. It is also efficient because it will only take you 10 to 15 minutes to completely review 2 or 3 days' worth of class notes.

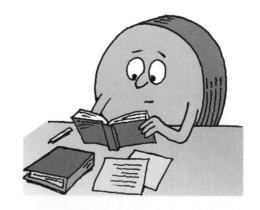

When to Review.

The first review of your notes should be performed within 2 days of the lecture. If the lecture has taken place on Monday, your review should occur on Tuesday or Wednesday. Do not wait more than 2 days. Studies have repeatedly shown that we forget nearly 50% of what we learn in the first 24 hours after we learn it. The reworking process will slow the forgetting process, but it will not stop it. The longer you wait to review your notes, the more time it will take and the more difficult it will be when you finally do it.

When to do a second, third, or any additional reviews depends on the success of the previous review. Review each day until you find that you remember and understand 80% or more of the material (you have to be the judge). When this is accomplished, the next review can wait for 3 or 4 days. If you find that after the first review you recall or understand only 70% of the material (an average amount), then the next review should occur within 2 or 3 days. If the amount you remember is less than 70%, you should review the material the next day. You must assess your own performance on each review to determine how soon to schedule another review. There are no hard and fast rules for this. A good review does not mean you have mastered the material forever, and what you remember clearly at one review may be the very thing you forget the next time around. **The only rule is to review frequently.** By doing this you will be well prepared for quizzes, tests, or any other measure of your learning.

How to Review.

To review your notes, **cover the right-hand column** (class notes) with a blank sheet of paper. Look at the topics, vocabulary, and further notes that you added to the left-hand column during the reworking process. These will serve as your study guide for review. Look at the first topic heading you have written. It might be something like "Hypnotics." Turn that heading into one or more questions. What are hypnotics? When are they used? What are the side effects? Are there persons for whom hypnotics are inappropriate? Ask these questions aloud; do not just think them. **Framing questions orally is what makes this review active**. Now that you have asked a question, the next step is obvious. Answer it without looking at the covered notes. Say the answer aloud. This oral question-and-answer process forces you to state the information in your own words and style. In addition, you are relying on more faculties in your learning than just the visual one of rereading. You are speaking and listening, which is more active than just looking at the words. **Recall is strongly enhanced when you express the information in your own words.**

Another benefit of this review process is that it **helps identify what you do not know.** If you ask a question and find yourself struggling to respond, then it will be clear that this is something you have not yet mastered. When this happens, uncover the class notes pertaining to that topic and read what is needed. Sometimes only three or four words will be needed to trigger recall. When this happens, immediately cover the notes and resume your oral response. Sometimes you will have to read a large portion of the notes to trigger your memory. The reading is now focused on material that you have clearly identified as unknown. This means that your review time will be much more productive. Instead of reading everything known and unknown, you will now be concentrating on reinforcing the known material and studying the unknown. **The best way to prepare for a test is to take a test.** By using the question-and-answer model, you are creating and taking your own test. You may discover that many of the questions you asked yourself also appear in some form on the classroom test covering that same material. If you have already answered the question several times for yourself, it will be easy to answer it on the test.

Two-Page Split-Note Variation.

There is a variation of the split-page note paper format that some students find works better for them. If you find that the 6-inch-wide right-hand column is too narrow for taking class notes, simply take your class notes on the right-hand page in your notebook and use the left-hand page for the reworking process. This allows more room for the charts, diagrams, or complex formulas that are often part of the lecture material in courses such as pharmacology. This two-page method will also allow you to incorporate text notes. To do this, divide the left-hand page into two columns of equal width. Use the right-hand column for the reworking of class notes and the left-hand column for text notes on the same topic.

On-the-Run Action.

Record the information you find to be most difficult to remember on 3″ × 5″ cards and carry them with you in your pocket or purse. When you are waiting in traffic or for an appointment, just pull out the cards and review again. This "found" time may add points to your test scores that you have lost in the past.

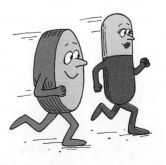

CHOOSE TO MASTER YOUR TEXTBOOKS

Many students find themselves falling asleep while reading their textbooks. Text material can be long, complex, sometimes confusing, and often highly technical. It can seem as though the more you read, the more there is to learn and the less you understand. Close the book and everything you have just read evaporates from your memory. If you feel like this, just remember—you are not alone. Every student feels this way. However, there are effective ways to maximize your learning and memory and maybe even reduce the time it takes to do this.

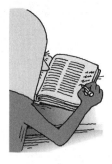

Many different study systems have been devised to aid in the mastery of textbook material, and each has worked for some students. The model presented here is a combination of the best elements of this multitude of systems and the best one for dealing with the subject matter in this pharmacology text.

Getting the most from a lecture requires active listening. The same active process applies to the reading of a textbook. Several techniques promote active reading. A good study system such as the PURR method presented in this textbook is one part of the process, but a good study system can be enhanced by reading with a pencil. Making text notations will help you concentrate and also make future review of the material more productive.

There are three notation systems:

■ Highlighting-underlining
■ Marginal notation
■ Written text notes

Each of these notation systems has certain advantages and disadvantages. No single one will work perfectly all the time. Just as you must use different techniques to meet the different needs of your patients, you also need to use different techniques of text notation to meet the different needs you have as a learner. First, though, let's discuss two general guidelines that apply to the different systems of text notation.

General Guidelines

1. **Read first.** Before you begin to make any text notations, you must first read the material. The objective of text notations is to identify the important ideas, facts, and terms just as this is the objective of listening during a lecture. If you attempt to mark text while reading it for the first time, everything will seem important and you will find yourself making far too many notations or highlighting far too much material.

2. **Be selective.** Be very selective. The objective of text notation is much like that of taking notes during a lecture—to pick out the important ideas for immediate learning and for future review. If you have ever looked at a used textbook, you are sure to have seen that the previous owner has highlighted nearly every line on some pages. Excessive marking means the reader was not discerning the important ideas as he or she was reading. If you are taking separate handwritten notes, you should **limit what you write down** to the major headings and subheadings, important and unfamiliar vocabulary, and no more than two sentences of personal notes for each paragraph. The object is not to rewrite the chapter but to distill the important information. If you are highlighting, limit the material marked to no more than 20% to 25% of the total material. This is not to say that you must impose this limit on every paragraph, but it should be an overall goal.

Text Notation Systems
Text Conventions

As you read and prepare for making text notations, be aware of certain conventions used throughout the text. These help the reader focus on what the authors consider important. By now you have noticed the use of headings in this study tips chapter. Look back at some of them and you will also notice that they are styled differently—some are all capitals; others have only the first letter of each word capitalized. These represent main topics and subtopics. Now look at a chapter in your text. Examine the way headings and bold facing draw your eyes to certain words, phrases, and portions of the page. These are text conventions provided by the authors to help you understand the organization of the material and the relationships within the text content. Other text conventions that you should note are numbered lists, bulleted lists, special display material, and the like.

Language Conventions

Another important aspect of text notation is to become language sensitive. In a class lecture, when you hear a professor say, for instance, "One of the most important first-generation anesthetics was …," the words *most important* are a direct cue that this is a significant point for your notes. The same type of cueing often occurs in the text. The authors want to make certain that their important ideas are communicated to you, the reader. Because the authors cannot speak to you face to face, however, they must rely on a certain written style to get important points across. This means that you must become aware of that style so that you can identify these important ideas. For example, in a sentence saying "Opioids can be classified into four main categories," the phrase *four main categories* is the author's way of telling you not only what is coming but also what you should be taking note of.

Pay attention if a paragraph begins with the phrase "The most significant effects …." Whenever an author uses words or phrases such as these, it tells you that something important is being discussed. When you highlight text, phrases such as *most important, four main categories,* and *most significant* are the cues you should look for to help identify the most important information. The combination of text conventions and language conventions helps make the reading and marking of text more successful.

How to Highlight and Underline

Text marking is done to help in future review. This means that text marking is a personal process and should be used to point out only the most important information. The previous two sections on conventions gave you some concrete ideas on what to mark in your textbook. The main point is **read before your mark.**

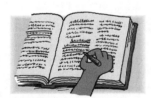

It is essential that you read meaningful blocks of text before you do any marking. A meaningful block may be as little as a single paragraph but never less. It may be as much as an entire chapter. In a text such as *Pharmacology and the Nursing Process,* in which the material is highly technical and challenging, it is unlikely that you will want to read more than a section of the chapter at a time before going back to highlight.

Look at Chapter 12. The first paragraph mentions the boldfaced terms *sedatives* and *hypnotics.* As you read this paragraph the first time, do not mark anything. Instead **read for a general understanding of the content.** After this, go back to the beginning of the section and note the following language conventions: *two basic elements, different stages, summarized, is known as,* and *four distinct stages.* These are all words and phrases that point out important information that should

be highlighted. You may not actually need to highlight all the information flagged by these words and phrases. Some of it is probably already familiar to you because of earlier courses you have taken or earlier chapters you have read in this text. Avoid highlighting information you have already mastered.

Review
When

How soon after you have done some form of text notation should you review what you have highlighted? Ideally review should begin within 24 to 48 hours after the initial learning has occurred. Psychologists have studied learning, memory, and forgetting and have found that we forget approximately 50% of what we learn after the first day or two. Therefore, the sooner you begin to review, the easier it is to move learning from short-term memory (quickly learned and quickly forgotten) to long-term memory.

How

The process for reviewing any text notations follows the same general principles that apply to lecture notes. The intent is to make your review an active process in which real learning takes place. For example, if you have written questions in the text's margins, try to answer these questions without rereading the text. If you are able to answer the question to your satisfaction, then move on to the next question. If you have highlighted terms and definitions, cover the definition and try to define the term without looking at the text. If you are able to do this, you have effectively moved material into long-term memory. If you cannot define the term, then read the text definition. As you read, think about the meaning and think about strategies you might use to help you remember the term and definition the next time. You will find additional memory strategies in the later section on studying for exams. The key is always to focus on being an active learner.

How Often

How often you review is a personal matter. The best way to judge is to be aware of your success, or lack of it, in the current review session. If you do very well at recalling information, then you can probably wait 3 to 4 days for the next review. If the review goes okay, then the next session should take place within 2 days. If you find yourself reviewing your own notations with little understanding and limited memory, then the next review should take place the following day. Each time you review, it will get easier and faster, and as you practice this approach to reviewing your text notations, you will gradually acquire a good sense of how often you need to review to maintain mastery of the material.

CHOOSE TO PASS EXAMS

You can pass your exams by **applying the recommendations and strategies** offered in this section. Start by following the dozen basic rules of exam success.

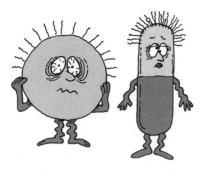

Rules for Success on Exams

1. Accept your anxiety as normal. Tests are important, both in the short term, from the standpoint of grades and successful completion of this course, and also in the long term, from the standpoint of completing the program and getting your degree and eventually the job you want. This fact can cause stress.

2. Reduce your stress by **studying often, not long.** The most important rule in preparing for exams is simple—spend at least 15 minutes every day (Saturdays, Sundays, and holidays included) in reviewing the "old" material. The more time you can find for this each day, the better, but spend at least 15 minutes. This one action will do more to reduce test anxiety than anything else you do. The more time you devote to reviewing past material learned, the more confident you will feel about your knowledge of the topic. This confidence will accompany you into the classroom on the exam day, and it will help you get the test score you want and of which you are capable. Just remember—**start the review process on the first day of the semester** and do some review every single day until the final exam.

3. Balance your review time between your lecture notes, textbook notes or highlighting, and any handouts you may have been given.

4. Ask your instructor about the exam. If he or she says the test is mostly on the lecture, then you may want to spend more time reviewing your class notes. Ask about the type of questions that will be on the exam. Will the test consist entirely of multiple-choice questions? Will it have true-or-false items? Will there be matching, short-answer, or essay questions? You should not study any differently for a multiple-choice exam than you should for a short-answer or essay exam. However, knowing the type or types of questions that will be on the test will help you develop a strategy for quizzing yourself.

5. Work with your study group to create practice tests. For example, if you know the test will consist of multiple-choice questions, then as you do your review, think of the kinds of questions you would ask if you were composing the test. Consider what would be a good question, what would be the right answer, and what would be other answers that would appear right but would in fact be incorrect.

6. Take the practice tests in each chapter and on the Companion CD. Practice writing out the answers of short-answer or essay questions. **The best way to prepare for a test is to take one.**

7. **Study wisely, not hard.** Use the study strategies offered in this guide so you can save time and be able to get a good night's sleep the night before your exam. Cramming is not smart, and it is hard work that increases stress while reducing learning. When you cram, your mind is more likely to go blank during a test. When you cram, the information is in your short-term memory so you will need to relearn it before a comprehensive exam. Relearning takes more time. The stress caused by cramming may interfere with your sleep. Your brain needs sleep to function at its best.

8. Prepare for exams when and where you are most alert and able to concentrate. **Use your personal prime time,** which was discussed earlier in the time management section. If you are most alert at night, study at night. If you are most alert at 2 AM, study in the early morning hours. Study where you can focus your attention and avoid distractions. This may be in the library or in a quiet corner of your home. The key point is to keep on doing what is working for you. If you are distracted or falling asleep, you may want to change when and where you are studying.

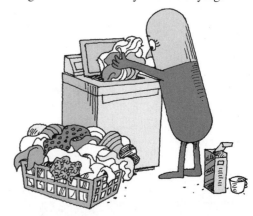

9. **Relax the last hour before an exam.** Your brain needs some recovery time to function effectively.

10. Survey the test before you start answering the questions. Plan how to complete the exam in the time allowed. Read the directions carefully and answer the questions you know for sure first.

11. Before turning in the exam, make sure that you have answered all of the questions. If you are to fill in the boxes on an answer sheet that will be read electronically, be sure you have put only one answer per line and that you have answered each question. If you must make a correction, be sure to erase carefully and thoroughly.

12. Celebrate your success. Congratulate yourself for choosing to pass your exam by applying the exam preparation and exam-taking skills that have been proven to work.

Strategies for Reviewing Class Notes

Look at your class notes. If you have been using the split-page model described earlier, you have made your own topic headings in the left-hand column beside the class notes. Cover the class notes and turn each heading into one or more questions. Think carefully about the answers and then answer aloud. By answering questions aloud, you are forcing yourself to think about what you know and organizing that knowledge in the way that is most meaningful to you. If you can answer your questions, then you have demonstrated that you know the material, and there is no immediate need to reread that section of notes. If you cannot answer one of your questions, then you know you need to review that material more intensively. Uncover the notes and read the pertinent ones. You are now using your review time effectively, because instead of just rereading everything, which invites boredom—or, worse yet, daydreaming—the rereading is directed at the material of which you are unsure. The result is more efficient use of your time and more effective learning.

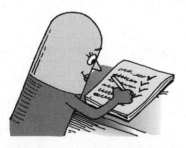

Strategies for Reviewing the Textbook

The technique you used for studying your class notes will also work for studying text material. As mentioned, in this book the authors have provided you with a variety of features that can help enormously. First, look at the objectives at the beginning of each chapter to be studied. Even if you have been assigned only small portions of the chapter, it is important to consider the objectives for the chapter as a whole. Ask yourself whether you have met these objectives. This is a quick way of assessing how much review may be necessary. If you feel confident that you have accomplished most of the objectives, then the review should go quickly. If you feel uncertain about many of them, then the review is going to take more time.

The next task is to consider the topic headings and language conventions. Use them in the same way as you have used the labels in your notes. Turn them into questions and answer these questions aloud. If you can answer them, then there is no need to reread. If you cannot, then you will need to reread the pertinent text.

Again, this way of reviewing is focusing your time and energy mostly where it is needed—on the material you have not yet mastered. Each time you review the text (or class notes), the sections of material you reread may differ. This is to be expected. You cannot remember everything forever, but if you spend time each day doing this type of review, you will remember more and for longer periods of time.

Strategies for Reviewing Terminology

One aspect of nursing that can seem overwhelming is the terminology. It is highly technical and specialized. Learning it poses the same kind of challenge as learning a foreign language. In fact, it almost *is* a foreign language. However, for the concepts and ideas to be mastered, the terms must be mastered. One of the best ways to go about doing this is to use a technique you probably learned in grade school—flash cards. Put each term on one side of a 3″ × 5″ note card and the definition or other essential information about the term on the back. Group together cards containing terms that have common word elements (e.g., terms beginning with *cardio*) or that concern common concepts (e.g., terms to do with renal function). The more relationships you can establish between words, the easier it will be to learn and remember them.

On-the-Run Action

Get in the habit of carrying a deck of 10 to 15 of these cards with you. When you have a few minutes, review as many cards as time allows. Sometimes start with the term side of the card and try to recall what is written on the back. Other times look at the definition on the back of the card and try to recall the term. Do not focus exclusively on term-to-definition learning because you may be given definitions or some variation on the exam and be asked to provide the terms.

Exam Time

This is it. The culmination of all your work—lectures, notes, flash cards, textbook readings, and handouts. **It is time to relax.** Test anxiety interferes with test performance. If you have put to use the learning techniques described in this chapter, you are ready for the exam. You have mastered the material, and you can do well on the exam. If you continue to experience test anxiety in spite of preparing thoroughly for the exam, it might be a good idea to visit a professional counselor on your campus.

Avoid cramming and remain confident in the learning techniques you have chosen to apply. This can usually control normal nervousness. Besides these learning techniques, however, techniques are also available for dealing with the various types of exam questions, and these are discussed in this section. None of these strategies can guarantee a 10-point jump in your test score. Only the degree to which you have mastered the material can make that sort of difference. However, each of the strategies described in this section may help you answer one or two questions correctly that you might otherwise have missed. **These test-taking strategies are not intended to replace regular study** and mastery; however, they are intended to enhance your test performance. If you use these strategies, you will see a positive gain in your test performance.

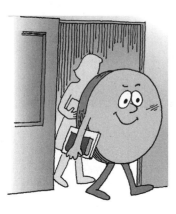

When the teacher passes out the exam, all your work and preparation are about to pay off, but do not just leap into the test. Take a couple of minutes to put yourself in a frame of mind for doing well on the test. At this point, you have a perfect test score—you have not answered any questions incorrectly yet. It is likely that you will get some answers wrong, but do not start out by making mistakes that cost you points which you should not have lost.

First, look over the entire test. Do not read it, but turn the pages and look at a question here and a question there. How many items are there on the test? Are all the questions of one type, or is there a mixture of types? Knowing in advance the length of the test and the types of questions helps you plan your strategy for taking the test.

Second, read the directions. This is the first opportunity you have to make a mistake that could cost points. Some directions for true-or-false questions may ask you to correct the statement and make it true. Others may ask you to justify your answer. When you respond with just a *T* or an *F,* you have lost important points because you did not read the directions.

Third, create a plan to complete the test in the time allowed. For example, if the test has 50 multiple-choice questions and the time limit is 40 minutes, then you know you will have to average a little better than one item per minute. Obviously you will need to allocate more time to essay questions if they are on the exam. Plan to glance at your watch or the classroom clock occasionally during the exam to make sure you are not losing time or going too quickly. Pace yourself. If you are answering questions quickly and are confident that the answers are right, do not worry about being ahead of schedule. If you spend too much time on individual questions, you may try to decide the answers to the last questions quickly, and this increases your chances of making errors. Planning a strategy for finishing the test within the time allowed helps you maintain a sharp focus on the task and enables you to do the best job possible.

Fourth, start answering the questions. If the test consists of only one type of question, then start with the first question. However, if the test has multiple-choice, true-or-false, and short-essay questions, for example, you must decide where it is best for you to start. If you find essay questions easy to do, then perhaps you should start with these. There is no reason you have to begin with the multiple-choice questions. On the other hand, if you find essay questions a challenge, then do not start with them. **Begin the test in a way that will give you confidence.**

Tips for Answering the Questions

- Start with the first question or with those types of questions you feel most confident answering. Wherever you choose to start, there is a strategy you can use that can improve your test performance.
- Read the question carefully, and if you know the answer, indicate it and move on to the next question. If you cannot immediately think of the answer, give it a few seconds of thought. If the answer comes, indicate it and move on. If the answer still does not come or if the question is confusing, then skip to the next question.
- In the first pass through the exam, answer what you know and skip what you do not know. Answering the questions you are sure of increases your

confidence and saves time. This is buying you time to devote to the questions with which you have more difficulty.

■ Notice that the subjects of the questions on a particular exam are related, that the answers to questions you have skipped may be provided by other questions on the test, or that a later question may trigger recall of the correct answer. Skipping questions of which you are unsure offers one more opportunity to get the correct answer.

■ After you have gone through the entire test completing the questions to which you are confident you know the answers, go back to the items you skipped. First check the time, however, so you know how much time you have left to answer these questions. On this second pass through the exam, you will often be surprised at how many questions you now can answer that drew a complete blank before.

■ Answer every question. A question without an answer is the same as a wrong answer. *Go ahead and guess.* You have studied for the test and you know the material well. You are not making a random guess based on no information. You are guessing based on what you have learned and your best assessment of the question.

■ When you have answered all the questions on a page, put a check in the upper right corner of this page. Avoid going back and second guessing yourself. There is nothing worse than changing right answers to wrong ones. Have confidence in your own knowledge and let go of the test. If you are the first person to complete a test but are sure of what you did, then turn it in. At the same time, do not let what others in the class are doing affect your test strategy. If you are the last person to turn the test in, it does not mean you know less than those who were faster. It simply means that you are a careful, thoughtful test taker.

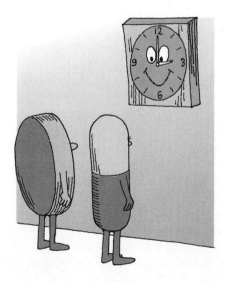

Strategies for Specific Types of Questions

For each type of question there are particular strategies you can use that can help prevent incorrect responses. Many times students miss questions not because of a lack of information but because of a poor strategy. Sometimes the error stems from misreading a question, for instance, overlooking a key word such as *not,* or from choosing an answer that does not quite fit the question asked. Errors like these can be costly. Expect to find some questions on a test to which you do not remember the answer or that are worded in a confusing way. A perfect test score is a great goal, but be realistic and accept the fact that perfect scores may be few and far between. At the same time, do not lose points because of careless and preventable errors.

Strategy for Multiple-Choice Questions

Multiple-choice questions can be challenging, because students think that they will recognize the right answer when they see it or that the right answer will somehow stand out from the other choices. This is a dangerous misconception. The more carefully the question is constructed, the more each of the choices will seem like the correct response. The successful student can do several things to improve performance on multiple-choice questions.

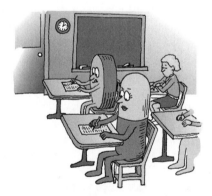

Before the strategies for analyzing multiple-choice questions are discussed, it is important to understand each part of a question and its purpose. There are three parts to a multiple-choice question: stem, distractors, and the correct choice.

First, there is the **question stem.** This is the complete question that one, or more, of the response choices will answer.

EXAMPLE:
If excessive amounts of water-soluble vitamins are ingested, what usually happens?

Notice that this could just as easily be a short-answer question. In this case, the stem is a complete sentence that should be answered by one of the response choices. The stem can also be an incomplete statement that one or more of the response choices completes correctly.

EXAMPLE:
The likelihood that a drug will have therapeutic effects increases dramatically when

This statement is incomplete, and you must pick out the response choice that best completes it.

The second part of multiple-choice questions is the **distractors.** These are the response choices that do not best answer or complete the stem. They are known as distractors because that is their purpose, to distract you from the best choice. Good distractors are usually very similar to the **best choice.** If you have not studied enough, a good distractor will be a very tempting choice, but you must reduce the allure of distractors.

The third and final part of all multiple-choice questions is the best choice. This is the choice you want to pick. Notice that it is the "best" choice. In many multiple-choice questions there may be more than one response choice that appears to answer the stem, and the differences between the responses may be slight. Your task is therefore to identify the option that **best** answers the stem, not necessarily the only right choice.

Recall.
The most reliable way to ensure that you select the correct response to a multiple-choice question is to recall it. Depend on your learning and memory to furnish the answer to the question. To do this, read the stem, and then *stop!* Do not look at the response options yet. Try to recall what you know and, based on this, what you would give as the answer. After you have taken a few seconds to do this, then look at all of the choices and select the one that most nearly matches the answer you recalled. It is important that you consider all the choices and not just choose the first option that seems to fit the answer you recall. Remember the distractors. Choice B may look okay, but choice D may be worded in a way that makes D a slightly better choice. If you do not weigh all the choices, you are not maximizing your chances of correctly answering each question.

Once you have decided on an answer, there is one more important step before you mark it. Look at the stem again. Does your choice answer the question that was asked? If the question stem asks "why," be sure the response you have chosen is a reason. If the question stem is singular, then be sure the option is singular, and the same for plural stems and plural responses. Many times, checking to make sure that the choice makes sense in relation to the stem will reveal the correct answer.

This is the most reliable technique to use for answering multiple-choice questions. If you do this for every multiple-choice question on the test, your accuracy

rate will be very high, and you will not need any further strategy. Unfortunately, however, recall does not always work, and when it does not, there are some additional strategies you can apply to improve your chances of picking the correct answer.

Recognition and Elimination.
Read each of the answer options carefully. Usually at least one of them will be clearly wrong. Eliminate this one from consideration. Now you have reduced the number of response choices by one and improved the odds. Continue to analyze the options. If you can eliminate one more choice in a four-option question, you have reduced the odds to 50/50, the same as the odds of correct random guessing for true-or-false questions. There are still some strategies that will help you pick the best choice. In addition, while you are eliminating the wrong choices, recall often occurs. One of the options may serve as a trigger that causes you to remember what a few seconds ago had seemed completely forgotten.

Look-Alike Answers.
After you have eliminated one or more choices, you may discover that two of the options are very similar. This can be very helpful, because it may mean that one of these look-alike answers is the best choice and the other is a very good distractor. Test both of these options against the stem. Ask yourself which one completes the incomplete statement grammatically and which one answers the question more fully and completely. The option that best completes or answers the stem is the one you should choose. Here, too, pause for a few seconds, give your brain time to reflect, and recall may occur.

Absolutes.
The presence of absolute words and phrases can also help you determine the correct answer to a multiple-choice item. If an answer choice contains an absolute (e.g., *none, never, must, cannot*), be very cautious. Remember that there are not many things in this world that are absolute, and in an area as complex as pharmacology, an absolute in an option may be reason to eliminate it from consideration as the best choice. This is only a guideline and should not be taken to be true 100% of the time; however, it can help you reduce the number of choices.

Negatives and Exceptions.
In the stem "A drug reaction could include all but which of these symptoms?" the phrase *all but* tells you to choose the response that is an exception. *All but one* of the choice options is a symptom. In this case, the option that is *not* a symptom is the best choice. If you look at the options and see several that seem correct, look at the stem again. It may be that you have overlooked an exception phrase such as

all but or *all but one*. A similar stem wording that can throw you off is a negative or negative prefix. The stem "It is generally *not* a good idea to administer adult dosages to…" is asking you to select the answer that names the inappropriate, not appropriate, recipient of a medication. The word *not* helps identify the answer.

All these strategies can help you analyze the response choices so that you have the best possible chance of selecting the correct choice. When you are ready to mark the answer, keep in mind that the final step is always to test your response against the stem.

If, after you have tried all of these strategies, you find yourself still unable to choose a response, there is one final strategy. Ask the instructor for clarification of the question. There is nothing to lose by asking and everything to gain. The worst that can happen is that the instructor will tell you that he or she cannot answer your question. The best that can happen is that the instructor will rephrase the question in a way that resolves the problem for you.

When asking for such clarification, try to phrase your question in a way that encourages a response. Do not simply state that you do not understand the question. This is generally not the approach that invites an answer. If you are having trouble with a term in the stem or response choices, ask for a definition. If there is a phrase that is unclear or a response choice that is confusing, ask for clarification. Anything you do to make your question more specific increases the likelihood that the instructor will answer it.

After all other avenues have been exhausted, remember the final rule. **Never leave a question unanswered.** Even if answering is no more than an educated guess on your part, go ahead and mark an answer. You might be right, but if you leave it blank, you will certainly be wrong and lose precious points.

Strategy for Short-Answer and Essay Questions

Notice that this strategy applies to both short-answer and essay questions. Both types of questions require careful thought and planning before you write an answer. It is helpful to get into the habit of regarding short-answer questions as short-essay questions. Too often students lose points on short-answer questions by being too brief. A short answer should usually consist of three or four sentences, but frequently students interpret "short answer" to mean four or five words.

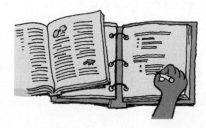

Start answering these questions by analyzing the question carefully and then framing a response that will fully answer it. Assume that the reader—in this case, the course instructor—does not know anything and that you have to explain it all. Short-answer and essay questions require you to show what you know. Do not assume that the instructor can read your mind or read between the lines of your response to discern what you knew but did not include. It is better to have a little more than was needed in your answer than not enough. Extra information will not hurt, but missing information will always cost points. Once again, remember that the idea is to gain a point here and there throughout the test, which will result in a higher score and a better grade for the course.

Two Key Issues

1. In writing answers to short-answer and essay questions, it is essential to answer exactly the question that is asked. This means that you must understand the question before you do any writing. Unlike with true-or-false and multiple-choice questions, which you should try to answer using every possible strategy before seeking help, with these questions you should ask for help before doing anything. The first opportunity you have to lose points in an essay question occurs with the first reading of the question. If you misread the question, you may write an excellent answer but not the right one. Such a mistake can be costly.

2. A good answer must be organized so that it is clear and logical to the reader. Do not read a question and start writing down whatever ideas spring to mind. Spend a minute or two thinking and planning the structure of the answer so that your ideas are clearly stated and the supporting details relate directly to each idea. Your instructor, the reader, will have a difficult time grading your essay if he or she has to read it two or three times to figure out what you were trying to say. Organization and clarity of expression really pay off in essay exams.

Five Steps to Good Essay Answers

1. **Read the questions carefully.** As was discussed earlier, misreading the question can result in a high-quality answer that does not address the question asked. Read and think about the question's major focus. Do not jump on the first familiar phrase or term and start writing without further thought.

2. **Decide on an approach.** Telling you to read the question carefully is good advice, but without some strategy to apply to the reading it might be difficult advice to carry out. Here is a strategy to help you read carefully

and begin to plan your answer. Look at the question as you read, and identify the words and phrases that tell you what to do. Some standard "what-to-do" words and phrases are used consistently in essay questions, such as *discuss, compare, contrast, explain, tell why,* and *analyze.* Circle each of these words or phrases as you read the question. The second part of the decision step is to underline what you are to write about. This circling and underlining will force a careful reading of the question and help you begin the process of organizing the answer. The sample question that follows is marked to show the circle and underline strategy.

SAMPLE QUESTION:

(Discuss) the <u>ways</u> in which <u>pediatric and elderly</u>

<u>patients</u> are <u>alike</u> in <u>determining</u> appropriate dosage.

(Explain) <u>why adult dosage</u> may be <u>inappropriate and</u> the

<u>dangers</u> in <u>using adult dosage</u> in these special populations.

3. **Compile a brief written outline.** Before you start writing your answer, take a few minutes to organize the points you want to cover. This should not be an elaborate outline with roman numerals, capital letters, and arabic numbers, but rather a quick sketch of the question and the points you want to make in the answer. The circle-and-underline step described earlier will help make this easy to do.

SAMPLE OUTLINE*:
Discuss
- Pediatric and elderly patients' similarity with regard to drug dosage
  - Body weight factor
  - Organ function

Explain
- Reasons adult dosage inappropriate
  - Drugs not tested on pediatric and elderly population
- Dangers of adult dosage
  - Possible organ damage
  - Increased absorption and possible side effects

Sketching out an outline like this will organize your ideas, speed your writing, and ensure that you are answering the question asked.

*This is a model of the process of the Decision and Outline Steps. It is not to be viewed as an accurate outline of pharmacologic content.

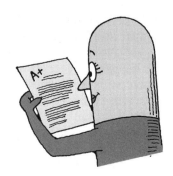

4. **Write an answer.** With the question analyzed and a quick outline in place, it is time to put your answer on paper. The basic structure of an exam essay or answer to a short-answer question is the same as that for an in-class composition on an assigned topic. Every rule on which composition teachers insist for writing assignments should be followed in writing essay answers.

Any answer of more than four or five sentences should follow the basic three-part essay structure of introduction, body, and conclusion.

The **introduction** should be only one or two sentences long. It tells the reader what you are going to present in your answer. There is a relatively simple way to write an essay introduction. State the question positively and add a few words that show the main points you intend to make in your answer.

SAMPLE INTRODUCTION:
Pediatric and elderly patients have a number of similarities that must be considered in determining drug dosage. Two of the most important are body weight and organ function, and these factors can make adult dosages inappropriate for these two populations.

These two sentences tell the reader exactly what you plan to discuss. From this point on, it becomes your task to explain why those two are important and how they affect drug dosage. You have told the reader what to expect, and you have begun to organize your answer.

The **body** is the most important part of any essay answer. In it you want to state the ideas, concepts, and points that you believe answer the question. These should be stated clearly and positively. Do not ramble on trying to cover all the possible variations that might fit into an answer. Decide on the most important, most significant points you have to make. Then state them and support and explain with relevant details that show how and why your points answer the question. For short-answer questions where three to five sentences are expected, drop the introduction and conclusion, and put all of your energy into a clear, concise body.

For the **conclusion,** there should be a concluding sentence or two to let the reader know that you have finished. Like the introduction, it should be brief and direct.

Restate the question, and summarize the key points made in your answer.

SAMPLE CONCLUSION:

It is evident that elderly and pediatric patients are very similar in their responses to drug dosages. Clearly the factors of body weight and organ function will play a major role in determining the appropriate dosages for these two groups.

5. **Read the answer.** The writing has been completed. Before you turn in the paper, take another minute or two and read over what you have written. Look for errors that would make the reader pause, question what you have said, or be unable to read a word or phrase. Sometimes the mind works much faster than the pen, and a word or phrase is left out in writing. Use a caret (∧) and insert the word or phrase where it belongs. If your writing got a little sloppy and a word is hard to read, cross it out and print it clearly right above. Proofreading and correcting small errors like these will make the answer easier to read and understand. Anything that contributes to the overall quality of an answer will influence the grade in a positive manner. You will not have time to rewrite an answer, but you should correct obvious errors.

Strategy for True-or-False Questions

True-or-false items outwardly appear to be fairly simple. After all, the statement is either true or false. The odds of answering correctly are 50/50, and if all else fails, a coin toss can decide the issue. Appearances are deceiving, however, and true-or-false questions can be very challenging to answer. Good test strategy should be applied to answer all types of questions, because the object is to get the best score you can, and this represents the total points for all correct answers.

Read the Question.
Reading the question may seem like such an obvious part of all test-taking strategies that it may appear absurd even to be told to do this. If you do not pay careful attention to the wording of true-or-false statements, however, then you are increasing the odds of making an otherwise avoidable error. Take the time to read and understand the statement. Read it all the way through to the end. Do not jump to conclusions based on half the statement.

Assume That the Statement Is True.
As you read each true-or-false statement, begin with the assumption that the statement is true. The idea behind this strategy is that it will cause you to read the statement carefully, which will result in your choosing the

correct answer. This approach to reading the statement makes the reading an active process, because you are then reading to confirm the truth in the statement. You will be analyzing the statement as you read, looking for any information that would contradict or change the statement from true to false. You will also be choosing your answer as you read rather than waiting to the end to decide whether the statement was true or false. Obviously not every statement will be true, but this step makes you a much more thoughtful reader, and that encourages better test performance.

Remember one other important rule when analyzing true-or-false statements. **If any part of the statement is false, then the entire statement is false.** There may be only one altered word or prefix (such as *un-* or *anti-*) that changes a statement from true to false, but that is all that is required.

Strategies for Analysis.
Sometimes, no matter how carefully you have read the question, the answer is not immediately obvious. When that happens, there are a number of strategies you can use to analyze the question. Using these strategies will not guarantee that you will get the correct answer, but they will often help you see something about the statement you might have overlooked and assist you in identifying the correct answer.

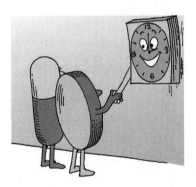

Absolutes and Qualifiers.
Absolutes are words such as *none, never, all,* or *always.* These words mean that there are absolutely no exceptions to the statement. For instance, the statement "All birds fly" means just that. Every bird, past, present, and future, has flown or does fly. If there is or has been just one bird that has not flown or does not fly, then the statement is false. *All* in this statement is an absolute. True-or-false statements that contain such absolutes are usually false. In an area as complex as pharmacology, it is unlikely that there are many absolutes. If you are struggling with a question that has you stumped, look for absolute words. They may help you determine the answer.

On the other hand, there are words that suggest the possibility of exceptions. Such words or phrases are called qualifiers; examples of these are *some, possibly, in most cases,* and *will generally.* "Most birds can fly" is an example of a qualified statement. The word *most* tells you that some not precisely specified number of all birds can fly. This makes it more probable that the statement is true.

Stated in the Negative.

A true-or-false statement that is rendered in the negative can be very difficult to answer. To draw on the earlier example, "It is not true that all birds can fly" is such a statement. The word *not* in this statement can make it much more complex to read and answer. There is a relatively simple way to deal with this type of statement. Read it as though the negative were not included, so that it becomes "It is true that all birds can fly." This statement is clearly false. Because the word *not* reverses the meaning of the statement, this makes the statement "It is not true that all birds can fly" true. Simply put, if the statement is true without the negative, then it becomes false with the negative. Similarly, if it is false without the negative, then it is true with the negative.

Strings.

A string is a true-or-false statement that requires careful attention. It is a statement that contains a list of several words or phrases, but often one or more of the words or phrases is false. It is easy to read the statement and see that the first two or three words or phrases are true but then to overlook the one that is incorrect, with the consequence that you mark the answer as true when it is actually false. An example of a string is "Many warm-weather crops, such as tomatoes, can be grown year-round in southern California, southern Florida, South America, and South Dakota."

As you read this statement, it is easy to be lured by the words *southern* and *South* into thinking that the statement is true without noting the fact that South Dakota is a northern state with fairly harsh winters and that there are parts of South America where the climate is very cold. The statement is false, but the string can trick you into thinking that the statement is true.

These strategies for analyzing true-or-false items can help you increase the number of correct answers, but they are not intended to replace study and learning. The best way to perform well on any test is to know the answers based on your own learning. When the answer does not immediately come to mind, however, apply these strategies. Although they will not necessarily lead to a 10-point difference in your score, they may help you add 2 points to your score. Better scores mean better course grades, and of course, this results in improved self-confidence and improved chances of success.

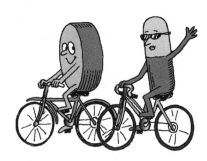

CONCLUSION

Remember: These study tips are only as valuable as you make them!

Chapter 1
The Nursing Process and Drug Therapy

CHAPTER REVIEW

Choose the best answer for each of the following.

1. Which phase of the nursing process requires the nurse to establish a comprehensive baseline of data concerning a particular patient?
   a. Assessment
   b. Planning
   c. Implementation
   d. Evaluation

2. The nurse may revise or eliminate unrealistic goals during which phase of the nursing process?
   a. Assessment
   b. Planning
   c. Implementation
   d. Evaluation

3. Prescribed medications are prepared and administered during which phase of the nursing process?
   a. Assessment
   b. Planning
   c. Implementation
   d. Evaluation

4. Which of the following must occur for a goal statement to be patient centered?
   a. Family input must be considered in developing the goal.
   b. The patient must be involved in establishing the goal.
   c. The nurse must develop the goal.
   d. The physician must be involved in establishing the goal.

5. Which of the following is part of a complete medication history?
   a. Use of "street" drugs
   b. Current laboratory work
   c. Past history of surgeries
   d. Family history

6. During which phase of the nursing process does the nurse prioritize the nursing diagnoses?
   a. Assessment
   b. Planning
   c. Implementation
   d. Evaluation

7. Below is a list of data gathered during an assessment of Ms. Biehle, a young woman visiting your clinic with what she describes as "maybe an ulcer." Label each item as either objective data (O) or subjective data (S).

   _____ Ms. Biehle tells you that she smokes a pack of cigarettes a day.

   _____ She is 5 feet 5 inches tall and weighs 135 pounds.

   _____ You find that her pulse rate is 68 beats/min and her blood pressure is 128/72 mm Hg.

   _____ Her stool was tested for occult blood by a laboratory technician; the results were negative.

   _____ Ms. Biehle says that she does not experience nausea, but she reports pain and heartburn, especially after eating popcorn—something she and her husband have always done while watching TV before bedtime.

   _____ She experiences occasional increases in stomach pain, a "feeling of heat" in her abdomen and chest at night when she lies down, and increased incidents of heartburn.

CRITICAL THINKING AND APPLICATION

Answer the following questions on a separate sheet of paper.

8. Identify the "Five Rights" of drug administration and specify ways to ensure that each of these rights is addressed.

9. The following items will help you review the nursing process:

   Data are collected during the (a) _____ phase of the nursing process.

   Data can be classified as (b) _____ or (c) _____.

   To formulate the nursing diagnosis, the nurse must first (d) _____ the information collected.

   The planning phase includes identification of (e) _____ and (f) _____.

   The (g) _____ phase consists of initiation and completion of the nursing care plan.

   The (h) _____ phase is ongoing and includes monitoring the patient's response to medication and determining the status of goals.

10. Discuss one of the "other rights" described in the text and how it fits in with the nursing process.

CASE STUDY

Read the scenario and answer the following questions on a separate sheet of paper.

A 69-year-old woman has been admitted to the hospital due to nausea and vomiting. She also has a diagnosis of hepatitis C. She says she stopped drinking 3 years ago but has had increasing problems with peripheral edema and shortness of breath and has had trouble getting out of bed or a chair by herself. Laboratory results show that her liver enzyme levels are elevated; her sodium and potassium levels are decreased. Her blood pressure is 160/98 mm Hg, her pulse rate is 98 beats/min, and her respiratory rate is 24 breaths/min. She is afebrile and states that she is having slight abdominal pain.

1. From the brief facts given, what information will be important to consider when obtaining a drug history?

2. From the nursing diagnoses in Box 1-3, choose at least two current and two "risk for" nursing diagnoses for this patient. What priority would you assign to your nursing diagnoses?

3. The physician wrote the following drug order:

   November 4, 2007

   Give Lasix now.

   Charles Simmons, MD

Patient's Name: Jane Doe	F	Age: 73
Medical Record No: 1234567	Date of Birth: 1/16/34	

   What elements, if any, are missing from the this medication order? What should you do next?

4. After the order is clarified, the pharmacy sends up furosemide (Lasix), 80-mg tablets, but the patient is unable to swallow them because of her nausea. Your colleague suggests giving the Lasix to her as an intravenous injection. What should you do next?

5. After the patient receives the dose of Lasix, what should you do?

Chapter 2
Pharmacologic Principles

CHAPTER REVIEW

Provide the best answer for each of the following.

1. Number the following drug forms in order of speed of dissolution and absorption, with 1 being the fastest and 4 being the slowest:
   a. Capsules
   b. Enteric-coated tablets
   c. Elixirs
   d. Powders

2. When considering the various routes of drug elimination, the nurse is aware that elimination occurs mainly from the
   a. renal tubules and skin.
   b. skin and lungs.
   c. bowel and renal tubules.
   d. lungs and gastrointestinal tract.

3. The nurse is aware that excessive drug dosages, poor circulation, impaired metabolism, or inadequate excretion may result in which drug effect?
   a. Tolerance
   b. Cumulative effect
   c. Incompatibility
   d. Antagonistic effect

4. Drug half-life is defined as the amount of time required for 50% of a drug to
   a. be absorbed by the body.
   b. reach a therapeutic level.
   c. exert a response.
   d. be eliminated by the body.

5. The nurse recognizes that drugs given by which route will be altered by the first-pass effect?
   a. Oral
   b. Sublingual
   c. Subcutaneous
   d. Intravenous

6. If a drug binds with an enzyme and thereby prevents the enzyme from binding to its normal target cell, it will produce an effect known as which of the following?
   a. Receptor interaction
   b. Enzyme stimulation
   c. Enzyme interaction
   d. Nonspecific interaction

Match each field of study with the corresponding job description of a person working in that field.

7. _____ Pharmaceutics

8. _____ Pharmacokinetics

9. _____ Pharmacodynamics

10. _____ Pharmacogenetics

11. _____ Pharmacotherapeutics

12. _____ Pharmacognosy

13. _____ Toxicology

14. _____ Teratology

15. _____ Prophylactic therapy

a. Lisa is researching botanical and zoologic sources of drugs to treat multiple sclerosis. She is part of a university research team that is currently experimenting with varying the biochemical composition and therapeutic effects of several possible new drugs.

b. Jeffrey works for a pharmaceutical corporation. One of its new drugs looks very promising, and Jeffrey's company is experimenting with dosage forms for this investigational new drug. He is responsible for measuring the relationship between the physiochemical properties of the dosage form and the clinical therapeutic response.

c. Meiko examines case studies of patients with similar conditions and drug therapies to determine similarities based on clinical observations.

d. Hamische researches various poisons and is particularly concerned with the detection and treatment of the effects of drugs and other chemicals in certain mammals.

e. Steven represents a research firm that subcontracts with the Food and Drug Administration to observe and report on drug-induced congenital anomalies and the toxic effects drugs can have on the developing fetus.

f. Diane and Phil have spent the last 3 years gathering family histories, legal case reports, and current clinical data to identify possible genetic factors that influence individuals' responses to meperidine and related drugs.

g. David works on a study that is gathering data on the use of two different drugs for the treatment of rheumatoid arthritis.

h. Michelle's research has taken her to Southeast Asia and Australia to participate in worldwide research on the treatment of a neoplastic disease that is more prevalent in the populations of those two regions.

i. Leslie's laboratory monitors drug distribution rates between various body compartments, from absorption through excretion. Recently, her laboratory was able to suggest a positive change in the dosage regimen for an injectable drug, bringing her firm a prestigious award.

j. Gregory's research unit recently recommended two new contraindications for the use of a newly marketed drug after discovering previously unknown biochemical and physiologic interactions of this drug with another unrelated drug.

CRITICAL THINKING AND APPLICATION

Answer the following questions on a separate sheet of paper.

16. Mr. Cullen enters the trauma center in some distress. He is experiencing symptoms that demand quick absorption of a drug. If presented with the following choices, which route of administration would you use: subcutaneous or intramuscular? Mr. Cullen's physician asks you to further increase absorption—mechanically. How can you do this?

17. Ms. Clark has had ovarian cancer for over a year. She is now in the late stages of her illness and in severe pain. She has been admitted to a hospice unit and is receiving morphine through a patient-controlled analgesia pump. This is an example of which type of drug therapy: acute, maintenance, supplemental, or palliative? Explain your answer.

CASE STUDY

Read the scenario and answer the following questions on a separate sheet of paper.

A 65-year-old man with liver cirrhosis is admitted to the medical-surgical unit with nausea and vomiting. He also has a diagnosis of heart failure. You note that his serum albumin level is low. The physician has written admission orders, and you are trying to make the patient comfortable. He is to take nothing by mouth except for clear liquids. An intravenous infusion of dextrose 5% in water at 50 mL/hr has been ordered, and the nurses have had difficulty inserting his intravenous line.

1. One of the drugs ordered is known to reach a maximum level in the body of 200 mg/L and has a half-life of 2 hours. If this maximum level of 200 mg/L is reached at 4 PM, then what will the drug's level in the body be at 10 PM?

2. Describe how factors identified in the patient's history would affect the following:
    a. Absorption
    b. Distribution
    c. Metabolism
    d. Excretion

3. Placement of a peripherally inserted central catheter is ordered. The physician writes an order for a dose of an intravenous antibiotic to be given before this procedure is carried out. What is the reason for this order?

4. This patient is also receiving digoxin (Lanoxin) for heart failure. This drug is known to have a low therapeutic index. Explain this concept.

Chapter 3
Life Span Considerations

CHAPTER REVIEW

Choose the best answer for each of the following.

1. Which physiologic factor is most responsible for the differences in the pharmacokinetic and pharmacodynamic behavior of drugs in neonates and adults?
   a. Infant's stature
   b. Infant's smaller weight
   c. Immaturity of neonatal organs
   d. Adult's longer exposure to toxins

2. When considering drug therapy in pediatric patients, the nurse recognizes that which group of drugs is the most toxic for children?
   a. phenobarbital, morphine, and aspirin
   b. phenobarbital, codeine, and atropine
   c. theophylline, atropine, and digoxin
   d. morphine, atropine, and digoxin

3. Most drug references recommend that pediatric dosages be based on which of the following?
   a. Total body water content
   b. Fat–to–lean mass ratio
   c. Height measured in centimeters
   d. Milligrams per kilogram of body weight

4. When considering drug dosages in elderly patients, the nurse recognizes that drug dosages in the elderly should be based
   a. more on age than on height or weight.
   b. more on weight than on age.
   c. on the total body water content.
   d. on the glomerular filtration rate.

5. When giving medications to the elderly, the nurse should keep in mind the changes that occur due to aging. Which of the following statements regarding changes in the elderly patient are true? Select all that apply.
   a. Total body water content is increased as body composition changes.
   b. Gastric pH is less acidic because of reduced hydrochloric acid production.
   c. Protein albumin binding sites are reduced because of decreased protein.
   d. Fat content is increased because of decreased lean body mass and altered total body water.
   e. The absorptive surface area of the gastrointestinal tract is increased due to flattening and blunting of the villi.

Match each pregnancy safety category with its corresponding description.

6. _____ Category A

7. _____ Category B

8. _____ Category C

9. _____ Category D

10. _____ Category X

a. Possible fetal risk in humans is reported; however, the potential benefits may, in selected cases, outweigh the risks and warrant the use of these drugs in pregnant women.

b. Studies indicate no risk to animal fetus; information for humans is not available.

c. Fetal abnormalities are reported, and positive evidence of fetal risk in humans is available from animal and/or human studies.

d. Studies indicate no risk to the fetus.

e. Adverse effects are reported in animal fetuses; information for humans is not available.

CRITICAL THINKING AND APPLICATION

Answer the following questions on a separate sheet of paper.

11. You are a nurse at a community clinic frequented by a number of elderly patients. Mrs. Milner comes to your clinic complaining of dizziness and nausea. As you take her medication history, she shows you her "pill box." Inside you see almost a dozen different pills, all to be taken at noon. How could this happen? How could she possibly need so many medications at the same time?

12. The physician confirms that Mrs. Milner's "new symptoms," as she refers to them, are a result of polypharmacy. She protests, telling you, "Honey, I've got news for the doctor. I've had to take lots of drugs at the same time all my life. It never bothered me before. Why would it now when I'm even more used to it?" Explain at least three physiologic changes that occur with aging and the way in which these changes affect pharmacokinetics and pharmacodynamics.

CASE STUDY

Read the scenario and answer the following questions on a separate sheet of paper.

You are performing telephone triage in a pediatric clinic. A mother calls about her 28-month-old toddler, who has had chickenpox for 2 days. She wants to give aspirin because the toddler's fever is 101° F (38.3° C) but is unsure because her toddler "hates to take pills."

1. Should the mother use aspirin for this fever? Check a drug reference, if needed, for developmental considerations in this situation.

2. The mother states that her husband is going to the drugstore for some medicine. What advice would you give her regarding the dosage form of an antipyretic for her toddler?

3. When the husband returns from the store, he shows the mother the bottle of Children's Tylenol Suspension Liquid that was recommended by the store's pharmacist. He wonders, though, why the pharmacist would need to know the toddler's weight before suggesting this medication. Explain.

4. The toddler receives a dose of 1 teaspoon per the directions for a child of his weight of 28 lb. Later, when his 5-year-old sister needs a dose, she receives 1.5 teaspoons because of her weight of 45 lb. If the drug contains 160 mg per teaspoon, then how much medication did the 5-year-old receive in her dose?

5. What should the parents look for when evaluating the children's response to a dose of acetaminophen?

Chapter 4
Cultural, Legal, and Ethical Considerations

CHAPTER REVIEW

Choose the best answer for each of the following.

1. When reviewing drug classifications, the nurse knows that drugs classed as category C-I, which are to be dispensed "only with an approved protocol," include
   a. codeine, cocaine, and meperidine.
   b. heroin, LSD, and marijuana.
   c. phenobarbital, chloral hydrate, and benzodiazepines.
   d. cough preparations and diarrhea control drugs.

2. When a health care provider is writing a prescription for a drug, he or she is not permitted to mark a refill on the prescription if the drug falls into which category?
   a. C-II
   b. C-III
   c. C-IV
   d. C-V

3. The nurse is aware that the ethical principle of "Do no harm" is known as
   a. autonomy.
   b. beneficence.
   c. confidentiality.
   d. nonmaleficence.

4. Which legal act required drug manufacturers to establish the safety and efficacy of a new drug before its approval for use?
   a. Federal Food and Drugs Act of 1906
   b. Federal Food, Drug, and Cosmetic Act of 1938
   c. Kefauver-Harris Amendments of 1962
   d. Durham-Humphrey Amendment of 1951

5. Which of the following is the correct definition for *placebo?*
   a. An investigational drug used in a new drug study
   b. An inert substance that is not a drug
   c. A legend drug that requires a prescription
   d. A substance that is not approved as a drug but is used as an herbal product

6. During an admission assessment, which of the following would be part of the findings of a cultural assessment?
   a. The patient uses aspirin as needed for pain.
   b. The patient has a history of hypertension.
   c. The patient is allergic to shellfish.
   d. The patient does not eat pork products for religious reasons.

Match each investigational drug study phase with its corresponding description.

7. _____ Phase I

8. _____ Phase II

9. _____ Phase III

10. _____ Phase IV

a. A study using small numbers of volunteers who have the disease or disorder that the drug is meant to diagnose or treat. Subjects are monitored for drug efficacy and adverse effects.

b. Postmarketing studies conducted by drug companies to obtain further proof of the drug's therapeutic effects.

c. A study that involves a large number of patients at research centers designed to monitor for infrequent adverse effects and to identify any associated risks. Double-blind, placebo-controlled studies eliminate patient and researcher bias.

> d. A study that uses small numbers of healthy volunteers, as opposed to volunteers with the target ailment, to determine dosage range and pharmacokinetics.

Match each cultural group with its corresponding cultural practice.

11. _____ Asian

12. _____ Hispanic

13. _____ Native American

14. _____ African American

a. Some may seek a balance between the body and mind through the use of "cold" remedies or foods for "hot" illnesses, and vice versa.

b. Some may use folk medicine, protective bracelets, and laying on of hands.

c. Some believe that opposing forces of negative and positive energy lead to health or illness depending on whether the forces are balanced.

d. Some believe in the need for a balance among body, mind, and environment to maintain health and harmony with nature.

CRITICAL THINKING AND APPLICATION

Answer the following questions on a separate sheet of paper.

15. Identify a cultural group in your area and explore the health belief practices for that group.
    a. Are there any barriers to adequate health care?
    b. What is the attitude toward Western medicines and health treatments?
    c. What questions should you ask in your cultural assessment?

CASE STUDY

Read the scenario and answer the following questions on a separate sheet of paper.

You work in an outpatient treatment clinic for patients with human immunodeficiency virus (HIV) infection. During a recent staff meeting, the medical director discussed a new drug that has shown good results in clinical trials in another country. This drug has not yet been tested in the United States. She stated that she hopes to start clinical trials of that drug in the HIV clinic.

The following week, you are asked to start a new drug regimen for four patients with HIV infection. One of the drugs is new to you, and when you ask about it, the medical director replies, "Oh, that's the new drug I mentioned last week! One of my colleagues in that country sent me some samples, so we're going to try it here. The Food and Drug Administration has already started trials here in the United States. We will be comparing how these four patients do compared with four other patients who are in the same stages of HIV infection. The patients won't even know about this change."

1. Should you give the drugs as requested? If not, what should be done to correct the situation?

2. What ethical principle(s) guide your decision?

3. One of the potential study patients, brought in by his brother, seems reluctant to answer questions and says he "doesn't need any drugs." Upon further questioning, you find out that he would prefer to take some home remedies that his mother has made for him. How should you handle this situation?

4. When you meet with potential study patients, several mention that they fear others will find out about their illness if they participate in the study. What should you tell these patients?

Chapter 5

Medication Errors: Preventing and Responding

CHAPTER REVIEW

Provide the best answer for each of the following.

1. A(n) _____ is defined as any preventable adverse drug event that involves inappropriate medication use by a patient or health care professional. It may or may not cause harm to the patient.

2. A(n) _____ reaction is defied as an abnormal and unexpected response to a medication, other than an allergic reaction, that is peculiar to an individual patient.

3. A(n) _____ is any undesirable effect of a medication that is expected or anticipated to occur in patients who receive a given medication.

4. A(n) _____ is a type of adverse drug event that is defined as any unexpected, unintended, or excessive response to a medication.

5. A(n) _____ is an undesirable occurrence related to administration of or failure to administer a prescribed medication.

6. True or false: All adverse drug reactions are adverse drug events.

7. True or false: All adverse drug events are caused by medication errors.

8. Identify six ways to avoid medication errors.

9. Name at least four of the classes of medications that are considered "high alert" drugs.

10. The National Coordinating Council for Medication Error Reporting and Prevention recommends that certain terms be written out in full instead of being abbreviated. Write out the full meaning of each abbreviated word or phrase that appears in bold in the following list.

Digoxin 125 **mcg** PO now	
Lasix 40 mg IV **qd**	
d/c all meds	
NPH insulin 12 **u** SQ **ac** breakfast **qd**	
Floxin Otic 1 **gtt AD** bid	
Levothyroxine 125 **μg** every morning	

CASE STUDY

Read the scenario and answer the following questions on a separate sheet of paper.

A nursing student discovers that she has given her patient two aspirin tablets instead of the one-tablet daily dose that was ordered for antiplatelet effects. She is upset and talks to her fellow students, who tell her to keep quiet about it. "One extra aspirin won't hurt your patient," they tell her.

1. What should the nursing student do first? Describe other appropriate actions after this.

2. How could the student have prevented this error?

3. Should the patient be told about it? Explain your answer.

4. If the patient was not hurt by this incident, then is it considered a medication error? Explain.

5. The student has decided to inform her instructor. The instructor helps the student complete a report to the U.S. Pharmacopeia Medication Errors Reporting Program. Explain the reason for this report. Will the student's name be reported?

Chapter 6
Patient Education and Drug Therapy

CRITICAL THINKING AND APPLICATION

Answer the following questions on a separate sheet of paper.

1. You are to present information regarding antihypertensive drug therapy to two patients, a 40-year-old and a 78-year-old. Describe the differences in interventions you would use in your teaching strategies related to possible alterations in thought processes and sensory-perceptual status in these two patients.

2. You are to present information to a young mother on how to help her 8-year-old child use a metered-dose inhaler. Neither the mother nor her child speaks English. Discuss strategies to use in developing a teaching plan for them.

3. Your patient has been taking oral hypoglycemics for 1 month, and her blood glucose readings are still very high. On assessment, you discover a possible reason for these high readings. Develop a nursing diagnosis for this patient based on the following:

   a. The patient says that no one has ever told her about required dietary restrictions.

   b. The patient tells you that she only takes the medication if she feels ill.

4. For each of the following medications, develop a measurable goal and specific outcome criteria related to teaching a patient about the medication therapy. Use later chapters in the textbook for reference.

   a. Oral contraceptives

   b. Diuretic therapy with furosemide

   c. digoxin

   d. Transdermal nitroglycerin patches

   e. indomethacin

5. Develop a patient teaching plan for a 55-year-old patient who will be receiving warfarin therapy after discharge. Refer to the appropriate chapter in the text for information. Include the following:

   a. Assessment—the objective and subjective data that would be needed

   b. Nursing diagnosis

   c. Planning—a measurable goal and outcome criteria

   d. Implementation—specific educational strategies

   e. Evaluation—means for validating that learning had occurred

CASE STUDY

Read the scenario and answer the following questions on a separate sheet of paper.

A 77-year-old male, accompanied by his wife, visits the office for a 3-month checkup. He has been treated for hypertension and has a history of angina. While in the office, he pulls a small bottle of sublingual nitroglycerin tablets from his pants pocket and states, "I never go anywhere without these." He says he "gets along okay" with his medicines at home and that it "doesn't hurt anything" if he misses a day or two of his medications. His blood pressure today is 130/92 mm Hg, pulse rate is 88 beats/min, and respiratory rate is 12 breaths/min. Previously, his blood pressure readings have been 160/98, 152/92, and 148/94 mm Hg.

After the patient is evaluated by the physician, new medication orders are written as follows:

- HCTZ 25-mg tablet, once a day
- Slow-K, 1 tablet daily
- Diltiazem 60-mg tablet, three times a day
- Prevacid, 15-mg capsule, before breakfast and dinner
- nitroglycerin sublingual tablets, as needed for chest pain

1. Based on your assessment, what nursing diagnosis would you suggest for this situation?

2. State a goal and outcome criteria for your nursing diagnosis.

3. Describe the teaching strategies you would use when teaching this patient about how to take his medications correctly.

4. How would you evaluate the effectiveness of the education process in this situation?

Chapter 7

Over-the-Counter Drugs and Herbal and Dietary Supplements

DOUBLE PUZZLE

Unscramble each of the clue words. Then take the letters that appear in the circles and unscramble them for the final message.

LAIREANV

RCGIAL

FEFREEVW

TS. NOJH'S TWRO

KONIGG

WAS OLTATPEM

NISGGNE

NAAHICCEE

LAOE

SOADELNEGL

| | | | B | | | | | | | | | | Y | |

CHAPTER REVIEW

Choose the best answer for each of the following.

1. Classifications of drugs commonly used as over-the-counter (OTC) remedies include which of the following? Choose all that apply.
   a. Nonsteroidal antiinflammatory drugs
   b. Cold remedies
   c. Antibiotics
   d. Smoking deterrent systems
   e. Topical antiviral ointments
   f. Histamine-2 (H_2) blockers

2. Advantages of OTC remedies include which of the following?
   a. Third-party health insurance payers usually cover the costs.
   b. Patients can feel better faster when self-medicating.
   c. There are fewer drug interactions.
   d. Patients can self-treat minor ailments and reduce physician visits.

3. In the United States, the Food and Drug Administration does which of the following regarding the manufacture of herbal products?
   a. Enforces standards of herbal product quality and safety
   b. Requires the manufacturers of herbal products to prove efficacy
   c. Sets standards for quality control
   d. Defines herbal products as dietary supplements

4. Tachyphylaxis may develop in patients who use which of the following herbal products?
   a. Aloe
   b. Echinacea
   c. Feverfew
   d. Kava

5. The nurse is admitting a patient who has a diagnosis of right lower lobe pneumonia. Upon assessment, the nurse learns that the patient is wearing an herbal pack on her chest. What should the nurse do first?
   a. Remove the pack immediately.
   b. Report the pack to the physician.
   c. Ask the patient about the herbal pack.
   d. Document the presence of the herbal pack.

CRITICAL THINKING AND APPLICATION

Answer the following questions on a separate sheet of paper.

6. Review the herbal boxes for garlic, ginger, flaxseed, saw palmetto, ginkgo, glucosamine and chondroitin, and valerian in the appropriate chapters. (See the list of herbal boxes located inside the back cover of the textbook.) Which of these herbal products may have serious interactions with anticoagulants such as warfarin and heparin?

7. List the types of individuals who may have more frequent adverse reactions to OTC drugs.

8. List contraindications to the use of herbal products.

9. Identify an OTC product or herbal or dietary supplement that you (or a family member) take and review the indications, drug interactions, contraindications, and adverse effects. Did you find any concerns?

CASE STUDY

Read the scenario and answer the following questions on a separate sheet of paper.

A 30-year-old woman is in the clinic for her yearly gynecologic checkup. She is not pregnant but would like to have children soon and states that she and her husband are trying to conceive. She says that she is "very concerned" about her health, and watches her diet and exercises regularly to stay in shape. She has a family history of heart disease but no other health concerns. Her physical assessment reveals no abnormalities or health problems.

> On her medical history sheet, she writes that she takes several drug and herbal products as follows:
> Echinacea, from September to March, to prevent the flu
> Adult aspirin, one tablet every day, to prevent a heart attack
> Garlic tablets twice a day for my heart
> Kava tea as needed for relaxation
> One glass of red wine with dinner
> Valerian capsules for sleep as needed (usually three or four times a week)

1. Are there any drug or herbal interactions in this listing?

2. Do any of these products have a potential for problems if used over the long term?

3. Is there any specific information on which you should focus in taking the patient's history or performing an assessment given that she is using these drugs and herbal products?

4. She tells you that she thinks the herbal products are "safe" because the government would not allow them to be sold if they were not. Is this true?

5. What would you emphasize when teaching her about the use of herbal products and OTC drugs?

Chapter 8
Substance Abuse

CHAPTER REVIEW

Match each drug with its corresponding description.

1. _____ cocaine

2. _____ ecstasy

3. _____ phenobarbital

4. _____ heroin

5. _____ disulfiram

6. _____ nicotine

7. _____ naltrexone

8. _____ bupropion (Zyban)

9. _____ opium

10. _____ "roofies"

a. A nicotine-free treatment for nicotine dependence

b. Known as the "date rape" drug

c. The source plant for heroin

d. The addictive chemical in tobacco products

e. An opioid that is injected by "mainlining" or "skin popping"

f. Used in managing withdrawal from barbiturates

g. Used to deter the use of alcohol during alcohol abuse treatment

h. A stimulant that is either "snorted" through the nasal passages or injected intravenously

i. A stimulant that is popular at "raves" with college-age students

j. An opioid antagonist used for opioid abuse or dependence

Choose the best answer for each of the following.

11. A patient who has been taking disulfiram (Antabuse) therapy for 3 months has been off the therapy for 2 days. He decides to go out with friends to have a beer. What effects may he experience?
    a. No ill effects
    b. Diarrhea
    c. Vomiting
    d. Euphoria

12. The most common drug effects leading to abuse of opioids include
    a. hallucinations.
    b. sleep.
    c. stimulation.
    d. relaxation and euphoria.

13. Which medications may be used to manage opioid withdrawal? Select all that apply.
    a. disulfiram (Antabuse)
    b. clonidine (Catapres)
    c. methadone
    d. bupropion (Zyban)
    e. naltrexone (ReVia).

14. When teaching a patient about drug interactions, the nurse is aware that combining benzodiazepines with ethanol or barbiturates may lead to death due to which of the following?
    a. Cardiac dysrhythmia
    b. Convulsions
    c. Respiratory arrest
    d. Stroke

15. A patient with a known history of chronic excessive ingestion of ethanol has developed memory problems and comes to the health clinic with hard-to-believe stories of what has happened to him. The nurse recognizes that these symptoms are associated with which disorder?
    a. Cerebrovascular accident
    b. Korsakoff's psychosis
    c. Narcolepsy
    d. Bipolar disorder

CRITICAL THINKING AND APPLICATION

Answer the following questions on a separate sheet of paper.

16. Describe how nicotine is used to ease withdrawal from nicotine use. How is bupropion (Zyban) used in smoking cessation programs?

17. How is medication therapy different for mild, moderate, and severe alcohol withdrawal?

CASE STUDY

Read the scenario and answer the following questions on a separate sheet of paper.

A 19-year-old male, Mr. C., is admitted to the emergency department after he collapsed at a fraternity party. The paramedics state that there were beer-drinking contests at the party, and it is unknown how much Mr. C. had to drink. His friend says that Mr. C. was upset over losing a girlfriend, and he has worried about how heavily Mr. C. has been drinking in the past 2 weeks.

Mr. C. is semiconscious but unable to answer questions coherently, and his speech is slurred. His blood pressure is 100/58 mm Hg, his pulse rate is 110 beats/min, and his breathing is heavy with a respiratory rate of 16 breaths/min. He vomited on the way to the hospital.

1. Is ethanol considered a central nervous system stimulant or depressant?

2. What are the effects of severe alcoholic intoxication on the cardiovascular and respiratory systems?

3. The patient is admitted to the medical unit for observation. For what should the nurse be observant at this time?

4. The next evening Mr. C. is more alert but still unsteady in his gait. He says he wants to go home, but you notice fine tremors of his hands. Should he be discharged at this time? Explain.

5. If Mr. C. continues the pattern of heavy drinking, what effects could the chronic ingestion of ethanol have on his body?

Chapter 9
Photo Atlas of Drug Administration

CHAPTER REVIEW

Choose the best answer for each of the following.

1. To expel air bubbles after drawing fluid from an ampule, remove the needle, hold the syringe with the needle pointing up, and do which of the following?
   a. Draw back slightly on the plunger, tap the side of the syringe to cause bubbles to rise toward the needle, and push the plunger upward to eject air.
   b. Tap the side of the syringe to cause bubbles to rise toward the needle, draw back slightly on the plunger, and push the plunger upward to eject air.
   c. Tap the side of the syringe to cause bubbles to rise toward the needle, draw back slightly on the plunger, push the plunger upward to eject air, and eject a small amount of fluid.
   d. Draw back slightly on the plunger, tap the side of the syringe to cause bubbles to rise toward the needle, and push the plunger upward to eject air; do not eject fluid.

2. When giving intradermal injections, the nurse will remember to do which of the following?
   a. Massage the site lightly after the injection
   b. Have the patient massage the site until the pain diminishes
   c. Avoid massaging the site
   d. Apply heat to the site after the injection

3. When medication is administered by intravenous push, the correct way to occlude the intravenous line is to do which of the following?
   a. Pinch the tubing just above the injection port
   b. Pinch the tubing at least 2 inches above the injection port
   c. Fold the tubing just above the injection port
   d. Do not occlude the line because it is not necessary to occlude the tubing for this procedure

4. When more than one medication is to be added to a solution, which action is correct?
   a. Use an equal volume of each medication.
   b. First assess the two drugs for compatibility.
   c. Always add the drugs at least 1 hour apart.
   d. Use the same needle for both medications.

5. When oral medications are administered, which action is correct?
   a. If a patient cannot swallow medications, crush all the medications together and administer with applesauce.
   b. Give oral medications with meals to avoid gastrointestinal upset.
   c. Stay with the patient until each medication has been swallowed.
   d. Give all medications on an empty stomach to facilitate absorption.

6. When administering eardrops, which action by the nurse is correct?
   a. Press a cotton ball firmly into the ear canal after giving the drops.
   b. Have the patient sit up and tilt the head for 2 to 3 minutes.
   c. Gently massage the tragus of the ear.
   d. Have the patient remain in the side-lying position for 20 minutes.

7. Which position is correct when the nurse administers nasal drops for the frontal or maxillary sinuses?
   a. Tilt the patient's head backward and facing toward the left side.
   b. Tilt the patient's head back over the edge of the bed with the head turned toward the side treated.
   c. Place a pillow under the patient's shoulders and tilt the head back.
   d. Tilt the patient's head to the side opposite the side treated.

8. Which action by the nurse is correct when administering drugs via a nasogastric tube?
    a. Allow the fluid to flow via gravity.
    b. Use gentle but consistent pressure when forcing the fluid into the tube.
    c. Shake the tube gently to facilitate the movement of fluid in the tube.
    d. Confirm placement of the tube after the medication is given.

9. Z-track intramuscular injections are indicated in which of the following situations?
    a. When there is insufficient muscle mass in the landmarked area
    b. Whenever massaging the area after medication administration is contraindicated
    c. With medications that are known to be irritating, painful, and/or staining to tissues
    d. With any injection that is given into the dorsogluteal muscle

10. When giving sublingual medications, the nurse recalls that medications given by this route have which advantage?
    a. They are immediately absorbed.
    b. They are excreted rapidly.
    c. They are metabolized immediately.
    d. They are distributed equally.

11. The dosage of a prochlorperazine (Compazine) rectal suppository is twice what has actually been ordered. The nurse's most appropriate intervention would be which of the following?
    a. Cut the suppository in half.
    b. Call the physician for clarification.
    c. Administer another type of suppository.
    d. Instruct the patient to retain the suppository for only 5 minutes.

12. Which of the following is a contraindication to the administration of rectal suppositories?
    a. Vomiting
    b. Fever
    c. Constipation
    d. Rectal bleeding

13. The nurse applies a transdermal patch to a site that is
    a. hairy.
    b. nonhairy.
    c. moist.
    d. within a skinfold.

14. Which of the following is important to tell the patient when teaching about the instillation of nasal drops?
    a. Clear the nasal passages by blowing the nose gently before administering the medication.
    b. Clear the nasal passages by blowing the nose gently after administering the medication.
    c. Sit in a semi-Fowler's position for 5 minutes after the instillation of the medication.
    d. Place the nose dropper approximately ½ inch into the nostril when instilling drops.

15. Which of the following is true regarding the administration of ophthalmic medications? Select all that apply.
    a. Have the patient look upward while instilling the medication.
    b. Instill the prescribed number of drops into the conjunctival sac.
    c. Have the patient close his or her eyes tightly after the drop has been instilled.
    d. Apply gentle pressure to the patient's nasolacrimal duct for 30 to 60 seconds after instilling the drops.
    e. Apply ointment to the conjunctival sac starting at the outer canthus and working toward the inner canthus.

CRITICAL THINKING AND APPLICATION

Answer the following questions on a separate sheet of paper.

16. Describe how to assess injection sites for each of the following:

    a. Subcutaneous injections *should be given @ a 90° angel, do not massage site after injection; 45° for child or overly thin person*

    b. Intramuscular injections *should be done at a 90° angle, don't massage*

    c. Intradermal injections *should be given at 5°-15° angel, 3 to 4 fingers widths below the antecubital space do not massage site after.*

17. Describe the proper technique of needle insertion for each of the following:

    a. Subcutaneous injections *same as c. when giving in abdomen, be sure to choose a site @ least 2in away from umbilicus*

    b. Intramuscular injections *1st assess size and integrity of muscle to fit amout of injection; Palpate for hardness or tenderness note bruising or infection*

    c. Intradermal injections *Avoid areas of bruising, rashes or inflammation, edema of discoulation*

18. You are administering an intramuscular injection to your patient. After the needle enters the site, you grasp the lower end of the syringe barrel with your nondominant hand and slowly pull back on the plunger to aspirate the drug. Blood appears in the syringe. What do you do? *remove the needle, dispose of syringe and prepare another medication*

19. You are preparing a liquid medication for a patient. How does the usual procedure change when the volume of medication required is less than 5 mL? *draw it into a calibrated oral syringe*

20. A patient has been given a new inhaler that contains 250 doses of medication. The order specifies that the patient is to take "one puff four times a day." How many days will this inhaler last before it becomes empty? *1 puff 4x a day   62 days to empty.*

CASE STUDY

Read the scenario and answer the following questions on a separate sheet of paper.

A mother comes to a family practice office with her 2-year-old daughter and 8-month-old son. She is planning a trip abroad and needs to obtain immunizations for herself and her children before she leaves.

1. The mother and the infant each need to be given an intramuscular immunization. Describe the differences in choosing sites and giving an intramuscular injection in the mother and the infant. *Both will have injection in the vastus lateralis*

2. The 2-year-old daughter has an ear infection, and the physician has prescribed eardrops. What should you teach the mother about giving these eardrops to her child? *when giving mom should pull up and back down pinna, and keep on side for 5-10min*

3. Two days later, the mother brings the infant back to the office because she has developed a high fever. You prepare to give the infant a liquid oral antipyretic and note that the dose is 4 mL. How do you measure this medication? *with a disposable oral-dosing syringe, place in mouth besides the tounge.*

4. The mother wants to add the medication to her baby's bottle. How would you administer this liquid medication to the infant? *say you can not add to formula, but an empty nipple may be used and only administer small amouts each time*

Chapter 10
Analgesic Drugs

CRITICAL THINKING CROSSWORD

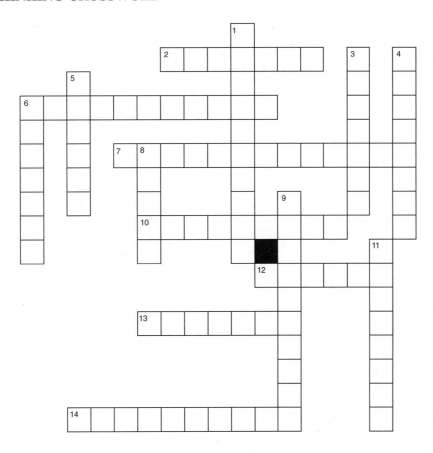

Across

2. Any drug that binds to a receptor and causes a response has _____ properties.
6. Mrs. G. is experiencing pain and itching due to a severe case of poison ivy on the skin of her arms and legs. She is experiencing _____ pain.
7. Mr. R., described in 12 Across, is recovering. He requires continued pain management but is able to take less powerful doses of medication now. Every day he tells you that he finds he can "do more and more normal things, even though there is still some pain there." Mr. R. is describing his level of _____ (two words).

Down

1. Mr. D.'s drug binds to a receptor but causes an effect opposite to that of the type of drug discussed in 13 Across. He is taking a drug with _____ properties.
3. Mrs. H. has experienced back pain "for years." She says that it is worse in the late afternoon and at night but that "really, even when it lessens somewhat, it is there all the time in some form." Mrs. H. is experiencing _____ pain.

10. Ms. L. was in an auto accident and injured her leg. In assessing the level of a stimulus applied to her toe that results in a perception of pain, you are testing her pain _____.

12. Mr. R. is brought to the emergency department in tremendous pain. The emergency department team recognizes the need to immediately bring the pain under some control to make assessment, diagnosis, and treatment more manageable. After assessing that it is not contraindicated, the attending physician initiates administration of a very strong and addicting pain reliever. This is no doubt a(n) _____ analgesic.

13. Ms. T. is taking a drug that binds to part of a receptor and causes effects that are not as strong as those of a pure agonist. She is taking a(n) _____ agonist.

14. Mr. Y. is experiencing the effects of withdrawal from an opioid analgesic; he had become physically dependent on the drug, and now that he no longer has access to it, he is suffering withdrawal, or opioid _____ syndrome.

4. Mr. E. paces the floor all night, holding his side. The pain is so severe that he is sick to his stomach. His wife brings him to the emergency department, where it is quickly discovered that Mr. E. has a kidney stone. The type of pain he has been experiencing is _____ pain.

5. This word is often used interchangeably with the term *opioid*.

6. Mr. J. has injured his ankle in a friendly basketball game with his peers after work. His wife brings him to the urgent care center several hours later because of the pain. Mr. J. is probably experiencing _____ pain.

8. Mrs. M. had breast reduction surgery yesterday and is complaining of pain around her incisions. Mrs. M. is experiencing _____ pain.

9. Mr. C. has entered a treatment center to help him overcome a psychologic dependence on a cocaine derivative. He is seeking help for a _____ use of this drug, characterized by a continuous craving that is not pain related.

11. Mr. V. is already taking an opioid pain reliever. When his pain increases, the drug is not as effective. He is given a second analgesic drug in addition to the first drug. "Two pain killers?" he asks you. "Is that safe?" You explain that the second drug is not a primary analgesic but has properties that will add to the analgesic effects of the opioid. It is being used, then, as a(n) _____ drug.

CHAPTER REVIEW

Choose the best answer for each of the following.

1. During a marathon, a runner had to drop out after 16 miles because of severe muscle spasms. This type of pain is classified as which of the following?
   a. Chronic pain
   b. Somatic pain
   c. Visceral pain
   d. Superficial pain

2. A young man has been taken to the emergency department because of a suspected overdose of morphine tablets. Which drug may be used to treat this overdose?
   a. meperidine (Demerol)
   b. naproxen (Naprosyn)
   c. aspirin
   d. naloxone HCl (Narcan)

3. An anticonvulsant drug has been ordered as part of a patient's pain management program. The purpose of the anticonvulsant in this case is to
   a. produce sleep.
   b. prevent seizures.
   c. relieve neuropathic pain.
   d. reduce anxiety.

4. Moderate to severe pain is best treated with which of the following?
   a. acetaminophen (Tylenol)
   b. Opioid antagonists
   c. Benzodiazepines
   d. Opioid analgesics

5. Which of the following should be included in an assessment before giving an opioid analgesic? Choose all that apply.
   a. Blood clotting times
   b. The level of pain rated on a scale
   c. Prior analgesic use (time, type, amount, and effectiveness)
   d. Dietary history
   e. Allergies

Match each type of pain with its corresponding description.

6. _____ Acute pain

7. _____ Chronic pain

8. _____ Somatic pain

9. _____ Visceral pain

10. _____ Superficial pain

11. _____ Vascular pain

12. _____ Neuropathic pain

13. _____ Phantom pain

14. _____ Psychogenic pain

15. _____ Central pain

a. Pain that is due to psychologic factors, not physical conditions or disorders

b. Pain that is thought to account for most migraine headaches

c. Pain that relates to a body part that has been removed

d. Pain that originates from the skin or mucous membranes

e. Pain that occurs with tumors, trauma, or inflammation of the brain

f. Persistent or recurring pain that is often difficult to treat

g. Pain that is sudden and usually subsides when treated

h. Pain that originates from the organs or smooth muscles

i. Pain that originates from the skeletal muscles, ligaments, or joints

j. Pain that results from injury or damage to the peripheral nerve fibers

CASE STUDY

Read the scenario and answer the following questions on a separate sheet of paper.

A 58-year-old woman has been admitted for surgery to remove a small growth from her lower back, just under the skin. That evening she asks for pain medication. Upon assessment, you find that she rates her pain level as "8" and that her pain is located mainly in the immediate area around her incision. You prepare to give her an intravenous dose of morphine sulfate.

1. What type of pain is she experiencing?

2. What nonpharmacologic intervention may be used to reduce her pain?

3. Within an hour of receiving the morphine, the patient complains that her skin feels "itchy" but she cannot see any hives. What do you tell her?

4. What serious adverse effect is possible if she receives too much morphine sulfate? What, if anything, can be given to treat this?

5. Two days later she is ready to be discharged home. Her physician writes a prescription for Vicodin. The patient sees the generic label and asks why the medication contains Tylenol. Explain the purpose of the acetaminophen (Tylenol) in this medication and for her pain treatment.

Chapter 11
General and Local Anesthetics

CRITICAL THINKING CROSSWORD

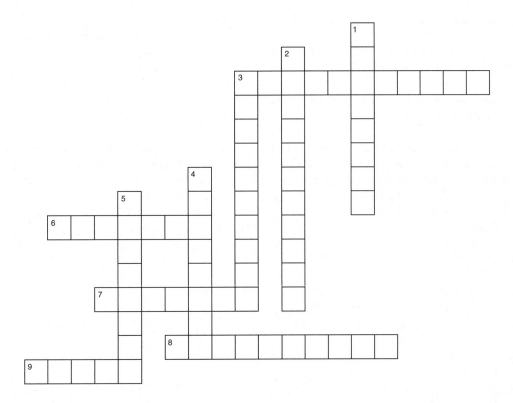

Across

3. A commonly used, long-acting, nondepolarizing neuromuscular blocking agent (NMBA).
6. Anesthetic drugs that alter the central nervous system (CNS), resulting in loss of consciousness and deep muscle relaxation, are termed _____.
7. _____ anesthetics are applied directly to the skin and mucous membranes.
8. Drugs used in combination with anesthetics to control the adverse effects of anesthetics.
9. Drugs that render a specific portion of the body insensitive to pain without affecting consciousness are called _____ anesthetics.

Down

1. An anticholinergic drug given preoperatively to dry secretions.
2. A broad term for drugs that depress the CNS.
3. Anesthetics administered directly into the CNS by various spinal injection techniques are examples of _____ anesthetics.
4. The practice of using combinations of drugs to produce general anesthesia rather than using a single drug.
5. Another name for 9 Across.

CHAPTER REVIEW

Choose the best answer for each of the following.

1. Examples of adjunctive drugs used with anesthesia include which of the following? Select all that apply.
   a. Sedatives-hypnotics
   b. Anticonvulsants
   c. Anticholinergics
   d. Inhaled gas
   e. Opioid analgesics

2. Lidocaine is frequently used for which of the following?
   a. Spinal anesthesia
   b. Local anesthesia
   c. Intravenous anesthesia
   d. General anesthesia

3. The nurse monitoring a patient after surgery keeps in mind that the primary concern with use of an NMBA is which of the following?
   a. Respiratory arrest
   b. Headache
   c. Bradycardia
   d. Hypertension

4. To decrease the possibility of a headache after spinal anesthesia, the nurse should instruct the patient to do which of the following?
   a. Sit in high Fowler's position
   b. Lie flat in bed
   c. Limit fluids
   d. Engage in activity

5. Local anesthesia is indicated for which of the following? Select all that apply.
   a. Cardioversions
   b. Suturing a skin laceration
   c. Diagnostic procedures
   d. Long-duration surgery
   e. Dental procedures

6. A sudden elevation in body temperature in a patient who has just returned from surgery may indicate which of the following?
   a. A normal temperature change after surgery
   b. Malignant hypertension
   c. Malignant hyperthermia
   d. Fever

7. A patient is receiving an NMBA. Indicate the order in which the following areas become paralyzed once this drug is given (1 = first, 3 = last).
   ___ a. Limbs, neck, trunk muscles
   ___ b. Intercostal muscles and diaphragm
   ___ c. Small, rapidly moving muscles, such as those of the fingers and eyes

CRITICAL THINKING AND APPLICATION

Answer the following questions on a separate sheet of paper.

8. Henry is a student nurse who has assisted the nurse anesthetist in surgery on prior occasions. Today, however, he is nervous because it is a child who will undergo general anesthesia. Why might this make Henry more nervous than usual?

9. Mr. Smith is being administered an NMBA while he is receiving mechanical ventilation. What is important to remember when working with him while he is receiving this therapy?

10. Mrs. Edwards will undergo cardioversion this afternoon, and the nurse anesthetist has explained to her that she will not be asleep but that she will not remember the procedure. Mrs. Edwards asks you, "How can this be?" What is your explanation?

CASE STUDY

Read the scenario and answer the following questions on a separate sheet of paper.

You are a nursing student, and today you are assigned to an observation day in the operating room, with a certified registered nurse anesthetist (CRNA) as your contact for the day. The first case is a patient undergoing a right lower lung lobectomy due to lung cancer. The patient has a history of paraplegia from an old automobile accident. The patient's blood pressure has been maintained at 120/72 mm Hg, and the pulse has ranged from 100 to 110 beats/min during the surgery. The patient's body temperature has lowered to 96.2° F (35.7° C) after surgery. The patient's respiration has been maintained by ventilator.

1. Before the surgery, the CRNA explained that the patient will undergo "balanced anesthesia." What is meant by this term?

2. What is the purpose of administering the drug succinylcholine during anesthesia?

3. As your patient goes to the postanesthesia care unit (PACU), the CRNA asks you to monitor for signs of succinylcholine toxicity. Why would this be of concern at this time?

4. What can be done if the patient has received too much succinylcholine?

5. Another patient is undergoing a procedure performed using local anesthesia. Are there advantages of this type of anesthesia over general anesthesia?

6. In the PACU, what are the main concerns of the nurse monitoring the patient recovering from anesthesia?

Chapter 12

Central Nervous System Depressants and Muscle Relaxants

CHAPTER REVIEW

Choose the best answer for each of the following.

1. A hypnotic is a drug that
   a. produces sleep.
   b. slows the destruction of dopamine.
   c. prevents nausea and vomiting.
   d. relieves pain.

2. A patient who has been taking a benzodiazepine for 5 weeks has been instructed to stop the medication. The best way to discontinue the medication is to
   a. stop taking the drug immediately.
   b. plan a gradual reduction in dosage.
   c. overlap this medication with another drug.
   d. take the medication every other day for a number of weeks.

3. A patient will be undergoing a brief surgical procedure to obtain a biopsy from a superficial mass on his arm. The nurse expects that which type of barbiturate will be used at this time?
   a. Ultrashort
   b. Short
   c. Intermediate
   d. Long

4. While monitoring a patient who took an overdose of barbiturates, the nurse keeps in mind that the cause of death would be which of the following?
   a. Tachycardia
   b. Hypertension
   c. Dyspnea
   d. Respiratory arrest

5. A patient with back muscle spasms is being treated with a skeletal muscle relaxant. These drugs are most effective when used with
   a. benzodiazepines.
   b. moist heat.
   c. physical therapy.
   d. aspirin.

6. The nurse is providing care for a patient who has accidentally taken an overdose of benzodiazepines. Which drug would be used to treat this patient?
   a. methamphetamine
   b. xanthines
   c. flumazenil
   d. naloxone

CRITICAL THINKING AND APPLICATION

Answer the following questions on a separate sheet of paper.

7. A 19-year-old college freshman is brought into the emergency department with a suspected barbiturate overdose. What symptoms would you expect to see? How is overdose treated?

8. Jackie is taking benzodiazepines to treat her insomnia. Today she visits your clinic and states that she is going to Europe for 2 months and wants a prescription that will allow her to take enough medication along for her entire stay. The physician declines. She is a little insulted and asks you why the physician refused her request. "Does my doctor think I'm an addict or something?" What do you explain to her? What other options are possible for her?

9. Mrs. Alexander, who is 81 years of age, weighs significantly more than her 47-year-old daughter, yet she is given a lower dosage of medication for insomnia of a similar degree. Why? Is this a dosage calculation error?

10. You have been asked to take a patient history for William, who will be given a benzodiazepine.

    a. What conditions or disorders should you ask about?

    b. What drug intake should you be most concerned about?

    c. What if William were an infant? A great-grandfather? Would this additional information matter? Why or why not?

11. Mr. Palmer is recovering from an automobile accident and has received a prescription for cyclobenzaprine for painful muscle spasms.

    a. What patient teaching should he receive about this medication?

    b. What other measures should be included in addition to this drug therapy?

12. Define tachyphylaxis and name one drug that can cause it. Is it an advantage or disadvantage? Why?

CASE STUDY

Read the scenario and answer the following questions on a separate sheet of paper.

A 44-year-old woman has had problems with insomnia "off and on for a few years" and has tried over-the-counter medications, herbal remedies, and prescription drugs. She likes to drink a glass of wine each night before going to bed. Today she is visiting the clinic for a checkup and asks for a prescription for secobarbital (Seconal) because that was the last drug she tried several years ago. She says she can't understand why the pharmacy won't refill her prescriptions for Seconal. The physician prescribes zaleplon (Sonata) instead.

1. Why did the physician change her prescription?

2. What are the consequences of long-term use of barbiturates?

3. What interactions should she be cautioned about while she is taking Sonata?

4. What other patient teaching is important for this patient?

Chapter 13
Antiepileptic Drugs

CRITICAL THINKING CROSSWORD

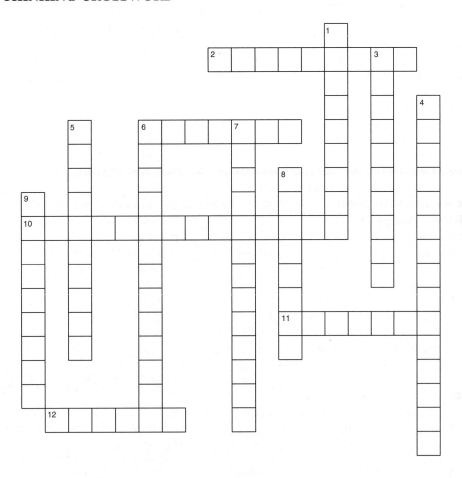

Across

2. Status epilepticus is considered a life-threatening
   _____.
6. A type of epilepsy with an unknown cause.
10. A potentially fatal adverse effect of valproic acid.
11. A brief episode of abnormal electrical activity in
    the nerve cells of the brain.
12. Intravenously administered antiepileptic drugs
    should be delivered this way to avoid serious
    adverse effects.

Down

1. A type of epilepsy with a distinct cause.
3. An involuntary spasmodic contraction of voluntary
   muscles throughout the body.
4. These drugs are among the first-line drugs for the
   treatment of status epilepticus.
5. Another term for 6 Across.
6. A barbiturate used primarily to control tonic-clonic
   and partial seizures.
7. The metabolic process that occurs when the metabolism of a drug increases over time, which leads to
   lower than expected drug concentrations.
8. Recurrent episodes of convulsive seizures.
9. A first-line antiepileptic drug, the long-term use of
   which can cause gingival hyperplasia.

CHAPTER REVIEW

Choose the best answer for each of the following.

1. A teenaged girl has seizures characterized by temporary lapses in consciousness that last only a few seconds. Her teachers have said that she "daydreams too much." These types of seizures are known as which of the following?
   a. Simple seizures
   b. Complex seizures
   c. Partial seizures
   d. Generalized seizures

2. Which condition is a life-threatening emergency in which patients typically do not regain consciousness?
   a. Status epilepticus
   b. Tonic-clonic convulsion
   c. Epilepsy
   d. Secondary epilepsy

3. Which of the following is true about intravenous infusion of phenytoin? Select all that apply.
   a. It should be injected quickly.
   b. It should be injected slowly.
   c. It should be followed by an injection of sterile saline.
   d. Continuous infusion should be avoided.

4. Which of the following is a possible adverse effect of phenobarbital therapy?
   a. Constipation
   b. Gingival hyperplasia
   c. Drowsiness
   d. Dysrhythmias

5. Which drug is considered the first choice for the treatment of status epilepticus?
   a. phenobarbital
   b. diazepam
   c. valproic acid
   d. phenytoin

6. A patient who is experiencing neuropathic pain tells the nurse that the physician is going to start him on a new medication that is generally used to treat seizures. The nurse anticipates that which drug will be ordered?
   a. phenobarbital
   b. phenytoin
   c. gabapentin
   d. tiagabine

CRITICAL THINKING AND APPLICATION

Answer the following questions on a separate sheet of paper.

7. What is meant by autoinduction in a drug? Identify at least one antiepileptic drug that undergoes autoinduction.

8. Jeremy, an 8-year-old boy, has resisted his oral doses of topiramate, which has made compliance with the drug regimen difficult. His mother calls and says that she has found a way to get him to take it: she crushes the tablet and sprinkles it on flavored gelatin. She is delighted. What is your response?

CASE STUDY

Read the scenario and answer the following questions on a separate sheet of paper.

Four-year-old Mattie has started preschool. Today the teacher called Mattie's mother to tell her that she noticed that Mattie seems to have a problem with "daydreaming." She explained that Mattie seemed inattentive during group work and was staring out into space several times a day. She was also worried because she saw Mattie's eyes move back and forth rapidly during these episodes. These "spells" lasted a minute or two, and then Mattie seemed fine. The mother has brought Mattie to the pediatric office to have her checked. The physician suspects that Mattie is experiencing a type of seizure disorder and has ordered some diagnostic testing.

1. What type of seizure is Mattie experiencing?

2. After the diagnostic testing is performed, what medication is most likely to be prescribed for Mattie?

3. This medication comes in a syrup at a concentration of 250 mg/5 mL. What is important to teach the mother regarding administration of this type of medication?

4. What should the mother be taught to monitor while Mattie is taking this medication?

5. After a year, Mattie's mother is pleased that the seizures have "disappeared" and wants to take Mattie off the medication. What is your response?

Chapter 14
Antiparkinsonian Drugs

CHAPTER REVIEW

Choose the best answer for each of the following.

1. A patient with Parkinson's disease has difficulty performing voluntary movements. This is known as
   a. akinesia.
   b. dyskinesia.
   c. chorea.
   d. dystonia.

2. Which drug may be used early in the treatment of Parkinson's disease but eventually loses effectiveness and must be replaced by another drug?
   a. amantadine
   b. levodopa
   c. selegiline
   d. tolcapone

3. When teaching a patient who is taking levodopa for Parkinson's disease, what should the nurse tell the patient about vitamin supplements?
   a. Vitamin supplements should not be taken at this time.
   b. Vitamin supplements should be taken twice a day to ensure that the patient receives enough nutrients.
   c. The patient should avoid supplements that contain vitamin B_6 (pyridoxine).
   d. The patient should not take more than the recommended amount of calcium.

4. A patient who is newly diagnosed with Parkinson's disease and beginning medication therapy with entacapone, a catechol ortho-methyltransferase inhibitor (COMT), asks the nurse, "How soon will improvement occur?" The nurse's best response is which of the following?
   a. "That varies from patient to patient."
   b. "You should discuss that with your physician."
   c. "You should notice a difference right away."
   d. "It may take several weeks before you notice any degree of improvement."

5. Anticholinergic drugs administered during treatment of Parkinson's disease are given to control or minimize which of the following symptoms? Select all that apply.
   a. Drooling
   b. Constipation
   c. Muscle rigidity
   d. Bradykinesia

6. A patient who has been taking levodopa for 4 months has been instructed by the health care provider to take a "drug holiday" for 10 days. The patient should be prepared for which of the following?
   a. A reduction in symptoms of Parkinson's disease
   b. Withdrawal effects while the drug is stopped
   c. The need to take higher dosages when the drug is resumed
   d. A possible stay in the hospital during the time he is not taking the drug

CRITICAL THINKING AND APPLICATION

Answer the following questions on a separate sheet of paper.

7. Mr. Hicks is about to have levodopa added to his carbidopa treatment regimen.

    a.   Why must dopamine be administered in the form of levodopa?

    b.   What problems are avoided when carbidopa is given with levodopa?

    c.   How does the carbidopa work when given with levodopa?

8. Mrs. Reynolds, a 35-year-old new mother, has experienced slowing movements, cogwheel rigidity, and pill-rolling tremor. Sadly, she has been diagnosed with Parkinson's disease, a somewhat rare occurrence in someone her age. In addition to the usual history questions, what must you ask in anticipation of dopaminergic therapy in Mrs. Reynolds's specific situation?

9. Jane, age 45, is taking benztropine in addition to a dopaminergic drug for Parkinson's disease. Her 76-year-old neighbor comments that he cannot take benztropine because it is too risky for his heart and kidneys. Jane calls and asks why this is not a concern in her case. What do you say?

CASE STUDY

Read the scenario and answer the following questions on a separate sheet of paper.

Alexander, a 54-year-old man, has been diagnosed with Parkinson's disease and is about to start drug therapy. His symptoms are mild, yet he has some akinesia that interferes with his ability to type at work. The physician explains that Alexander may have to take a variety of drugs as the disease progresses.

1. What is the underlying pathologic defect in Parkinson's disease?

2. What is the aim of drug therapy for Parkinson's disease?

3. The first drugs prescribed for Alexander are amantadine (Symmetrel) along with levodopa-carbidopa (Sinemet CR). What is the purpose of taking the amantadine at this time?

4. The physician tells Alexander that the amantadine may be helpful in the early stages but will need to be changed at a later date. Why is this true?

5. What is the "on-off phenomenon" that may occur with the use of levodopa? How does the carbidopa affect this phenomenon?

Chapter 15

Psychotherapeutic Drugs

CHAPTER REVIEW

Choose the best answer for each of the following.

1. Patients taking the newer antipsychotic drugs such as quetiapine (Seroquel) should be cautioned about which problem when beginning this therapy?
   a. Mood swings
   b. Diarrhea
   c. Postural hypotension
   d. Anorexia

2. When giving hydroxyzine intramuscularly, the nurse should be sure to do which of the following?
   a. Use the Z-track method
   b. Use a large-gauge needle
   c. Apply an ice pack to the site for 20 minutes
   d. Divide the dose into two injections

3. The wife of a patient who has started taking antidepressant therapy asks, "How long will it take for him to feel better?" How should the nurse respond?
   a. "Well, depression rarely responds to medication therapy."
   b. "He should be feeling better in a few days."
   c. "It may take 4 to 6 weeks before you see an improvement."
   d. "You may not see any effects for several months."

4. Extrapyramidal effects of drugs include which of the following? Select all that apply.
   a. Tremors
   b. Elation and a sense of well-being
   c. Painful muscle spasms
   d. Motor restlessness
   e. Bradycardia

5. The nurse instructs a patient who is undergoing therapy with monoamine oxidase inhibitors (MAOIs) to avoid tyramine-containing foods. What medical emergency may occur if the patient eats these foods while taking MAOIs?
   a. Gastric hemorrhage
   b. Toxic shock
   c. Cardiac arrest
   d. Severe hypertensive crisis

Match each term with its corresponding definition or description.

6. _____ sertraline

7. _____ tyramine

8. _____ Tricyclics

9. _____ Psychosis

10. _____ Mania

11. _____ diazepam

12. _____ amitriptyline

13. _____ risperidone

14. _____ Benzodiazepines

15. _____ lithium

16. _____ Anxiety

17. _____ Affective disorders

18. _____ Depression

19. _____ phenelzine

20. _____ Bipolar affective disorder

a. The unpleasant state of mind in which real or imagined dangers are anticipated and/or exaggerated.

b. A state characterized by an expansive emotional state (including symptoms of extreme excitement and elation) and hyperactivity.

c. A group of psychotropic drugs prescribed to alleviate anxiety.

d. Emotional disorders characterized by changes in mood.

e. A major psychologic disorder characterized by episodes of mania or hypomania, cycling with depression.

f. Classified as an MAOI.

g. Patients taking MAOIs need to be taught to avoid foods that contain this substance.

h. Antidepressant drugs that block reuptake of amine neurotransmitters.

i. An abnormal emotional state characterized by exaggerated feelings of sadness, melancholy, and worthlessness out of proportion to reality.

j. A frequently prescribed benzodiazepine.

k. The most widely used tricyclic antidepressant.

l. An atypical antipsychotic drug used to treat schizophrenia.

m. A second-generation antidepressant.

n. A main treatment for mania.

o. A term used to describe a major emotional disorder that impairs the mental function of the affected individual to the extent that the individual cannot participate in everyday life.

CRITICAL THINKING AND APPLICATION

Answer the following questions on a separate sheet of paper.

21. Carl, a 26-year-old unemployed electrician, is brought to the emergency department by his sister. He is extremely drowsy and confused, his breathing is slow and shallow, and he smells strongly of whiskey. The sister tells you that Carl has been seeing a psychiatrist for his "anxiety."
    a. What do you suspect might be wrong with Carl?
    b. How will he likely be treated?

22. Mr. Delvini, a 49-year-old restaurant owner, has been prescribed the MAOI phenelzine (Nardil). After the physician leaves the room but before you have a chance to discuss Mr. Delvini's medication regimen with him, he turns to his wife and says, "I'm sure this medicine will work. Let's have a bottle of wine tonight to celebrate."
    a. What should you say?
    b. A few weeks later, Mr. Delvini is brought to the emergency department with a severe headache, stiff neck, sweating, and elevated blood pressure. His wife says his symptoms started a few minutes after they ate at their restaurant. What is wrong with Mr. Delvini, and what probably caused it?

23. Beth has been diagnosed with depression. Why might the physician prescribe a second-generation antidepressant instead of a first-generation antidepressant?

24. A young adult has been admitted to the emergency department with a suspected overdose of an antidepressant. The physicians are monitoring his cardiac status closely. Why is this?

CASE STUDY

Read the scenario and answer the following questions on a separate sheet of paper.

Gene, a 38-year-old businessman, mentions during a checkup that he has felt very anxious and upset over the past few months. He discusses the pressures of his business and states that he has had trouble sleeping at night, which makes him more irritable. Lately he has been very worried over a contract proposal presentation that will take place in a few months. The physician gives him a prescription for alprazolam, 0.25 mg three times a day.

1. Gene is concerned about potential adverse effects of this medication. What should you tell him?

2. What other measures should be taken for Gene at this time?

3. After 3 months, Gene is back in the office for a follow-up appointment. He is upset because a friend told him about another friend who was taking that same medication but died due to an overdose. Gene wants to stop taking the alprazolam immediately. Is this recommended? If not, why not?

4. What are the symptoms of alprazolam overdose, and what is the antidote, if any?

5. Six months later, Gene is no longer taking alprazolam but comes back to the office because he still feels anxious. The physician gives him a prescription for buspirone, 30 mg twice a day. Gene questions why he is given a different drug. What are the advantages, if any, of taking buspirone instead of alprazolam?

Chapter 16

Central Nervous System Stimulants and Related Drugs

CHAPTER REVIEW

Choose the best answer for each of the following.

1. Which statement best describes a common use for doxapram?
   a. To control increased respiration caused by other drugs
   b. To treat respiratory insufficiency associated with chronic obstructive pulmonary disease
   c. To treat postoperative respiratory excitation
   d. To stimulate respirations in patients with head injury

2. Which of the following are results of stimulation of the central nervous system (CNS) by stimulant drugs? Select all that apply.
   a. Increased fatigue
   b. Decreased drowsiness
   c. Increased respiration
   d. Bradycardia
   e. Euphoria

3. Caffeine should be avoided by patients who have a history of which of the following?
   a. Cardiac dysrhythmias
   b. Asthma
   c. Diabetes mellitus
   d. Gallbladder disease

4. Serotonin agonists are newer CNS stimulants used to treat which of the following?
   a. Attention deficit hyperactivity disorder (ADHD)
   b. Hypertension
   c. Migraine headaches
   d. Narcolepsy

5. The physician has ordered orlistat (Xenical). The nurse recognizes that this drug is used to treat which of the following?
   a. Anorexia
   b. Malnutrition
   c. Narcolepsy
   d. Obesity

6. When a child is taking drugs for ADHD, the nurse should instruct the caregivers to closely monitor the child's
   a. blood glucose levels.
   b. physical growth, especially weight.
   c. grades at school.
   d. respiratory rates.

CRITICAL THINKING AND APPLICATION

Answer the following questions on a separate sheet of paper.

7. Stacey, age 35, reports that she falls asleep unexpectedly at work, in class, and even while singing in her city's madrigal choir.

   a. What is wrong with Stacey?

   b. What might be the drug of choice for Stacey?

   c. Describe the therapeutic effects of such drugs.

   d. Draw up a patient teaching plan for Stacey. Offer guidelines for (1) dosage alterations and (2) substances she might be wise to avoid.

8. Five-year-old Jeffrey is taking atomoxetine (Strattera) for ADHD. What specific precautions must be taken with children who are taking ADHD drugs? Why?

9. What nutritional counseling is needed for patients taking orlistat (Xenical)?

10. Sadie experiences migraine headaches about four times a year and has a new prescription for a triptan antimigraine medication. She tells you that she hopes that the medication will prevent her "awful headaches." What do you tell her?

CASE STUDY

Read the scenario and answer the following questions on a separate sheet of paper.

Nancy, a 44-year-old accountant, has had an increasing number of headaches in the past year. When she has these headaches, she often is nauseated and vomits. She has been to her physician, who has ordered several diagnostic tests. As a result, Nancy has been diagnosed with migraine headaches and will be given a prescription for a serotonin agonist.

1. How do serotonin agonists work in the treatment of migraine headaches?

2. What dosage form(s) would be helpful for Nancy's situation?

3. If the physician decides to write a prescription for sumatriptan (Imitrex), Nancy's history should be assessed for which conditions?

4. What foods may be associated with the development of migraine headaches?

5. What else should be included in the treatment regimen for Nancy's migraine headaches?

Chapter 17
Adrenergic Drugs

CHAPTER REVIEW

Choose the best answer for each of the following.

1. Another name for adrenergic drugs is
   a. anticholinergic drugs.
   b. parasympathetic drugs.
   c. central nervous system drugs.
   d. sympathomimetic drugs.

2. Adrenergic drugs produce which of the following effects? Select all that apply.
   a. Urinary retention
   b. Glycogenolysis
   c. Decreased respiratory rate
   d. Increased heart rate

3. The nurse is aware that adrenergic drugs may be used to treat which of the following conditions? Select all that apply.
   a. Asthma
   b. Glaucoma
   c. Hypertension
   d. Nasal congestion
   e. Seizures
   f. Nausea and vomiting

4. A woman has just been stung by a bee, and she is upset because she is allergic to bees. She reaches for her bee-sting kit, which would most likely contain which of the following?
   a. epinephrine
   b. methylphenidate HCl
   c. dopamine
   d. norepinephrine

5. A 13-year-old girl was diagnosed with asthma 2 years ago. Today her physician wants to start her on salmeterol administered via inhaler. The nurse needs to remember to include which statement when teaching the girl and her family about this drug?
   a. "It should be taken at the first sign of an asthma attack."
   b. "The dosage is two puffs every 4 hours or any time needed for asthma attacks."
   c. "Don't use this for an asthma attack; it is supposed to help with long-term management of your symptoms."
   d. "Be sure to take your steroid inhaler first."

CRITICAL THINKING AND APPLICATION

Answer the following questions on a separate sheet of paper.

6. The mother of 3-year-old Kyle is giving him phenylephrine drops as a nasal decongestant.

   a. How does this medication help with nasal congestion?

   b. Kyle's mother comes back to the clinic and complains that after a week his congestion is worse, not better. What possible explanation can you offer?

7. Mr. Dickens, who has had a history of problems with a hormonal imbalance, has been admitted for septic shock, and the physician prescribes dopamine. However, something tells you that you should double-check whether he should take this drug. What makes you think to do this?

8. Mr. Ganaden and Mr. Cowan are both on dopamine infusions. Mr. Ganaden's infusion is being administered at a low rate, and Mr. Cowan's at a high rate. Can you explain why these infusion rates might be different?

9. A patient in the intensive care unit has received too high a dose of epinephrine. For what should the nurse monitor, and what should the nurse expect to do for this patient?

10. Greg, a 49-year-old construction worker, is in the urgent care center for treatment of a leg laceration. Just after receiving an intravenous antibiotic, he starts to wheeze and says, "Oh, I just remembered. I'm allergic to penicillin!"

    a. What is happening?

    b. What should the nurse do first?

    c. What drug do you think will be given in this situation?

CASE STUDY

Read the scenario and answer the following questions on a separate sheet of paper.

Sixteen-year-old Maureen, who plays soccer on her high school team, has been treated for asthma for a year. Her symptoms have been controlled with an inhaled steroid and occasional use of an albuterol metered-dose inhaler. This afternoon, though, her mother brings her into the urgent care center because Maureen has had trouble "getting her breath" after a particularly rough game. Maureen complains of a feeling of "tightness" in her chest and wants to sit up. She appears anxious and has a nonproductive cough. Her respiratory rate is 28 breaths/min, and her peak expiratory flow is 70% of normal. Chest auscultation reveals a short inspiratory period with prolonged expiratory wheezes in both lungs.

1. The physician orders albuterol to be given through a nebulizer. What should the nurse assess before giving this medication? During and after administration?

2. Why is the albuterol given via inhalation rather than orally?

3. After the nebulizer medication treatment is completed, Maureen complains of feeling "shaky and jittery." What do you tell her?

4. The physician gives Maureen a prescription for a salmeterol inhaler. What is important to teach Maureen and her mother about this medication?

Chapter 18
Adrenergic-Blocking Drugs

CHAPTER REVIEW

Choose the best answer for each of the following.

1. Adrenergic blockade at the α-adrenergic receptors leads to which of the following effects? Select all that apply.
   a. Vasodilation
   b. Decreased blood pressure
   c. Increased blood pressure
   d. Constriction of the pupil
   e. Tachycardia

2. The nurse discovers that the intravenous infusion of a patient who has been receiving an intravenous vasopressor has infiltrated. The nurse will expect which drug to be used to reverse the effects of the vasopressor in the infiltrated area?
   a. phentolamine
   b. prazosin
   c. ergotamine
   d. metoprolol

3. A patient with migraine headaches is being evaluated. One potential treatment is ergotamine tablets. The nurse notes that the patient has the following conditions. Which would be a contradiction to the use of ergotamine?
   a. Asthma
   b. Hypertension
   c. Pregnancy
   d. Hypothyroidism

4. A patient has been given prazosin as treatment for benign prostatic hypertrophy. Which instruction is important to include when teaching him about the effects of this medication?
   a. Avoid caffeine
   b. Change position slowly to avoid orthostatic changes
   c. Watch for weight loss of 2 lb within 2 weeks
   d. Take extra supplements of calcium

5. A patient who has been taking a β-blocker for 6 months tells the nurse during a follow-up visit that she wants to stop taking this medication. She is wondering if there is any problem with stopping the medication all at once. The nurse's best response is which of the following?
   a. "No, there are no ill effects if this medication is stopped."
   b. "There should be only minimal effects if you stop this medication."
   c. "You may experience orthostatic hypotension if you stop this medication abruptly."
   d. "If you stop this medication suddenly, there is a possibility you may experience chest pain or rebound hypertension."

CRITICAL THINKING AND APPLICATION

Answer the following questions on a separate sheet of paper.

6. Mrs. Wong, a patient on your hospital floor, is receiving a dopamine intravenous infusion. When you first come on the late-night shift, she seems just fine. However, the next time you check on her you notice that the intravenous line has dislodged and the infusion has infiltrated. What could happen as a result? Is this serious? What kind of treatment do you recommend? Describe the unusual injection process and its rationale.

7. Mr. Cortis has had a myocardial infarction (MI). He is told that he will be prescribed a "cardioprotective drug." He asks you to explain. Why can some β-blockers be said to "protect" the heart?

8. Ms. Clarkson has been prescribed a β-blocker. She is about to be released from the hospital, but first her nurse gives her instructions about taking her apical pulse for 1 full minute, as well as her blood pressure. Why? What should she be looking for? Is there anything she should be instructed to report to her physician?

9. Mr. Sniders, a 78-year-old widower, has a new prescription for prazosin because of a new diagnosis of benign prostatic hypertrophy. What concern, if any, is there with this drug? What teaching will he need?

CASE STUDY

Read the scenario and answer the following questions on a separate sheet of paper.

Bruce, a 58-year-old accountant, is in the hospital after having an MI. The physician has told him that damage to his heart was minimal, and the patient has started post-MI rehabilitation and education. The patient has discussed having to "mend his ways," because in addition to the MI he has had asthma for years that has been managed poorly. The physician discusses starting Bruce on a β-blocker to "protect his heart" and gives him a prescription for atenolol (Tenormin).

1. What type of β-blocker is appropriate for Bruce, and why?

2. Discuss how atenolol helps in this situation.

3. What adverse effects should Bruce be taught about when he starts this medication?

4. At his 3-month checkup, Bruce tells you that he wants to stop taking this medication. Should this medication be stopped abruptly?

Chapter 19
Cholinergic Drugs

CHAPTER REVIEW

Match each definition with its corresponding term. (Note: Not all terms will be used.)

1. _____ Antidote for overdose of a cholinergic drug

2. _____ Cholinergic drugs that act by making more acetylcholine (ACh) available at the receptor site, which thus allows ACh to bind to and stimulate the receptor

3. _____ Cholinergic drugs that bind to cholinergic receptors and activate them

4. _____ Receptors located postsynaptically in the effector organs (smooth muscle, cardiac muscle, the glands) supplied by the parasympathetic fibers

5. _____ Receptors located in the ganglia of the parasympathetic nervous system (PSNS) and the sympathetic nervous system

6. _____ A description of the action of the PSNS

7. _____ The neurotransmitter responsible for the transmission of nerve impulses to the effector cells in the PSNS

8. _____ The enzyme responsible for breaking down ACh

a. cholinesterase

b. Muscarinic

c. catecholamine

d. "Fight or flight"

e. "Rest and digest"

f. Direct-acting cholinergic drugs

g. Indirect-acting cholinergic drugs

h. atropine

i. acetylcholine

j. Nicotinic

Choose the best answer for each of the following.

9. The desired effects of cholinergic drugs come from stimulation of which receptors?
   a. Cholinergic
   b. Nicotinic
   c. Muscarinic
   d. Ganglionic

10. The undesirable effects of cholinergic drugs come from stimulation of which receptors?
    a. Cholinergic
    b. Nicotinic
    c. Muscarinic
    d. Ganglionic

11. When a patient mentions bethanechol when asked about his medication history, the nurse recognizes that this drug is used for the treatment of which of the following?
    a. Diarrhea
    b. Urinary retention
    c. Urinary incontinence
    d. Bladder spasms

12. When caring for a patient with a diagnosis of myasthenia gravis, the nurse can expect that which of the following drugs is used for symptomatic treatment of this disease?
    a. bethanechol
    b. tacrine
    c. donepezil
    d. physostigmine

13. A 62-year-old woman has started taking donepezil for early-stage Alzheimer's disease. Her daughter expresses relief that "there is finally a pill to cure Alzheimer's disease." The nurse's best response would be which of the following?
    a. "She should expect reversal of symptoms within a few days."
    b. "The dosage should be increased if no improvement is noted."
    c. "This drug may help to improve symptoms, but it is not intended as a cure."
    d. "Yes, it has been a great help for many patients."

14. A patient has received an inadvertent overdose of a cholinergic drug. Early signs of a cholinergic crisis would include which of the following? Select all that apply.
    a. Dry mouth
    b. Salivation
    c. Flushing of the skin
    d. Abdominal cramps
    e. Constipation
    f. Dyspnea

15. The nurse will prepare to give which drug to a patient who is experiencing a cholinergic crisis?
    a. atropine
    b. tacrine
    c. donepezil
    d. physostigmine

CRITICAL THINKING AND APPLICATION

Answer the following questions on a separate sheet of paper.

16. List the effects of cholinergic poisoning by using the acronym SLUDGE.

17. Mrs. Sibanda has recently had abdominal surgery, and she is resting well except that she is unable to void her urine. She has some distention in her lower abdomen over the symphysis pubis.

    a. What drug is likely to be the drug of choice?

    b. Mrs. Sibanda is still unable to void her urine. Her urinary retention worsens and becomes painful, and when her physician is contacted, he recommends radiography to determine whether a stone is present in her urinary tract; his suspicions are confirmed. How much can the physician increase her dosage?

18. Mr. Keegan has been determined to have a high potential for a negative reaction to the cholinergic prescribed to him. However, his physician believes that the potential benefits are worth the risk.

    a. For what reaction should you be closely monitoring Mr. Keegan?

    b. In addition to close monitoring, what else can you do to be prepared?

19. Ms. Bethke has recently been diagnosed with myasthenia gravis and is taking medication for the treatment of symptoms associated with the disease. She asks you, "How much success can I expect?"

   a.   What will you say?

   b.   What kind of negative effects should she should report to a physician?

CASE STUDY

Read the scenario and answer the following questions on a separate sheet of paper.

Arthur, a 68-year-old retired banker, has been diagnosed with early-stage Alzheimer's disease. He has remained active in his church activities and likes to golf every week. He is in the office today with his son and is asking about the "new drugs that are available to reverse Alzheimer's disease." Arthur has had no serious health problems except a mild case of hepatitis A 1 year earlier.

1. What drugs are available to "reverse Alzheimer's disease?" Explain.

2. The physician is considering either galantamine (Reminyl) or rivastigmine (Exelon) for Arthur. Is there anything in his history that may influence the choice of medication?

3. Describe the different mechanisms of action of direct-acting and indirect-acting cholinergic-blocking drugs.

4. Arthur is given a prescription for rivastigmine. What adverse effects should be expected, and what should he and his son be told regarding ways to manage these adverse effects?

Chapter 20
Cholinergic-Blocking Drugs

CHAPTER REVIEW

Choose the best answer for each of the following.

1. Before giving an anticholinergic drug, the nurse should check the patient's history for which of the following?
   a. Glaucoma
   b. Osteoporosis
   c. Thyroid disease
   d. Diabetes mellitus

2. Adverse effects to expect from anticholinergic drugs include which of the following? Select all that apply.
   a. Dilated pupils
   b. Constricted pupils
   c. Dry mouth
   d. Urinary retention
   e. Urinary frequency
   f. Diarrhea

3. In reviewing the medication orders for a newly admitted patient, the nurse recognizes that an indication for atropine sulfate includes which of the following?
   a. Myasthenia gravis
   b. Reduction of secretions preoperatively
   c. Tachycardia due to sinoatrial node defects
   d. Narrow-angle glaucoma

4. During patient teaching for a 70-year-old man who will be taking an anticholinergic drug, the nurse should reinforce that this medication places the patient at higher risk for which of the following?
   a. Angina
   b. Fluid overload
   c. Heat stroke
   d. Hypothermia

5. A 28-year-old woman is preparing to take a cruise and has asked for a prescription drug to prevent motion sickness. The physician orders Transderm-Scop (scopolamine) patches. The nurse should include which statement when teaching the patient about this drug?
   a. "The patch can be applied anywhere on the upper body."
   b. "Apply the patch 4 to 5 hours before travel."
   c. "Apply the patch just before boarding the ship"
   d. "Be sure to change the patch daily."

CRITICAL THINKING AND APPLICATION

Answer the following questions on a separate sheet of paper.

6. A patient is given atropine sulfate before surgery. Describe how this drug is helpful during the perioperative period. What other drug can be used for this purpose?

7. Mr. Miller is brought into the emergency department conscious but with an overdose of a cholinergic blocker.

   a. Describe how Mr. Miller will be treated.

   b. How should you respond if Mr. Miller begins having hallucinations related to the overdose?

8. Mr. Hansen is taking dicyclomine (Bentyl) for irritable bowel syndrome. He calls the clinic and tells you that he would like to get his doctor's permission to take an antihistamine for his cold. What drug interactions might he expect?

9. How does atropine work in the following situations?

   a. A patient is experiencing severe bradycardia, with a heart rate of 38 beats/min, and he is losing consciousness.

   b. A crop duster pilot has been exposed to an organophosphate insecticide in an industrial accident.

CASE STUDY

Read the scenario and answer the following questions on a separate sheet of paper.

Mrs. Walsh, age 63, is in the outpatient clinic today for a physical. During history taking, she admits to having a "terrible problem" with her bladder. She describes having sudden urges to urinate and is "ashamed to say" that, at times, she has lost control of her bladder. She has had no other health issues except for "some eye problems" off and on for the past year. The physician is considering starting Mrs. Walsh on tolterodine (Detrol).

1. What are the contraindications for this medication? Are there any potential concerns given Mrs. Walsh's history?

2. What are the advantages of using tolterodine rather than other drugs with similar actions?

3. Mrs. Walsh enjoys working outside in her yard. What special precautions should she take?

4. After a week of therapy, she calls the clinic to complain of a dry mouth. She said she didn't think this was supposed to happen with this drug. What advice do you give to her?

Chapter 21
Positive Inotropic Drugs

CHAPTER REVIEW

Choose the best answer for each of the following.

1. When monitoring patients who are taking digoxin, the nurse keeps in mind that the serum digoxin level should be which of the following?
   a. 0.1 to 0.5 ng/mL
   b. 0.5 to 2.0 ng/mL
   c. 2.0 to 5.0 ng/mL
   d. 5.0 to 8.4 ng/mL

2. A patient is experiencing digitalis toxicity. The nurse would expect an order for which drug?
   a. vitamin K
   b. atropine
   c. digoxin immune Fab
   d. potassium

3. Before giving oral digoxin, the nurse discovers that the patient's radial pulse is 55 beats/min. The nurse's next action should be to
   a. give the dose.
   b. delay the dose until later.
   c. hold the dose and notify the physician.
   d. check the apical pulse for one minute.

4. Which statement regarding digoxin therapy and potassium levels is correct?
   a. Low potassium levels increase the chance of digoxin toxicity.
   b. High potassium levels increase the chance of digoxin toxicity.
   c. Digoxin reduces the excretion of potassium in the kidneys.
   d. Digoxin promotes the excretion of potassium in the kidneys.

5. When infusing amrinone, the nurse should keep in mind which of the following?
   a. The medication should be mixed in saline before administration.
   b. The true color of intravenous amrinone is clear yellow.
   c. The drug may cause reddish discoloration of the extremities.
   d. Hypertension is the primary effect seen with excessive doses.

6. When caring for a patient who is taking digoxin, the nurse should monitor for signs and symptoms of toxicity, including which of the following? Select all that apply.
   a. Anorexia
   b. Diarrhea
   c. Visual changes
   d. Nausea and vomiting
   e. Headache
   f. Bradycardia

CRITICAL THINKING AND APPLICATION

Answer the following questions on a separate sheet of paper.

7. You are caring for Mrs. Chin, who is undergoing cardiac glycoside therapy. She begins to vomit and complains of a headache and fatigue. Diagnostic studies reveal short episodes of ventricular tachycardia on the ECG and a serum potassium level of 6 mEq/L. What action might you expect to be taken?

8. Mr. Davis has atrial fibrillation and flutter, and the physician initially prescribes digoxin intravenously at 1.5 mg/day. What is the purpose of this dosage, and how does it compare with the dosage on which Mr. Davis will be maintained?

9. How does the concept of a therapeutic window relate to the monitoring of patients taking cardiac glycosides?

10. While monitoring Mr. Ferris after oral digoxin administration, you note increased urinary output, decreased dyspnea and fatigue, and constipation. Mr. Ferris complains to you that if he were allowed to eat bran as often as he used to, he wouldn't be constipated. What do your findings indicate? What is your response to Mr. Ferris?

11. Mr. Montgomery is experiencing heart failure that has not responded well to diuretic and digoxin therapy. The physician changes his medication to amrinone.

    a.   What effect does amrinone have on cardiac muscle contractility and the blood vessels?

    b.   What advantage does this phosphodiesterase inhibitor have over the cardiac glycosides?

    c.   What is the most worrisome adverse effect of amrinone?

CASE STUDY

Read the scenario and answer the following questions on a separate sheet of paper.

A 68-year-old woman is admitted to the hospital with a diagnosis of mild left-sided heart failure. At rest she is comfortable, but she has noticed that she has symptoms when she tries to get dressed or do simple housework. She becomes short of breath with activity, tires easily but cannot sleep at night, and feels "generally irritable." She also has diffuse bilateral crackles that do not clear with coughing and a third heart sound. She has slight pedal edema. The physician has ordered therapy with intravenous digoxin (Lanoxin).

1. Digoxin has several effects. Explain the meaning of each of the following:

    • Positive inotropic effect

    • Negative chronotropic effect

    • Negative dromotropic effect

2. As a result of these effects, what would you expect to see with regard to each of the following?

    • Stroke volume

    • Venous blood pressure and vein engorgement

    • Coronary circulation

    • Diuresis

3. After 3 days of therapy she complains of feeling nauseated and has no appetite. She also wonders why the lights are so bright and blurry. Her radial pulse rate is 52 beats/min. When you check the results of her laboratory work, you note that her digoxin level from that morning is 3.5 ng/mL. What should you do?

Chapter 22
Antidysrhythmic Drugs

CHAPTER REVIEW

Choose the best answer for each of the following.

1. The antidysrhythmic drug lidocaine is used mainly to treat which of the following?
   a. Atrial fibrillation
   b. Bradycardia
   c. Complete heart block
   d. Ventricular dysrhythmias

2. When monitoring a patient who is taking quinidine, the nurse recognizes that which of the following is a possible adverse effect of this drug?
   a. Weakness
   b. Tachycardia
   c. Gastrointestinal upset
   d. Hypertension

3. When administering amiodarone, the nurse should monitor for which of the following adverse effects?
   a. Pulmonary toxicity
   b. Hypertension
   c. Urinary retention
   d. Visual halos

4. A primary use of verapamil is to treat which of the following conditions?
   a. Cardiac asystole
   b. Heart block
   c. Ventricular dysrhythmia, including premature ventricular contraction
   d. Recurrent paroxysmal supraventricular tachycardia (PSVT)

5. A patient is experiencing a rapid dysrhythmia, and the nurse is preparing to administer adenosine. Which is the correct administration technique for this drug?
   a. It should be given as a fast intravenous push.
   b. It should be given intravenously, slowly, over at least 5 minutes.
   c. It should be taken with food or milk.
   d. It should be given as an intravenous drip infusion.

6. If a drug has a prodysrhythmic effect, then the nurse must monitor the patient for which of the following?
   a. Decreased heart rate
   b. New dysrhythmias
   c. A decrease in dysrhythmias
   d. Reduced blood pressure

7. **Match the site to its correct intrinsic rate:**

   a. Sinoatrial node _____
   b. Atrioventricular node _____
   c. Purkinje fibers _____

   (1) 40 to 60 beats/min
   (2) 40 or fewer beats/min
   (3) 60 to 100 beats/min

CRITICAL THINKING AND APPLICATION

Answer the following questions on a separate sheet of paper.

8. Mr. Killian, who has been diagnosed with hypertension, is hospitalized after a myocardial infarction (MI).

   a. To reduce the risk of sudden cardiac death in Mr. Killian, the physician prescribes a drug from which class? Why?

   b. How would a history of asthma in Mr. Killian affect the drug choice?

9. Mr. Needham has a life-threatening ventricular tachycardia that has been resistant to treatment, and the physician has now prescribed what she calls a "last resort" drug. To what drug is she referring, and why is it considered a drug of last resort?

10. Mr. Maxwell is a 50-year-old schoolteacher being treated with lidocaine after an MI.

    a. He is very upset and says that he hates injections; he wants to know why he can't just take a pill. What do you tell him?

    b. If Mr. Maxwell has a history of cirrhosis, would the dosage of the lidocaine be affected?

11. Mrs. Inez calls the health clinic complaining of chest pain and dizziness. She says she cannot remember whether she took her quinidine yesterday and wants to know whether she should take two doses today, especially because she is feeling so bad. What do you tell Mrs. Inez?

CASE STUDY

Read the scenario and answer the following questions on a separate sheet of paper.

Jack, age 39, is taking diltiazem as part of his treatment for occasional PSVT. He also has a history of seizures.

1. How do calcium channel blockers such as diltiazem work?

2. What therapeutic effects are expected?

3. Is there a possible concern with drug interactions?

4. After 4 months of therapy, Jack experiences dizziness, dyspnea, and a very rapid heart rate and is taken to the emergency department. He is diagnosed with sustained PSVT, and intravenous verapamil does not help. What do you think would be tried next?

Chapter 23
Antianginal Drugs

CHAPTER REVIEW

Choose the best answer for each of the following.

1. The purpose of antianginal drug therapy is to
   a. increase myocardial oxygen demand.
   b. increase blood flow to peripheral arteries.
   c. increase blood flow to ischemic cardiac muscle.
   d. decrease blood flow to ischemic cardiac muscle.

2. A patient taking nitroglycerin should be taught that a common adverse effect of this drug is
   a. blurred vision.
   b. dizziness.
   c. headache.
   d. weakness.

3. Nitroglycerin is available in which of the following forms? Select all that apply.
   a. Continuous intravenous drip
   b. Intravenous bolus
   c. Sublingual spray
   d. Oral dosage forms
   e. Topical ointment
   f. Rectal suppository

4. For a patient using transdermal patches, the nurse recognizes that the best way to prevent tolerance to nitrates is to do which of the following?
   a. Leave the old patch on for 2 hours when applying a new patch
   b. Apply a new patch every other day
   c. Leave the patch off for 24 hours once a week
   d. Remove the patch at night for 8 hours and then apply a new patch in the morning

5. Patients who are taking β-blockers for angina need to be taught that these drugs
   a. are for long-term prevention of angina episodes.
   b. should be taken as soon as angina pain occurs.
   c. should be discontinued if dizziness is experienced.
   d. should be carried with them at all times in case angina occurs.

6. Which type of antianginal medication is most effective for the treatment of coronary artery spasms?
   a. β-blockers
   b. Calcium channel blockers
   c. Nitrates
   d. Nitrites

CRITICAL THINKING AND APPLICATION

Answer the following questions on a separate sheet of paper.

7. You are playing racquetball at a community center when you notice a commotion at a gathering of senior citizens in a nearby room. You rush in to find a man lying unconscious on the floor. Several people say that he is having a "heart attack." One man hands you a pill bottle and asks, "Would it help to give him one of my heart pills?" A woman agrees, saying, "Yes! Can't you put it under his tongue?" You see that the medication bottle is labeled *Isordil* (isosorbide dinitrate). What do you know about this medication, and what should you do?

8. Ms. Vickers is a 70-year-old woman seen in the emergency department for a laceration to her thumb. During your assessment, Ms. Vickers tells you that she has been "tired and depressed" and has been having "nightmares" since her physician prescribed heart medicine for her angina. Which drug do you suspect Ms. Vickers is taking? Why do you think so?

9. During your home visit with Theresa, she shows you a journal entry describing the duration, time of onset, and severity of a recent angina attack. She reports no adverse effects to her nitroglycerin and shows you where she keeps the tablets, in a clear plastic pillbox on the kitchen windowsill. What do you discuss with Theresa?

CASE STUDY

Read the scenario and answer the following questions on a separate sheet of paper.

While playing handball, 59-year-old Gideon experiences chest pain. He has had angina before and has sublingual nitroglycerin in his gym bag.

1. What type of angina is he experiencing?

2. What should he do to treat this episode of angina?

3. After he takes the nitroglycerin tablets, the chest pain does not subside. He wants his handball partner to drive him to the hospital. Is this what he should do at this time?

4. Other than nitroglycerin, which class of drugs is typically good for this type of angina?

Chapter 24
Antihypertensive Drugs

CRITICAL THINKING CROSSWORD

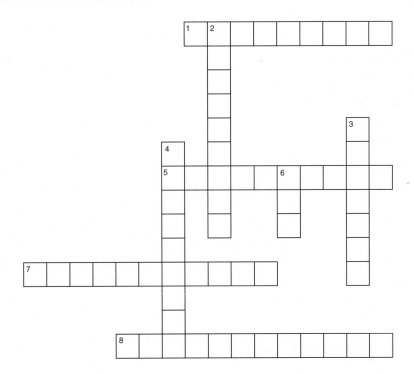

Across

1. High blood pressure associated with diseases such as renal, pulmonary, endocrine, and vascular diseases is known as _____ hypertension.
5. Another term for 3 Down.
7. A common adverse effect of adrenergic drugs involving a sudden drop in blood pressure when patients change position is known as _____ hypotension.
8. These drugs are used in the management of hypertensive emergencies.

Down

2. Another term for 3 Down.
3. Elevated systemic arterial pressure for which no cause can be found is known as _____ hypertension.
4. The primary effect of these drugs is to decrease plasma and extracellular fluid volumes.
6. Drugs that are often used as first-line drugs in the treatment of both heart failure and hypertension are known by the acronym _____ inhibitors.

CHAPTER REVIEW

Choose the best answer for each of the following.

1. A 46-year-old man has been taking clonidine for 5 months. For the last 2 months, his blood pressure has been normal. During this office visit, he tells the nurse that he would like to stop taking the drug. The nurse's best response would be which of the following?
   a. "I'm sure the doctor will stop it—your blood pressure is normal now."
   b. "Your doctor will probably have you stop taking the drug for a month, and then we'll see how you do."
   c. "This drug should not be stopped suddenly; let's talk to your doctor."
   d. "It's likely that you can stop the drug if you exercise and avoid salty foods."

2. When administering angiotensin-converting enzyme (ACE) inhibitors, the nurse keeps in mind that adverse effects include which of the following? Select all that apply.
   a. Diarrhea
   b. Fatigue
   c. Restlessness
   d. Headaches
   e. A dry cough
   f. Tremors

3. A patient with type 2 diabetes mellitus has developed hypertension. The nurse knows that the blood pressure goal for this patient would be which of the following?
   a. Less than 110/80 mm Hg
   b. Less than 120/80 mm Hg
   c. Less than 130/84 mm Hg
   d. Less than 140/90 mm Hg

4. A patient is being treated for a hypertensive emergency. The nurse expects which drug to be used?
   a. sodium nitroprusside
   b. losartan
   c. captopril
   d. prazosin

5. A patient in her eighth month of pregnancy has preeclampsia. Her blood pressure is 210/100 mm Hg this morning. This type of hypertension is classified as which of the following?
   a. Primary
   b. Idiopathic
   c. Essential
   d. Secondary

CRITICAL THINKING AND APPLICATION

Answer the following questions on a separate sheet of paper.

6. Mr. Quester, 61 years of age, comes to the emergency department at night with symptoms of severe hypertensive emergency. The emergency department resident on call initiates therapy with sodium nitroprusside. The patient is transferred to the intensive care unit and monitored. Hours later, his blood pressure falls to 100/60 mm Hg, and he is lethargic and complaining of feeling dizzy. What should the nurse do?

7. A patient has had an average blood pressure reading of 124/86 mm Hg for the last 3 months. He has a history of type 2 diabetes mellitus and had a myocardial infarction 6 months ago.

   a. Is this patient's hypertension considered normal? Explain your answer.

   b. Will drug therapy be ordered? Explain your answer.

8. Indicate which ACE inhibitor would be best for the following patients. Explain your answers.

   a. Irene, who has liver dysfunction, has high blood pressure, and is seriously ill

   b. Kory, who has a history of poor compliance with his medication regimen

9. Mr. Bass will be starting prazosin for hypertension. What should he be taught before he takes even the first dose of this medication?

10. White and African American patients are known to react differently to antihypertensive agents.

    a. Which antihypertensives are considered more effective in white patients than in African American patients?

    b. Which antihypertensives are considered more effective in African American patients than in white patients?

CASE STUDY

Read the scenario and answer the following questions on a separate sheet of paper.

John, a 44-year-old African American man, has been seen twice in the last month for "blood pressure problems." At the first visit, his blood pressure was 144/90 mm Hg; at the second visit, his blood pressure was 154/96 mm Hg. The physician is preparing to start antihypertensive therapy.

1. According to the 2003 *Seventh Report of the Joint National Committee on Prevention, Detection, Evaluation, and Treatment of High Blood Pressure* (see Table 24-1 in the textbook), into which classification would he fall according to his blood pressure reading?

2. What initial drug therapy would be appropriate for him? What factors are considered when choosing which drug to use?

3. If John also has a history of diabetes mellitus, what would be the blood pressure goal? Why?

4. John tells you that he hopes this medication will not "slow him down" because he likes to "jump out of bed and get started" with his day. What teaching should you provide for him to help him adjust to his blood pressure medication?

Chapter 25

Diuretic Drugs

CHAPTER REVIEW

Match each term with its corresponding definition.

1. _____ Diuretics

2. _____ Potassium-sparing diuretics

3. _____ Kaliuretic diuretics

4. _____ Osmotic diuretics

5. _____ Thiazides

6. _____ Ascites

7. _____ CAIs

8. _____ Loop diuretics

9. _____ Nephron

10. _____ GFR

a. Potent diuretics that act along the ascending limb of the loop of Henle; furosemide is an example.

b. Abbreviation for the term that describes an index of how well the kidneys are functioning as filters.

c. A general term for drugs that accelerate the rate of urine formation.

d. The main structural unit of the kidney.

e. A term for diuretics that cause the body to lose potassium.

f. Diuretics that result in the diuresis of sodium and water and the retention of potassium; spironolactone is an example.

g. Diuretics that act on the distal convoluted tubule, where they inhibit sodium and water resorption; HCTZ is an example.

h. Abbreviation for a class of diuretics that inhibit the enzyme carbonic anhydrase; acetazolamide is an example.

i. Drugs that induce diuresis by increasing the osmotic pressure of the glomerular filtrate, which results in a rapid diuresis; mannitol is an example.

j. An abnormal intraperitoneal accumulation of fluid.

Choose the best answer for each of the following.

11. Which of the following are indications for the use of diuretics? Select all that apply.
    a. To increase urine output
    b. To reduce uric acid levels
    c. To treat hypertension
    d. To treat open-angle glaucoma
    e. To treat edema associated with heart failure

12. When providing patient teaching to a patient who is taking a potassium-sparing diuretic such as spironolactone (Aldactone), the nurse should include which dietary guidelines?
    a. There are no dietary restrictions with this medication.
    b. The patient should consume foods high in potassium, such as bananas and orange juice.
    c. The patient should avoid foods high in potassium.
    d. The patient should drink 1 to 2 L of fluid per day.

13. When teaching a patient about diuretic therapy, the nurse notes that which of the following is the best time of day to take these medications?
    a. Morning
    b. Midday
    c. Bedtime
    d. Time of day does not matter

14. When monitoring a patient for hypokalemia related to diuretic use, the nurse looks for which possible symptoms?
    a. Nausea, vomiting, and anorexia
    b. Diarrhea and abdominal pain
    c. Orthostatic hypotension
    d. Muscle weakness and lethargy

15. A patient with severe heart failure has been started on therapy with a carbonic anhydrase inhibitor (CAI), but the nurse mentions that this medication may be stopped in a few days. Which of the following is the reason for this short treatment?
    a. CAIs are not the first choice for treatment of heart failure.
    b. CAIs lose their diuretic effect in 2 to 4 days because metabolic acidosis develops.
    c. It is expected that the CAIs will dramatically reduce the fluid overload related to the heart failure.
    d. Allergic reactions to the CAIs are common.

CRITICAL THINKING AND APPLICATION

Answer the following questions on a separate sheet of paper.

16. Ms. Andersen is a 62-year-old retired teacher who is being treated for diabetes and open-angle glaucoma. The physician has prescribed a diuretic as an adjunct drug in the management of Ms. Andersen's glaucoma.

    a. Which diuretic drug was probably prescribed?

    b. What undesirable effect of the drug does the physician need to consider?

17. You are about to administer mannitol to Arthur, who is in early acute renal failure.

    a. What is the significance of Arthur's renal blood flow and glomerular filtration in this situation?

    b. By what means do you administer the mannitol? What special guidelines do you follow?

    c. Arthur later complains of a headache and chills. Should the mannitol therapy be ended? Explain your answer.

18. Mr. Ferrara has been admitted to your unit for treatment of ascites. He also has some renal impairment and a history of heavy drinking.

    a. Which diuretic drug do you expect to be administered to Mr. Ferrara?

    b. What monitoring will be performed frequently? Why?

19. Brendan, a 39-year-old bricklayer, is taking thiazide for hypertension. During a follow-up visit, he tells you that he thinks the drug is affecting his "love life."

  a. To what adverse effect of thiazide therapy is Brendan probably referring?

  b. While you are talking, you notice a package of licorice in Brendan's coat pocket. He tells you he eats the candy "for energy," especially because he has been feeling so tired the past couple of days. What do you tell Brendan?

20. You receive a call from Mrs. Hill, who recently started diuretic therapy for hypertension. Mrs. Hill is concerned because her neighbor, who also takes medication for hypertension, has told her not to eat a lot of bananas or other foods containing potassium. "But you told me to eat foods high in potassium," Mrs. Hill says to you. "What's going on?" What is your response to Mrs. Hill?

CASE STUDY

Read the scenario and answer the following questions on a separate sheet of paper.

Lily has been taking furosemide (Lasix) for 3 months as part of her treatment for heart failure. At this time she is complaining that she is feeling tired and has muscle weakness and no appetite; her blood pressure is 100/50 mm Hg.

1. What do her symptoms suggest? How did this happen?

2. What dietary measures could she have taken to prevent this problem?

The physician switches her medication to spironolactone (Aldactone).

3. How does this drug differ from furosemide?

4. For what drug interactions should you check before she begins taking spironolactone?

Chapter 26

Fluids and Electrolytes

CHAPTER REVIEW

Choose the best answer for each of the following.

1. Common uses of crystalloids include which of the following? Select all that apply.
   a. Fluid replacement
   b. Promotion of urinary flow
   c. Transport of oxygen to cells
   d. Replacement of electrolytes
   e. As maintenance fluids
   f. Replacement of clotting factors

2. The intravenous order for a newly admitted patient calls for "Normal saline to run at 100 mL/hr." The nurse will choose which concentration of normal saline?
   a. 0.33%
   b. 0.45%
   c. 0.9%
   d. 3.0%

3. A patient has been admitted with severe dehydration after working outside on a very hot day. The nurse expects which intravenous fluid to be ordered for rapid fluid replacement?
   a. Albumin
   b. Hetastarch
   c. Fresh frozen plasma
   d. 3% sodium chloride

4. When giving intravenous potassium, which of the following is important for the nurse to remember?
   a. Intravenous doses are preferred over oral dosage forms.
   b. Intravenous solutions should contain at least 50 mEq/L.
   c. It must always be given in diluted form.
   d. It should be given by slow intravenous bolus.

5. When a patient is receiving blood products, the nurse monitors for signs of a possible transfusion reaction, such as which of the following?
   a. Subnormal temperature and hypertension
   b. Apprehension, restlessness, fever, and chills
   c. Decreased pulse and respirations and fever
   d. Headache, nausea, and lethargy

6. Which product is used to increase clotting factor levels in patients with a demonstrated deficiency rather than for routine fluid resuscitation?
   a. Plasma protein fraction
   b. Fresh frozen plasma
   c. Packed red blood cells
   d. Albumin

CRITICAL THINKING AND APPLICATION

Answer the following questions on a separate sheet of paper.

7. Name advantages and disadvantages of using crystalloids to replace fluid in patients with dehydration.

8. Some fluids are known as *oxygen-carrying resuscitation fluids*.

   a. Which class of fluids is given this designation?

   b. Why are these fluids able to carry oxygen?

   c. Why are they the most expensive of the three types of fluids, and why is their origin a potential problem for a recipient?

9. Tanya, a 16-year-old student, is brought to the clinic by her mother, who says that Tanya has been on "some sort of fad diet." The mother is concerned because Tanya is tired and weak. During your assessment, Tanya admits that she has been using laxatives and eating very little during the past few weeks.

   a. What electrolyte imbalance is Tanya probably experiencing?

   b. Assuming that laboratory studies show the problem to be mild, how can it be corrected?

10. Mr. Sanchez, a 45-year-old mail carrier, has come to the emergency department sweating profusely and complaining of stomach cramps and diarrhea. He says that he has been "miserable" from the heat the past few days. His serum sodium level is 128 mEq/L.

    a. What electrolyte imbalance do you suspect?

    b. The physician prescribes an oral medication and then asks you to discuss dietary considerations with Mr. Sanchez. What do you tell Mr. Sanchez?

    c. What adverse effect of sodium may be of special concern for Mr. Sanchez?

11. Victor is receiving a transfusion of a blood product.

    a. You observe Victor, knowing that an adverse reaction to the transfusion may be manifested by what signs and symptoms?

    b. Victor's wife is crying and says, "People get AIDS from transfusions. What happens if Victor gets AIDS?" What do you tell her?

    c. The transfusion for Victor seems to be progressing smoothly. How often do you check Victor's vital signs while he is receiving the transfusion?

    d. After 45 minutes, Victor is restless, and his pulse rate has increased. What do you do?

CASE STUDY

Read the scenario and answer the following questions on a separate sheet of paper.

An elderly man was admitted to the unit with hypoproteinemia caused by chronic malnutrition. You note that he has some edema over his body, and his total protein level is 4.8 g/dL.

1. What is the normal total protein level? What is the relationship between his serum total protein level and the edema you have noted?

2. You are preparing to give him 1 unit of 5% albumin. How does albumin work in this situation?

3. What advantages does albumin have over crystalloids in this situation?

4. For what adverse effects should you monitor him while he is receiving albumin?

Chapter 27
Coagulation Modifier Drugs

CHAPTER REVIEW

Match each definition with its corresponding term. (Note: Not all terms will be used.)

1. _____ A drug that prevents the lysis of fibrin, thereby promoting clot formation

2. _____ The termination of bleeding by mechanical or chemical means

3. _____ A substance that prevents platelet plugs from forming

4. _____ A drug that dissolves thrombi

5. _____ The general term for a substance that prevents or delays coagulation of the blood

6. _____ A laboratory test used to measure the effectiveness of heparin therapy

7. _____ A test used, along with another measure, to evaluate the effectiveness of warfarin sodium therapy

8. _____ A standardized measure of the degree of coagulation achieved by drug therapy with warfarin sodium

9. _____ A substance that reverses the effect of heparin

10. _____ A substance that reverses the effect of warfarin sodium

11. _____ Naturally occurring tissue plasminogen activator secreted by vascular endothelial cells

12. _____ A blood clot that dislodges and travels through the bloodstream

a. Prothrombin time

b. Activated partial thromboplastin time (APTT)

c. International normalized ratio (INR)

d. streptokinase

e. alteplase (Activase)

f. Thrombus

g. Embolus

h. vitamin K

i. protamine sulfate

j. Antiplatelet drug

k. Antifibrinolytic

l. Thrombolytic drug

m. Anticoagulant

n. Hemostasis

Choose the best answer for each of the following.

13. For which of the following conditions is the use of anticoagulants appropriate? Select all that apply.
    a. Atrial fibrillation
    b. Thrombocytopenia
    c. Myocardial infarction
    d. Presence of mechanical heart valve
    e. Aneurysm
    f. Leukemia

14. During teaching of a patient who will be taking warfarin sodium (Coumadin) at home, which statement by the nurse is correct regarding over-the-counter drug use?
    a. "Choose nonsteroidal antiinflammatory drugs as needed for pain relief."
    b. "Aspirin products may result in increased anticoagulant effect."
    c. "Vitamin E therapy is recommended to improve the effect of the Coumadin."
    d. "Mineral oil is the laxative of choice while taking anticoagulants."

15. Which drug has antiplatelet properties?
    a. aspirin
    b. warfarin sodium
    c. heparin
    d. streptokinase

16. When administering subcutaneous heparin, the nurse should remember to do which of the following?
    a. Use the same sites for injection to reduce trauma
    b. Use a 1-inch needle for subcutaneous injections
    c. Inject the medication without aspirating for blood return
    d. Massage the site after the injection to increase absorption

17. During thrombolytic therapy, the nurse monitors for bleeding. Which symptoms may indicate a serious bleeding problem? Select all that apply.
    a. Hypertension
    b. Hypotension
    c. Decreased level of consciousness
    d. Increased pulse rate
    e. Restlessness

18. Which drug is indicated for the prevention and treatment of deep vein thrombosis after knee or hip replacement surgery?
    a. Antiplatelet drugs, such as aspirin
    b. Adenosine diphosphate (ADP) inhibitors, such as clopidogrel (Plavix)
    c. Anticoagulants, such as warfarin sodium (Coumadin)
    d. Low-molecular-weight heparins, such as enoxaparin (Lovenox)

CRITICAL THINKING AND APPLICATION

Answer the following questions on a separate sheet of paper.

19. Mrs. Washington, a 60-year-old homemaker, is receiving subcutaneous heparin therapy for prevention of deep vein thrombosis. After you give Mrs. Washington her injection, she complains of pain and begins to rub the site. Is that a problem?

20. During cardiopulmonary bypass for heart surgery, Mr. Wong was intentionally given a large dose of heparin. The surgeon then determines that the effects of the heparin need to be reversed quickly.
    a. How will this be done?
    b. How will the amount of antidote be determined?
    c. What is the most commonly used test for determining the effects of heparin therapy?

21. Vitamin K is a reversal drug for warfarin sodium. How can its use cause a problem in a patient experiencing warfarin toxicity?

22. Following surgery, Mr. Thurman has a chest tube in place. The site has been bleeding excessively. What type of drug might the physician prescribe in this situation and why?

23. William, a 38-year-old writer who has von Willebrand's disease, has undergone emergency surgery after an automobile accident. What drug is used in the management of bleeding in patients like William? What is its effect?

24. Tobias has been given alteplase (Activase) during his treatment for acute myocardial infarction.

    a.   Do you expect Tobias to have an allergic reaction to the drug? Explain your answer.

    b.   A few minutes later, Tobias suffers a reinfarction. What drug should Tobias receive now?

25. Ursula, an inpatient on your unit, is on anticoagulant therapy. You enter her room to find that she is restless and confused.

    a.   Why are these findings significant?

    b.   In this case, what other problems might you expect to find?

    c.   What should you do?

CASE STUDY

Read the scenario and answer the following questions on a separate sheet of paper.

After experiencing transient ischemic attacks, Doug has been started on clopidogrel (Plavix). He has had a history of atherosclerotic heart disease and has had problems with peptic ulcer disease.

1. He asks, "Why am I taking this fancy medicine? Why can't I just take an aspirin a day, like they say on television?" What do you tell him?

2. What should he be taught to report to his health care provider while he is taking this drug?

3. What precautions should he follow while he is taking this drug?

4. What herbal products should he avoid while he is taking this drug?

Chapter 28

Antilipemic Drugs

CHAPTER REVIEW

Choose the best answer for each of the following.

1. Patients taking cholestyramine may experience which of the following adverse effects?
   a. Blurred vision and photophobia
   b. Drowsiness and difficulty concentrating
   c. Diarrhea and abdominal cramps
   d. Belching and bloating

2. Dietary measures for the patient on antilipemic therapy include which of the following? Select all that apply.
   a. Taking supplements of fat-soluble vitamins
   b. Taking supplements of B vitamins
   c. Increasing fluid intake
   d. Choosing foods that are lower in cholesterol and saturated fats
   e. Increasing the intake of raw vegetables, fruit, and bran

3. In reviewing the history of a newly admitted cardiac patient, the nurse recognizes that which of the following conditions she notes is a contraindication to antilipemic therapy?
   a. Liver disease
   b. Renal disease
   c. Coronary artery disease
   d. Diabetes mellitus

4. A woman is being screened in the cardiac clinic for risk factors for coronary artery disease. Which of the following would be considered a negative, or favorable, risk factor for her?
   a. High-density lipoprotein (HDL) cholesterol level of 30 mg/dL
   b. HDL cholesterol level of 75 mg/dL
   c. Early menopause
   d. Age of 57 years

5. A patient who has started taking niacin complains that he "hates the side effects." Which statement by the nurse is most appropriate?
   a. "You will soon build up tolerance to these side effects."
   b. "You should take the niacin on an empty stomach."
   c. "You can take the niacin every other day if the side effects are bothersome."
   d. "Try taking a small dose of ibuprofen or another nonsteroidal antiinflammatory drug 30 minutes before taking the niacin."

6. Which lipoprotein is often called the "good cholesterol?"
   a. Very-low-density lipoprotein (VLDL)
   b. Low-density lipoprotein (LDL)
   c. High-density lipoprotein (HDL)
   d. Triglycerides

CRITICAL THINKING AND APPLICATION

Answer the following questions on a separate sheet of paper.

7. For each of the following drugs, name the antilipemic category and briefly describe how the drug lowers lipid levels.

   a. gemfibrozil (Lopid)

   b. niacin

   c. lovastatin (Mevacor)

   d. cholestyramine (Questran)

8. Mr. Harris is a 46-year-old business executive who travels frequently. He is slightly overweight "from all that room service," but he did quit smoking 6 years ago. During a routine checkup, Mr. Harris is found to have an LDL cholesterol level of 230 mg/dL. He says, "I'm a busy man! Just give me some pills. I've got a plane to catch!" Will the physician prescribe an antilipemic for Mr. Harris? Explain your answer.

9. Mr. Jahnke is a 49-year-old farmer. During assessment, you discover the following: Mr. Jahnke's mother is living, but his father "dropped dead of a heart attack" at 53 years of age. Mr. Jahnke is a smoker with mild asthma and some arthritis in his hands. His blood pressure today is 122/78 mm Hg, and laboratory studies show an HDL cholesterol level of 77 mg/dL. Discuss Mr. Jahnke's risk factors for high cholesterol levels.

10. Mrs. Kim has been treated with cholestyramine for type IIa hyperlipidemia for the past 2 months. She tells you that she "can't stand being so irregular" and that she has developed another "embarrassing problem" as well. What is wrong with Mrs. Kim, and how can you help her?

11. Justus is a 55-year-old attorney being treated with lovastatin for his hyperlipidemia. His current health status includes mild hypertension and a peptic ulcer. You know that niacin is frequently prescribed as an adjunct to other antilipemic drugs. Would niacin be helpful for Justus? Explain your answer.

12. You are visiting Mrs. Nguyen, a homebound patient who is being treated for hyperlipidemia and hypertension. During your visit, Mrs. Nguyen takes her antihypertensive medication and then begins stirring her dose of cholestyramine into a glass of orange juice. What patient teaching does Mrs. Nguyen require?

CASE STUDY

Read the scenario and answer the following questions on a separate sheet of paper.

Mr. Miller has been diagnosed with type IIa hyperlipidemia and has been given a prescription for atorvastatin (Lipitor). He acts thrilled with the news, and says, "Great! Now I don't have to worry about watching my diet because I'm on this medicine!"

1. Is he right? What type of dietary guidelines should he follow while on this therapy?

2. What therapeutic effects do you hope to see as a result of his taking this medication?

3. After 2 months of therapy, you note that his liver enzyme levels are slightly elevated. Is this a concern? What other laboratory values should be monitored while Mr. Miller is taking atorvastatin?

4. Mr. Miller calls the office to complain about some muscle pain. He thought he had pulled a muscle during a tennis match, but the pain has not lessened in 3 days. Is this a concern?

Chapter 29
Pituitary Drugs

CHAPTER REVIEW

1. **Complete the following table.**

Hormone	Function	Mimicking Drug(s)
Adrenocorticotropics hormone (ACTH, corticotropin)	Targets adrenal gland; mediates adaptation to stressors; promotes synthesis of the following three hormones: a.	b.
Growth hormone	c.	d.
e.	Increases water resorption in distal tubules and collecting duct of nephron; concentrates urine; potent vasoconstrictor	f.
Endogenous oxytocin	g.	h.

Choose the best answer for each of the following.

2. Corticotropin is used for which of the following? Select all that apply.
   a. Treatment of diabetes insipidus
   b. Treatment of multiple sclerosis
   c. Stimulation of skeletal growth
   d. Prevention of carcinoid crisis
   e. Reduction of antiinflammation
   f. Diagnosis of adrenocortical insufficiency

3. A nurse is administering octreotide to a patient who has a metastatic carcinoid tumor. The patient asks about the purpose of this drug. The nurses best response would be which of the following?
   a. "This drug helps to reduce the size of your tumor."
   b. "This drug works to prevent the spread of your tumor."
   c. "Octreotide is given to reduce the nausea and vomiting you are having from the chemotherapy."
   d. "This drug helps to control the flushing and diarrhea that you are experiencing."

4. Which nursing diagnosis is most appropriate for a patient who is receiving a pituitary drug?
   a. Constipation
   b. Disturbed body image
   c. Impaired physical mobility
   d. Impaired skin integrity

5. The nurse should instruct a patient taking desmopressin acetate as a nasal spray for the treatment of diabetes insipidus to do which of the following to obtain maximum benefit from the drug?
   a. Clear the nasal passages after spraying the medication
   b. Inhale the spray for full drug effect
   c. If nasal congestion occurs, take an over-the-counter preparation to control mucus
   d. Administer the nasal spray at the same time every day

6. During assessment, the nurse discovers that a patient on corticotropin therapy is experiencing tremors and slight tetany. The nurse recognizes that these findings may indicate the development of which of the following?
   a. Hypokalemia
   b. Hyperkalemia
   c. Hypocalcemia
   d. Hypernatremia

CRITICAL THINKING AND APPLICATION

Answer the following questions on a separate sheet of paper.

7. A 44-lb child experiencing growth failure is to receive somatrem (Protropin) therapy. The dosage ordered is 0.3 mg/kg per week, to be given as a series of 6 daily injections.

   a. What is the dose per week that this child will receive?

   b. What is the dose per injection?

8. Alexis has multiple sclerosis. She is experiencing pain associated with inflammation.

   a. What drug might the physician recommend for Alexis?

   b. For what cautions and/or contraindications should you assess before this drug is administered?

   c. What else might you include in assessing Alexis before treatment?

   d. Alexis is determined to be an appropriate candidate for this drug of choice. Draw up an appropriate patient teaching plan.

9. You have recently begun working in a specialized endocrinology clinic. Your first patient, Patricia, a second-grader, is not growing at the rate that is expected. The physician has determined that Patricia is a candidate for somatropin therapy. Her parents are nervous about giving injections to Patricia. What should be emphasized when teaching her parents about giving this drug?

10. Jack, a 25-year-old man, has come to the clinic asking for "growth hormone." He heard that a cousin, who was diagnosed with dwarfism, is taking the hormone to "get taller" and Jack wants to take this hormone too. He is 5 feet, 5 inches tall. What do you tell him?

CASE STUDY

Read the scenario and answer the following questions on a separate sheet of paper.

Mr. Collins has been experiencing severe thirst, which he reports "of course makes me go to the bathroom all the time, it seems." He is also dehydrated, despite the large amounts of water he has been drinking.

1. Predict Mr. Collins's probable disorder and two likely drugs of choice for Mr. Collins.

2. How will you assess Mr. Collins before administering these drugs?

3. As a result of your assessment, it has been determined that Mr. Collins should do well with desmopressin therapy. Indicate how you would describe the treatment and its therapeutic effects (that is, how it mimics the natural hormone) to the patient.

4. Following your explanation, Mr. Collins says, "Okay, okay, but what does it do for me?" Explain the physical improvements Mr. Collins should be able to see.

Chapter 30
Thyroid and Antithyroid Drugs

CRITICAL THINKING CROSSWORD

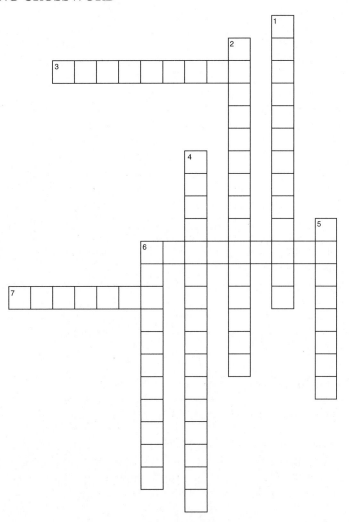

Across

3. The type of hypothyroidism that results from insufficient secretion of thyroid-stimulating hormone (TSH) from the pituitary gland
6. The principal thyroid hormone that influences the metabolic rate
7. The type of hypothyroidism that is due to the inability of the thyroid gland to perform a function

Down

1. The most commonly prescribed synthetic thyroid hormone
2. Excessive secretion of thyroid hormones
4. A drug used to treat hyperthyroidism
5. The type of hypothyroidism that stems from reduced secretion of thyrotropin-releasing hormone from the hypothalamus
6. Another name for TSH

CHAPTER REVIEW

Choose the best answer for each of the following.

1. Patients who begin therapy with levothyroxine should be told to expect effects from the medication
   a. immediately.
   b. within a few days.
   c. within a few weeks.
   d. within a few months.

2. A patient wants to switch brands of levothyroxine. The nurse's best response would be which of the following?
   a. "If you do this, you should reduce the dosage of your current brand before starting the new one."
   b. "Levothyroxine has been standardized, so there is only one brand."
   c. "It shouldn't matter if you switch brands; they are all very much the same."
   d. "You should check with your physician before switching brands."

3. Patient teaching for a patient taking antithyroid medication should include the need to avoid which foods?
   a. Soy products and seafood
   b. Bananas and oranges
   c. Dairy products
   d. Processed meats and cheese

4. Which of the following is a true statement that might be included in the nurse's teaching of patients taking thyroid medications?
   a. Keeping a log or journal of individual responses and a graph of pulse rate, weight, and mood would be helpful.
   b. The medication should be discontinued if the adverse effects become too strong.
   c. The medication should be taken at the same time every day.
   d. Nervousness, irritability, and insomnia may be a result of a dosage that is too high.

5. A patient is scheduled for a radioactive isotope study. Upon review of his medications, the scheduling nurse notes that he takes levothyroxine daily. Which statement is correct regarding the use of this medication before a radioactive isotope study?
   a. The patient should continue to take the medication as ordered.
   b. The patient should skip the medication on the morning of the test.
   c. The patient should stop the medication about 4 weeks before the test.
   d. The patient should reduce the dosage 1 week before the test.

CRITICAL THINKING AND APPLICATION

Answer the following questions on a separate sheet of paper.

6. Mrs. Westin, age 43, comes into the clinic complaining of hair loss, lethargy, and constipation. "I just can't eat anything," she says. As you take her blood pressure, you notice that her skin feels thickened. She also seems to have a lump in her neck. Which of the disorders discussed in this chapter is Mrs. Westin most likely to have? Suggest several possible appropriate medications. Which of those is generally preferred? Why?

7. Ms. Hilton has had Graves' disease for 3 years. Today she reports symptoms of diarrhea, muscle weakness, fatigue, and palpitations. Also, she says that despite the diarrhea, she often has an increased appetite. She is also having trouble sleeping and wonders whether she is undergoing menopause because she suffers flushing, heat intolerance, and altered menstrual flow. As you ask her questions about these symptoms, you note that she seems irritable. This is understandable given her multiple symptoms; however, you have known Ms. Hilton since she began treatment for Graves' disease, and she has never acted this way before, no matter how bad she felt. What's going on here?

8. After undergoing a thyroidectomy as treatment for a thyroid tumor that turned out to be benign, Rebecca is given a prescription for levothyroxine. "I thought I would be cured after this surgery!" she exclaimed. "Why do I have to take a pill every day?" What do you explain to Rebecca?

CASE STUDY

Read the scenario and answer the following questions on a separate sheet of paper.

Goldie, a 38-year-old teacher, has come to the clinic complaining of having "no energy or appetite" and yet her weight has increased by 15 lb in the last month. You note that her hair is thin and her skin is dull. Laboratory work reveals an elevated level of TSH.

1. What do Goldie's symptoms suggest? What medication do you expect to be ordered for her?

2. Explain the concept of "euthyroid" as it would relate to Goldie's condition.

3. One month after therapy has begun, Goldie calls the office to complain that she "can't sleep at all" since she started taking the medication. She says she tries to take it at the same time every morning but often forgets and takes it at dinnertime. What teaching, if any, does she need to help her with this problem?

Chapter 31

Antidiabetic Drugs

CHAPTER REVIEW

Choose the best answer for each of the following.

1. When administering insulin, the nurse must keep in mind that the most immediate and serious adverse effect of insulin therapy is which of the following?
   a. Hyperglycemia
   b. Hypoglycemia
   c. Bradycardia
   d. Orthostatic hypotension

2. A dose of long-acting insulin has been ordered for bedtime for a diabetic patient. The nurse expects to give which type of insulin?
   a. regular
   b. Lente
   c. NPH
   d. glargine

3. A patient is to be placed on an insulin drip to control his high blood glucose levels. The nurse knows that which of the following is the only type of insulin that can be given intravenously?
   a. regular
   b. Lente
   c. NPH
   d. Ultralente

4. While monitoring a patient who is receiving insulin therapy, the nurse observes for signs of hypoglycemia, such as which of the following?
   a. Decreased pulse and respiratory rates and flushed skin
   b. Increased pulse rate and a fruity, acetone breath odor
   c. Weakness, sweating, and confusion
   d. Increased urine output and edema

5. When giving oral acarbose (Precose), the nurse should administer it at what time?
   a. 15 minutes before a meal
   b. 30 minutes before a meal
   c. With the first bite of a meal
   d. 1 hour after eating

6. A patient taking rosiglitazone (Avandia) tells the nurse, "There's my insulin pill!" The nurse describes the mechanism of action of rosiglitazone by explaining that this drug is not insulin but works by
   a. stimulating the beta cells of the pancreas to produce insulin.
   b. decreasing insulin resistance.
   c. inhibiting hepatic glucose production.
   d. decreasing intestinal absorption of glucose.

7. The sliding-scale insulin order reads: "Do bedside glucose testing before meals. For glucose results over 150 mg/dL, give regular (Humulin R) insulin, 1 unit for every 20 mg/dL over 150 mg/dL." If the blood glucose level is 238 mg/dL, the patient will receive _____ unit(s) of insulin.

CRITICAL THINKING AND APPLICATION

Answer the following questions on a separate sheet of paper.

8. Explain the mechanism of action of

   a. pramlintide

   b. exenatide

9. Alice has mild hypoglycemia. Her physician has recommended dietary modifications to treat the condition.

   a. What general dietary guidelines should she follow?

   b. You know that one of the early signs of hypoglycemia is irritability. Why is this true?

   c. If Alice experiences hypoglycemia at home, what are the treatment options?

10. Your co-worker Bill is in the medication room preparing a dose of Novolin-R to administer to a patient.

    a. Before he administers the medication, how should Bill verify the order?

    b. When you enter the room, you notice that the insulin is cloudy. When you tell Bill to discard it, he says, "Insulin is supposed to look this way." Who is right, you or Bill?

    c. You examine the vial. A date on the label indicates that it has been on the shelf in this room for 2 months. Is this a problem?

11. Alec is a 20-year-old student at a private Jewish university in a large city. He has been diagnosed with type 1 diabetes. The physician determines that Alec would best be treated with an insulin product that has an onset of action of 1 or 2 hours and a duration of action of 10 to 18 hours.

    a. What type of insulin does Alec require?

    b. What else might the physician need to consider when choosing a specific drug for Alec?

12. Mrs. Franklin, a 48-year-old homemaker, is 5 feet tall and weighs 180 lb. During a routine physical, laboratory studies indicate an elevated blood glucose level. Your assessment of Mrs. Franklin reveals that she is a smoker with mild hypertension. The physician suspects type 2 diabetes.

    a. What initial treatment is indicated for Mrs. Franklin? Explain your answer.

    b. At a follow-up visit 3 months later, Mrs. Franklin's blood glucose level is still elevated. She has quit smoking, however, and has been walking for exercise. What treatment is indicated now?

13. Dennis is a 40-year-old taxicab dispatcher who takes chlorpropamide (Diabinese). He comes to the emergency department late one Sunday evening complaining that he feels weak, he vomited earlier, he has a headache, and his face "feels hot." You note that Dennis has profound flushing and is sweating.

    a. What do Dennis's signs and symptoms indicate?

    b. What may have caused this? How can you tell?

14. Your patient is taking insulin every morning with sliding-scale coverage. The specified dosages are:
    NPH insulin, 20 units, every morning before breakfast, and regular insulin, sliding-scale coverage, before meals and at bedtime, as follows:
    Blood glucose level lower than 200 mg/dL: no additional coverage
    Blood glucose level 200 to 249 mg/dL: 2 units regular (Humulin R) insulin
    Blood glucose level 250 to 299 mg/dL: 4 units regular (Humulin R) insulin
    Blood glucose level 300 to 349 mg/dL: 6 units Regular (Humulin R) insulin
    Blood glucose level higher than 350 mg/dL: call for orders

    How much insulin will your patient receive in the following circumstances?
    a. Before breakfast, if her blood glucose level is 275 mg/dL
    b. Before lunch, if her blood glucose level is 199 mg/dL
    c. Before dinner, if her blood glucose level is 328 mg/dL

CASE STUDY

Read the scenario and answer the following questions on a separate sheet of paper.

The physician is planning to prescribe glipizide (Glucotrol) for Mr. Dressel, a 50-year-old financial advisor with a history of renal failure. In particular, Mr. Dressel requires treatment for the short-term elevation in blood glucose level that occurs after he eats.

1. Why did the physician choose a second-generation sulfonylurea rather than, for example, chlorpropamide?

2. Why would glipizide be a good choice for Mr. Dressel?

3. When should he take this drug?

4. A few weeks later Mr. Dressel comes down with the flu. He is vomiting and has been unable to eat all day. What should he do, and why?

Chapter 32
Adrenal Drugs

CHAPTER REVIEW

Choose the best answer for each of the following.

1. A 50-year-old man has been taking prednisone following a severe reaction to poison ivy. He notices that the dosage of the medication decreases. During a follow-up office visit, he asks the nurse why he must continue the medication and why he cannot just stop taking it now that the skin rash is better. The nurse knows that
   a. sudden discontinuation of this medication may cause an adrenal crisis.
   b. he would experience withdrawal symptoms if the drug were discontinued abruptly.
   c. Cushing's syndrome may develop as a reaction to a sudden drop of serum cortisone levels.
   d. he can stop taking the medication if his rash is better.

2. Which medication is the preferred oral glucocorti-coid for antiinflammatory or immunosuppressant purposes?
   a. fludrocortisone
   b. dexamethasone
   c. prednisone
   d. hydrocortisone

3. When monitoring a patient who is taking corticosteroids, the nurse observes for adverse effects, including which of the following? Select all that apply.
   a. Fragile skin
   b. Increased glucose levels
   c. Nervousness
   d. Hypotension
   e. Weight loss
   f. Drowsiness

4. A patient has Cushing's syndrome. The nurse expects which drug to be used to inhibit the function of the adrenal cortex in the treatment of this syndrome?
   a. dexamethasone
   b. aminoglutethimide
   c. hydrocortisone
   d. fludrocortisone

5. A patient who has been taking corticosteroids has developed a "moon face" and facial redness, and has many bruises on her arms. The most appropriate nursing diagnosis would be which of the following?
   a. Risk for infection
   b. Imbalanced nutrition (less than body requirements)
   c. Deficient fluid volume
   d. Disturbed body image

6. Because corticosteroids may cause sodium retention, the nurse should closely monitor patients with which condition when administering corticosteroids?
   a. Diabetes mellitus
   b. Seizure disorders
   c. Heart failure
   d. Hyperthyroidism

CRITICAL THINKING AND APPLICATION

Answer the following questions on a separate sheet of paper.

7. Ms. Rivera, a 30-year-old hospital receptionist, is receiving glucocorticoid therapy after a kidney transplant. You are reviewing her drug regimen with her when she tells you that she frequently uses aspirin or ibuprofen to treat problems like headaches or menstrual cramps. She also mentions that she enjoys walking for exercise and likes to visit sick children on the hospital's pediatric ward when she has time. What issues do you discuss with Ms. Rivera?

8. Peter, a 21-year-old mechanic, has developed a severe skin rash after a camping trip. The physician is planning to prescribe prednisone. Your nursing assessment reveals that Peter has type 1 diabetes.

   a. Does that finding affect Peter's treatment? Explain your answer.

   b. To help minimize gastrointestinal effects, what advice do you have for someone taking an oral form of a systemic adrenal drug?

9. You are watching a student nurse prepare to apply a topical glucocorticoid to a patient's skin rash. After donning gloves, she places some of the medication on her finger. Should you intervene, or is the student nurse doing fine so far? What other consideration is involved in determining the technique for applying a topical drug?

10. Nina has been prescribed a steroid drug delivered via inhaler. What special instructions do you give her?

CASE STUDY

Read the scenario and answer the following questions on a separate sheet of paper.

Julie is in the urgent care center because of an exacerbation of asthma. She is usually able to control it with inhaled bronchodilators, but the physician decides to give her a short course of prednisone in a dose that started high and then tapered down over a week's time.

1. Why is the dose tapered instead of just discontinued after a week?

2. What are potential effects of long-term therapy?

3. Is this drug a glucocorticoid or mineralocorticoid? Explain the difference.

4. What time of day should she take this drug? Explain.

Chapter 33
Women's Health Drugs

CHAPTER REVIEW

Choose the best answer for each of the following.

1. When reviewing the health history of a patient who wants to begin taking oral contraceptives, the nurse recalls that contraindications include which of the following? Select all that apply.
   a. Multiple sclerosis
   b. Pregnancy
   c. Thrombophlebitic disorders
   d. Breast cancer
   e. Abnormal vaginal bleeding

2. When the nurse is teaching patients about postmenopausal estrogen replacement therapy, which statement is correct?
   a. "The smallest dose that is effective will be prescribed."
   b. "Oral forms should be taken on an empty stomach for best absorption."
   c. "Estrogen therapy should be long term to prevent menopausal symptoms."
   d. "If estrogen is taken, supplemental calcium will not be needed."

3. When combination oral contraceptives are given to provide postcoital emergency contraception, the nurse should remember which of the following facts?
   a. They are not effective if the woman is already pregnant.
   b. They should be taken within 12 hours of unprotected intercourse.
   c. They are given in one dose.
   d. They are intended to terminate pregnancy.

4. When reviewing an order for dinoprostone cervical gel, the nurse recalls that this drug is used for which of the following purposes?
   a. To induce abortion during the third trimester
   b. To improve cervical inducibility ("ripening") near term for labor induction
   c. To soften the cervix in women who are experiencing infertility problems
   d. To reduce postpartum uterine atony and hemorrhage

5. A pregnant woman is experiencing contractions. The nurse remembers that drugs such as terbutaline are used to prevent contractions
   a. before the twentieth week of gestation.
   b. between the twentieth and thirty-seventh weeks.
   c. after the thirty-seventh week.
   d. at any time during the pregnancy if delivery is not desired.

6. What patient teaching is appropriate for a patient taking alendronate (Fosamax)? Select all that apply.
   a. Take on an empty stomach.
   b. Take at night just before going to bed.
   c. Take with an 8-oz glass of water.
   d. Take with a sip of water.
   e. Take first thing in the morning upon arising.
   f. Do not lie down for at least 30 minutes after taking.

CRITICAL THINKING AND APPLICATION

Answer the following questions on a separate sheet of paper.

7. Isabelle is a 48-year-old woman exhibiting symptoms of menopause. Assessment of Isabelle reveals a history of depression and mild arthritis.

    a. What do you need to ask Isabelle, and why?

    b. The physician decides to prescribe estrogen therapy. At this time, what do you know about the dose and the length of time it will be administered?

8. Ms. Keller is a 25-year-old paralegal with diabetes. She is at the physician's office today because her menstrual periods have ceased. The physician has decided to prescribe a hormonal drug.

    a. Which drug will the physician likely prescribe?

    b. What adjustments to Ms. Keller's existing drug regimen might need to be made?

9. Jacklyn receives a prescription for Ortho-Novum for birth control purposes. At a follow-up visit 4 months later, she tells you, "I'm really messing up. I take the pills for 3 weeks, but when I'm off them for a week, sometimes I don't remember to start again!"

    a. What might you suggest to help Jacklyn?

    b. Jacklyn then expresses concern that her menstrual bleeding, now that she is taking birth control pills, is "nothing compared with what it used to be." She asks you whether she is okay. What do you tell Jacklyn?

10. Ms. Jones, a sales associate in a bookstore, is being treated for fertility problems. She is currently on a drug regimen that includes chorionic gonadotropin and Pergonal.

    a. Why is Ms. Jones taking two fertility drugs?

    b. After the first course of treatment, Ms. Jones does not become pregnant. Describe her next course of treatment.

11. Mrs. Ingalls has been taking estrogen therapy for several weeks. During a routine checkup, she sheepishly tells you that she has not been able to quit smoking yet. She also mentions that she is going to Aruba for a vacation the next month. What patient teaching does Mrs. Ingalls require?

12. Mrs. Simmons, age 33, comes in for her yearly gynecologic examination, and the physician recommends alendronate (Fosamax), 5 mg daily. Mrs. Simmons experienced early menopause last year and asks you, "Why did the doctor wait until now to start me on estrogen? I didn't need it before."

    a. What do you explain about the purpose of this medication?

    b. What risk factors might Mrs. Simmons have to support therapy with alendronate?

13. Other than its intended effects in the prevention of osteoporosis, what is a possible benefit of the drug ibandronate?

CASE STUDY

Read the scenario and answer the following questions on a separate sheet of paper.

Ms. O'Hara, a 34-year-old computer programmer, is having mild contractions. She is in the thirtieth week of gestation, and the physician determines that she is experiencing premature labor.

1. What drug is the physician likely to prescribe, and how does it work?

2. In what position do you place Ms. O'Hara before starting the intravenous infusion. Why?

3. Ms. O'Hara's contractions stop, and she is sent home on maintenance ritodrine therapy. At a follow-up visit, her blood glucose and electrolyte levels are checked. Why?

4. During her thirty-ninth week of gestation, her contractions return. Will she receive this same therapy?

Chapter 34
Men's Health Drugs

CHAPTER REVIEW

Choose the best answer for each of the following.

1. A 19-year-old college football player asks his friend's mother, who is a nurse, about taking steroids to help him "beef up" his muscles. Which of the following is true?
   a. There should be no problems as long as he does not exceed the recommended dosage.
   b. Long-term use may cause a life-threatening liver condition.
   c. He would need to be careful to watch for excessive weight loss.
   d. These drugs also tend to increase the male's sperm count.

2. In which of the following situations would androgens be prescribed for a woman? Select all that apply.
   a. Development of secondary sex characteristics
   b. Fibrocystic breast disease
   c. Ovarian cancer
   d. Treatment of endometriosis
   e. Postmenopausal osteoporosis prevention
   f. Metastatic breast cancer

3. A patient will be receiving testosterone therapy for male hypogonadism and has a new prescription for Testoderm patches. The nurse needs to include which teaching about the use of this medication?
   a. The patch should be applied only to the scrotum.
   b. The patch should not be applied to the scrotum.
   c. If the adverse effects become bothersome, the patient should stop using the patch.
   d. The patch should be applied to a different area of the upper body each day.

4. Before a patient begins therapy with finasteride, the nurse should make sure that which laboratory test has been performed?
   a. Blood glucose level
   b. Complete blood count
   c. Urinalysis
   d. Prostate specific antigen (PSA) level

5. A patient is taking finasteride for the treatment of benign prostatic hypertrophy. His wife, who is 3 months pregnant, is worried about the adverse effects that may occur with this drug. Which statement by the nurse is the most important at this time?
   a. "Gastric upset may be reduced if he takes this drug on an empty stomach."
   b. "You should notice therapeutic effects of increased libido and erection within 1 month."
   c. "This medication should not even be handled by pregnant women because it may harm the fetus."
   d. "You may experience transient hair loss while taking this medication."

6. Which drug is used, in low dosages, for androgenetic alopecia in men?
   a. finasteride (Propecia)
   b. vardenafil (Levitra)
   c. danazol (Danocrine)
   d. oxandrolone (Oxandrin)

CRITICAL THINKING AND APPLICATION

Answer the following questions on a separate sheet of paper.

7. Mr. Michaels is being treated for hypogonadism. He has been taking intramuscular injections of testosterone cypionate but has complained about the pain caused by the injections. Today he will be switched to an oral dosage form. He expects to get "testosterone pills." However, you remember the poor performance of the drug when given via that route, and you tell him that it will probably not be testosterone itself.

   a. Mr. Michaels is skeptical of switching drugs and asks for more information. Explain specifically why oral testosterone does not work well.

   b. What do you predict Mr. Michaels will receive instead?

   c. Discuss potential contraindications that might apply to this patient.

8. Mr. Michaels is administered methyltestosterone buccally. He reports that he gets "tired" of waiting for the buccal tablet to dissolve and asks whether he can swallow or chew it, at least after it is mostly dissolved.

   a. If Mr. Michaels does let most of the tablet dissolve on its own, is it acceptable to compromise, for the sake of patient compliance, by letting him chew or swallow the rest?

   b. "And while we're on the subject," Mr. Michaels says, "I'm going on a fishing trip next week. I'd like not to have to bother with the pills. Can we work something out so that I stop temporarily and pick back up with the treatment as soon as I get back?" What do you say?

9. Mr. Olafson has been prescribed finasteride for his benign prostatic hypertrophy. He asks, "How does it work?" You explain that it will cause his prostate to decrease in size and alleviate discomfort.

   a. "No," he says. "You don't understand. I'm not a pharmacist, but I am a chemist. Tell me how it works." Tell him everything you know about how finasteride works.

   b. What are the most important things to include in his patient teaching plan?

10. Compare the application methods for the following forms of testosterone: Testoderm patch, Androderm patch, and AndroGel.

CASE STUDY

Read the scenario and answer the following questions on a separate sheet of paper.

Mr. Edward, age 72, has asked the physician for "help with a private matter." He tells the physician that he would like to try Viagra, "that drug that helps with a certain problem."

1. What assessment findings may contraindicate the use of sildenafil (Viagra) by Mr. Edward?

2. If he is a candidate for therapy with Viagra, what patient teaching should he receive?

3. What concerns would there be about his liver function? About his vision?

4. When should he take this medication?

Chapter 35

Antihistamines, Decongestants, Antitussives, and Expectorants

CHAPTER REVIEW

Choose the best answer for each of the following.

1. Which of the following are correct statements to include in patient teaching about antihistamine use? Select all that apply.
   a. Antihistamines are best tolerated when taken with meals.
   b. The patient can suck on hard candy or chew gum if he or she experiences dry mouth.
   c. The main adverse effect of antihistamines is drowsiness.
   d. Over-the-counter medications are generally safe to use with antihistamines.

2. A patient asks the nurse for advice about one of the newer antihistamines that does not cause drowsiness. Which of these drugs is appropriate?
   a. loratadine (Claritin)
   b. diphenhydramine (Benadryl)
   c. dimenhydrinate (Dramamine)
   d. meclizine (Antivert)

3. Which drugs are considered first-line drugs for the treatment of nasal congestion?
   a. Antihistamines such as diphenhydramine
   b. Decongestants such as naphazoline
   c. Antitussives such as dextromethorphan
   d. Expectorants such as guaifenesin

4. When giving an antitussive, the nurse remembers that they are used primarily to
   a. relieve nasal congestion.
   b. thin secretions to ease removal of excessive secretions.
   c. stop the cough reflex when the cough is nonproductive.
   d. suppress productive and nonproductive coughs.

5. Which teaching is appropriate for the patient receiving an expectorant?
   a. Avoid fluids for 30 to 35 minutes after the dose.
   b. Force fluids, unless contraindicated, to aid in expectoration of sputum.
   c. Avoid driving or operating heavy machinery while taking this medication.
   d. Expect secretions to become thicker.

6. A patient has been self-medicating with diphenhydramine to help her sleep. She calls the clinic nurse to ask, "why do I feel so tired during the day after I take this pill? I get a good night's sleep!" Which statement by the nurse is correct?
   a. "You are probably getting too much sleep."
   b. "You are taking too much of the drug."
   c. "This drug is not really meant to help people sleep."
   d. "This drug often causes a 'hangover effect' during the day after taking it."

CRITICAL THINKING AND APPLICATION

Answer the following questions on a separate sheet of paper.

7. Why are histamine-1 (H_1) blockers most beneficial when given early in a histamine-mediated reaction?

8. Do the traditional antihistamines have any advantages over the newer, nonsedating antihistamines? Explain your answer.

9. Mrs. Ling was seen in the office several days ago with a common cold. She has been on decongestant therapy with naphazoline nasal spray since that time. Today she calls to say, "I thought I was getting over this, but suddenly my nose is more stuffed up than ever." Does Mrs. Ling possibly need a stronger dosage of the decongestant? Explain your answer.

121

10. Keith has been using a topical nasal decongestant for the past few days. He calls the physician's office to report that he is feeling nervous and dizzy and that his heart seems to be racing. What might be the cause of Keith's symptoms?

11. How does benzonatate differ from other antitussive drugs in its mechanism of action? In its drug interaction profile?

12. One day you encounter your neighbor Irene as you are returning home from work. She is on her way to the drugstore, she tells you, because she has been experiencing a nonproductive cough and wants to get a cough medicine "to loosen things up." You recall that Irene mentioned a few months ago that she has problems with her thyroid. Do you wish Irene good luck and continue on your way? Explain your answer.

13. Lisa is a 5-year-old patient who has bronchitis accompanied by a nonproductive cough. The physician has prescribed Robitussin DM for the cough. Lisa's father tells you that his 11-year-old son was prescribed Robitussin A-C several months earlier for a severe cough. He asks you whether his son's cough medicine would help Lisa because "there's plenty left in the bottle." What do you tell him?

14. Justin calls the nurse at the office because he experiences "palpitations and a racing heart" every morning after breakfast. Upon questioning, he states that he has been taking a decongestant for a cold and has been drinking an extra cup of coffee in the morning "to get going" because the cold has kept him from sleeping well. What could be his problem?

CASE STUDY

Read the scenario and answer the following questions on a separate sheet of paper.

James, a 35-year-old electrician, is seen in the emergency department with a rash on his arms and hands that appeared after he was working in his yard. You suspect that the physician will prescribe topical diphenhydramine, but during the nursing assessment, James tells you that he has diabetes.

1. How does James's diabetes affect his possible treatment with diphenhydramine?

2. If James does receive a topical diphenhydramine preparation, what other drug might be found in combination with it?

The topical medication did not help his rash, and James has been switched to oral diphenhydramine. He tells you that he expects to return to work tomorrow and hopes this medication "does the trick."

3. What cautions, if any, should James be aware of while taking this medication?

4. Are there any concerns with drug interactions?

Chapter 36

Bronchodilators and Other Respiratory Drugs

CHAPTER REVIEW

Choose the best answer for each of the following.

1. Frequent use of bronchodilators may cause which adverse effects? Select all that apply.
   a. Blurred vision
   b. Increased heart rate
   c. Decreased heart rate
   d. Nausea
   e. Nervousness
   f. Tremors

2. For patients taking a leukotriene antagonist, the nurse should include which of the following in patient teaching?
   a. If a dose is missed, the patient may take a double dose to maintain blood levels.
   b. The patient should gargle or rinse the mouth after using the inhaler.
   c. The medication should be taken at the first sign of bronchospasm.
   d. Improvement should be seen within a week of use.

3. Which drug acts by blocking leukotrienes and thus reducing inflammation in the lungs?
   a. albuterol (Proventil)
   b. cromolyn (Intal)
   c. theophylline (Theo-Dur)
   d. montelukast (Singulair)

4. A patient in status asthmaticus has not yet responded to epinephrine. The nurse will expect which of the following drugs to be used next?
   a. albuterol (Proventil)
   b. aminophylline
   c. cromolyn (Intal)
   d. montelukast (Singulair)

5. When a patient is taking parenteral xanthine derivatives, such as aminophylline, the nurse should monitor for which adverse effect?
   a. Decreased respirations
   b. Hypotension
   c. Tachycardia
   d. Hypoglycemia

6. A patient who is taking a β-adrenergic agonist for bronchodilation may also take which type of inhaled drug for its antiinflammatory effects?
   a. Corticosteroid
   b. Anticholinergic
   c. Xanthine derivative
   d. Antileukotriene

CRITICAL THINKING AND APPLICATION

Answer the following questions on a separate sheet of paper.

7. Describe briefly how idiopathic asthma differs from allergic asthma.

8. Tom, a 70-year-old retiree who smoked for 40 years, has been diagnosed with chronic obstructive pulmonary disease (COPD); the treatment regimen prescribed includes theophylline. After a few weeks, Tom tells you that he is experiencing nausea and "bad heartburn at night." The laboratory studies show the level of theophylline in his blood to be 30 mcg/mL. What might be wrong with Tom, and how can it be corrected?

9. Willie is a 9-year-old boy who is brought to the emergency department by his aunt because he is having an acute asthma attack. The physician orders epinephrine intravenously. How do you calculate the dosage for Willie?

10. Sylvia has come to the clinic today complaining of nausea, palpitations, and anxiety. She says that her heart feels "as if it's going to fly out of my chest." Physical examination confirms an increased heart rate. Sylvia's records indicate that she has asthma for which she uses an albuterol inhaler. What do you suspect might be wrong with Sylvia, and what do you advise her to do?

11. Mrs. Voss, a 65-year-old office manager, has arthritis, glaucoma, and emphysema. The physician is planning prophylactic treatment for her emphysema.

    a. What three types of drugs might be considered for treatment of COPD?

    b. What factor must the physician keep in mind when determining the best drug for Mrs. Voss?

12. Several months ago the physician prescribed an orally administered corticosteroid for Mr. Zoller, who has chronic bronchial asthma.

    a. What are the disadvantages of administering the corticosteroids orally?

    b. Today the physician adds Beclovent to Mr. Zoller's drug regimen and also reduces the dosage of the oral corticosteroid. Is that safe?

13. Sam is a 10-year-old girl who is to be treated with theophylline for her asthma.

    a. What particular effect will have to be watched for, and why?

    b. Sam's mother asks whether she can crush the tablets to make them easier for Sam to swallow. Is that advisable?

14. Alice has been treated for asthma for several months and has the following inhalers: albuterol (Proventil) and fluticasone (Flovent). Which one should she choose if she experiences an asthma attack? Explain your answer.

CASE STUDY

Read the scenario and answer the following questions on a separate sheet of paper.

Jennie has been treated for adult-onset asthma for 3 years. Today she has started taking montelukast (Singulair), one 10-mg tablet daily.

1. How does this medication differ from traditional antiasthma drugs?

2. Jennie says, "I hope this medicine works better than the other one I took when I had an asthma attack." What should be your reply?

3. Jennie takes ibuprofen on occasion for arthritic pain. What should you advise about taking this medication with montelukast?

4. After 3 months, Jennie stops taking the montelukast. She says, "My symptoms are better, and I don't want to take medicine unless I need it." Is this appropriate?

Chapter 37
Antibiotics Part 1

CRITICAL THINKING CROSSWORD

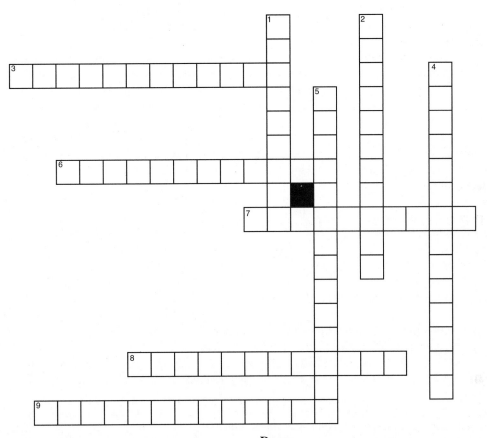

Across

3. Antibiotics taken before exposure to an infectious organism in an effort to prevent the development of infection
6. The classification for the drug doxycycline
7. An antibiotic derived from a fungus or mold often seen on bread or fruit
8. Antibiotics that kill bacteria
9. The classification for the drug cefazolin

Down

1. The classification for the drug erythromycin
2. The classification for the drug sulfisoxazole
4. Antibiotics that inhibit the growth of bacteria
5. An infection that occurs during antimicrobial treatment for another infection and involves overgrowth of a nonsusceptible organism

CHAPTER REVIEW

Choose the best answer for each of the following.

1. A drug interaction occurs between penicillins and which of the following? Select all that apply.
   a. Alcohol
   b. Oral contraceptives
   c. Digoxin
   d. Nonsteroidal antiinflammatory drugs
   e. Warfarin
   f. Anticonvulsants

2. Which intervention is important for the nurse to perform before beginning antibiotic therapy?
   a. Obtain a specimen for culture and sensitivity
   b. Give with an antacid to reduce gastrointestinal (GI) upset
   c. Monitor for adverse effects
   d. Restrict oral fluids

3. The nurse will instruct a patient who is taking a tetracycline antibiotic to
   a. take it with milk.
   b. take it with 8 oz of water.
   c. take it 30 minutes before taking iron preparations.
   d. use an antacid to decrease GI discomfort.

4. A patient is to receive antibiotic therapy with a cephalosporin. When assessing the patient's drug history, the nurse recognizes that an allergy to which type of drug may be a possible contraindication to cephalosporin therapy?
   a. Cardiac glycosides
   b. Thiazide diuretics
   c. Penicillins
   d. Macrolides

5. When asked about drug allergies, a patient says, "I can't take sulfa drugs because I'm allergic to them." Which question should the nurse ask next?
   a. "Do you have any other drug allergies?"
   b. "Who prescribed that drug for you?"
   c. "How long ago did this happen?"
   d. "What happened when you took the sulfa drug?"

CRITICAL THINKING AND APPLICATION

Answer the following questions on a separate sheet of paper.

6. Mr. Renville, a 50-year-old banker, is scheduled for colorectal surgery tomorrow. The surgeon is planning to administer a prophylactic antibiotic. What drug is frequently used for this purpose, and why?

7. Sean is a 19-year-old college freshman who has been diagnosed with gonorrhea. The physician has prescribed doxycycline therapy. During your nursing assessment, you and Sean discuss his diet, which includes "lots of meat, milk, and veggies." Sean also tells you that he jogs frequently and is a member of the tennis team.

   a. In addition to instruction about sexually transmitted diseases, what patient teaching does Sean require?

   b. A few days later Sean calls and complains of an upset stomach and diarrhea. What do you suspect might be wrong with Sean?

8. Sandra, a 59-year-old homemaker, has bronchitis and has been taking an antibiotic for 1 week. She calls the nurse and complains of severe itching and a whitish discharge in her vaginal area. What has happened, and what caused it?

CASE STUDY

Read the scenario and answer the following questions on a separate sheet of paper.

A 78-year-old patient, admitted to the hospital with a stroke 2 days earlier, has developed a urinary tract infection. His Foley catheter is draining urine that is cloudy and dark yellowish orange with a strong odor. Strands of pus are also visible in the urine. He is receiving an intravenous heparin infusion and has a history of type 2 diabetes. The physician orders co-trimoxazole (Bactrim).

1. What should be assessed before giving this medication?

2. Are there any potential drug interactions?

3. Why was this particular antibiotic chosen?

4. Is this antibiotic bactericidal or bacteriostatic? Explain.

Chapter 38
Antibiotics Part 2

CHAPTER REVIEW

Choose the best answer for each of the following.

1. When patients are receiving aminoglycosides, the nurse must monitor for tinnitus, which may indicate which of the following?
   a. Cardiotoxicity
   b. Hepatotoxicity
   c. Ototoxicity
   d. Nephrotoxicity

2. A patient is being prepared for colon surgery and will be receiving neomycin tablets during the day before surgery. He asks the nurse why he needs to take this medicine before he even has surgery. The nurse's best response is which of the following?
   a. "This medicine helps to clear out your bowels before surgery."
   b. "It helps to reduce the number of bacteria in your intestines before surgery."
   c. "It is given to sterilize your bowel before surgery."
   d. "It is given to prevent an infection after surgery."

3. A patient has been admitted to the unit with a stage IV pressure ulcer. After 2 days, the wound culture results come back positive for methicillin-resistant *Staphylococcus aureus* (MRSA). The nurse knows that the drug of choice for the treatment of MRSA infection is
   a. vancomycin.
   b. an aminoglycoside, such as gentamicin.
   c. ciprofloxacin.
   d. dapsone.

4. A patient who is receiving vancomycin therapy should notify the nurse immediately if which of the following effects are noted? Select all that apply.
   a. Ringing in the ears
   b. Dizziness
   c. Hearing loss
   d. Fullness in the ears

CRITICAL THINKING AND APPLICATION

Answer the following questions on a separate sheet of paper.

5. Angie has a severe infection and is receiving an aminoglycoside once a day. She says, "They tell me I have a terrible infection. Why am I not getting the antibiotic more than once a day? I don't understand!" What should you tell her?

6. Explain the concept of "trough" levels during aminoglycoside therapy and the way in which renal function is monitored.

7. Greg has been taking amiodarone for a heart rhythm problem. He has developed an infection from an open wound, and the sensitivity report indicates that levofloxacin is the best choice to fight this infection. Are there any concerns?

8. Nitrofurantoin has been ordered for a patient who has a severe urinary tract infection caused by *Escherichia coli*. Explain why this drug is used for this type of infection. You note that the following order has also been written for this patient: "Force fluids to 2000 mL/day." Explain the reason for forcing fluids.

CASE STUDY

Read the scenario and answer the following questions on a separate sheet of paper.

Virgil has been admitted to your unit and placed on aminoglycoside therapy as part of treatment for a urinary tract infection with *Pseudomonas*. He is 65 years old, awake and alert, but anxious about his problem and wants to "hurry up and get better."

1. What two serious toxicities for which will you monitor, what are their symptoms, and how can they be prevented?

2. The physician adds penicillin to Virgil's drug regimen. Explain the reason for this.

3. Virgil's "trough" aminoglycoside level is 3.0 mcg/mL, and his serum creatinine level is increased from 2 days earlier. Are these results a concern? What should you do? Explain.

Chapter 39
Antiviral Drugs

CHAPTER REVIEW

Choose the best answer for each of the following.

1. Acyclovir is considered the drug of choice for treatment of infection with which of the following?
   a. Cytomegalovirus (CMV)
   b. Human immunodeficiency virus (HIV)
   c. Respiratory syncytial virus (RSV)
   d. Varicella-zoster virus (VZV)

2. When administering ganciclovir, the nurse keeps in mind that the main dose-limiting toxicity for this drug is which of the following?
   a. Renal failure
   b. Gastrointestinal disturbances
   c. Peripheral neuropathy
   d. Bone marrow suppression

3. When reviewing the health history of a patient who is to receive foscarnet, the nurse knows that which condition would be a contraindication to its use?
   a. Renal toxicity
   b. CMV retinitis
   c. Asthma
   d. Immunosuppression

4. Amantadine would be used most appropriately in which of the following patients?
   a. A 29-year-old man who tests positive for HIV
   b. A 22-year-old woman who is in her eighth month of pregnancy and tests HIV positive
   c. A heart transplant patient who is to receive prophylaxis for influenza A
   d. Elderly patients who require prophylaxis for influenza B

5. A patient calls the clinic nurse to ask for oseltamivir (Tamiflu) "because I was exposed to the flu over the weekend at a family reunion." The nurse knows that Tamiflu is indicated for which of the following? Select all that apply.
   a. Prevention of infection after exposure to influenza virus types A and B
   b. Reduction of the duration of influenza by several days in adults
   c. Treatment of topical herpes simplex virus infections
   d. Reduction of the severity of shingles symptoms

CRITICAL THINKING AND APPLICATION

Answer the following questions on a separate sheet of paper.

6. Why are so few antiviral drugs available? Why are viruses so difficult to kill?

7. Amy is 12 weeks into her pregnancy when she discovers that she is HIV positive. Amy is very upset and says, "I won't live long enough to have this baby. We're both going to die." Is it possible to treat Amy and/or the fetus? Explain your answer.

8. Bailey, a 53-year-old teacher with osteoporosis, has shingles.

   a. What drug do you expect the physician to prescribe?

   b. What instructions will you give Bailey regarding any dietary considerations?

   c. Several months later, Bailey calls the office to say that her symptoms have returned. What action do you expect to be taken now?

9. Brenda is a 5-year-old who has bronchopneumonia caused by RSV.

   a. What antiviral drug is used to treat RSV?

   b. Brenda's mother wonders whether the treatment will be completed before Brenda's birthday, which is just 2 weeks away. What do you tell her?

10. Eduardo, a 25-year-old translator, has acquired immunodeficiency syndrome (AIDS). He was treated with zidovudine (AZT) for several months, but now the physician has switched him to didanosine powder.

    a. What frequently is the reason that patients are switched from AZT to another anti-HIV drug?

    b. What instructions do you give Eduardo regarding administration of the didanosine?

    c. Should Eduardo discontinue the antacid he has been taking? Explain your answer.

11. You overhear a co-worker explaining to a student nurse the procedure for administering acyclovir intravenously. After the acyclovir is diluted in sterile water, your co-worker says, "We'll administer this over at least an hour." Should you intervene? Explain your answer.

12. Stacy has had flu symptoms for 4 days and feels miserable. She calls the nurse practitioner in the clinic to ask for "that medicine, Tamiflu, that is supposed to make the flu symptoms better." Should Stacy receive this medication at this time? Explain.

CASE STUDY

Read the scenario and answer the following questions on a separate sheet of paper.

Mr. C., a 30-year-old stockbroker, has been diagnosed with genital herpes simplex type 2 (HSV-2) infection. The physician has prescribed topical acyclovir (Zovirax).

1. What patient teaching do you provide to Mr. C. regarding administration of this drug?

2. Mr. C. asks you how long it will take for the Zovirax to cure his herpes. What is your reply?

3. What else should you discuss with Mr. C., who is married?

4. HSV-2 is closely related to which other viruses?

Chapter 40
Antitubercular Drugs

CHAPTER REVIEW

Choose the best answer for each of the following.

1. During isoniazid therapy, the nurse will closely monitor results of which laboratory tests?
   a. Liver enzyme levels
   b. Hematocrit and hemoglobin level
   c. Creatinine level
   d. Platelet count

2. The nurse should include which of the following information in the teaching plan for a patient who is taking isoniazid?
   a. Urine and saliva may be reddish orange.
   b. Pyridoxine may be needed to prevent neurotoxicity.
   c. Injection sites should be rotated daily.
   d. The medication should be taken with an antacid to reduce gastric distress.

3. Patients who are in the initial period of treatment for tuberculosis need to be taught to do which of the following? Select all that apply.
   a. Wash their hands and cover their mouths when coughing or sneezing to reduce the spread of tuberculosis
   b. Throw away dirty tissues with care
   c. Be sure to get adequate rest, nutrition, and relaxation
   d. Skip medication doses occasionally if gastric distress occurs

4. A patient with newly diagnosed tuberculosis asks the nurse for how long he will need to take "all this medicine." The nurse replies that drug therapy for active tuberculosis may need to last for as long as
   a. 6 months.
   b. 12 months.
   c. 24 months.
   d. a lifetime.

5. Why are multiple medications used in the drug regimen for tuberculosis?
   a. It reduces the possibility of the organism's becoming drug-resistant.
   b. It ensures a cure of the disease.
   c. This regimen will reduce symptoms immediately.
   d. Patient compliance is better with multiple medications.

CRITICAL THINKING AND APPLICATION

Answer the following questions on a separate sheet of paper.

6. Diane, a 33-year-old proofreader, has been prescribed prophylactic isoniazid treatment.

   a. What laboratory studies should be performed before the start of therapy? Why?

   b. After Diane has taken isoniazid for 2 months, the physician significantly reduces her dosage of the drug. Why might that be?

7. Ms. Innes is undergoing antitubercular therapy that includes streptomycin.

   a. How is streptomycin administered?

   b. For what adverse effects will you monitor?

   c. Ms. Innes takes an oral contraceptive. Is that a concern given Ms. Innes's streptomycin therapy? Explain your answer.

8. Why would an eye examination be performed before instituting antitubercular therapy?

9. Mr. Fiore, a 42-year-old marketing executive, is on antitubercular therapy. During his first follow-up visit, he is evasive when you ask him about his compliance with his therapy regimen. He does tell you that he has been very busy lately, entertaining various clients "at everything from cocktail parties to big sit-down dinners."

   a. What issues should you discuss with Mr. Fiore?

   b. Several weeks later, Mr. Fiore returns for another follow-up visit. On examination, you see no apparent signs of the tuberculosis. How can Mr. Fiore's therapeutic response be confirmed?

10. Frannie is a homeless 68-year-old woman who lives in a shelter some of the time. She was diagnosed at the community health clinic with tuberculosis, and antitubercular therapy has been instituted.

    a. What patient education issues are of particular concern in Frannie's case?

    b. Frannie is staying at the shelter and seems to be handling her medication regimen well, but one day she comes by the clinic to tell you that she is afraid the medication may be bad for her. "Whenever I go to the bathroom, everything is reddish-orange," she says. What do you suspect is going on, and what do you tell Frannie?

CASE STUDY

Read the scenario and answer the following questions on a separate sheet of paper.

George, a 73-year-old retired plant foreman, has been diagnosed with tuberculosis. Nursing assessment reveals a history of gout and diabetes. He also has a history of heavy drinking.

1. What considerations will the physician keep in mind when deciding on a first-line drug for George?

2. George tells you that he has been told that he has a "liver problem." His medical record mentions that he is a slow acetylator. How does this affect his therapy?

3. How will his history of "heavy drinking" affect his therapy?

4. You instruct George about taking vitamin B_6 along with the isoniazid therapy. When he asks you why this is necessary, what do you tell him?

Chapter 41
Antifungal Drugs

CHAPTER REVIEW

Match each definition with the corresponding term.

1. _____ Single-celled fungi that reproduce by budding

2. _____ One of the major groups of antifungal drugs; includes amphotericin B and nystatin

3. _____ A very large, diverse group of eukaryotic, thallus-forming microorganisms that require an external carbon source

4. _____ One of the major groups of antifungal drugs; includes ketoconazole, miconazole, and clotrimazole

5. _____ A term for yeast infection of the mouth

6. _____ One of the older antifungal drugs that acts by preventing susceptible fungi from reproducing

7. _____ The oldest antifungal drug

8. _____ An antifungal drug commonly used to treat candidal diaper rash

9. _____ An infection caused by fungi

10. _____ Multicellular fungi characterized by long, branching filaments called hyphae, which entwine to form a mycelium

a. Thrush

b. Molds

c. griseofulvin

d. Mycosis

e. Polyenes

f. Fungi

g. Imidazoles

h. amphotericin B

i. nystatin

j. Yeast

Choose the best answer for each of the following.

11. An infant has thrush. The nurse knows that which of these drugs is appropriate for the treatment of thrush?
    a. amphotericin B
    b. fluconazole
    c. nystatin
    d. miconazole

12. During an infusion of amphotericin B, the nurse monitors for adverse effects, which may include which of the following? Select all that apply.
    a. Abdominal pain
    b. Fever
    c. Malaise
    d. Diarrhea
    e. Chills
    f. Rash

13. A patient calls the gynecologic clinic because she has begun to menstruate while taking medication for a vaginal infection. She asks the nurse, "What should I do about taking this vaginal medicine right now?" Which of the following would be the nurse's best response?
    a. "You should stop the medication until the menstrual flow has stopped."
    b. "Just take the medication at night only."
    c. "You should stop the medication for 3 days, then start it again."
    d. "It's okay to continue to take the medication."

14. Which medication is often used as a one-dose treatment for vaginal candidiasis?
    a. ketoconazole
    b. fluconazole
    c. griseofulvin
    d. imidazole

15. Which is the drug of choice for treatment of many severe systemic fungal infections?
    a. amphotericin B
    b. fluconazole
    c. griseofulvin
    d. flucytosine

CRITICAL THINKING AND APPLICATION

Answer the following questions on a separate sheet of paper.

16. Why are there so few oral and parenteral drugs to treat mycotic infections?

17. Mr. Kim has been diagnosed with cryptococcal meningitis, and the physician has prescribed fluconazole (Diflucan).

    a. Why did the physician choose this drug rather than one of the other imidazoles?

    b. The results of Mr. Kim's cerebrospinal fluid culture eventually come back negative. When he hears the good news, he says, "Great! I'm tired of taking this medicine." What is your response?

18. The physician is planning intravenous amphotericin B therapy for James.

    a. What guidelines do you follow in diluting the drug?

    b. What adverse effects do you expect James to experience?

    c. Should you stop the infusion if those effects occur? Explain your answer.

19. Lewis has a severe fungal infection for which the physician has prescribed griseofulvin. During your nursing assessment, Lewis tells you that he hopes the infection will clear up soon because he is going on a cruise in a week and he plans to "party every night!" What patient teaching issues should you discuss with Lewis?

20. Chrissie has thrush and has a prescription for nystatin oral troches. After a few days, she calls the physician to report that her mouth is not better. "I've been chewing them slowly every time I take one. I don't understand why it's not working!" she says. What is your response?

CASE STUDY

Read the scenario and answer the following questions on a separate sheet of paper.

Sally, a 68-year-old hospital volunteer, has been diagnosed as having pneumonia with invasive aspergillosis. She has been treated for 2 weeks without showing much improvement, and the physician is considering starting voriconazole (Vfend) therapy. Sally is also receiving a medication for treatment of a cardiac dysrhythmia.

1. What is the reason for starting voriconazole therapy now rather than earlier?

2. What consideration may arise depending on the cardiac medication she is taking?

3. What should be monitored while she is taking voriconazole?

Chapter 42

Antimalarial, Antiprotozoal, and Anthelmintic Drugs

CHAPTER REVIEW

Choose the best answer for each of the following.

1. Before beginning antiprotozoal therapy, the nurse should assess for which possible contraindications?
   a. Underlying renal, cardiac, thyroid, or liver disease and pregnancy
   b. Porphyria and glucose-6-phosphate dehydrogenase (G6PD) eficiency
   c. Glaucoma, cataracts, anemia, and petechiae
   d. Constipation, gastritis, and lactose intolerance

2. The nurse should warn the patient taking thiabendazole about which possible adverse effect?
   a. Reddish orange urine
   b. Urine with an asparagus-like odor
   c. "A metallic taste in the mouth
   d. Severe halitosis

3. A patient is taking quinine therapy for a mild case of malaria. The physician has decided to add a sulfonamide or tetracycline drug along with the quinine. When the nurse gives the patient the prescription for this new medication, the patient is upset about having to take "another pill." What is the nurse's best explanation for the second drug?
   a. "The antibiotic treats bacterial infections that accompany malaria."
   b. "The antibiotic reduces the severe adverse effects of quinine."
   c. "The antibiotic will help the quinine to work more effectively against the malaria."
   d. "The antibiotic therapy is also needed to kill the parasite that causes malaria."

4. Which drug is used mainly for the management of *Pneumocystis jirovecii* (formerly *Pneumocystis carinii*) pneumonia? Select all that apply.
   a. metronidazole
   b. pentamidine
   c. primaquine
   d. pyrantel
   e. atovaquone

5. Which of the following is true regarding anthelmintic therapy?
   a. The medication can be stopped once symptoms disappear.
   b. Anthelmintics are more effective in their parenteral forms.
   c. Anthelmintics are broad in their actions and can be substituted easily for one another if a given medication is not well tolerated.
   d. The medication must be taken exactly as ordered for the length of time ordered.

6. Which patient is at the highest risk of dying from a protozoal infection?
   a. A teenager with no health problems
   b. A patient with diabetes mellitus
   c. A patient who has had a kidney transplant
   d. A patient with a history of myocardial infarction

CRITICAL THINKING AND APPLICATION

Answer the following questions on a separate sheet of paper.

7. Professor Henson has just returned from a research sabbatical in Africa where she did not adequately protect herself from mosquito exposure; thus, she has contracted malaria. What kind of parasite causes malaria? Which drug is recommended if the parasite is in the exoerythrocytic phase of development? What exactly is the exoerythrocytic phase?

8. Professor Henson's physician would like to prescribe the drug you identified in your answer to question 7. You should assess this patient for which kind of contraindications?

9. Professor Henson's husband, who accompanied her on her trip, has even more recently begun to develop signs of malaria. He is given chloroquine, a 4-aminoquinoline derivative. Unlike his wife, however, Mr. Henson sees no diminishing of his symptoms. His strain of malaria appears to be chloroquine-resistant. What alternative(s) can you suggest for Mr. Henson?

10. The medical clinic in which you work has a full waiting room this morning. Patient A is being seen for an intestinal disorder that he acquired after swimming in Lake Michigan. Patient B is a patient with acquired immunodeficiency syndrome (AIDS) who is showing early signs of pneumonia. Patient C is being treated and evaluated on a regular basis for a sexually transmitted disease. Here's your challenge: All three patients have something in common in terms of the causes of their disorders. Describe what that could be. Second, based on that commonality, predict what disorder, of those discussed in this chapter, each patient may have. (Hint: One patient has giardiasis.) Third, select the drug you feel the physician is likely to prescribe for each patient.

CASE STUDY

Read the scenario and answer the following questions on a separate sheet of paper.

Sandra, age 15, has been diagnosed with an infestation of intestinal roundworms, specifically ascariasis, after a visit to another country. You are preparing to medicate her with pyrantel.

1. How is this infestation diagnosed?

2. What are the contraindications to therapy with pyrantel?

3. The recommended dosage for pyrantel is 11 mg/kg, up to a maximum of 1 g, in a one-time dose. If Sandra weighs 57 kg, what dose should she receive?

4. What are expected adverse effects of this medication?

Chapter 43

Antiseptic and Disinfectant Agents

CRITICAL THINKING CROSSWORD

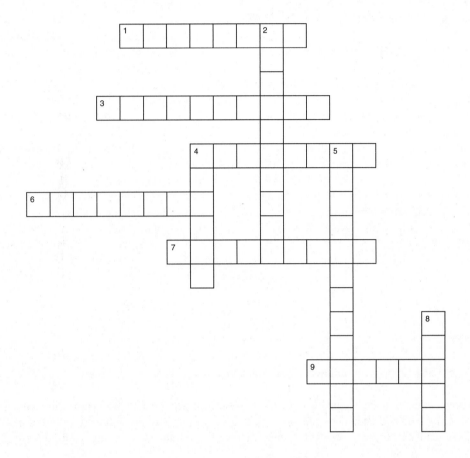

Across

1. A surface-active drug, also known as benzalkonium chloride
3. A type of infection also known as a "hospital-acquired" infection
4. The classification of Cidex
6. An iodine drug widely used as an antiseptic
7. Chlorhexidine gluconate
9. A sodium hypochlorite solution

Down

2. A substance that inhibits the growth and reproduction of microorganisms without necessarily killing them
4. An acid used in a 5% solution for killing microorganisms
5. A chemical applied to nonliving objects to destroy microorganisms
8. An example of a phenolic compound

CHAPTER REVIEW

Choose the best answer for each of the following.

1. During a class on nosocomial infections, several facts are shared. Which of the following statements about nosocomial infections are true? Select all that apply.
   a. They are contracted in the home or community.
   b. They are contracted in a hospital or institution.
   c. They are more difficult to treat.
   d. The organisms that cause these infections are more virulent.

2. Which statement accurately describes the action of antiseptics?
   a. They are used to kill organisms on nonliving objects.
   b. They are used to kill organisms on living tissue.
   c. They are used to sterilize equipment.
   d. They are used to inhibit the growth of organisms on living tissue.

3. When preparing an area of skin before a procedure, the nurse knows that which strength of isopropanol (isopropyl alcohol) is most effective against microorganisms?
   a. 25%
   b. 50%
   c. 70%
   d. 95%

4. Before using povidone-iodine (Betadine) solution to prepare skin for surgery, the nurse should ask the patient about allergies to which of the following?
   a. Seafood
   b. Penicillin
   c. Mercury
   d. Milk

5. If a patient is allergic to povidone-iodine, the nurse may use which agent as a surgical scrub?
   a. Acetic acid
   b. Hibiclens
   c. Gentian violet
   d. Phenol

6. Which agent is used to disinfect surgical instruments?
   a. 5% acetic acid
   b. hydrogen peroxide
   c. glutaraldehyde (Cidex)
   d. Gentian violet

CASE STUDY

Read the scenario and answer the following questions on a separate sheet of paper.

A patient has been admitted to the hospital with an infected surgical wound in his groin area. The initial orders call for irrigating twice a day with hydrogen peroxide, then packing with gauze soaked with tincture of iodine. The hospital's wound care nurse reads this order, assesses the patient, then tells you that she is going to call the physician for another order.

1. Why is the wound care nurse questioning this order?

2. The new order calls for irrigation with Dakin's solution, then wet-to-dry packing with saline. What is Dakin's solution, and what concentration is appropriate for topical wound care?

3. Your patient says, "That has a familiar smell. Why are you bleaching my wound?" What do you tell him?

4. What should you do after the dressing procedure is completed?

Chapter 44

Antiinflammatory, Antirheumatic, and Related Drugs

CHAPTER REVIEW

Choose the best answer for each of the following.

1. When teaching a patient about the common adverse effects of therapy with nonsteroidal antiinflammatory drugs (NSAIDs), the nurse should mention which of the following?
   a. Dizziness
   b. Heartburn
   c. Palpitations
   d. Diarrhea

2. A 13-year-old teen has the flu, and her mother is concerned about her fever of 103° F (39.4° C). Which medication should the nurse suggest the mother use to treat the teen's fever?
   a. aspirin
   b. acetaminophen
   c. indomethacin
   d. naproxen

3. A patient is receiving treatment with allopurinol for an acute flare-up of gout. Which statements should be included in the patient teaching? Select all that apply.
   a. "Be sure to avoid alcohol and caffeine."
   b. "Take the medication with meals to prevent stomach problems."
   c. "You need to take this medication on an empty stomach to improve absorption."
   d. "You need to increase fluid intake to up to 3 L a day."

4. When reviewing the health history of a patient who is to receive NSAID therapy, the nurse keeps in mind that contraindications for the use of these drugs include which of the following?
   a. Pericarditis
   b. Osteoarthritis
   c. Bleeding disorders
   d. Juvenile rheumatoid arthritis

5. A patient receiving gold injections as treatment for arthritis should be told which of the following?
   a. Injections will be given via the intravenous route.
   b. The medication is more effective if fluids are restricted.
   c. Relief from symptoms can be expected in a few days.
   d. Relief from symptoms may take 3 to 4 months.

6. A young man is in the urgent care center after experiencing a severe ankle sprain during a basketball game. The nurse expects that which pain reliever will be ordered for this patient?
   a. ketorolac (Toradol)
   b. aspirin
   c. indomethacin (Indocin)
   d. meloxicam (Mobic)

CRITICAL THINKING AND APPLICATION

Answer the following questions on a separate sheet of paper.

7. Ms. Bailey is brought into the emergency department exhibiting the following symptoms: tinnitus, hearing loss, dimming vision, and dizziness. She is also very thirsty and sweating profusely, and has had severe nausea and vomiting. On examination you discover that she has an increased heart rate and is experiencing some confusion. At first she appears drowsy and then begins to hyperventilate. You suspect salicylism, but your colleague says, "No, this is acute salicylate intoxication." If he is correct, how was he able to tell? What causes each?

8. Ms. Bailey turns out to have acute toxicity stemming from a salicylate overdose. Describe an appropriate treatment plan.

9. Mr. Chestnut comes to the emergency department with symptoms that are similar to Ms. Bailey's but not as extensive. He is experiencing drowsiness, mental confusion, and disorientation, and had a seizure while en route to the hospital. What is wrong? What would you expect if the situation were allowed to progress?

10. How will Mr. Chestnut's treatment differ from Mrs. Bailey's?

11. Mr. Henry has come to the clinic complaining of a severe flare-up of his gout. He tells you that he does not take his medicine on a regular basis because it "kills" his stomach. He also says that he hates to take medicine but hates the gout more. He has a prescription for allopurinol and a follow-up appointment for next week. What patient teaching does Mr. Henry need?

12. Eileen has had arthritic joint pain for months, and her current pain management regimen has been less than successful. During a checkup today, she tells you that she has heard of a new drug, Toradol, that "works wonders." She wants to try it for "a couple of months" to see if it can help her. What do you tell her?

13. Your neighbor calls you over to "check out this aspirin bottle" that she found in her medicine cabinet. It has a strong vinegary odor. She wants to know if she can still take it for her headaches. What do you tell her?

CASE STUDY

Read the scenario and answer the following questions on a separate sheet of paper.

Sadie has been taking indomethacin as part of therapy for osteoarthritis but lately has noticed that it has been less effective. Her physician has decided to try celecoxib (Celebrex). Sadie has a history of hepatitis (15 years earlier).

1. What advantages might there be to treatment with celecoxib rather than indomethacin?

2. What potential adverse effects should you warn Sadie about before she takes this medication? What should she report?

3. She asks you if she can drink her usual glass of wine each evening while taking this medication. What do you tell her?

Chapter 45

Immunosuppressant Drugs

CHAPTER REVIEW

Choose the best answer for each of the following.

1. When monitoring patients on immunosuppressant therapy, the nurse must keep in mind that the major risk factor for patients taking these drugs is which of the following?
   a. Severe hypotension with potential renal failure
   b. Increased susceptibility to opportunistic infections
   c. Decreased platelet aggregation
   d. Increased bleeding tendencies

2. A patient is experiencing rejection of a transplanted organ. The nurse expects which drug to be given to manage this?
   a. azathioprine
   b. cyclosporine
   c. muromonab-CD3
   d. tacrolimus

3. A patient who is taking cyclosporine calls the office to say that he has heard that some food can increase the effectiveness of this drug. The nurse recognizes that he is talking about which of the following?
   a. Dairy products
   b. Orange juice
   c. Grapefruit juice
   d. Red wines

4. When teaching patients who are taking oral doses of immunosuppressants, the nurse should instruct the patient to take them
   a. with food to minimize gastrointestinal upset.
   b. on an empty stomach to increase absorption rate.
   c. only when adverse effects are tolerable.
   d. with antacids.

5. Patient teaching for those taking immunosuppressants should include which of the following? Select all that apply.
   a. The mouth and tongue should be inspected carefully for white patches.
   b. Allergic reactions to these drugs are rare.
   c. Patients should avoid crowds to minimize the risk of infection.
   d. Patients should report any fever, sore throat, chills, or joint pain.

6. Which of the following is the only immunosuppressant currently indicated for the treatment of multiple sclerosis?
   a. glatiramer acetate (Copaxone)
   b. azathioprine (Imuran)
   c. basiliximab (Simulect)
   d. daclizumab (Zenapax)

CRITICAL THINKING AND APPLICATION

Answer the following questions on a separate sheet of paper.

7. Mrs. Flick is about to undergo kidney transplant surgery. The physician plans for her to start taking daclizumab.

   a. Mrs. Flick asks you why. Explain how you will answer her.

   b. Describe the laboratory studies to be performed and documented. How often should they be performed? What purpose do they serve?

   c. Three days before her surgery, an oral antifungal drug is added to Mrs. Flick's regimen. "Why do I have to take this, too?" she asks. Explain how you will answer.

8. A patient on cyclosporine (Neoral) therapy is convinced that the cyclosporine is upsetting his stomach. What can be done to alleviate this problem?

9. Tess has had a renal transplant. She is being given muromonab-CD3 intravenously, 5 mg/day in a single bolus. On the second day, she begins to exhibit chest pain, dyspnea, and wheezing. Her leukocyte count is 4000/mm^3. What is happening?

10. John has relapsing-remitting multiple sclerosis and is in the hospital because of an acute exacerbation. The physician talks to him about a "different type" of therapy with an immunosuppressant drug. What drug will be used, and how can it help John?

CASE STUDY

Read the scenario and answer the following questions on a separate sheet of paper.

Mr. K. had renal transplant surgery 6 months ago and so far has had no problems with organ rejection. He is taking cyclosporine in a maintenance dose. He wants to go back to work and is in for a checkup before approval is given for a return to his job.

1. He asks if he will have to continue the cyclosporine. What is your response?

2. He complains of difficulty swallowing, and as you examine his mouth, you look for signs of oral candidiasis. What findings would indicate that he has this condition?

3. After 2 weeks at work, Mr. K. calls to report that he has the flu. He has a sore throat, chills, and achy joints, and he is very tired. What is your advice?

4. When you receive his most recent white blood cell count, you note that the results are 2900/mm^3. Is this a concern, and what action, if any, will be taken?

Chapter 46

Immunizing Drugs and Biochemical Terrorism

CHAPTER REVIEW

1. **Complete the following chart by filling in all missing information.**

Drug	Active or Passive?	Purpose
a.	b.	Chicken pox
Hib	c.	d.
e.	Active	Hepatitis B prophylaxis
f.	g.	Postpartum antibody suppression
BCG vaccine	h.	i.
DTaP	j.	k.
Tetanus immune globulin	l.	m.
Td	n.	o.

Choose the best answer for each of the following.

2. The immunity that is passed from a mother to her nursing infant through antibodies in breast milk is known as which type of immunity?
    a. Artificially acquired passive immunity
    b. Naturally acquired passive immunity
    c. Active immunity
    d. Genetic immunity

3. Which of the following contain substances that trigger the formation of antibodies against specific pathogens?
    a. Antivenins
    b. Serums
    c. Toxoids
    d. Vaccines

4. When reviewing various immunizing drugs, the nurse recalls that some products provide long-lasting immunity against a particular pathogen. An example would be
    a. poliovirus vaccine, live oral.
    b. tetanus immune globulin.
    c. $Rh_0(D)$ immune globulin.
    d. black widow spider antivenin.

5. The nurse is preparing to give a second dose of DTaP vaccine to a 6-month-old infant. The infant's mother tells the nurse that the last time he received this vaccination, the injection site on his leg became warm, slightly swollen, and red. The nurse's best response would be
    a. to explain that these effects can be expected and give the medication.
    b. to give half the prescribed dose this week and the other half next week if tolerated well.
    c. to skip the dose and notify the physician.
    d. to wait 6 months and then administer the dose.

6. A nurse has been stuck by a used needle while starting an intravenous line. Which preparation is used as prophylaxis against disease after exposure to blood and body fluids?
    a. Hib vaccine
    b. $Rh_0(D)$ immune globulin
    c. Hepatitis B immune globulin
    d. Hepatitis antitoxin

CRITICAL THINKING AND APPLICATION

Answer the following questions on a separate sheet of paper.

7. Jim, a cabinetmaker, is cut by a woodworking tool and comes to the clinic for stitches. When the nurse asks him about his tetanus vaccination history, he says, "I have no idea when my last tetanus shot was—I thought once I had all the shots for school that I was set for life! Surely I don't need any more." What do you explain to Jim?

8. Mrs. Tims, an 82-year-old widow, is in the office for a follow-up appointment to evaluate her emphysema. The physician recommends that she have an influenza virus vaccine. As you prepare the injection, Mrs. Tims says, "I had a flu shot last year—why do I need another one this year?" What is your explanation to her?

9. Mr. Smythe brings his toddler, Carl, in for a 12-month well-child checkup. Before you give the measles-mumps-rubella (MMR) vaccine injection, what adverse effects do you tell Mr. Smythe to watch for in Carl's response to the immunization? What can be done to relieve these adverse effects?

10. There have been news reports about anthrax threats. Your neighbor is worried and asks you which type of anthrax is the most deadly. What does he mean by "which type," and what is the answer to his question?

11. Paul has received several immunizations in preparation for an overseas trip. He expected to feel some soreness at the injection sites, but the next morning he wakes up with swelling of the face and tongue, difficulty breathing, shortness of breath, nausea and vomiting, and a fever of 102° F (38.9° C). What is happening, and what should he do?

CASE STUDY

Read the scenario and answer the following questions on a separate sheet of paper.

You are volunteering at a local animal shelter and helping to care for a sick dog that has just been admitted. During the examination the dog nipped both you and the veterinarian. A little later, the veterinarian tells you that she fears that the dog has rabies and that both of you have been exposed. The veterinarian tells you that she has received a vaccine for rabies but that you will need to be vaccinated immediately.

1. Is rabies a virus or a bacteria?

2. Did the vaccine the veterinarian received previously give her active or passive immunization? Explain.

3. Will the vaccine you receive give you active or passive immunization? Explain why this particular type of vaccine is preferred in your situation.

4. How will your vaccine(s) be given?

Chapter 47

Antineoplastic Drugs Part 1: Cancer Overview and Cell Cycle–Specific Drugs

CRITICAL THINKING CROSSWORD

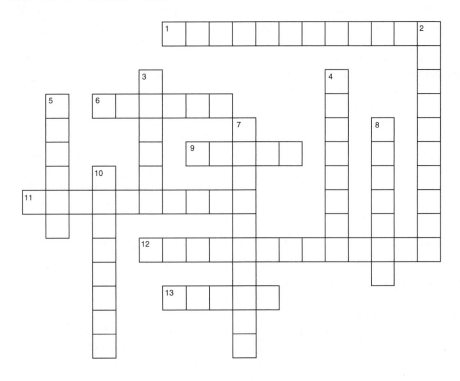

Across

1. During a pharmacology lecture, the instructor explains that some of the antineoplastic drugs have two reactive alkyl groups to alkylate two cancer cell DNA molecules. Thus, they are _____ drugs.
6. Mr. Kilpatrick's physician is not surprised to find that methotrexate is killing the cells of Mr. Kilpatrick's stomach, which results in nausea and vomiting; the methotrexate therapy is displaying a strong _____ potential in this patient.
9. Your patient is receiving methotrexate. Your instructor asks for a full description of its mechanism of action, so you explain that it will inhibit dihydrofolic reductase from converting _____ acid to a reduced folate and thus ultimately prevent the synthesis of DNA and cell reproduction. The result, you explain, is that the cell will die.

Down

2. Mr. Kellogg has been treated with methotrexate for its folate-antagonistic properties. Now, however, he seems to be experiencing a toxicity reaction. The treatment he will receive will be _____ rescue.
3. Ms. Lilliankamp recently underwent biopsy of a lump near her breast. Several days later, her physician calls and tells her that the lump is noncancerous and therefore is not an immediate threat to life. She is pleased to hear, then, that it is

   _____.

4. Ms. Hart has a malignant neoplasm of the blood-forming tissues. Her bone marrow is being rapidly replaced with proliferating leukocyte precursors; she also has abnormal numbers (and forms) of immature white blood cells in her circulation, and even her lymph nodes, spleen, and liver are being infiltrated. Ms. Hart's type of cancer is known as

   _____.

11. Ms. Patchett had a biopsy performed on the same day that Ms. Lilliankamp (3 Down) did. When her biopsy specimen is analyzed, however, the results are the opposite of Ms. Lilliankamp's; that is, her lump is a(n) _____.

12. Mr. Bronte has just undergone a series of chemotherapeutic treatments when it is discovered that the antineoplastic drug has leaked into surrounding tissues; in other words, _____ of the drug has occurred.

13. Mr. Cunningham is very interested in his chemotherapeutic process. As you are discussing a drug's action, he hears you use the term _____, and he asks you what it means. You explain that this is the point at which the lowest neutrophil count occurs after administration of a chemotherapy agent that causes bone marrow suppression.

5. Mr. Harris is told that his cancer has metastasized. His physician explains to him that this means it has _____ to other areas of his body.

7. Mr. Harris has been diagnosed with chronic lymphocytic leukemia; Ms. Fehrers has multiple myeloma. Both patients will need treatment with an drug that can generate a reaction called _____, which, when it involves a cellular constituent such as DNA, will interfere with the mitosis and cell division of the cancer cells.

8. Your patient is receiving an antineoplastic drug that has the ability to interfere with the process of cancer cell reproduction, which, if not halted, would result in the formation of two genetically identical daughter cancer cells containing the diploid number of chromosomes needed for its proliferation. In other words, the drug will interfere with the cancer cells' _____ and cell division.

10. Ms. Fehrers has been given her first chemotherapy treatment. However, it soon becomes apparent that the adverse effects she is experiencing prevent her from being given dosages that will be high enough to be effective. These are dose-_____ adverse effects.

CHAPTER REVIEW

Choose the best answer for each of the following.

1. When administering antineoplastic drugs, the nurse needs to keep in mind that the general adverse effects of these drugs include which of the following? Select all that apply.
   a. Bone marrow suppression
   b. Infertility
   c. Diarrhea
   d. Urinary retention
   e. Nausea and vomiting
   f. Stomatitis

2. A patient will be receiving chemotherapy with paclitaxel. What should the nurse expect to do along with administering this drug?
   a. Administer platelet infusions
   b. Provide acetaminophen as needed
   c. Keep the patient on "nothing-by-mouth" status because of expected nausea and vomiting
   d. Premedicate with a steroid and antihistamine

3. As the nurse is preparing to give the patient chemotherapy, the patient asks the nurse why more than one drug is used. The nurse should explain that combinations of chemotherapeutic drugs are used to
   a. prevent drug resistance.
   b. reduce the incidence of adverse effects.
   c. decrease the cost of treatment.
   d. reduce treatment time.

4. If extravasation of a neoplastic drug occurs, what should the nurse do first?
   a. Remove the intravenous catheter immediately
   b. Stop the drug infusion without removing the intravenous catheter
   c. Aspirate residual drug or blood from the tube if possible
   d. Administer the appropriate antidote

5. During chemotherapy, the nurse should monitor the patient for symptoms of stomatitis, such as which of the following?
   a. Indigestion and heartburn
   b. Severe vomiting and anorexia
   c. Ulcerations of the mouth
   d. Diarrhea and perianal irritation

CASE STUDY

Read the scenario and answer the following questions on a separate sheet of paper.

Allen, a 40-year-old physician, has been diagnosed with acute lymphocytic anemia and will be receiving chemotherapy with methotrexate. He is scheduled to receive his first treatment today.

1. What is methotrexate's classification, and how does it work?

2. What laboratory test results should be checked before he receives this medication?

3. Allen tells you that he often has problems with ankle pain from an old injury and takes ibuprofen (Motrin) for relief. Is this a concern?

4. What other medications may be given along with the methotrexate chemotherapy, and why?

Chapter 48

Antineoplastic Drugs Part 2: Cell Cycle–Nonspecific and Miscellaneous Drugs

---

CHAPTER REVIEW

Choose the best answer for each of the following.

1. While hanging a new infusion bag of a chemotherapy drug, the nurse accidentally spills a small amount of solution on the floor. The nurse's best action would be which of the following?
   a. Let it dry then mop the floor
   b. Wipe the area with a paper towel
   c. Use a spill kit to clean the area
   d. Ask the housekeeping department to wipe the floor

2. A patient is receiving leucovorin as part of his chemotherapy regimen. The nurse expects that the patient is receiving which antineoplastic drug?
   a. bleomycin
   b. cisplatin
   c. dactinomycin
   d. methotrexate

3. A patient receiving chemotherapy for a testicular tumor complains of hearing a "loud ringing sound" in his ears. The nurse expects that which of the following will happen next?
   a. The therapy will continue as ordered.
   b. The therapy will be stopped until the patient's hearing is evaluated.
   c. The therapy will be withheld for a day, then resumed.
   d. The therapy will be stopped until renal studies are performed.

4. When teaching a patient who is receiving outpatient chemotherapy about potential problems, the nurse needs to mention signs and symptoms of an oncologic emergency, which include which of the following? Select all that apply.
   a. Swollen tongue
   b. Alopecia
   c. Blood in the urine
   d. Nausea and vomiting
   e. Temperature of 100° F (37.8° C) or higher
   f. Chills

5. The nurse monitors very closely for signs of liver toxicity when which antineoplastic drug is given?
   a. doxorubicin
   b. cisplatin
   c. bevacizumab
   d. hydroxyurea

6. A patient who has cancer is to receive a course of chemotherapy with doxorubicin. Which coexisting condition will require very close monitoring while the patient is taking this drug?
   a. Hypertension
   b. Diabetes mellitus
   c. Gout
   d. Cardiomyopathy

CRITICAL THINKING AND APPLICATION

Answer the following questions on a separate sheet of paper.

7. Describe the concept of *cytoprotection* and provide some examples of how this may be accomplished during chemotherapy.

8. Mrs. Smythe has been receiving bleomycin to treat a lung tumor, and lately she has been experiencing increased difficulty breathing. She tells you, "I guess this cancer is getting worse. The medicine is not working." Do you agree or is there another possible concern?

9. Mr. Ward has a brain tumor and is facing surgery. His oncologist tells him that during his surgery, wafers of the chemotherapy drug carmustine will be placed. Mr. Ward asks you, "How does this drug work if I don't have to swallow it?" Explain how you will answer him.

10. During a busy evening shift, a physician tells you that he wants to start Mrs. Nexter's chemotherapy immediately. The physician asks you to mix the drug as soon as possible and start the infusion. Should you do this? Explain your answer.

11. Mr. Gill, who had been receiving an infusion of mechlorethamine, has an infiltrated intravenous site. He wants you to pull out the intravenous line immediately because "it hurts so much." What will you do? How will this extravasation be treated?

CASE STUDY

Read the scenario and answer the following questions on a separate sheet of paper.

Dottie, age 63, has been diagnosed with mid-stage ovarian cancer and will be receiving chemotherapy with cisplatin after surgery. She is understandably anxious about the therapy but says she wants to "beat the cancer."

1. Cisplatin is associated with three main toxicities. Describe each one.

2. Before she receives the therapy, what should be assessed?

3. During therapy, Dottie complains of an "odd tingling" in her toes. Is this a concern? Explain.

4. Dottie tells you that she'd rather "drink nothing" when she is feeling nauseated. Is this a concern? Explain what you need to teach her about fluids.

Chapter 49
Biologic Response–Modifying Drugs

CHAPTER REVIEW

Match each definition with its corresponding term. (Note: Not all terms will be used.)

1. _____ A type of cytokine that promotes resistance to viral infection in uninfected cells

2. _____ Cytokines that regulate the growth, differentiation, and function of bone marrow stem cells

3. _____ Cytokines that are produced by sensitized T lymphocytes upon contact with antigen particles

4. _____ An immunoglobulin that binds to antigens to form a special complex

5. _____ A substance that is foreign to the human body

6. _____ The primary functional cells of the cell-mediated immune system

7. _____ The specific cells of the humoral immune system

a. Colony-stimulating factors

b. Antibody

c. B lymphocytes (B cells)

d. T lymphocytes (T cells)

e. Interferons

f. Lymphokine-activated killer cells

g. Lymphokines

h. Antigen

i. Memory cells

Choose the best answer for each of the following.

8. When giving interferon drugs, the nurse knows that the best time to administer them is
   a. in the morning, before the patient rises.
   b. at mealtimes.
   c. between meals.
   d. at bedtime.

9. A patient with a critically low hemoglobin level and hematocrit is to receive a drug that will stimulate the production of red blood cells. The nurse expects that the patient will receive which of the following?
   a. filgrastim (Neupogen)
   b. epoetin alfa (Epogen)
   c. sargramostim (Leukine)
   d. oprelvekin (Neumega)

10. While teaching a patient about the possible adverse effects of the interferons, the nurse should mention which of the following? Select all that apply.
    a. Myalgia
    b. Fever
    c. Diarrhea
    d. Fatigue
    e. Chills
    f. Dizziness

11. A patient is starting therapy with adalimumab (Humira) after a course of therapy with methotrexate failed to improve the patient's condition. The nurse recognizes that this patient is being treated for which of the following?
    a. Advanced-stage cancer
    b. Multiple sclerosis
    c. Severe rheumatoid arthritis
    d. Systemic lupus erythematosus

CRITICAL THINKING AND APPLICATION

Answer the following questions on a separate sheet of paper.

12. Sonja is to receive interferon therapy as part of the treatment for cancer. Sonja is very athletic and participates in sports activities on a regular basis. The physician explains that there is a dose-limiting adverse effect of this type of drug that may have a huge effect on her daily activities. What is this adverse effect, and how will it concern Sonja?

13. Trevor is receiving chemotherapy as part of his treatment for Hodgkin's disease. As he begins therapy, he tells the nurse, "I've seen those commercials about the drugs that increase your white blood cell count. Can't I start taking one of them now to keep my counts from getting so low?" What are the drugs he is referring to, and what is your answer?

14. Brittany has received chemotherapy, and the results of today's laboratory work have indicated a critically low platelet count. She has received 2 units of platelets, but the physician has decided to give her a medication to improve her platelet counts. What drug will be given, how will it be given, and what concerns are there while her platelet count is so low?

CASE STUDY

Read the scenario and answer the following questions on a separate sheet of paper.

Connie, a 58-year-old cashier, is in the hospital because of extreme weakness. She has received hemodialysis three times a week for chronic renal failure for the last 2 years. The laboratory results revealed a critically low hematocrit and hemoglobin level, and the physician has ordered a transfusion of 2 units of packed red blood cells. However, Connie states that she cannot accept the blood transfusion because of her religious beliefs. As a result, there are orders to begin therapy with epoetin alfa (Epogen).

1. How does epoetin work?

2. What laboratory test results should be monitored while she is taking this medication, and why?

3. Connie is concerned about the source of this drug. What can you tell her about this?

4. She is going to be taking this drug at home. What is the route by which it will be given?

5. When Connie realizes that she will be giving herself injections up to three times a week, she complains, "Isn't there something else I can take? I don't want that many shots!" Is there an alternative?

Chapter 50

Gene Therapy and Pharmacogenomics

CHAPTER REVIEW

Match each definition with its corresponding term. (Note: Not all terms will be used.)

1. _____ A structure in the nucleus that contains a linear thread of DNA that transmits genetic information

2. _____ A term for all of the chromosomal material within a cell

3. _____ The biologic unit of heredity

4. _____ The complete set of genetic material of any organism

5. _____ The study of genomes, including the way genes and their products work in both health and disease

a. Allele

b. Gene

c. Genome

d. Genomics

e. Genetics

f. Chromatin

g. Chromosome

CRITICAL THINKING AND APPLICATION

Answer the following questions on a separate sheet of paper.

6. What is DNA, and what is its primary purpose?

7. What was the goal of the Human Genome Project?

8. Name two effects of the Human Genome Project.

9. What is recombinant DNA, and how is this technology useful in pharmacology?

10. Explain the purpose of gene therapy. Has it been approved in the United States for routine treatment of disease?

Chapter 51
Acid-Controlling Drugs

CHAPTER REVIEW

Match each definition with its corresponding term. (Note: Not all terms will be used.)

1. _____ Drugs known as H$_2$ blockers that reduce stimulated acid secretion

2. _____ Drugs that block all acid secretion in the stomach

3. _____ A cytoprotective drug

4. _____ The cells responsible for producing and secreting hydrochloric acid in the stomach

5. _____ A type of antacid that can cause diarrhea

6. _____ Antacids that have constipating effects

7. _____ The cause of many peptic ulcers

8. _____ Drugs used to relieve the painful symptoms associated with gas

9. _____ A type of antacid that may contribute to the development of kidney stones

10. _____ A drug that can result in systemic alkalosis

a. Aluminum-containing antacids

b. Calcium-containing antacids

c. Magnesium-containing antacids

d. Antiflatulents

e. Proton pump inhibitors

f. *Helicobacter pylori*

g. Sodium bicarbonate

h. Histamine type 2 receptor antagonists

i. Sucralfate

j. Chief cells

k. Parietal cells

Choose the best answer for each of the following.

11. A patient with renal failure wants to take an antacid for "sour stomach." The nurse needs to consider that some antacids may be dangerous when taken by patients with renal failure and should recommend which type of antacid?
    a. Activated charcoal
    b. Aluminum-containing antacids
    c. Calcium-containing antacids
    d. Magnesium-containing antacids

12. A patient with peptic ulcer disease will be starting medication therapy. He tells the nurse that he smokes and wonders if that will affect his treatment. The nurse's best response would be which of the following?
    a. Smoking has no effect on these medications.
    b. The actions of antacids are less potent when the patient smokes.
    c. Smoking has been shown to decrease the effectiveness of H_2 blockers.
    d. Smoking has been shown to increase the adverse effects of H_2 blockers.

13. Which drug class would be used as first-line therapy for gastroesophageal reflux disease (GERD) that has not responded to customary medical treatment?
    a. H_2 blockers
    b. Antacids
    c. Mucosal protectants
    d. Proton pump inhibitors

14. Which of the following statements about proton pump inhibitors are true? Select all that apply.
    a. They should be taken 1 hour before antacids.
    b. They should be taken 30-60 minutes before meals.
    c. They should be taken with meals.
    d. They are part of the treatment of patients with *H. pylori* infections.
    e. There are very few adverse effects with these drugs.

CRITICAL THINKING AND APPLICATION

Answer the following questions on a separate sheet of paper.

15. Your neighbor, Mr. Medley, comes over to get advice on antacids. He says he has taken Maalox "for years" for indigestion, but it is no longer helping. He asks, "Can you recommend another antacid or one of those expensive, fancy pills that the pharmacy sells? Or should I just take baking soda?" What is your response?

16. Mrs. Knopf is advised to take omeprazole to treat her severe case of GERD; nothing else has worked. Develop a patient teaching plan that will instruct Mrs. Knopf in how this medication should be taken.

17. Mr. McKinney has called to ask which antacid he should take. He has been to the store and is confused by the great variety on the shelves. He says he needs something for "occasional heartburn" when he eats something too spicy. He has a history of heart failure and is taking antihypertensive drugs. What type of antacid should he take, and what other instructions would he need?

18. Mr. Simmons is taking enteric-coated aspirin for mild arthritis symptoms. He tells you that he plans to take the aspirin with his favorite antacid, Maalox, because he does not want any stomach problems. What should you tell him?

19. Frank has been diagnosed with a peptic ulcer caused by *H. pylori* infection. He has been told that he will be started on Regimen 1 drug therapy for this disease. What does this mean?

CASE STUDY

Read the scenario and answer the following questions on a separate sheet of paper.

Edna, age 78, has been self-treating with antacids for "heartburn" for 6 months. After an upper gastrointestinal tract endoscopy, she has been diagnosed with GERD. The decision has been made to start treatment with cimetidine (Tagamet). Edna has been generally healthy except for a history of asthma. She says that she does not smoke but that she enjoys going to a Bingo session every Saturday for a few hours where there is smoking, beer, and pizza.

1. When Edna sees the prescription for cimetidine, she asks, "Why do I need a prescription? I can buy this over the counter!" What do you say in reply?

2. How will the cimetidine help her GERD?

3. What cautions, if any, are associated with the use of cimetidine?

4. Will staying in a smoke-filled room affect her therapy? Explain.

Chapter 52
Antidiarrheals and Laxatives

CRITICAL THINKING CROSSWORD

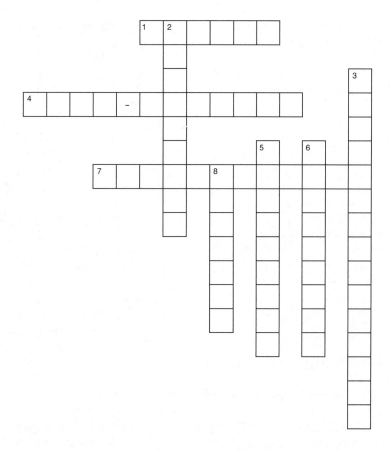

Across

1. Laxatives that increase osmotic pressure in the small intestine, increasing water content and resulting in distention
4. Laxatives that absorb water into the intestine, increasing bulk and distending the bowel
7. A laxative that increases fecal water content in the large intestine, resulting in distention, increased peristalsis, and evacuation

Down

2. Acts by coating the walls of the gastrointestinal tract, binding to causative bacteria or toxin to allow elimination via the stool
3. Acts by decreasing peristalsis and muscular tone of the intestine and thus slowing the movement of substances through the gastrointestinal tract
5. Laxatives that softens the stool
6. A laxative that stimulates the nerves that supply the intestine, which results in increased peristalsis
8. Also act to decrease bowel motility

CHAPTER REVIEW

Choose the best answer for each of the following.

1. Bismuth subsalicylate (Pepto-Bismol) would be the treatment of choice for which patient?
   a. A 7-year-old child who has chickenpox
   b. A 23-year-old woman who has severe abdominal pain
   c. A 45-year-old man who is complaining of constipation
   d. A 58-year-old man who developed diarrhea after traveling out of the country

2. Because of the possibility of toxicity, a patient who is self-treating with Pepto-Bismol should be told to avoid
   a. aspirin.
   b. acetaminophen.
   c. calcium supplements.
   d. vitamin tablets.

3. A patient asks for a medication that will provide rapid relief of constipation. After ruling out possible contraindications, the nurse should suggest which of the following?
   a. psyllium (Metamucil)
   b. methylcellulose (Citrucel)
   c. docusate sodium (Colace)
   d. magnesium hydroxide (milk of magnesia)

4. A patient has been given PEG-3350 in a solution called GoLYTELY as preparation for a colonoscopy. He started having diarrhea after about 45 minutes. Two hours later, he tells the nurse that "the diarrhea has not stopped yet." What should the nurse do?
   a. Give him an antidiarrheal drug, such as loperamide (Lomotil)
   b. Give him another dose of the GoLYTELY to finish cleansing his bowel
   c. Remind him that it may take up to 4 hours to completely evacuate the bowel
   d. Report this to the physician

5. A 79-year-old woman visits the clinic today and tells the nurse that her "bowels just aren't right." She wants advice on the best laxative to take so that she can have a bowel movement every day. Which of the following is an appropriate response by the nurse? Select all that apply.
   a. "A normal bowel pattern does not necessarily mean that you will have a bowel movement every day."
   b. "Try taking Metamucil with sips of water."
   c. "You can try taking milk of magnesia every other day—it's a mild laxative."
   d. "Increasing fluids and fiber in your diet are better alternatives than laxative use."

CRITICAL THINKING AND APPLICATION

Answer the following questions on a separate sheet of paper.

6. Anna has called the health clinic in a panic. She says that she has been taking Pepto-Bismol for diarrhea and noticed this morning that her tongue "is a funny color." She asks, "Have I overdosed on this stuff? What should I do?" What do you tell Anna?

7. Mrs. Benedict is a 65-year-old retiree with osteoporosis and glaucoma. She has recently developed diarrhea, and the physician is considering antidiarrheal therapy. Mrs. Benedict tells you that her husband recently "had a bout of diarrhea" for which he took Donnatal. Mrs. Benedict wonders whether Donnatal would help in her case. What do you tell her?

8. Hillary has come to the physician's office complaining of constipation. During your assessment, Hillary mentions that she recently started graduate school and has not had time lately to keep up her usual exercise regimen and that her diet "is a disaster." She says that, on some days, all she has time to do is grab a milkshake at the student center. She also tells you that she has been taking antacids for "heartburn." What might be causing Hillary's constipation?

9. Ira, a 45-year-old accountant, has chronic constipation.

   a. What are the advantages of the bulk-forming laxatives in treating Ira's problem?

   b. The physician prescribes psyllium. What instructions do you give Ira regarding its administration?

10. Drake is a 5-year-old boy with constipation. The physician has ordered treatment with glycerin suppositories.

    a. Why is glycerin a good choice for Drake?

    b. For what adverse effects will you monitor?

11. Five-year-old Kyle has diarrhea for which the physician has ordered an antidiarrheal drug.

    a. How will the dosage likely be determined?

    b. The next day Kyle's mother calls to tell you that Kyle seems to be no better and that his abdomen "looks bloated" and is painful. What do you do?

CASE STUDY

Read the scenario and answer the following questions on a separate sheet of paper.

Charles, a 54-year-old accountant, recently completed a 2-week course of antibiotic therapy for pneumonia. He still has a slight cough and is now experiencing severe diarrhea.

1. What is the probable cause of his diarrhea?

2. What antidiarrheal drug is indicated for Charles?

3. How does this drug work?

4. Is this drug considered a drug or a dietary supplement? Explain.

Chapter 53

Antiemetic and Antinausea Drugs

CHAPTER REVIEW

Choose the best answer for each of the following.

1. Which drugs may cause drowsiness and drying of secretions when given to reduce nausea?
   a. Antihistamines
   b. Neuroleptics
   c. Serotonin blockers
   d. Tetrahydrocannabinoids

2. Which class of antinausea drugs has proven to be very effective in preventing chemotherapy-induced nausea and vomiting? Select all that apply.
   a. Antihistamines
   b. Neuroleptics
   c. Serotonin blockers
   d. Anticholinergics
   e. Tetrahydrocannabinoids

3. When reviewing the drugs used for nausea and vomiting, the nurse recalls that the drug which is a synthetic derivative of the major active substance in marijuana is known as
   a. ondansetron (Zofran).
   b. metoclopramide (Reglan).
   c. prochlorperazine (Compazine).
   d. dronabinol (Marinol).

4. A patient is undergoing chemotherapy. When giving antiemetics, the nurse will remember that these drugs are most effective against nausea when given
   a. before meals.
   b. at bedtime.
   c. before the chemotherapy begins.
   d. just after the chemotherapy begins.

5. When giving dronabinol to a patient with acquired immunodeficiency syndrome (AIDS), the nurse knows that this drug may also have what effect in addition to reducing nausea?
   a. Euphoria
   b. Enhanced appetite
   c. Reduced pain
   d. Enhanced sleep

CRITICAL THINKING AND APPLICATION

Answer the following questions on a separate sheet of paper.

6. Norman, who has Parkinson's disease, is experiencing nausea and vomiting. What class of antiemetic drug would *not* be a good choice for Norman, and why?

7. Petra has gastroesophageal reflux disease, and the physician has ordered oral metoclopramide.

   a. What instructions do you give Petra regarding administration of the medication?

   b. A few days later, Petra calls to say that she thinks the medication is "too strong." She also mentions that her evening routine includes "a couple of glasses of wine." What do you tell Petra?

8. Nellie, a patient on your unit, has been prescribed prochlorperazine (Compazine) via an intramuscular injection. She is on "nothing-by-mouth" status and has no intravenous access at this time. You are preparing the injection when Nellie says, "I hate shots. Can't I just take it by mouth?" What alternatives are there for this drug, and what should you do?

9. Chuck, a 33-year-old who is in a later stage of AIDS, has lost much weight and has no appetite. His physician has prescribed dronabinol. When Chuck finds out that this medication is derived from marijuana, he becomes very upset. "Why is the doctor giving me pot?" he asks. What do you explain?

CASE STUDY

Read the scenario and answer the following questions on a separate sheet of paper.

Mr. Ontkin has been prescribed ondansetron (Zofran) during his chemotherapy, which is daily for 2 weeks.

1. For what significant drug interactions should you assess before he takes the ondansetron?

2. Mr. Ontkin tells you that he still has nausea. He is puzzled because "I take the medicine for nausea as soon as I feel nauseated." What should you tell him?

3. One day Mr. Ontkin complains to you that he gets a headache every time the ondansetron is administered. What should you do?

Chapter 54

Vitamins and Minerals

CHAPTER REVIEW

Match each definition with the corresponding term.

1. _____ Specialized protein that catalyzes chemical reactions in organic matter

2. _____ A deficiency of cyanocobalamin

3. _____ A nonprotein substance that combines with a protein molecule to form an active enzyme

4. _____ A condition caused by a vitamin D deficiency that is characterized by soft, pliable bones

5. _____ An inorganic substance ingested and attached to enzymes or other organic molecules

6. _____ An organic compound essential in small quantities for normal physiologic and metabolic functioning of the body

7. _____ A condition resulting from an ascorbic acid deficiency that is characterized by weakness and anemia

8. _____ An essential organic compound that can be dissolved and stored in the liver and fatty tissues

9. _____ Biologically active chemicals that make up vitamin E compounds

10. _____ A disease of the peripheral nerves caused by an inability to assimilate thiamine

a. Beriberi

b. Coenzyme

c. Enzyme

d. Fat-soluble vitamin

e. Mineral

f. Pellagra

g. Pernicious anemia

h. Rickets

i. Scurvy

j. Tocopherols

k. Vitamin

l. Water-soluble vitamin

11. _____ An essential organic compound that can be dissolved in water but is not stored in the body for long periods of time

12. _____ A disease resulting from a niacin deficiency or a metabolic defect that interferes with the conversion of tryptophan to niacin

Choose the best answer for each of the following.

13. When giving vitamins, the nurse needs to remember that certain vitamins can be toxic if consumed in excess amounts. These include which of the following? Select all that apply.
    a. Vitamin A
    b. Vitamin C
    c. Niacin
    d. Vitamin D
    e. Vitamin K
    f. Folic acid

14. A patient believes that taking megadoses of vitamin C is healthy. The nurse should tell the patient that megadoses of vitamin C
    a. are usually nontoxic because vitamin C is water-soluble.
    b. can produce nausea, vomiting, headache, and abdominal cramps.
    c. can lead to scurvylike symptoms.
    d. may cause dangerous heart dysrhythmias.

15. If excessive amounts of water-soluble vitamins are ingested, what usually happens?
    a. The body will store them in muscle and fat tissue until needed.
    b. They are stored in the liver until needed.
    c. They circulate in the blood, bound to proteins, until needed.
    d. Excess amounts are excreted in the urine.

16. When reviewing the diet of a patient who has a calcium deficiency, the nurse recalls that efficient absorption of calcium in the diet requires adequate amounts of which of the following?
    a. Magnesium
    b. Intrinsic factor
    c. Coenzymes
    d. Vitamin D

CRITICAL THINKING AND APPLICATION

Answer the following questions on a separate sheet of paper.

17. Mrs. Steinman has developed vitamin D deficiency as a result of long-term use of lubricant laxatives. She is advised to take supplements for her vitamin D deficiency. However, the physician also advises her to get vitamin D through more natural sources, both dietary and endogenous. "What did he mean by 'endogenous'?" she asks you. Explain to Mrs. Steinman what is meant by an endogenous source and make her a list of foods rich in vitamin D as well.

18. Ms. Evans has recently undergone an ileal resection, which is understandably affecting her digestive functions. She is experiencing some signs of malabsorption. When routine laboratory tests are performed, you discover that she is mildly anemic.

    a. What type of anemia do you expect?

    b. What about her condition is contributing to this deficiency?

    c. Create a hand-held patient education card for Ms. Evans, concentrating on diet. Be sure to include a list of foods that contain the vitamin or vitamins of which she is most likely to suffer a deficiency.

19. Mr. Graham is hospitalized with severe hypocalcemia. Your colleague Jeffrey recommends immediately beginning a rapid infusion of intravenous calcium. The physician's order requires infusion of 1% procaine. Refute or defend the rationales of both Jeffrey and Mr. Graham's physician. In either case, what should you watch out for when giving intravenous calcium? Back up your response with your own data.

20. Mrs. Smith will be taking iron for treatment of anemia, and her physician instructed her to take it with orange juice. She asks you for an explanation of this. What do you tell her?

CASE STUDY

Read the scenario and answer the following questions on a separate sheet of paper.

After Mr. Wong is treated for colitis with a broad-spectrum antibiotic, he begins to show signs of vitamin K deficiency.

1. How did this happen? How will he receive supplements?

2. What function does vitamin K serve in the human body?

3. Despite the infrequent occurrence of this deficiency, what other patient populations can sometimes be at risk for it?

4. What dietary supplements can you recommend?

Chapter 55

Nutrition Supplements

CRITICAL THINKING CROSSWORD

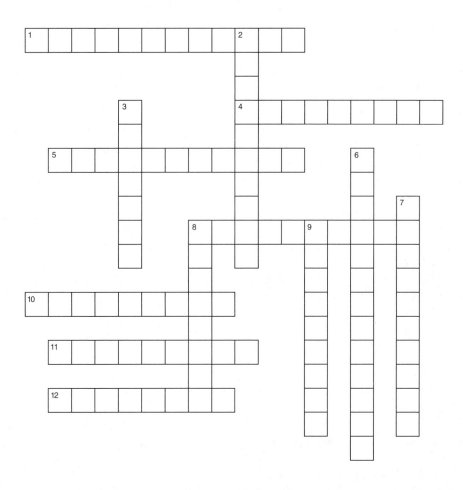

Across

1. Mr. George is receiving _____ when it is determined that he is going to need nutritional supplementation as well. When you see that he is taking this drug, however, you ask if the feeding can wait until his other drug therapy has run its course. You are concerned that the nutritional supplement will inactivate this drug because of high gastric acid content or prolonged emptying time.

4. Ms. Carter needs amino acids in nutritional supplements. The main use, or primary role, of amino acids is protein synthesis, or _____.

5. Mr. Harris is about to receive a _____, in which a feeding tube will be surgically inserted directly into his stomach.

Down

2. When Ms. Carter asks why she needs amino acid supplemental feedings, you explain that amino acids promote growth and help with wound healing. One of the principle ways they do so is by reducing or slowing the breakdown of proteins, or

_____.

3. The Johnsons recently appeared in a television commercial because they drink Ensure to meet a few extra nutritional needs they have experienced with aging. Their nephew recently had surgery; while recovering, he received nasogastric delivery of a modular formulation to supplement a polymeric feeding formulation he needed. When their grandson was an infant, his parents supplemented

8. Mrs. Page is worried about her husband, who has postsurgical nausea. She sees that his roommate is receiving total parenteral nutrition (TPN) and asks "Can't you do that for my husband, just while he's so nauseated?" TPN, you explain, is to be used only when enteral support is impossible or when the gastrointestinal tract's _____ or functional capacity is insufficient.

10. Ms. Cedaras comes to the clinic when a cut on her hand "just won't heal up." She also says that as long as she is here, she would like to report symptoms of hair loss and scaly dermatitis. She wants a prescription for her skin problem, but the physician says, "There's something more going on here." He runs a few tests and discovers that Ms. Cedaras also has a decreased platelet level and some evidence of possible fatty liver. He says he suspects that Ms. Cedaras has essential _____ (two words) deficiency.

11. Mr. Hill is having trouble getting and digesting enough dietary forms of amino acids. His physician explains that he needs nutritional supplementation through enteral nutrition to ensure that he gets enough of these amino acids, because they cannot be produced by his own body. Mr. Hill is suffering from a deficiency of _____ amino acids.

12. Craig, a college sophomore, takes a great deal of interest in the supplementary nutritional product he is receiving and asks to read the label. He says, "There are some amino acids missing from this. Why aren't you giving me all of them?" You explain that some amino acids, all but eight, are manufactured in the body, using _____ sources.

his breast-feeding with an infant nutritional formulation. Each member of the Johnson clan discussed here has received some form of _____ nutrition.

6. Lauren in 8 Down is receiving _____ amino acids.

7. You are explaining to Mrs. Glendale's family that the parenteral nutritional supplementation you are about to start will help her by bypassing the entire gastrointestinal system, eliminating the need for absorption, _____, and excretion.

8. Lauren, age 10, is going through a period of rapid growth. She is receiving enough essential amino acids in her diet, and her body has no problems producing its normal levels of nonessential amino acids. Nevertheless, she is to receive two amino acids that are not produced in large enough quantities to support this rapid growth spurt. Lauren is to receive a supplemental source of histidine and _____.

9. Mr. Kennedy has been receiving peripheral parenteral nutrition. One day something rather rare occurs: his vein becomes inflamed. You notify the physician. "Left untreated," she tells you, "this could have become really severe. He could even have lost his arm eventually if you hadn't caught this so quickly." Mr. Kennedy, of course, has _____.

CHAPTER REVIEW

Choose the best answer for each of the following.

1. The maximum concentration of dextrose in peripheral TPN infusions should be which of the following?
   a. 10%
   b. 20%
   c. 50%
   d. 100%

2. A patient has a need for a nutritional supplement that contains complex nutrients derived from proteins, carbohydrates, and fat. However, this patient is intolerant to milk. Which product would be most suitable for this patient?
   a. Casec
   b. Polycose
   c. Ensure
   d. Vivonex

3. When monitoring a patient who is receiving TPN through a central line, the nurse should observe for complications, including which of the following? Select all that apply.
   a. Pneumothorax
   b. Aspiration
   c. Hyperglycemia
   d. Infection
   e. Air embolus

4. A patient who is just starting to take enteral nutritional supplements should be taught that the most common adverse effect he or she may experience is which of the following?
   a. Anorexia
   b. Constipation
   c. Diarrhea
   d. Flatulence

5. When reviewing a patient's need for nutritional supplementation, the nurse remembers that peripheral TPN is most appropriate for which of the following?
   a. Patients who will receive short-term TPN (for less than 2 weeks)
   b. Patients who will receive long-term TPN (for longer than 2 weeks)
   c. Patients with severe nutritional problems
   d. Patients who wish to reduce their weight

6. Nursing interventions for patients receiving enteral feedings include which of the following?
   a. Checking gastric residual volumes once a day
   b. Starting the infusions at the maximum rate ordered
   c. Keeping the head of the bed flat
   d. Giving tube feeding formulas that are at room temperature

CRITICAL THINKING AND APPLICATION

Answer the following questions on a separate sheet of paper.

7. Ms. Schiller has one of the newer tubes for nasogastric feeding.

   a. What are the advantages and disadvantages of these newer tubes?

   b. What symptoms would she develop if she were lactose intolerant?

   c. Her tube feeding rate is 50 mL/hr. After 24 hours, you note that the residual amount is 120 mL. What should you do?

8. Mr. Robbins, who is on TPN therapy, has a weak pulse, hypertension, tachycardia, and decreased urine output. He seems somewhat confused, and you note, on examining him, that he exhibits pitting edema. What is wrong? Can you do anything about it? What could you have done differently to avoid this reaction?

CASE STUDY

Read the scenario and answer the following questions on a separate sheet of paper.

You are caring for Mrs. Thomas, who is receiving peripheral parenteral nutrition through an intravenous (IV) line in her right forearm. Your assessment shows that bag No. 3 is infusing at 100 mL/hr via an infusion pump, and the bag has about 300 mL remaining. The site is intact without redness or swelling.

1. Two hours later, Mrs. Thomas calls you because she accidentally pulled the IV line out of her arm. The remaining 300 mL of TPN has spilled on the floor. You have tried to reinsert the IV line but have not had success yet. What could occur if you cannot restart the infusion?

2. At last, the IV line has been reinserted, but you then discover that bag No. 4 has not yet been ordered from the pharmacy. What should you hang until TPN bag No. 4 is ready?

3. What else should you monitor while Mrs. Thomas is receiving peripheral parenteral nutrition?

Chapter 56
Blood-Forming Drugs

CHAPTER REVIEW

Choose the best answer for each of the following.

1. Three days after beginning therapy with oral iron tablets, a patient calls the office. "I'm very worried because my bowel movements are black!" What should the nurse do?
   a. Tell the patient to stop the iron tablets
   b. Tell the patient to take the tablets every other day instead of daily
   c. Ask the patient to come into the office for a checkup
   d. Explain to the patient that this is an expected effect of the medication

2. Patients who take iron preparations should be warned of the possible adverse effects, which may include which of the following?
   a. Dizziness and orthostatic hypotension
   b. Nausea, vomiting, and stomach cramps
   c. Drowsiness, lethargy, and fatigue
   d. Neuropathy and tingling in the extremities

3. What happens if folic acid is given to treat anemia without determining the underlying cause of the anemia?
   a. Erythropoiesis is inhibited.
   b. Excessive levels of folic acid may accumulate, causing toxicity.
   c. The symptoms of pernicious anemia may be masked, delaying treatment.
   d. Intestinal intrinsic factor is destroyed.

4. A patient is about to receive folic acid supplementation. The nurse knows that indications for folic acid supplementation include which of the following? Select all that apply.
   a. Megaloblastic anemia
   b. Tropical sprue
   c. Prevention of fetal neural tube defects
   d. Pernicious anemia

5. When teaching the patient about oral iron preparations, the nurse will include which of the following instructions? Select all that apply.
   a. Mix the liquid iron preparations with antacids to reduce gastrointestinal distress.
   b. Take the iron with meals if gastrointestinal distress occurs.
   c. Liquid forms should be taken through a straw to avoid discoloration of tooth enamel.
   d. Oral forms should be taken with juice, not milk.

6. A patient asks the nurse, "What foods are good sources of iron? I know meat contains iron, but what other choices are there?" The nurse should suggest which of the following?
   a. Apples
   b. Citrus fruits
   c. Wheat crackers
   d. Raisins

CRITICAL THINKING AND APPLICATION

Answer the following questions on a separate sheet of paper.

7. Mr. Dlugy is prescribed intramuscular iron dextran. However, before you can give him his first injection, the pharmacist suggests that you give him a smaller dose of 25 mg first. Why does she suggest this? How should intramuscular iron dextran be administered?

8. You are aware of the foods that contain iron. What other foods may either enhance the intake of iron or perhaps hinder it?

9. Four-year-old David has accidentally ingested an oral iron preparation, but he is not showing any adverse effects yet. Describe the treatment plan. If the serum iron concentration is higher than 300 mcg/dL, how is the treatment plan affected?

10. Describe the treatment of a child with more severe symptoms of iron intoxication than those seen in David (question 9). First describe the most severe symptoms of iron intoxication and then outline the treatment given.

CASE STUDY

Read the scenario and answer the following questions on a separate sheet of paper.

Maureen has been given ferrous fumarate capsules with instructions to take two capsules twice a day as part of her treatment for iron-deficiency anemia.

1. She asks you if she can take this drug with meals. What is your answer?

2. What else should you warn her to expect with this medication?

3. After a week, Maureen calls you because she does not like to swallow capsules. She says that her mother has iron tablets that are labeled *ferrous sulfate*. She wants to know if she can take those tablets instead. What do you tell her?

4. Because Maureen does not like the capsules, her iron preparation has been switched to an oral liquid suspension. While you are teaching her how to give herself the correct dosage, what else is important for you to tell her about liquid iron preparations?

Chapter 57
Dermatologic Drugs

CHAPTER REVIEW

Choose the best answer for each of the following.

1. Which of the following statements accurately describes antifungal therapy for topical infections?
   a. The length of treatment required to eradicate the organism may be from several weeks to as long as a year.
   b. Antifungal therapy works best when the affected area is exposed to sunlight.
   c. Oral drugs are the preferred drugs for treating topical fungal infections.
   d. Antifungal therapy is palliative only; fungi are rarely eradicated from topical areas.

2. When instructing a patient on how to use suppositories for vaginal yeast infections, the nurse should keep in mind that
   a. suppositories should be inserted every other day at bedtime for 1 week.
   b. suppositories should be inserted once daily at bedtime for 3 consecutive days.
   c. a one-time dose is administered in the morning.
   d. suppositories should be inserted every night at bedtime until symptoms stop.

3. A patient has a painful sunburn that covers a large area of her body. To enhance the patient's comfort, the nurse can suggest that which of the following formulations be used for this patient's topical medication?
   a. Aerosol spray
   b. Gel
   c. Oil
   d. Cream

4. A patient needs a medication that has excellent emollient properties. Because she works as a swimming coach, the medication prescribed should not wash off when it comes in contact with water. If each has the same healing properties, which of the following formulations would be preferred for this patient?
   a. Aerosol spray
   b. Oil
   c. Gel
   d. Cream

5. Which of the following statements about topical antiviral drugs are true? Select all that apply.
   a. Common adverse effects include stinging, itching, and rash.
   b. Topically applied acyclovir does not cure viral skin infections but does seem to decrease the healing time and pain.
   c. Topically applied acyclovir can cure viral skin infections if applied as soon as symptoms appear.
   d. Antiviral drugs are applied topically for the treatment of both initial and recurrent herpes simplex infections.

6. A 22-year-old woman is taking isotretinoin (Accutane) as part of the treatment for severe cystic acne. Which of the following is part of the patient teaching she will require?
   a. This drug reduces acne by causing skin peeling.
   b. Its use is contraindicated if she is allergic to erythromycin.
   c. She will need to apply it twice a day to her face, after washing her face thoroughly.
   d. She will need to use two forms of birth control while taking this medication.

CRITICAL THINKING AND APPLICATION

Answer the following questions on a separate sheet of paper.

7. Mr. Mugler has a topical skin infection. He is prescribed clindamycin. He has never used this drug before. You realize that it is a good idea to assess him for possible sensitivity or allergies. What precautions can you take?

8. You are getting ready to apply erythromycin to a patient's skin. The affected area of the skin is not oozing or even moist, but your supervisor still requires that you wear gloves. Why?

9. Mr. Lacroix's two children brought "something" home from school, and within a day, he had "it" too! He tells you that he has applied lindane to everyone's scalp, but he has come to the clinic to have his children and himself checked because he is not confident that he has "taken care of things properly." For what are Mr. Lacroix and his children being treated? Describe for him the basic steps in using lindane. What other measures should he take?

10. With a partner, develop two different case studies of acne patients. Assign one patient to take benzoyl peroxide and the other tretinoin. What differences in implementation and precautions do you come up with for the two patients?

11. A newly admitted patient has a stage III pressure ulcer that shows areas of exudate along with areas of healed granulation tissue. The orders for wound care include application of cadexomer iodine (Iodosorb). Explain what should be assessed before applying this medication and its purpose in wound care.

12. A patient with an infected pressure ulcer that contains an area of eschar needs to have the area surgically débrided, but instead the physician orders papain-urea (Accuzyme) treatment to the wound. What could be the reason for this order instead of surgery, and what is the purpose of this medication?

CASE STUDY

Read the scenario and answer the following questions on a separate sheet of paper.

Judy is in the clinic today because she burned her arm last evening while frying chicken. She has a second-degree burn over a 5-inch area of her forearm. She did not apply anything to it overnight, and the wound is reddened and peeling.

1. The physician tells you that he is going to apply silver sulfadiazine (Silvadene) cream to the site. What will he need to do before applying this cream?

2. He tells Judy that the area will need to be kept covered. Why is this necessary?

3. As the physician prepares to apply the cream, you notice that he is about to reach into the medication jar with his ungloved fingers. Is this okay?

4. Are there any adverse effects associated with this medication?

Chapter 58
Ophthalmic Drugs

CHAPTER REVIEW

Match each definition with the corresponding term. (Note: Not all terms will be used.)

1. _____ Adjustment of the lens of the eye to variation in distance

2. _____ Inflammation of the eyelids

3. _____ The clear, watery fluid that circulates in the anterior and posterior chambers of the eye

4. _____ An abnormal condition of the lens of the eye, characterized by loss of transparency

5. _____ Paralysis of the ciliary muscles, which prevents accommodation of the lens to variations in distance

6. _____ Excessive intraocular pressure caused by elevated levels of aqueous humor

7. _____ The mucous membrane that lines the eyelids

8. _____ Drugs that constrict the pupil

9. _____ The vascular middle layer of the eye, containing the iris, ciliary body, and choroid

10. _____ Drugs that dilate the pupil

a. Cycloplegia

b. Conjunctiva

c. Accommodation

d. Glaucoma

e. Mydriatics

f. Miotics

g. Uvea

h. Blepharitis

i. Vitreous humor

j. Aqueous humor

k. Cataract

Choose the best answer for each of the following.

11. When reviewing the medical record of a patient with a new order for a carbonic anhydrase inhibitor, the nurse knows that which condition would be a potential problem for a patient taking this drug?
    a. Glaucoma
    b. Ocular hypertension
    c. Allergy to sulfa drugs
    d. Allergy to penicillin

12. During an ophthalmic procedure, the patient receives ophthalmic acetylcholine. The nurse is aware that the purpose of this drug is
    a. to produce mydriasis for ophthalmic examination.
    b. to produce immediate miosis during ophthalmic surgery.
    c. to cause cycloplegia to allow for measurement of intraocular pressure.
    d. to provide topical anesthesia during ophthalmic surgery.

13. When giving latanoprost eyedrops, the nurse should advise the patient of which possible adverse effects?
    a. Temporary eye color changes, from light eye colors to brown
    b. Permanent eye color changes, from light eye colors to brown
    c. Photosensitivity
    d. Bradycardia and hypotension

14. A patient has come to the emergency department with an eye injury. After fluorescein is applied, the physician sees an area with a green halo. This indicates which of the following?
    a. A corneal defect
    b. A conjunctival lesion
    c. The presence of a hard contact lens
    d. A foreign object

15. When applying ophthalmic drugs, the nurse should follow which instructions? Select all that apply.
    a. Apply drops directly onto the cornea.
    b. Apply drops into the conjunctival sac.
    c. Apply pressure to the inner canthus for 1 minute after medication administration.
    d. Apply ointments in a thin layer.

16. To prevent gonorrheal eye infection, a newborn infant will receive
    a. dexamethasone (Maxidex) ointment.
    b. silver nitrate solution.
    c. erythromycin ointment.
    d. sulfacetamide (Cetamide) solution.

CRITICAL THINKING AND APPLICATION

Answer the following questions on a separate sheet of paper.

17. Jonathan has blue eyes; Julie has brown eyes. Why would the drug effects of the miotics on the iris be less pronounced in Julie?

18. Mrs. Ngo, a 60-year-old librarian, has open-angle glaucoma. The physician prescribes dipivefrin (Propine).

    a. Why might the physician have chosen that drug over epinephrine?

    b. What problems will you tell Mrs. Ngo to report?

    c. Do you expect any serious reactions to the drug? Explain your answer.

19. The physician prescribes a β-adrenergic blocker for Ned, who has ocular hypertension. Ned experiences what he calls "an allergic reaction" to the drug, and the physician changes Ned's medication to another β-blocking drug, timolol. Because both of these drugs are β-adrenergic blockers and Ned had a reaction to the first drug, why would the physician simply switch Ned to another drug in the same category?

20. Mrs. O'Rourke, who has acute narrow-angle glaucoma, has been scheduled for an iridectomy.

    a. What drug is indicated?

    b. Following administration of the drug, you find Mrs. O'Rourke sitting up in bed, complaining of a headache. How could her headache be diminished?

21. You are preparing to administer sulfacetamide to Tony, a patient with an eye infection.

    a. Why will you cleanse Tony's eye before administering the medication?

    b. Before using the sulfacetamide, you examine it and then throw the solution away and look for another container of sulfacetamide. Why did you do that?

22. Louisa has an inflammatory disorder of the eye for which the physician has prescribed a topical ophthalmic nonsteroidal antiinflammatory drug (NSAID). Why might the physician have chosen an NSAID over a corticosteroid?

23. Ms. Luna has been prescribed ophthalmic corticosteroid drops for an inflammation of her eye. The next day she calls the clinic and tells you, "These drops sting so much when I use them that I can't even put in my contacts." What is your advice?

CASE STUDY

Read the scenario and answer the following questions on a separate sheet of paper.

Mr. W. has developed a viral ocular infection—cytomegalovirus (CMV) retinitis—after being diagnosed with acquired immunodeficiency syndrome (AIDS) 6 months ago.

1. He is upset about the eye infection—he says he has been meticulous about his health and hygiene since his diagnosis and does not understand how he got this ophthalmic infection. What can you tell him?

2. What two methods of medication delivery are used to treat this infection?

3. The ophthalmologist decides to use ganciclovir to treat Mr. W.'s infection. How will this drug be started?

4. Mr. W. asks you how long this medication will be needed. What do you tell him?

Chapter 59

Otic Drugs

CHAPTER REVIEW

Choose the best answer for each of the following.

1. When assessing for otitis media, the nurse remembers that common symptoms of this condition include which of the following? Select all that apply.
   a. Pain
   b. Malaise
   c. Ear drainage
   d. Hearing loss
   e. Fever

2. A patient with a middle ear infection will generally require treatment with which of the following?
   a. Topical steroids
   b. Systemic steroids
   c. Topical antibiotics
   d. Systemic antibiotics

3. An elderly patient has a buildup of cerumen in his left ear. The nurse expects that this patient will receive which type of drug for this problem?
   a. Antifungal
   b. Wax emulsifier
   c. Steroid
   d. Local analgesic

4. Before giving eardrops, the nurse checks for contraindications to the use of otic preparations, such as which of the following?
   a. Eardrum perforation
   b. Infection
   c. Presence of cerumen
   d. Mastoiditis

5. In children, what usually precedes episodes of otitis media?
   a. Participation in a swim team
   b. Injury with a foreign object
   c. Upper respiratory tract infection
   d. Mastoiditis

CRITICAL THINKING AND APPLICATION

Answer the following questions on a separate sheet of paper.

6. A patient calls the physician's office complaining of severe pain in and drainage from his left ear. He also says he "had a little mishap" on his motorcycle yesterday. What do you tell him?

7. Why are antiinfective drugs frequently combined with steroids?

8. André, a 30-year-old teacher, has an ear infection and has a prescription for eardrops.

   a. What do you do before you instill the drops?

   b. What do you warn André might happen after the drops are instilled?

9. Mrs. Franz, a 52-year-old office manager, has come to the clinic today complaining of a painful, "itchy" left ear. The physician diagnoses an infection of the external auditory canal and prescribes a topical antibiotic.

   a.   What is the advantage of using a product containing hydrocortisone?

   b.   What would be a contraindication to Mrs. Franz's use of this type of drug?

10. Why do so many otic combination products contain local anesthetic drugs?

11. Ben is a 2-year-old who attends day care, and his brother Drew is a 6-year-old kindergartner. They both require otic drugs for ear infections.

    a.   What instructions do you give the boys' parents regarding instillation of the drops?

    b.   A few days after they are first seen, the boys' mother brings them back for a follow-up visit. Ben and Drew do not seem to be in pain, and there is no redness or swelling in either child's ears. What does this mean?

12. During a home visit, you observe Esther's husband preparing her eardrops. He puts a glass of water in the microwave, telling you that he will soak the bottle of eardrops in hot water to warm them up.

    a.   How is Esther's husband doing so far?

    b.   Later, immediately after her husband instills the drops, Esther sits up and asks you whether they are now doing everything right. What do you tell her?

CASE STUDY

Read the scenario and answer the following questions on a separate sheet of paper.

Mark, who is 45 years old, comes to the office complaining of a "heavy" feeling in his left ear, with slight pain and decreased hearing. When you walk into the examination room, you find Mark inserting a cotton-tipped applicator into his ear "to scratch it."

1. What do you suspect is the problem with his ears?

2. What can be done to address this problem?

3. You give Mark a container of carbamide peroxide (Debrox) drops. Before you continue, he asks you how many times a day he needs to take this medication and whether he can take it with meals. How is this medication given?

4. Why is there a combination of carbamide peroxide and glycerin in the Debrox?

Overview of Dosage Calculations

There are many important aspects to consider when doing calculations, but probably the most important one is common sense. If a drug dose calculation does not seem right, then most likely it is not. The administration of drugs to patients is a shared responsibility among the patient, physician, pharmacist, and nurse. All those involved have a moral, ethical, and legal responsibility to ensure that the administration takes place in a safe and effective way. The nurse has a legal and a professional responsibility to ensure that his or her patients receive the right dose of the right medication at the right time and in the right manner. There are many checks and balances in the system to guarantee that this happens. The necessary basic calculations involved in the safe and accurate administration of medications to patients are described in this section.

Calculating drug doses is one small part of the overall process of pharmacologic therapy. Before you actually calculate a drug dose, you must follow many steps. The nurse should evaluate the patient and the prescribed medication for the "5 rights": right patient, right drug, right dose, right time, and right route. Other principles to follow to decrease the likelihood of mistakes are to calculate doses systematically and to perform calculations consistently time after time so that the process becomes easier with each calculation. It also helps to have a peer check your calculations, especially if the dose seems unusual or the math is very difficult. Remember that common sense should prevail. If a calculation shows that you should give 25 mg of digoxin and the strongest strength is 0.25 mg, common sense should tell you that the patient should not be given 100 pills, especially since drug dosage forms are usually manufactured with the most commonly prescribed dosages in mind.

You must have basic arithmetic skills before beginning. The following basic principles may need to be reviewed:

➤ Basic multiplication
➤ Basic division
➤ Roman numerals
➤ Fractions (reducing to lowest terms, addition, subtraction, multiplication, division, mixed numbers)
➤ Decimals (adding, subtracting, multiplication, division)
➤ Ratios and percentages (changing a fraction to a percentage, changing a ratio to a percentage)
➤ Solving for "x" in a simple equation

RULES TO REMEMBER

❖ Before calculating a drug dose for a particular patient, you must first convert all units of measure to a SINGLE system, if this has not already been done. For example, do NOT attempt to guess a dosage if the drug is ordered in grains but the drug label is in milligrams. The best approach is to convert to the system used on the drug label. You may have to convert the patient's weight from pounds to kilograms if the medication is ordered to be given per kilogram of weight.

❖ **Rounding.** Always round your answers to the nearest dose that is measurable, after verifying that the dose is correct for that patient.

   • If a tablet is scored, you may round to the nearest half tablet.
     Example: 1.8 tablets, give 2 tablets
                    1.2 tablets, give 1 tablet

   • If a tablet is unscored, call the pharmacy. It is very difficult to cut an unscored tablet accurately. Remember that enteric-coated, sustained-release, or extended-release formulations cannot be cut or crushed!

   • Recheck your calculations if the dose is more than 1 or 2 tablets.

   • To round liquids, look at the equipment you plan to use. Some syringes are marked in tenths or hundredths of a milliliter. Larger syringes are marked in 0.2-mL increments. Tuberculin syringes are marked in hundredths. For liquid medications, NEVER round up to the nearest WHOLE number. If the answer is 1.8 mL, DO NOT round up to 2 mL. Rounding up in these situations may lead to overdosing. However, if you are using an electronic infusion pump, you will probably need to round to the nearest whole number.

   • To round to the nearest tenth, look at the hundredths column. If it is 0.5 or more, round UP to the next tenth.

Disclaimer: Please note that the drugs and dosages within this chapter are examples for educational purposes only; please refer to appropriate drug resources for dosage information.

Example: To round to the nearest tenth:
   1.78 or 1.75, round to 1.8
   1.32 or 1.34, round to 1.3

- A syringe calibrated in hundredths permits more exact measurement of small dosages. To round to the nearest hundredth, look at the thousandth column. If it is 0.005 or more, round UP to the next hundredth.
   Example: To round to the nearest hundredth:
      1.847, round to 1.85
      1.653, round to 1.65
- NOTE: Never round up liquid medications to the nearest whole number. If the answer is 1.6 mL, DO NOT round up to 2 mL! Such increases may lead to overdoses.
- PEDIATRIC DOSES are rounded to the TENTHS place, not whole numbers. Rounding to whole numbers may lead to overdoses.

❖ **Leading Zeros.** Always insert a zero (0) in front of decimals when the number is less than a whole number. This draws attention to the decimal and avoids potential errors.
   Example: 0.05 is CORRECT.
      .05 is NOT correct.

❖ **Trailing Zeroes.** Never place a lone zero after a decimal point. If the decimal is not noticed, a dangerous dosage error may occur.
   Example: 3 is CORRECT
      3.0 is NOT correct and may be mistaken for 30

❖ **Labeling.** Always label your answers with the appropriate unit. If the problem asked for a number of tablets, write "tablets." If you are to give an injection, use "mL." Heparin and insulin, however, use "units" instead of "mg" or "mcg." Intravenous drips will either be written in terms of "mL/hr" or "gtt/mL." Problems using an intravenous infusion pump are ALWAYS asking for mL/hr. THINK about what the question is asking, and then label your answer appropriately.

❖ **Common Sense.** Use common sense! Drug companies typically formulate medications that are close to the usual doses and medications that can provide the ordered dose with one or two tablets. If your answer indicates that you should give 60 mL intramuscularly, CHECK IT AGAIN! Remember, you can only give 2 to 3 mL intramuscularly, depending on institution policies, so a dosage of 60 mL would be inappropriate.

INTERPRETING MEDICATION LABELS

Medication labels contain a great amount of information—much of it in small print. The drug manufacturer prints some labels; others are prepared by pharmacy technicians or pharmacists for institutional use. The most important information is as follows:

- Generic name—the first letter is usually lowercase; this is the name used by all companies that produce the drug
- Trade, brand, or proprietary name—the first letter is usually capitalized; this name is used only by the manufacturer of the drug and may be followed by the "®" symbol
- Unit dose per milliliter, per tablet, per capsule, and so on
- Total amount in the container
- Route
- Directions for preparation, if needed
- Directions for storage
- Expiration date

Other information, such as a specification for adult or pediatric use, may be noted on the label.

Example:

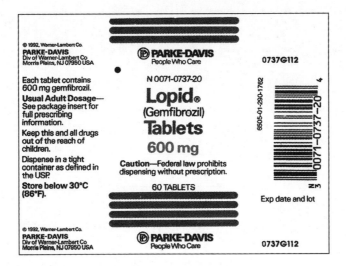

Generic name:	gemfibrozil
Trade name:	Lopid
Unit dose:	600 mg per tablet
Total amount in container:	60 tablets
Route:	(It is assumed that tablets are oral route.)

For the following labels, identify the information requested:

1.

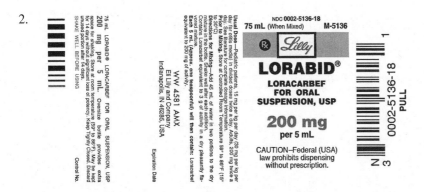

Generic name:	_____
Trade name:	_____
Unit dose:	_____
Total amount in container:	_____
Route:	_____

2.

Generic name:	_____
Trade name:	_____
Unit dose:	_____
Total amount in container:	_____
Route:	_____

3.

For IM use only	Upjohn NDC 0009-0626-01
See package insert for complete product information	2.5 mL Vial
Shake vigorously immediately before each use	Depo-Provera®
812 224 302	Sterile Aqueous Suspension sterile medroxyprogesterone acetate suspension, USP
The Upjohn Company Kalamazoo, MI 49001 USA	**400mg per mL**

Generic name: _____

Trade name: _____

Unit dose: _____

Total amount in container: _____

Route: _____

SECTION I: BASIC CONVERSIONS USING RATIO AND PROPORTION

A proportion is a way of stating a relationship of equality between two ratios. The first ratio listed is EQUAL to the second ratio listed. The double colon (::) that separates the two ratios means "is the same as." The numbers at each end of the ratio equation can be called the "outside," and the two numbers in the middle of the ratio (around the "::") can be called the "inside." Ratio and proportion problems can be used to calculate ONE of the numbers in the equation if it is not known. The simple rule to use is this:

The product of the outside terms equals the product of the inside terms.

If one of the terms is not known, it is designated as "x." The problem is then set up to solve for "x."

Example:

The problem "1 : 100 :: 4 : x" actually means:
"The relationship of 1 to 100 is the same as the relationship of 4 to x." The "x" is unknown.

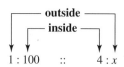

1 and x are the "outsides"; 100 and 4 are the "insides." To solve for "x," multiply the "outsides" ($1 \times x$) together, multiply the "insides" (100×4) together, and form an equation:

$(1 \times x) = (100 \times 4)$
$1x = 400$
$x = 400$

Proof: You may prove your equation as follows: Insert the answer for "x" in the original equation, then solve.

$1 \times 400 = 400$ (outsides)
$100 \times 4 = 400$ (insides)
$400 = 400$; the answer for "x" is correct.

Example:

5: 25:: 15: x
Multiply the "outsides" and the "insides" and form an equation; then solve for "x".
$(5 \times x) = (25 \times 15)$
$5x = 375$
$x = 375/5$
$x = 75$

Proof:

$5 \times 75 = 375$
$25 \times 15 = 375$
$375 = 375$

Calculating ratios is one of the major foundations of drug dosage calculations. When calculating a dosage, the nurse will use the medication on hand to calculate how much of it to give for a desired dosage. The nurse uses the principle of proportion to calculate accurately how much medication to give. The following chart provides a few common equivalents used in pharmacology. These equivalents are then used in ratio and proportion problems to calculate appropriate dosages.

BASIC EQUIVALENTS

Metric Equivalents	Other Equivalents
Weight 1 mg = 100 mcg (micrograms) 1 g = 1000 mg (milligrams) 1 kg (kilogram) = 1000 g (grams)	*Weight* 1 gr (grain) = 60 mg 1 g (gram) = 1000 mg = gr xv (15 grains) (approximately) 1 kg = 2.2 lb
Volume 1000 mL = 1 L (liter)	*Volume* 1 oz (ounce) = 30 mL 1 tsp (teaspoon) = 5 mL (milliliters) 1 tbsp (tablespoon) = 15 mL 2 tbsp = 30 mL

To find basic equivalents from one unit of measure to another, use the ratio and proportion approach.

Example 1: The drug dosage is 500 mg. You have scored tablets on hand that are 1 g each. How many tablets will you give?

You have *grams* on hand. You need to change the *milligrams* needed to the equivalent grams on hand.
Find the proper equivalents:
Equivalent: 1 g = 1000 mg
Next, set up the ratio and proportion equation.
On the LEFT side, put the ratio that you ***know:*** 1 g is 1000 mg
On the RIGHT side, put the ratio that you ***want to know:*** How many g ("*x*") is 500 mg?

Know   *Want to Know*
1 g : 1000 mg :: *x* g : 500 mg

Solve for *x*: $(1 \times 500) = (1000 \times x)$; $500 = 1000x$; $x = 500/1000$; $x = 0.5$
You will give 0.5 (half) of the 1-g tablet, which equals 500 mg.
To double-check your answer, substitute your answer for the *x* and solve. The "outsides" should equal the "insides."
$1 \times 500 = 500$; $1000 \times 0.5 = 500$; $500 = 500$

Example 2: Cough syrup, 45 mL, is ordered. The cough syrup comes in a 2-oz bottle. How many ounces do you give?

You have ounces on hand. You need to give 45 mL.
Equivalent: 1 oz = 30 mL
Know: 1 oz is 30 mL; ***want to know:*** How many ounces is 45 mL?

Know   *Want to Know*
1 oz : 30 mL :: *x* oz : 45 mL

$(1 \times 45) = (30 \times x)$; $45 = 30x$; $x = 45/30 = 1.5$ oz = 45 mL
Proof: $1 \times 45 = 45$; $30 \times 1.5 = 45$; $45 = 45$

Example 3: Mabel weighs 122 lb. How many kilograms does she weigh?

Equivalent: 1 kg = 2.2 lb

Know   ***Want to Know***
1 kg : 2.2 lb :: x kg : 122 lb

$(1 \times 122) = (2.2 \times x)$; $122 = 2.2x$; $122/2.2 = x$; $x = 55.45$ lb; round off to tenths: 55.5 lb
Proof: $1 \times 122 = 122$; $2.2 \times 55.45 = 121.99$ (rounds to 122)

Example 4: You have an injectable solution that is 50 mg strength. How many micrograms are in 50 mg?

Equivalent: 1 mg = 1000 mcg

Know   ***Want to Know***
1 mg : 1000 mcg :: 50 mg : x mcg

$(1 \times x) = (1000 \times 50)$; $1x = 50,000$; $x = 50,000$; therefore 50 mg = 50,000 mcg
Proof: $1 \times 50,000 = 50,000$; $1000 \times 50 = 50,000$

Example 5: Elixir is ordered as follows: "Give 2 tsp twice a day." How many milliliters would you give?

Equivalent: 1 tsp = 5 mL

Know   ***Want to Know***
1 tsp : 5 mL :: 2 tsp : x mL

$(1 \times x) = (5 \times 2)$; $1x = 10$; $x = 10$ mL
Proof: $1 \times 10 = 10$; $5 \times 2 = 10$; $10 = 10$
So, give 10 mL to equal 2 tsp.

Example 6: You have an injection that delivers 75 mcg. How many milligrams does it deliver?

Equivalent: 1 mg = 1000 mcg

Know   ***Want to Know***
1 mg : 1000 mcg :: x mg : 75 mcg

$(1 \times 75) = (1000 \times x)$; $75 = 1000x$; $x = 75/1000$; $x = 0.075$
So, 75 mcg = 0.075 mg. (Don't forget the leading zero!)
Proof: $1 \times 75 = 75$; $1000 \times 0.075 = 75$; $75 = 75$

PRACTICE PROBLEMS

Calculate the following conversions.

1. 600 mg   = _____ mcg   8. 750 mL   = _____ L

2. 1500 mg   = _____ mcg   9. 975 L   = _____ mL

3. 5000 mcg   = _____ mg   10. 500 mL   = _____ L

4. 5 g   = _____ mg   11. gr xvi   = _____ mg

5. 2.5 g   = _____ mg   12. 90 mg   = _____ gr

6. 900 mg   = _____ g   13. 4 tsp   = _____ mL

7. 8 kg   = _____ g   14. 60 mL   = _____ tsp

15. 90 mL = _____ tbsp   18. 90 kg = _____ lb

16. 3 oz = _____ mL   19. 150 lb = _____ kg

17. 6 mL = _____ oz   20. 11 kg = _____ lb

SECTION II: CALCULATING ORAL DOSES

To calculate oral dosages of medications, use the same ratio and proportion procedures described in Section I. Label all terms, and check your answers by proving them.

   The first step in doing medication dosage calculation problems is examining the order and the medication on hand. The units for both the order and the medicine on hand MUST be the same units (e.g., mg, mL). If they are not the same, then a conversion must first be done to change the ordered dose to the same units as the medication on hand.

Remember these rules:

- NEVER substitute one form of a medication for another, even if the dosage amount is the same. Parenteral forms of oral drugs are much stronger, and the resulting effects might be dangerous.
- Do not forget to place a zero in front of a decimal point (e.g., 0.75 mg). It reminds you that the number is a decimal, not a whole number.
- Are the medication ordered and the medication on hand in the same units? If not, convert the drug ordered to the units of the drug at hand.
- Place what you have on hand (what you know)—information from the label—on the LEFT side of the equation.
- Place what is ordered (what you want to know) on the RIGHT side of the equation.
- Solve the equation as described in Section I.
- ALWAYS label the units of your answer (tablets, capsules, mL, etc).

Example 1: The prescription reads, "Give 500 mg PO." The unit dose is 250 mg/tablet. How many tablets will you give?

   Ordered: 500 mg   **Unit dose:** 250 mg/tablet
   NOTE: Units match (mg).

   Know   *Want to Know*
   250 mg : 1 tablet :: 500 mg : x tablet

   $(250 \times x) = (1 \times 500)$; $250x = 500$; $x = 500/250 = 2$
   Answer: Give 2 tablets.
   Proof: $250 \times 2 = 500$; $1 \times 500 = 500$; $500 = 500$

Example 2: The order is to give 175 mg. The tablets on hand are 350-mg scored tablets. How many tablets will you give?

   Ordered: 175 mg   **Unit dose:** 350 mg/tablet
   NOTE: Units match (mg).

   Know   *Want to Know*
   350 mg : 1 tablet :: 175 mg : x tablet

   $(350 \times x) = (1 \times 175)$; $350x = 175$; $x = 175/350 = 0.5$
   Answer: Give 0.5 tablet (one half of the scored tablet).
   Proof: $350 \times 0.5 = 175$; $1 \times 175 = 175$; $175 = 175$

Example 3: You are asked to administer 100 mg of a drug. You have 0.05-g tablets on hand. How many tablets will you give?

   Ordered: 100 mg   **Unit dose:** 0.05 g/tablet
   NOTE: Units do not match (mg and g).
   First: Calculate: 100 mg = x g (equivalent: 1 g = 1000 mg)

Know   *Want to Know*

1 g : 1000 mg :: *x* g : 100 mg

$(1 \times 100) = (1000 \times x)$; $100 = 1000x$; $x = 100/1000 = 0.1$

100 mg = 0.1 g

Now that you have the ordered dose and the dose on hand in the same units, you can complete the problem.

Ordered: 0.1 g (100 mg)   **Unit dose:** 0.05 g/tablet

Know   *Want to Know*

0.05 g : 1 tablet :: 0.1g : *x* tablet

$(0.05 \times x) = (1 \times 0.1)$; $0.05 x = 0.1$; $x = 0.1/0.05 = 2$

Answer: Give 2 tablets.

Proof: $0.05 \times 2 = 0.1$; $1 \times 0.1 = 0.1$; $0.1 = 0.1$

Example 4: You are instructed to give 0.5 g of a drug. You have 250-mg tablets on hand. How many tablets will you give?

Ordered: 0.5 g   **Unit dose:** 250 mg/tablet

NOTE: Units do not match (g and mg).

First: Calculate: 0.5 g = *x* mg (equivalent: 1 g = 1000 mg)

Know   *Want to Know*

1 g : 1000 mg :: 0.5 g : *x* mg

$(1 \times x) = (1000 \times 0.5)$; $1x = 500$; $x = 500$

0.5 g = 500 mg

Now that you have the ordered dose and the dose on hand in the same units, you can complete the problem.

Ordered: 500 mg (0.5 g)   **Unit dose:** 250 mg/tablet

Know   *Want to Know*

250 mg : 1 tablet :: 500 mg : *x* tablet

$(250 \times x) = (1 \times 500)$; $250x = 500$; $x = 500/250 = 2$

Answer: Give 2 tablets.

Proof: $250 \times 2 = 500$; $1 \times 500 = 500$; $500 = 500$

Example 5: You are to administer 200 mg of guaifenesin syrup. You have a bottle labeled 100 mg/5 mL. How many mL will you give?

Ordered: 200 mg   **Unit dose:** 100 mg/5mL

NOTE: Units match (mg).

Know   *Want to Know*

100 mg : 5 mL :: 200 mg : *x* mL

$(100 \times x) = (5 \times 200)$; $100x = 1000$; $x = 1000/100 = 10$

Answer: Give 10 mL.

Proof: $100 \times 10 = 1000$; $5 \times 200 = 1000$; $1000 = 1000$

PRACTICE PROBLEMS

1. Dose ordered: ascorbic acid 0.5 g PO
   Dose on hand: 500-mg tablets
   How many tablets will you give? _____

2. Dose ordered: digoxin 0.5 mg PO
   Dose on hand: 250-mcg tablets
   How many tablets will you give? _____

3. Dose ordered: sulfisoxazole 0.25 g PO
   Dose on hand: 500-mg tablets
   How many tablets will you give? _____

4. Dose ordered: diphenhydramine syrup 50 mg PO
   Dose on hand: syrup 12.5 mg/5 mL
   How many milliliters will you give? _____

5. Dose ordered: 600 mg PO
   Dose on hand: gr v tablets
   How many tablets will you give? _____

6. Dose ordered: cefaclor 0.1 g PO
   Dose on hand: oral suspension 125 mg/5 mL
   How many milliliters will you give? _____

7. Dose ordered: zidovudine 0.3 g PO
   Dose on hand: 100-mg tablets
   How many tablets will you give? _____

8. Dose ordered: potassium chloride liquid 30 mEq PO
   Dose on hand: 20 mEq/15 mL
   How many milliliters will you give? _____

9. Dose ordered: 0.15 g PO
   Dose on hand: 50-mg capsules
   How many capsules will you give? _____

10. Dose ordered: 2 g PO
    Dose on hand: 500-mg tablets
    How many tablets will you give? _____

SECTION III: RECONSTITUTING MEDICATIONS

Many medications come in powder or crystal form and must be reconstituted by the addition of a diluent to create a liquid form. Many parenteral medications must be reconstituted before administration. Instructions for dissolving medications can be found in the literature that accompanies the medication or on the medication label. Most of the time, medications that need to be reconstituted are in delivery systems that match 50- or 100-mL IV bags, and reconstitution occurs as the nurse prepares the medication for use. However, there are still instances where you may be required to reconstitute a drug and then draw up the proper dose for parenteral use. These examples are for those instances.

For example, the instructions may read:

Add 1.2 mL normal saline to make 2 mL of reconstituted solution that yields 100 mg/mL.

This tells the user that the medication takes up 0.8 mL of space: 1.2 mL + 0.8 mL = 2 mL of medication solution. The label of the medication container will tell the user how many units, grams, milligrams, or micrograms are in each milliliter of the reconstituted drug. In this example, the dose on hand, after reconstitution, is 100 mg/mL.

Remember these rules:
- Read all instructions for reconstitution before doing anything! Be sure to ask a pharmacist if you have any questions.
- When reconstituting medications, be certain to use the exact *type* of diluent indicated, and add the exact *amount* of diluent as directed. Substitutions or inaccurate amounts of diluent can inactivate the medication or alter the concentration, thus altering the dose received by the patient.
- If the vial is a multiple-dose vial, the nurse who reconstitutes the medication must put the date, time, amount of diluent used, and his or her initials on the label. Follow the facility's policy for multi-dose vials.
- Many solutions are unstable after being reconstituted. Be sure to follow the directions on the label for proper storage of reconstituted medications. Follow the facility's policy for labeling the reconstituted solution.
- Make note of the time limit or expiration date for the reconstituted medication. Do not use the medication after it has expired.
- Ratio solutions indicate the number of grams of the medication per total milliliters of solution. For example, a medication that is designated 1:1000 has 1 g of medication per 1000 mL of solution.
  In order to avoid overdosing, it is essential that the nurse chooses the correct ratio solution!
- Percentage (%) solutions indicate the number of grams of the medication per 100 mL of solution. For example, a medication that is designated 10% has 10 g of drug per 100 mL of solution.
- COMPARE: "1:1000" indicates 1 g per 1000 mL
   "10%" indicates 10 g per 100 mL

As you calculate parenteral dosages:
- If the amount is greater than 1 mL, round *x* (the amount to be given) to tenths and use a 3-mL syringe to measure it.
- Small (less than 0.5 mL, or pediatric) dosages should be rounded to hundredths and measured in a tuberculin syringe. The tuberculin syringe is calibrated in 0.01-mL increments.

- THINK! For adults, the maximum volume of an IM injection is usually 3 mL. Sometimes the dose might have to be given in two divided doses; for example, a dose of 4 mL IM would usually be divided into two 2-mL doses. However, if your calculations yield an unusual number, such as 10 mL IM, look over your calculation and repeat your math! Double-check your calculations with a peer.

Always remember to note the route ordered. IM doses and IV doses are NOT always the same amount, and the drug formulations may differ; confusing the route may have fatal results.

Example 1: You receive an order for morphine 10 mg IM. The medication vial reads: 8 mg/mL.
How much morphine would you give?
Does this medication require reconstitution?
Would you use a 3-mL or a tuberculin syringe to measure this drug?
Ordered: 10 mg   **Unit dose:** 8 mg/mL

Know   *Want to Know*
8 mg : 1 mL :: 10 mg : x mL

$(8 \times x) = (1 \times 10)$; $8x = 10$; $x = 10/8 = 1.25$, rounded to 1.3
Answer: 1.3 mL measured in a 3-mL syringe. This medication does not require reconstitution.
Proof: $8 \times 1.3 = 10.4$ (rounds to 10); $1 \times 10 = 10$

Example 2: The ordered dose is 500 mg IV. The medication label reads:

> 500 mg MEDICATION FOR INJECTION
> For IM or IV use
> Add 2.7 mL sterile water for injection.
> Each 1.5 mL contains 250 mg medication.

How much medication would you give?
Does this medication require reconstitution?
Would you use a 3-mL or a tuberculin syringe to measure this drug?
Ordered: 500 mg   **Unit dose:** 250 mg/1.5 mL

Know   *Want to Know*
250 mg : 1.5 mL :: 500 mg : x mL

$(250 \times x) = (1.5 \times 500)$; $250x = 750$; $x = 750/250 = 3$
Answer: 3 mL measured in a 3-mL syringe. Reconstitute by adding 2.7 mL sterile water to the vial.
Proof: $250 \times 3 = 750$; $1.5 \times 500 = 750$; $750 = 750$

Example 3: You receive an order for penicillin G potassium 400,000 units IM. The medication label reads:

> ONE MILLION UNITS
> Penicillin G Potassium
> Use sterile saline as diluent as follows:
>
> | | Units per mL |
> | Add | reconstituted solution |
> | --- | --- |
> | 18.2 mL | 250,000 |
> | 8.2 mL | 500,000 |
> | 3.2 mL | 1,000,000 |

Which dilution would you choose for the ordered dose?
How much penicillin G potassium would you give?
Would you use a 3-mL or a tuberculin syringe to measure this drug?
Ordered: 400,000 units   **Unit dose:** Choosing the 8.2 diluent amount, unit dose is 500,000/mL.

Know   *Want to Know*

500,000 units : 1 mL :: 400,000 : x mL

$(500,000 \times x) = (1 \times 400,000)$; $500,000x = 400,000$; $x = 400,000/500,000 = 0.8$

Answer: 0.8 mL measured in either a 3-mL or tuberculin syringe.

Proof: $500,000 \times 0.8 = 400,000$; $1 \times 400,000 = 400,000$; $400,000 = 400,000$

NOTE: Choose the concentration that is close to the ordered dose. Choosing the 8.2 diluent amount allows for the injection amount to be small yet easily measured. If you had chosen the 18.2 diluent amount, the injection would have been 1.6 mL; choosing the 3.2 diluent would have made the injection amount very small: 0.04 mL.

Example 4: You receive an order for epinephrine 0.6 mg SC. The medication label reads:

> 1 mL ampule
> Epinephrine 1:1000
> For SC or IM use

What is the dose on hand?

How much epinephrine would you give?

Would you use a 3-mL or a tuberculin syringe to measure the drug?

First: Figure the dose on hand.

1:1000 = 1 g in 1000 mL = 1000 mg in 1000 mL = 1 mg in 1 mL

Then complete the problem:

Ordered: 0.6 mg   **Unit dose:** 1 mg/mL

Know   *Want to Know*

1 mg : 1 mL :: 0.6 mg : x mL

$(1 \times x) = (1 \times 0.6)$; $1x = 0.6$; $x = 0.6$

Answer: 0.6 mL measured in either a 3-mL or tuberculin syringe.

Proof: $1 \times 0.6 = 0.6$; $1 \times 0.6 = 0.6$; $0.6 = 0.6$

Example 5: Magnesium sulfate 5 g IV over 3 hours is the dosage ordered. The medication label reads:

> 10 mL vial
> Magnesium sulfate 10%
> For IM or IV use

What is the dose on hand?

How much magnesium sulfate would you give?

First: Figure the dose on hand.

10% = 10 g in 100 mL = 0.1 g per 1 mL

Then complete the problem:

Ordered: 5 g   **Unit dose:** 0.1 g/mL

Know   *Want to Know*

0.1 g : 1 mL :: 5 g : x mL

$(0.1 \times x) = (1 \times 5)$; $0.1x = 5$; $x = 5/0.1$; $x = 50$

Answer: 50 mL

Proof: $0.1 \times 50 = 5$; $1 \times 5 = 5$; $5 = 5$

PRACTICE PROBLEMS

1. Dose ordered: thiamine 200 mg IV
   On hand: 10-mL vial, 100 mg/mL
   How much will you give? _____

2. Dose ordered: gentamicin 60 mg IM
   On hand: 40 mg/mL
   How much will you give? _____

3. Dose ordered: heparin 8000 units SC
   On hand: 1-mL vial, 10,000 units/mL
   How much will you give? _____

4. Dose ordered: Medication 750 mg IV
   On hand: 1-g vial
   Instructions for reconstitution: Add 1.5 mL sterile water. Reconstituted solution will contain approximately 500 mg medication solution per mL.
   How much will you give? _____

5. Dose ordered: ampicillin 500 mg IV
   On hand: 1-g vial powder for injection
   Instructions for reconstitution: Add 66 mL sterile water. Reconstituted solution will contain 125 mg/5 mL.
   How much will you give? _____

6. Dose ordered: penicillin G potassium 300,000 units IM
   On hand: 1,000,000-units vial
   Instructions for reconstitution: Using only sterile water, add 9.6 mL to provide 100,000 units/mL, or 4.6 mL to provide 200,000 units/mL.
   Which concentration would you choose for this dose? _____
   How much will you give? _____

7. Dose ordered: epinephrine 750 mcg SC
   On hand: 1:1000
   How much will you give? _____

8. Dose ordered: Medication 0.2 mg
   On hand: 1:5000
   How much will you give? _____

9. Dose ordered: calcium gluconate 900 mg
   On hand: calcium gluconate 10%, 100-mL vial
   How much will you give? _____

10. Dose ordered: magnesium sulfate 4 g
    On hand: magnesium sulfate 50%, 10-mL vial
    How much will you give? _____

SECTION IV: PEDIATRIC CALCULATIONS

Doses used in pediatric patients must differ from those used in adults. The most common method for calculating doses for pediatric patients is weight-based (i.e., mg/kg). In some cases, dosages may be calculated using body surface area (BSA) calculations.

Body Surface Area Calculations

The BSA is a common method used to calculate therapeutic pediatric dosages. It requires the use of a chart called a West nomogram (see Figure 3-1 in your text) that converts weight to square meters (m^2) of BSA. The average adult is assumed to weigh 140 lb and have a BSA of 1.73 m^2. The BSA may be used to calculate the pediatric dose of certain medications.
- For a child of normal height and weight, find the m^2 for that weight on the shaded area of the nomogram chart.
  Example: Using Figure 3-1 in your text, find the BSA for a child who weighs 40 lb and is 38 inches tall (normal height for her weight). According to the nomogram, the BSA for 40 lb is 0.74 m^2.
- For a child who is underweight or overweight, the BSA is indicated at the point where a straight line connecting the height and weight intersects the unshaded surface area (SA) column.
  Example: Using Figure 3-1, find the BSA for a child who weighs 25 lb and has a height of 30 inches (underweight). According to the nomogram, the BSA for this child is 0.51 m^2.

There are two types of BSA problems.

1. The first type involves medications for which the literature provides recommended dosages in m^2.

   STEP 1: Check the order, and look up the recommended dose.
   The order is for 15 mg PO.
   The literature states that 40 mg/m^2 is safe for children.

STEP 2: Determine child's height and weight. Then consult the appropriate nomogram to obtain the BSA in m^2. This child weighs 22 lb and has a normal height of 70 cm. The BSA is approximately 0.46 m^2.

STEP 3: Calculate the recommended mg/m^2 dose (from the literature) using ratio and proportion. Then, for a safety check, compare it with the dose ordered.

For this calculation, what you know is the literature's recommendation (40 mg/m^2). What you want to know is the milligrams per the child's BSA (which is 0.46 m^2).

Know   *Want to Know*
40 mg : 1 m^2 :: x mg : 0.46 m^2

$(40 \times 0.46) = (1 \times x)$; $18.4 = 1x$; $x = 18.4$ (Pediatric doses are rounded to tenths place; do not round to whole numbers.)
Answer: 18.4 mg is the safe dose limit.
Decision: The order for 15 mg is safe.

Practice:

The medication ordered is 100 mg.
STEP 1: The literature recommends 50 mg/m^2 for children.

STEP 2: The child weighs 10 lb and has a normal height for his weight. The BSA is 0.27 m^2.

STEP 3: Calculate the dose for this child's BSA:

Know   *Want to Know*
50 mg : 1 m^2 :: x mg : 0.27 m^2

$(50 \times 0.27) = (1 \times x)$; $13.5 = 1x$; $x = 13.5$ (Pediatric doses are rounded to tenths place; do not round to whole numbers.)
Answer: 13.5 mg is the safe dose limit.
Decision: The order for 15 mg exceeds the safe dose limit and therefore is NOT safe. Notify the physician.

2. The second type of BSA involves situations when a recommended dose is cited in the literature for adults but not for children.
   STEP 1: Determine the BSA (m^2) of the child by dividing the adult dose by 1.73 m^2 (the average adult's BSA)

   STEP 2: Multiply the result by the average adult dose.

$$\frac{\text{Child's BSA (m}^2)}{\text{Average adult's BSA}} \times \text{Average adult dose of drug} = \text{Estimated child's dose}$$

Example: A 6-lb child has a BSA of 0.20 m^2, and the average adult dose of a drug is 300 mg. What would be the estimated safe dose for a child?

$$\frac{0.20\,m^2}{1.73\,m^2} \times 300\,mg = 34.68\,mg$$

Answer: 34.7 mg is the estimated safe dose for this child. (Round to tenths place for pediatric doses.)

Practice:

The average adult dose for a medication is 20 mg. The child has a BSA of 0.6 m^2.
What would be the estimated safe dose for a child?

$$\frac{0.6\,m^2}{1.73\,m^2} \times 20\,mg = 6.94\,mg$$

Answer: 6.9 mg is the estimated safe dose for this child. (Round to tenths place for pediatric doses.)

Weight-Based Calculations

When calculating the proper dose according to weight, **STEP 1** involves changing the weight from pounds to kilograms (if necessary).

- Be careful when converting ounces and pounds to kilograms. First, ounces must be converted to part of a pound (by dividing the ounces by 16). Remember, 16 ounces = 1 pound. Therefore 8 oz does not convert to 0.8 lb! Convert 8 ounces to pounds by dividing by 16: 8/16 = 0.5; 8 oz = 0.5 lb.
- Once you have converted ounces to pounds, then add the ounces to the pounds. For example, 10 lb 8 oz would equal 10.5 lb. You are now ready to convert pounds to kilograms.
- Remember: 1 kg = 2.2 lb. To convert 10.5 lb to kilograms, divide the pounds by 2.2.
- 1 kg : 2.2 lb :: x kg : 10.5 lb; $(1 \times 10.5) = (2.2 \times x)$; $10.5 = 2.2x$; $x = 10.5/2.2 = 4.8$ kg (rounded to tenths)
- DO NOT round pediatric weights to whole numbers!

Once you have converted the child's weight to kg, you are ready for STEP 2.

STEP 2 involves calculating the therapeutic dosage ranges for a child based on his or her weight. The nurse uses the child's weight (in kilograms) to calculate the low and high acceptable doses for that medication. This will give a range of dosage that this child could receive for this medication.

STEP 3 involves THINKING and comparing the ordered dose with the therapeutic dosage range that was calculated for that child. If the ordered dose is under or over the calculated therapeutic dosage range, then do not give the medication and notify the physician.

- **STEP 1:** Convert the child's weight from pounds to kilograms.
- **STEP 2:** Calculate therapeutic dose range (low and high).
- **STEP 3:** (1) Is the ordered dose safe (does not exceed the dosage range)?
    (2) Is the ordered dose therapeutic (falling within the recommended dosage range, not too low)?

Example 1: The ordered dose is 50 mg acetaminophen. The infant weighs 15 lb. The therapeutic dosage range for acetaminophen is 10 to 15 mg/kg/dose.

STEP 1: Convert pounds to kilograms by dividing 15 by 2.2.
15/2.2 = 6.82; 15 lb = 6.8 kg (Round pediatric weights to tenths, not to whole numbers.)

STEP 2: Calculate the therapeutic dosage range for this infant based on his weight.
Low dose: 10 mg/kg/dose × 6.8 kg = 68 mg/dose (note that the "kg" cancel out).
High dose: 15 mg/kg/dose × 6.8 kg = 102 mg/dose (note that the "kg" cancel out).
The therapeutic dosage range for this infant is 68 to 102 mg/dose for acetaminophen.

STEP 3: Compare the ordered dose with the therapeutic dosage range calculated in STEP 2.
Answer: The ordered dose of 50 mg is not therapeutic because it falls under the low recommended dose.

If the doctor orders 110 mg of acetaminophen for this infant, would that be a safe and therapeutic dose?
Answer: No, it would neither be safe nor therapeutic because it is higher than 102 mg.

Example 2: The ordered dose is amoxicillin 275 mg q8hr PO. The patient weighs 35 lb. The therapeutic dosage range for amoxicillin is 20 to 40 mg/kg/24 hr in divided doses.

STEP 1: Convert pounds to kilograms by dividing 35 by 2.2.
35/2.2 = 15.9; 35 lb = 15.9 kg

STEP 2: Calculate the therapeutic dosage range for this child based on his weight.
Low dose: 20 mg/kg/24 hr × 15.9 kg = 318 mg/24 hr
High dose: 40 mg/kg/24 hr × 15.9 kg = 636 mg/24 hr
NOTE: These ranges are for 24 hours! The dosage is every 8 hours, so dividing 24 hours by 8 tells us that there will be 3 doses within 24 hours. To figure out the single dosage for the low and high ranges, divide each 24-hour dose by 3:
318 mg/24 hr divided by 3 doses = 106 mg/dose
636 mg/24 hr divided by 3 doses = 212 mg/dose
Answer: The safe range for a single dose of amoxicillin for this child is 106 to 212 mg/dose.
(An alternate way to figure a single dose is to calculate the amount of medication the ordered dose would provide in 24 hours. In this example, knowing there are three doses given every 8 hours in a 24-hour period, multiplying the dose ordered by 3 would yield the ordered dose for 24 hours: 275 mg × 3 doses = 825 mg/24 hr.)

STEP 3: Is the ordered dose of 275 mg therapeutic for this child?

Answer: No, the ordered dose of 275 mg exceeds the therapeutic dosage range for this patient. Consult the physician. (Note also that the calculated 24-hour dose of 825 mg/24 hr exceeds the high range of 636 mg/24 hr calculated for this child.)

Many pediatric medications come in several concentrations. It is ESSENTIAL to use the correct concentration of medication to ensure accurate dosage and prevent accidental underdosage or overdosage.

Example: Acetaminophen comes in many forms, including:

        drops, 80 mg/0.8 mL
        elixir, 160 mg/5 mL
        liquid suspension, 160 mg/5 mL
        chewable tablet, 80 mg/tablet
        tablet, 325 or 500 mg/tablet
        suppository, 80, 120, 325, or 650 mg

A 4-month-old infant weighs 13 lb and has a fever of 101.5° F. What would be the therapeutic dosage range of acetaminophen this infant could receive? The recommended range is 10-15 mg/kg/dose.

STEP 1: 13 lb = 5.9 kg

STEP 2: Low dose: 10 mg/kg/dose × 5.9 = 59 mg/dose
          High dose: 15 mg/kg/dose × 5.9 = 88.5 mg/dose

Answer: The therapeutic dosage range for this infant is 59 to 88.5 mg/dose.

Referring to the forms of acetaminophen listed above, which form would you choose if this infant was to receive a 60-mg dose?

Answer: Choose the drops, 80 mg/0.8 mL, and administer 0.6 mL with a calibrated oral syringe or dropper. (80 mg : 0.8 mL :: 60 mg : x; $x = 0.6$ mL)

STEP 3: Is the ordered dose of 60 mg therapeutic for this infant?

Answer: Yes, the 60 mg dose falls within the 59 to 88.5 mg/dose range for this infant.

Why choose the drops? Remember, you are giving medication to an infant. The infant cannot take tablets; suppositories are not the first choice unless the infant cannot take oral medications, and rectal doses may be a little higher than oral doses. You should choose the medication form that is manufactured for infants and the form that will deliver the dose in an amount that is easily measured yet not too much for the infant to swallow. For example, if you chose the elixir or liquid suspension, 160 mg/5 mL, then you would need to give 2.5 mL. The 0.6 mL would be easier to administer to an infant. **NOTE:** Most liquid medication packages for infants and children have specific instructions for dosing and include the specific dropper to use for measuring liquids.

PRACTICE PROBLEMS

1. Your 6-year-old patient weighs 40 lb. Morphine sulfate via continuous infusion is ordered at 1 mg/hr. The therapeutic dosage range for continuous intravenous infusion is 0.025 to 2.6 mg/kg/hr.
    a. What are the low and high doses for this child?

    _____

    b. Is the ordered dose within a safe and therapeutic range? _____

2. A 5 year old weighs 33 lb. Ibuprofen is ordered at 120 mg PO q8hr. The therapeutic dosage range is 5 to 10 mg/kg/dose q6hr to q8hr, and the maximum dose is 40 mg/kg/24 hr.
    a. What are the low and high doses for this child?

    _____

    b. What is the maximum amount this child can receive in 24 hours? _____

    c. Is the ordered dose within a safe and therapeutic range? _____

3. A 10-year-old patient weighs 70 lb. Fortaz is ordered at 1.7 g q8hr IV. The therapeutic dosage range is 100 to 150 mg/kg/24 hr (divided q8hr IV).
   a. What are the low and high doses for this child in 24 hours? _____
   b. What are the low and high doses for this child per individual dose? _____
   c. Is the ordered dose within a safe and therapeutic range? _____

4. Your patient weighs 15 lb. The medication ordered is 150 mcg bid. The therapeutic dosage range of the medication is 0.02 to 0.05 mg/kg/day.
   a. What are the low and high doses for this child in 24 hours? _____
   b. What are the low and high doses for this child per individual dose? _____
   c. Is the ordered dose within a safe and therapeutic range? _____

5. A child weighs 34 lb. The medication ordered is 30 mg IM preoperatively. The therapeutic dosage range is 1 to 2.2 mg/kg.
   a. What are the low and high doses for this child per individual dose? _____
   b. Is the ordered dose within a safe and therapeutic range? _____

6. For a child weighing 50 lb, medication is ordered at 0.2 mg daily IV. The therapeutic dosage range is 4 to 5 mcg/kg/day.
   a. What are the low and high doses for this child per individual dose? _____
   b. Is the ordered dose within a safe and therapeutic range? _____

SECTION V: BASIC INTRAVENOUS CALCULATIONS

Intravenous (IV) fluids and medications are given over a designated period of time. For instance, the order may read:

Give 1000 mL normal saline over 8 hours IV.

For IVs that infuse with an infusion pump, the milliliters per hour is calculated (mL/hr).
For IVs that infuse by gravity, the rate at which an IV is given is measured in terms of drops per minute (gtt/min). To calculate mL/hr and gtt/min, we need to consider what the order contains and what equipment is used. In order to calculate drops per minute we need to know the drop factor of the IV tubing. The size of the drops delivered per milliliter can vary with different types of tubing. The drop factor of a certain tubing set is printed on the packaging label.
Adding to the above order:

The drop factor for the IV tubing is 15 gtt/mL.

The order now reads:

Give 1000 mL normal saline over 8 hours IV. The drop factor is 15 gtt/mL.

STEP 1: Calculate milliliters per hour.
We know that 1000 mL is to infuse over 8 hours. We want to know how much is to infuse over 1 hour. Set up the equation:

Know   ***Want to Know***
1000 mL : 8 hr :: x mL : 1 hr

$(1000 \times 1) = (8 \times x)$; $1000 = 8x$; $x = 8/1000$; $x = 125$ mL/hr
Rate: To give 1000 mL normal saline over 8 hours, give 125 mL/hr for 8 hours.
A quick way to determine the hourly rate is to divide the TOTAL VOLUME by the TOTAL TIME (if the time is in hours): 1000 mL ÷ 8 hr = 125 mL/hr.

STEP 2: Calculate the gtt/min.
To set up a gravity IV drip, further calculations are needed. To ensure the proper rate, one must count the drops per minute (gtt/min).
We know the rate is 125 mL/hr and the drop factor is 15 gtt/mL. Since we need to change from hours to minutes, another equivalent we'll need is 60 min = 1 hr.

When mL/hr is known, the formula for calculating gtt/min is as follows:

$$\frac{drop\,factor\,(gtt/mL)}{time\,(min)} \times hourly\,rate\,(mL/hr) = gtt/min$$

Plugging in what we know:

$$\frac{15\,gtt/mL*}{60\,min/hr} \times 125/hr = x\,gtt/min$$

*To make it easier to calculate, reduce the 15/60 fraction to 1/4 before multiplying by 125.
$1/4 \times 125 = 125/4 = 31.25$ (round mL/hr to whole numbers)
Answer: 31 gtt/min for a gravity drip

Points to remember:

- The drop factor varies per IV tubing set manufacturer. It can range from 10 to 60 gtt/min.
- Infusion sets that deliver 60 gtt/min are called microdrips.
- **STEP 1:** To calculate mL/hr, divide the TOTAL VOLUME by the TOTAL TIME (in hours).
- **STEP 2:** To calculate gtt/min when the hourly rate is known, use the formula:

$$\frac{drop\,factor\,(gtt/mL)}{time\,(min)} \times hourly\,rate\,(mL/hr) = gtt/min$$

- THINK! If you are using an infusion pump, you need to calculate milliliters per hour.
- THINK! Round off your answer to the nearest whole number. You cannot count a partial drop! Also, electronic infusion pumps will usually use the nearest whole number in mL. (Exceptions to this may occur in critical care or pediatric settings.)

Example 1: The order reads "200 mL to be infused for 1 hr." If the drop factor is 15 gtt/mL, how many gtt/min will be given?
Start at STEP 1 or STEP 2?
Start at STEP 1. You need to know the hourly rate in mL/hr.
STEP 1: Calculate mL/hr. Divide total volume by the total time (in hours).
200 mL over 1 hr = 200 mL/hr.
STEP 2: Calculate gtt/min using the formula:

$$\frac{drop\,factor}{time\,(min)} \times hourly\,rate = 15/60 \times 200 = 1/4 \times 200 = 50$$

Answer: 50 gtt/min

Example 2: The order is for 1000 mL to infuse at 150 mL/hr. The drop factor is 20 gtt/mL. How many gtt/min will be given?
Start at STEP 1 or STEP 2?
Start at STEP 2. The hourly rate, 150 mL/hr, has been given.
STEP 2: Calculate gtt/min using the formula:

$$\frac{drop\,factor}{time\,(min)} \times hourly\,rate = 20/60 \times 150 = 1/3 \times 150 = 50$$

Answer: 50 gtt/min

Example 3: You receive an order for 200 mL to be infused for 90 minutes. You have a microdrip set (60 gtt/mL). How many gtt/min will be given?
Start at STEP 1 or STEP 2?
Start at STEP 1. Calculate the hourly rate. Remember, 60 min = 1 hr.
STEP 1:

Know   **Want to Know**
200 mL : 90 min :: x mL : 60 min

$(200 \times 60) = (90 \times x)$; $12,000 = 90x$; $x = 12,000/90$ $x = 133.33$
Rate: 133 mL/hr (Round to nearest whole number.)
STEP 2: Calculate gtt/min using the formula:

$$\frac{\text{drop factor}}{\text{time (min)}} \times \text{hourly rate} = 60/60 \times 133 = 1 \times 133 = 133$$

Answer: 133 gtt/min
Short cut: For microdrips, when the drip factor is 60 and the time is 60 minutes, the "60s" cancel out to "1" and the result is that the ordered mL/hr = the gtt/min.

PRACTICE PROBLEMS

Calculate the following, and prove your answers.

1. Give 1000 mL lactated Ringer's solution over 6 hours. The drop factor is 15 gtt/mL.
   Start at STEP 1 or STEP 2?
   a. mL/hr: _____
   b. gtt/min: _____

2. Infuse 600 mL blood over 3 hours. The blood administration set has a drop factor of 10 gtt/mL.
   Start at STEP 1 or STEP 2?
   a. mL/hr: _____
   b. gtt/min: _____

3. Infuse 1000 mL normal saline over 12 hours, using tubing with a drop factor of 15 gtt/mL.
   Start at STEP 1 or STEP 2?
   a. mL/hr: _____
   b. gtt/min: _____

4. Infuse 200 mL D_5NS over 2 hours using a microdrip set.
   Start at STEP 1 or STEP 2?
   a. mL/hr: _____
   b. gtt/min: _____
   c. What is the drop factor? _____

5. Infuse D_5W at 75 mL/hr. The drop factor is 10 gtt/mL.
   Start at STEP 1 or STEP 2?
   gtt/min: _____

6. Infuse D_5W at 75 mL/hr. The drop factor is 15 gtt/mL.
   Start at STEP 1 or STEP 2?
   gtt/min: _____

7. Infuse D_5W at 75 mL/hr. The drop factor is 20 gtt/mL.
   Start at STEP 1 or STEP 2?
   gtt/min: _____

8. After looking at your answers for questions 5, 6, and 7, what observation can you make about the relationship between the drop factor and the resulting gtt/min?

9. Give 50 mL of an antibiotic over 30 minutes. You will be using an infusion pump.
   Start at STEP 1 or STEP 2?
   a. mL/hr: _____
   b. gtt/min: _____
   c. Do you need to calculate both mL/hr and gtt/min for this situation? _____

10. Infuse 500 mL normal saline over 4 hours, using tubing with a drop factor of 60 gtt/mL.
    Start at STEP 1 or STEP 2?
    a. mL/hr: _____
    b. gtt/min: _____

PRACTICE QUIZ

Convert the following.

1. 750 mcg = _____ mg

2. 8 g = _____ mg

3. 250 lb = _____ kg

4. 75 kg = _____ lb

5. 3 tsp = _____ mL

6. gr x = _____ mg

Calculate the following, and prove your answers.

7. Dose ordered: indomethacin (oral suspension) 50 mg qid
   Dose on hand: Oral suspension 25 mg/5 mL
   How much would you give per dose? _____

8. Dose ordered: procainamide 0.5 g q4hr PO
   Dose on hand: 500-mg tablets.
   How much would you give per dose? _____

9. Dose ordered: phenytoin 100 mg IV now
   Dose on hand: 5-mL ampule labeled "50 mg/mL"
   How much would you give per dose? _____

10. Dose ordered: lidocaine 50 mg IV now
    Dose on hand: lidocaine 1% in 5-mL ampule
    How much would you give? _____

11. Dose ordered: epinephrine 0.25 mg SC now
    Dose on hand: epinephrine 1:1000 ampule
    How much would you give? _____

12. Dose ordered: heparin 15,000 units IV bolus
    Dose on hand: heparin 10,000 units/mL
    (5-mL vial)
    How much would you give? _____

13. Dose ordered: polythiazide 1 mg PO daily
    Dose on hand: polythiazide 1-mg tablet
    Child's weight: 22 lb
    Therapeutic dosage range: 0.02 to 0.08 mg/kg once daily
    a. What is the safe and therapeutic range for this child? _____
    b. Is the ordered dose safe and therapeutic?
    _____

14. Ordered: Infuse normal saline 500 mL over 8 hours. The tubing drop factor is 15.
    a. What is the rate of the IV? _____
    b. What is the gtt/min? _____

15. Ordered: $D_5\frac{1}{2}NS$ to infuse at 50 mL/hr via an infusion pump.
    a. How will this be administered—mL/hr or gtt/min? _____
    b. What is the rate? _____

16. Ordered: 1000 mL D_5W to infuse over 24 hours. The tubing drop factor is 60.
    a. What is the rate of the IV? _____
    b. What is the gtt/min? _____

17. Ordered: MEDICATION 500 mg IVPB q6hr.
    Dose on hand: MEDICATION powder for injection (See label.)

1-g vial
MEDICATION
Add 5 mL sterile water for injection.
Solution will contain 200 mg/mL.

    a. How much does this vial contain?
    _____
    b. How much will you give for each dose?
    _____

18. Ordered: penicillin G 200,000 units IM qid
    Dose on hand: penicillin G 5,000,000 units
    The medication label reads:

FIVE MILLION UNITS multidose vial Penicillin G	
Use sterile saline as diluent as follows:	
	Units per mL
Add	reconstituted solution
23 mL	200,000
18 mL	250,000
8 mL	500,000
3 mL	1,000,000

    a. What concentration should you choose?
    _____
    b. How much sterile saline should you add to the vial to obtain this concentration?
    _____
    c. How much medication will you give?
    _____
    d. How do you label the vial? _____

19. A child weighs 31 lb.
    Dose ordered: ceftriaxone sodium 600 mg IV q12hr
    Dose on hand: See label.
    Maximum safe dose: Up to 100 mg/kg/day in two divided doses

    ```
    1 g
    ceftriaxone sodium
    DIRECTIONS: Add 9.6 mL sterile water
    for injection to equal 100 mg/mL.
    ```

    a. How much would you give for this dose? _____

    b. What is the maximum safe dose for this child (in 24 hours)? _____

    c. What is the maximum safe dose for this child (per dose)? _____

    d. Is the ordered dose within a safe and therapeutic range? _____

20. Dose ordered: digoxin 125 mcg daily
    Dose on hand: Pediatric elixir 0.05 mg/mL
    How much would you give? _____

Answers

WORKSHEETS

CHAPTER 1
The Nursing Process and Drug Therapy

Chapter Review/Critical Thinking and Application

1. a
2. d
3. c
4. b
5. a
6. b
7. S, O, O, O, S, S
8. Answers may vary slightly with each one but should include the following:
   - *Right drug:* Compare drug orders and medication labels. Consider whether the drug is appropriate for that patient. Obtain information about the patient's medical history and a thorough, updated medication history, including over-the-counter medications taken.
   - *Right dose:* Check the order and the label on the medication, and check for all of the Five Rights at least three times before administering the medication. Recheck the math calculations for dosages and contact the physician when clarification is needed.
   - *Right time:* Assess for a conflict between the pharmacokinetic and pharmacodynamic properties of the drugs prescribed and the patient's lifestyle and likelihood of compliance.
   - *Right route:* Never assume the route of administration or change it; always check with the physician or prescriber.
   - *Right patient:* Check the patient's identity before administering a medication. Ask for the patient's name, and check the identification band or bracelet to confirm the patient's name, identification
   - number, age, and allergies.
9. a. assessment
   b. objective
   c. subjective
   d. analyze
   e. goals

f. outcome criteria
g. implementation
h. evaluation
10. Answers may vary. Several additional rights are discussed in the Implementation section. These rights cover aspects of implementation such as ensuring safety, calculating dosages correctly, ensuring accuracy in drug transcription, and so on.

Case Study

1. See the discussion in Chapter 1 under Assessment. Important points include the following:
   - Use of prescription and over-the-counter medications
   - Use of home remedies, herbal treatments, vitamins
   - Intake of alcohol, tobacco, caffeine
   - Current or prior use of street drugs
   - Health history
   - Family history
   - Allergies
2. Answers will vary but may include the following:
   - Activity intolerance
   - Acute pain
   - Anxiety
   - Deficient knowledge
   - Fatigue
   - Ineffective breathing pattern
   - Ineffective health maintenance
   - Ineffective therapeutic regimen management
   - Noncompliance
   - Risk for aspiration
   - Risk for injury
   - Risk for falls

   Prioritization will depend on the nursing diagnoses chosen but should be developed with the patient's input.
3. The medication order is missing the *route* of delivery and the *dose* amount. You should contact the physician to clarify the incomplete order.
4. Once again, you should contact the physician and never change the medication route without an order.
5. After administering any drug, the nurse should evaluate the patient's response to the drug therapy. In this case, monitoring intake and output, monitoring vital signs, and watching for postural hypotension would be important.

CHAPTER 2
Pharmacologic Principles

Chapter Review/Critical Thinking and Application

1. 1 = c; 2 = d; 3 = a; 4 = b.
2. c
3. b
4. d
5. a
6. c
7. b
8. i
9. j
10. f
11. g
12. a
13. d
14. e
15. c
16. Because muscles have a greater blood supply than the skin, drugs injected intramuscularly are typically absorbed faster than those injected subcutaneously. Absorption can be increased by applying heat to the injection site or by massaging it, which increases the blood flow to the area and thus enhances absorption.
17. This is an example of palliative therapy—drug therapy that is not curative but is intended to make the patient as comfortable as possible.

Case Study

1. Half-life is the time it takes for one half of the original amount of a drug in the body to be eliminated and is a measure of the rate at which drugs are excreted by the body. If the half-life is 2 hours, then in this example the drug levels would be as follows:
   4 PM = 200 mg/L
   6 PM = 100 mg/L
   8 PM = 50 mg/L
   10 PM = 25 mg/L
2. a. He has nausea and vomiting and cannot take medications by mouth. His medications will need to be given parenterally.
   b. Because of his decreased serum albumin level, lesser amount of drugs that are usually protein bound will be bound to protein, and as a result, more free drug will be circulating and the duration of drug action may be increased. In addition, his heart failure may result in decreased cardiac output and thus decreased distribution.
   c. His liver failure will result in decreased metabolism of drugs.
   d. Because his liver may not be able to effectively metabolize drugs and convert them to water-soluble compounds, excretion through the kidneys may be decreased.
3. This situation illustrates prophylactic therapy to *prevent* illness or other undesirable outcome. Prophylactic intravenous antibiotic therapy may be used to prevent infection during a high-risk surgery or procedure, such as placement of the peripherally inserted central catheter.
4. Therapeutic index is the ratio between the toxic and therapeutic concentrations of a drug. A low therapeutic index means that the difference between a therapeutically active dose and a toxic dose is small. As a result, the drug has a greater likelihood of causing an adverse reaction. The nurse should monitor the patient's response carefully when a drug has a low therapeutic index.

CHAPTER 3
Life Span Considerations

Chapter Review/Critical Thinking and Application

1. c
2. a
3. d
4. b
5. b, c, d
6. d
7. b
8. e
9. a
10. c
11. Keep in mind that elderly patients take a greater proportion of both prescription and over-the-counter (OTC) medications, and they commonly take multiple medications on a daily basis. In addition, the elderly also have more chronic diseases than younger people. They may see several different specialists, each of whom may each prescribe his or her own set of medications. In addition, some patients self-administer OTC products to ease the discomfort of even more ailments. This use of multiple mediations is called *polypharmacy*.
12. Drawing on the information in the box Life Span Considerations: The Elderly Patient— Pharmacokinetic Changes, students may describe a variety of physiologic changes affecting the cardiovascular, gastrointestinal, hepatic, and renal systems.

Case Study

1. Children and teenagers should not take aspirin to treat chickenpox or flulike symptoms because Reye's syndrome, a rare but serious illness, has been associated with aspirin use at these ages. It is important to check for precautions when giving any medication to children.
2. If the toddler does not like or cannot take pills, have the parent ask the pharmacist for a liquid form of the medication, which may be flavored and better accepted by the child than a pill.
3. The most common dosage calculation method for children is the milligrams per kilogram formula. However, for OTC preparations, the manufacturer will convert kilograms to pounds to make dosing by the parents easier.
4. The 5-year-old child received 240 mg (at 160 mg/tsp, 1.5 tsp = 240 mg).
5. The parents should monitor the children's fever—the expected response is that the fever will go down. In addition, because the medication also has analgesic effects, signs of discomfort may decrease. The parents should also monitor for any adverse effects of the medication or worsening of the child's illness.

CHAPTER 4
Cultural, Legal, and Ethical Considerations

Chapter Review/Critical Thinking and Application

1. b
2. a
3. d
4. c
5. b
6. d
7. d
8. a
9. c
10. b
11. c
12. a
13. d
14. b
15. Answers will vary depending on the group identified.
    a. Barriers may include language, poverty, access, pride, and beliefs regarding medical practices.
    b. Attitudes will vary depending on the group identified.
    c. Questions may include the following topics: health beliefs and practices, past use of medicine, folk remedies, home remedies, use of over-the-counter drugs and treatments,

usual responses to illness, responsiveness to medical treatments, religious practices and beliefs, and dietary habits.

Case Study

1. You should not give the drugs until it is established that the study has been reviewed by an institutional review board and that the patient has given informed consent. As a professional, the nurse has the responsibility to provide safe nursing care, and it is within the nurse's realm of practice to provide information and assist the patient in facing decisions regarding health care. The nurse also has the right to refuse to participate in any treatment or aspect of a patient's care that violates personal ethical principles.
2. Principles include the following:
    • Autonomy—the patient's right to self-determination. The nurse supports this by ensuring informed consent.
    • Beneficence—the duty to do good. Will the patient be best served by this course of action?
    • Nonmaleficence—the duty to do no harm.
    • Veracity—the duty to tell the truth, especially with regard to investigational new drugs and informed consent.
3. Some patients believe strongly in using home remedies instead of medications. You should assess and consider health beliefs and practices at the beginning of the therapeutic relationship.
4. The issue of confidentiality should be discussed. The researchers have a duty to respect privileged information about a patient. Measures that the researchers will use to ensure the confidentiality of participants should be discussed.

CHAPTER 5
Medication Errors: Preventing and Responding

Chapter Review/Critical Thinking and Application

1. medication error
2. idiosyncratic
3. side effect
4. adverse drug reaction (ADR)
5. adverse drug event (ADE)
6. True
7. False
8. To avoid medication errors: Follow the Five Rights! Carefully read all drug labels and confirm the Five Rights of medication administration. Repeat a verbal order and spell the drug name out loud. Never assume a route of administration; if an order is unclear or incomplete, clarify the order with the prescriber. Always read the label three times and

check the medication order before administering the medication. See text for other possible answers.

9. Refer to Box 5-1. Antibiotics; anticoagulants; antidiabetic drugs, particularly insulin; antineoplastic drugs; cardiovascular drugs; central nervous system–active drugs; vaccines.

10. digoxin 125 micrograms PO now
Lasix 40 mg IV daily
Discontinue all meds
NPH insulin 12 units SQ with breakfast daily
Floxin otic 1 drop right ear bid
levothyroxine 125 micrograms every morning

Case Study

1. The nursing student should immediately inform her instructor of the error. Then together they should monitor the patient's response and follow the institution's procedure for reporting a medication error. Reporting medication errors is a professional and ethical responsibility.

2. By checking the Five Rights before giving this medication. In this situation, she missed the right dose. In addition, if the student had understood the rationale for the medication (i.e., the low dose needed for antiplatelet therapy), then she may have avoided this error. One must be knowledgeable about medications and the rationale for their use in a particular patient before administering them.

3. According to Chapter 5, the recommendation is that the patient be told of the error both as ethical practice and because of the legal implications.

4. Yes. A medication error is defined as "any preventable adverse drug event involving inappropriate medication use by a patient or health care professional"; it may or may not cause harm to the patient.

5. The U.S. Pharmacopeia Medication Errors Reporting Program (USPMERP) exists to gather and disseminate safety information regarding medications. By reporting this error, the student contributes to the USPMERP database of medication errors and their causes. This service is confidential.

CHAPTER 6
Patient Education and Drug Therapy

Critical Thinking and Application

1. Refer to the information in Chapter 24 for specific information about antihypertensive drug therapy. In addition, Table 6-1 provides information relevant to the development of teaching strategies for the 78-year-old patient.

2. Refer to Box 6-2. Ideally, a health care professional who speaks the mother's language

should do the teaching. Some strategies include using pictures and illustrations, demonstrating by example, and finding an interpreter. In addition, the patient should be provided with detailed written instructions in her native language.

3. a. Answers will vary, but this nursing diagnosis should address deficient knowledge.
   b. Answers will vary, but this nursing diagnosis should address noncompliance.

4. Answers will vary, depending on the type of medication. Refer to the appropriate chapters for specific patient and family teaching and possible goals and expected outcomes.

5. Teaching plans will vary somewhat in format, but each should contain the following information:
   a. Some of the assessment items listed in the text in the section Assessment of Learning Needs Related to Drug Therapy.
   b. Deficient knowledge.
   c. A measurable goal with outcome criteria related to the nursing diagnosis.
   d. Specific educational strategies for providing the information needed.
   e. Specific questions designed to validate whether learning has occurred.

Case Study

1. Both "Deficient knowledge" and "Noncompliance" are possible answers. In this case, "Deficient knowledge" is probably the most correct, because this nursing diagnosis exists when the patient has a lack of or limited understanding about his or her medications. For example, nitroglycerin tablets should not be stored in one's pants pockets because the body heat may destroy the active compounds in the tablets. In addition, the patient was not aware of the importance of not missing doses of antihypertensive medication. Noncompliance exists when the patient does not take the medication as directed or at all, and the data collected indicate that the patient's condition has reoccurred or has not resolved. In this case, his blood pressure has improved from previous readings, despite what he has said about taking his medications.

2. Answers may vary. A goal for the nursing diagnosis of "Deficient knowledge" in this case may be the following: "The patient self-administers his prescribed medications on schedule without missing doses." Outcome criteria may include the following: "The patient is able to describe the schedule of medications that are ordered. The patient is able to state the rationale for consistent dosing of antihypertensive medications. The patient is able to state the proper storage and administration of sublingual nitroglycerin tablets. The patient is able

to identify potential side effects of the prescribed medications and knows when to report them."

3. Again, answers may vary. Refer to Box 6-2. Suggestions include the following:
   - A teaching session regarding medication administration should be held with both the patient and his wife in attendance. If necessary, find out whether they have any children or neighbors nearby who may be able to assist with medications as needed.
   - Assist the patient in developing a daily time calendar for taking the medications prescribed.
   - Suggest the use of a daily or weekly pill container that can assist in reminding when doses are due. If necessary, a neighbor or the patient's son or daughter can come over periodically to fill this container.
   - Discuss and provide written literature on the purposes and side effects of each medication ordered and on other important issues regarding these medications.

4. Confirm whether learning has occurred by asking the patient and his wife questions related to the teaching session. Assess their understanding of the time calendar and the concept of using pill containers. Follow-up can be accomplished via telephone as needed, and a return visit to review medications can be scheduled. In addition, the patient must keep return appointments to the office so that the therapeutic outcomes of the drug therapy (i.e., blood pressure readings) can be measured.

CHAPTER 7
Over-the-Counter Drugs and Herbal and Dietary Supplements

Double Puzzle

Valerian
Garlic
Feverfew
St. John's wort
Ginkgo
Saw palmetto
Ginseng
Echinacea
Aloe
Goldenseal
Herbal therapy

Chapter Review/Critical Thinking and Application

1. a, b, d, f
2. d
3. d
4. b
5. c

6. Garlic, ginger, ginkgo, flaxseed, glucosamine and chondroitin.
7. Elderly adults; children; patients with single and/or multiple acute and chronic illnesses; patients who are frail or in poor health; patients who are debilitated and nutritionally deficient; patients who are immunocompromised. In addition, those who have a history of renal, hepatic, cardiac, or vascular disorders may have problems with over-the-counter (OTC) medications.
8. Contraindications to use of herbal products include renal, liver, or cardiac disorders; platelet or clotting disorders; stroke or cerebral bleeding of any type; hypertension; peptic ulcers; gastrointestinal bleeding; and any other type of abnormal bleeding. Specific contraindications exist for specific herbal products; see the text for more information.
9. Answers will vary.

Case Study

1. The aspirin and garlic tablets may interfere with platelet and clotting functions. If the wine is taken with the kava and/or valerian, central nervous system depression may occur.
2. The Food and Drug Administration (FDA) has recently issued a warning about the use of kava and possible liver toxicity. Also, tachyphylaxis may develop in patients who use echinacea for longer than 8 weeks.
3. Because she is trying to conceive, she needs to consider the fact that the herbal drugs have not been tested or proved safe for use in pregnancy. Also, aspirin use is contraindicated in pregnancy because of its antiplatelet effects.
4. Herbal products are not required by the FDA to be proven safe or effective. They are classified as dietary supplements and are not subject to the same rules as are drugs. Therefore, the patient must receive adequate information about the herbal products, including their risks, side effects, and possible benefits.
5. Many patients believe that if a product is "natural" then it is safe. Each product should be discussed with the patient, and the patient should be instructed about possible contraindications, safe use, frequency of dosing, specifics about how to take the product, and the way to monitor for both therapeutic effects and complications or toxic effects.

CHAPTER 8
Substance Abuse

Chapter Review/Critical Thinking and Application

1. h
2. i
3. f

4. e
5. g
6. d
7. j
8. a
9. c
10. b
11. c
12. d
13. b, c, e
14. c
15. b
16. The nicotine transdermal system (patch) and nicotine polacrilex (gum) can be used to supply nicotine without the carcinogens in tobacco. The patches provide a stepwise reduction in delivery and work by gradually reducing the nicotine dose over time. With the gum, rapid chewing releases an immediate dose of nicotine, but this dose is about half of what the average smoker receives from one cigarette, and the onset of action is longer than with smoking. Therefore, the reinforcement and self-reward effects of smoking are minimized. Zyban is a sustained-release form of the antidepressant bupropion and is the first nicotine-free prescription medicine used to treat nicotine dependence.
17. For all three levels of ethanol withdrawal, benzodiazepines such as diazepam (Valium), lorazepam (Ativan), and chlordiazepoxide (Librium) are used in various doses and frequencies. The doses are lower for "mild" withdrawal; for "moderate" ethanol withdrawal, higher doses of the benzodiazepines are used and dosage is tapered over 5 days as needed. For "severe" withdrawal, also known as *delirium tremens,* the dosages of diazepam, lorazepam, or chlordiazepoxide are at their highest until the patient's agitation has subsided. In addition, thiamine injections may be given.

Case Study

1. Ethanol causes central nervous system depression.
2. Acute severe alcoholic intoxication may cause cardiovascular depression, and long-term excessive use has largely irreversible effects on the heart. Moderate amounts may either stimulate or depress respiration, but large amounts produce lethal respiratory depression.
3. First, the nurse should monitor the patient's respiratory and cardiovascular status and prevent injury from falling or aspiration from vomiting. In addition, the nurse should be alert to the patient's behavior and mental status to identify changes in his condition. Withdrawal from alcohol can lead to serious conditions such as delirium

tremens (see question 4). Careful assessment of vital signs and mental status is imperative at this time, because early withdrawal symptoms may be an increase in blood pressure and pulse with an altered mental status.
4. Mr. C. should stay in the hospital for observation for and possible treatment of delirium tremens, which may begin with tremors and agitation and progress to hallucinations and sometimes death. See Box 8-6 for information on treatment of ethanol withdrawal.
5. Chronic excessive ingestion of ethanol is directly associated with several serious mental and neurologic disorders. Nutritional and vitamin B deficiencies can occur, which result in conditions such as Wernicke's encephalopathy, Korsakoff's psychosis, polyneuritis, and nicotinic acid deficiency encephalopathy. Seizures may also occur. In addition, long-term ingestion of ethanol may result in alcoholic hepatitis or liver cirrhosis.

CHAPTER 9
Photo Atlas of Drug Administration

Chapter Review/Critical Thinking and Application

1. b
2. c
3. a
4. b
5. c
6. c
7. b
8. a
9. c
10. a
11. b
12. d
13. b
14. a
15. a, b, c, e
16. a. Palpate sites for masses or tenderness, and assess the amount of subcutaneous tissue.
    b. Note the integrity and size of the muscle and palpate for tenderness.
    c. Note any lesions or discoloration of the forearm.
17. See the descriptions under Figure 9-37 for each type of injection.
18. Remove the needle and ensure that the site is not bleeding. Discard the medication and syringe, draw up new medication, and repeat the procedure in a different location.
19. Rather than pouring it into a medication cup, draw small volumes of liquid medications into a calibrated oral syringe.

20. 250 divided by 4 (4 puffs/day) would equal 62.5 days.

Case Study

1. For the adult, the ventrogluteal site is the preferred injection site. If the woman is of average size, choose a needle that is 1½ inches long and 21 to 25 gauge and insert the needle at a 90-degree angle. For the infant, the preferred site is the vastus lateralis site. The needle should be of the correct length to ensure that it reaches muscle tissue, not the subcutaneous layer.

2. For an infant or child younger than 3 years of age, the pinna of the ear should be pulled down and back before the drops are administered. The drops should be directed along the sides of the ear rather than directly onto the eardrum. The drops should be taken out of refrigeration about 30 minutes before administering them. The mother should stay with her child and ensure that she lies on her side for 5 to 10 minutes. Gentle massage of the tragus area of the ear with her finger will help distribute the medication down the ear canal.

3. Liquid medication doses under 5 mL should be drawn up in a calibrated oral syringe.

4. Liquids are usually ordered because infants cannot swallow pills or capsules. A plastic disposable oral dosing syringe is recommended for measuring small doses of liquid medications. Position the infant so that the head is slightly elevated. Place the plastic dropper or syringe inside the infant's mouth, beside the tongue, and administer the liquid in small amounts while allowing the infant to swallow each time. Take great care to prevent aspiration. A crying infant can easily aspirate medication. Do not add the medication to a bottle of formula. The infant may refuse the feeding or may not drink all of the bottle and, as a result, would not get the entire dosage of medication.

CHAPTER 10
Analgesic Drugs

Critical Thinking Crossword

Across
2. Agonist
6. Superficial
7. Pain tolerance
10. Threshold
12. Opioid
13. Partial
14. Abstinence

Down
1. Antagonist
3. Chronic
4. Visceral
5. Opiate
6. Somatic
8. Acute
9. Compulsive
11. Adjuvant

Chapter Review

1. b
2. d
3. c
4. d
5. b, c, e
6. g
7. f
8. i
9. h
10. d
11. b
12. j
13. c
14. a
15. e

Case Study

1. Superficial pain, which originates from the skin or mucous membranes.

2. A back rub. Massage to the affected area often decreases the pain. When an area is rubbed or liniment is applied, large sensory fibers from peripheral receptors carry impulses to the spinal cord. This causes impulse transmission to be inhibited and the gate to be closed. This in turn reduces recognition of the pain impulses arriving by means of the small fibers. This is the same pathway that the opioid analgesics use to alleviate pain.

3. All opioids cause some histamine release. It is thought that this histamine release is responsible for many of the unwanted side effects, such as itching.

4. The most serious side effect of opioids is central nervous system depression, which may lead to respiratory depression. Naloxone (Narcan), an opioid reversal drug, may have to be administered to reverse severe respiratory depression.

5. The use of a nonopioid analgesic with an opioid is known as adjuvant analgesic therapy. This allows the use of smaller doses of opioids, which accomplishes two important functions. First, it diminishes some of the side effects that are seen with higher doses of opioids, such as respiratory depression, constipation, and urinary retention. Second, it

approaches the pain stimulus by another mechanism of action and has a resulting synergistic beneficial effect in reducing the pain.

CHAPTER 11
General and Local Anesthetics

Critical Thinking Crossword

Across
3. Pancuronium
6. General
7. Topical
8. Adjunctive
9. Local

Down
1. Atropine
2. Anesthetics
3. Parenteral
4. Balanced
5. Regional

Chapter Review/Critical Thinking and Application

1. a, c, e
2. b
3. a
4. b
5. b, c, e
6. c
7. 1 = c; 2 = a; 3 = b
8. Pediatric patients are more susceptible to problems such as central nervous system depression, toxicity, atelectasis, pneumonia, and cardiac abnormalities because their hepatic, cardiac, respiratory, and renal systems are not fully developed or fully functional.
9. These drugs cause paralysis but not sedation. The patient is still able to hear you and feel your touch. It is important to remain professional at all times and to take the time to reassure the patient and orient him to his surroundings, to what noises mean, and to what you are going to be doing to him.
10. She will be given a combination of intravenous medications that will produce analgesia and also amnesia of the procedure, but she will still be alert enough to breathe on her own and follow verbal directions as needed. In some cases, local anesthesia will be used to enhance patient comfort. This type of sedation is called *moderate sedation;* it is associated with fewer complications than general anesthesia and a shorter recovery time.

Case Study

1. In balanced anesthesia, minimal doses of a combination of anesthetic drugs (both intravenous and inhaled) are given to achieve the desired level of anesthesia for the surgical procedure. Adjunctive drugs may also be used and commonly include sedative-hypnotics, narcotics, and neuromuscular blocking drugs (NMBAs) (depolarizing drug such as succinylcholine and the nondepolarizing or competitive drugs such as pancuronium or d-tubocurarine). Combining several different drugs makes it possible for general anesthesia to be accomplished with smaller amounts of anesthetic gases and thereby reduces the side effects.
2. The main therapeutic use of the NMBA succinylcholine is to maintain controlled ventilation during surgical procedures. When respiratory muscles are paralyzed by NMBAs, mechanical ventilation is easier because the body's drive to control respirations is eliminated by the drug; this allows the ventilator to have total control of the respirations.
3. Multiple medical conditions (listed in Box 11-4) can predispose an individual to toxicity. These conditions increase the sensitivity of an individual to NMBAs and prolong their effects. Because the patient's temperature has decreased, hypothermia may lead to an increased sensitivity to the medication. In addition, the history of paraplegia is another condition that may predispose this patient to toxicity.
4. Anticholinesterase drugs such as neostigmine, pyridostigmine, and edrophonium are antidotes and are used to reverse muscle paralysis.
5. Local anesthesia is most commonly used in settings in which loss of consciousness, whole-body relaxation, and loss of unresponsiveness are either unnecessary or unwanted. A lower incidence of toxic effects is associated with the use of local anesthetics, because very little of these drugs is absorbed systemically.
6. Regardless of the type of anesthesia a patient is receiving, one of the most important nursing considerations during this time is close and frequent observation of the patient and all body systems, with specific attention to the ABCs of nursing care (*a*irway, *b*reathing, and *c*irculation) and vital signs. Resuscitative equipment, as well as any drug antidote, should be kept nearby in case of cardiorespiratory distress or arrest. Other nursing actions include monitoring all aspects of body functions (including attention to the ABCs of care), instituting safety measures, and implementing the physician's orders.

CHAPTER 12
Central Nervous System Depressants and Muscle Relaxants

Chapter Review/Critical Thinking and Application

1. a
2. b
3. a
4. d
5. c
6. d
7. Answers should reflect the discussion under Toxicity and Management of Overdose in the textbook. The priority of care would be to maintain the ABCs (*a*irway, *b*reathing, and *c*irculation), especially respirations, because respiratory depression is likely.
8. These drugs can be taken for insomnia only if their use is limited to the short term (less than 2 to 4 weeks). With long-term use, rebound insomnia and severe withdrawal can develop. If Jackie needs to take something to help her sleep while she is on her trip, the nonbenzodiazepine hypnotics may be an option; and, of course, you could provide patient teaching on nonpharmacologic methods to aid sleep.
9. Elderly patients should be started on lower dosages because they generally experience a more pronounced effect from benzodiazepines.
10. a. Ask about allergies, central nervous system (CNS) disorders, sleep disorders, diabetes, addictive disorders, personality disorders, thyroid conditions, and renal and liver function.
    b. Alcohol and CNS depressants, but also all prescribed or over-the-counter medications
    c. The patient's age matters, because these drugs have increased effects in elderly persons and small children.
11. a. Patient teaching should include information about potential side effects and potential drug interactions. In addition, safety measures to prevent injury stemming from decreased sensorium must be emphasized.
    b. These medications are most effective when used in conjunction with rest and physical therapy.
12. Tachyphylaxis is the rapid appearance of a progressive decrease in response to a pharmacologically or physiologically active substance after its repetitive administration. Chloral hydrate, an older nonbarbiturate sedative-hypnotic drug, has this characteristic. The occurrence of tachyphylaxis is a disadvantage because it makes the drug useful for only short-term therapy.

Case Study

1. Barbiturates are considered controlled substances because of the potential for misuse and the severe effects that result if they are not used appropriately. Other hypnotic drugs are now used more frequently than barbiturates because they have fewer side effects and are safer than the older barbiturates. They also do not suppress rapid eye movement (REM) sleep to the same extent as do barbiturates.
2. Barbiturates deprive people of REM sleep (dreaming sleep), and long-term use can result in agitation and inability to deal with normal stress. In addition, when the barbiturate is stopped, the returning REM sleep may be more intense than before and lead to nightmares (a rebound effect). Barbiturates are habit forming, they have a low therapeutic index, and severe withdrawal effects may occur when the medication is stopped. Other drugs have been shown to be safer to use for treatment of insomnia.
3. Other CNS depressants, especially alcohol, should be avoided. There may also be an additive effect when the herbal product valerian is taken.
4. Zaleplon is indicated for the short-term treatment of insomnia and has been shown to be effective for up to 5 weeks. It has a very short half-life, so the patient should be taught that if sleep difficulties include early awakenings, a dose can be taken as long as it is at least 4 hours before the patient must arise. In addition, the patient should explore other nonpharmacologic options for the treatment of insomnia and try to find the cause of the sleep problems. See Box 12-1 for information on nonpharmacologic measures to promote sleep.

CHAPTER 13
Antiepileptic Drugs

Critical Thinking Crossword

Across
2. Emergency
6. Primary
10. Hepatotoxicity
11. Seizure
12. Slowly

Down
1. Secondary
3. Convulsion
4. Benzodiazepines
5. Idiopathic
6. Phenobarbital
7. Autoinduction
8. Epilepsy
9. Phenytoin

Chapter Review/Critical Thinking and Application

1. d
2. a
3. b, c, d
4. c
5. b
6. c
7. Carbamazepine undergoes autoinduction, the process by which the metabolism of a drug increases over time, which leads to lower than expected drug concentrations.
8. Jeremy's mother should be told that topiramate should be taken whole and should not be crushed, broken in half, or chewed. It does have a very bitter taste and seems to be better tolerated when taken with food. She can still give it with gelatin, as long as the dosage form remains whole.

Case Study

1. Generalized seizures, more specifically, absence seizures. These are most often seen in children.
2. The succinimide ethosuximide (Zarontin) is indicated for treatment of absence seizures in children. See Table 13-1.
3. She needs to be sure to measure the dose carefully with an exact graduated device or oral syringe, rather than using a household teaspoon, and to give the medication at the same time daily. She should report excessive sedation, confusion, lethargy, or decreased movement. See Patient Teaching Tips for more information.
4. She should be encouraged to keep a journal to record Mattie's signs and symptoms before, during, and after any seizure activity to measure the therapeutic effectiveness of the medication.
5. A therapeutic response to antiepileptic drugs does not mean that the patient has been cured of the seizures but only that seizure activity is decreased or absent. Further evaluation will be needed before a decision is made to stop the medication. Treatment may need to last for years or may be lifelong.

CHAPTER 14
Antiparkinsonian Drugs

Chapter Review/Critical Thinking and Application

1. b
2. a
3. c
4. c
5. a, c
6. d

7. a. Dopamine must be given in this form because exogenously administered dopamine cannot pass through the blood-brain barrier; levodopa can.
   b. The addition of carbidopa avoids the high peripheral levels of dopamine and unwanted side effects induced by the very large dosages of levodopa necessary when the drug is given alone.
   c. Carbidopa does not cross the blood-brain barrier and thus prevents levodopa breakdown in the periphery. This, in turn, allows levodopa to reach and cross the blood-brain barrier. Once in the brain, the levodopa is then broken down to dopamine, which can be used directly.
8. You must ask whether Mrs. Reynolds is lactating; if so, use of amantadine is contraindicated.
9. Elderly patients, especially men with benign prostatic hypertrophy, are at risk for urinary retention. Jane's neighbor may or may not have that condition, but his age is a major factor. Jane's age is not a concern at this time. This drug may also cause palpitations.

Case Study

1. The primary cause of Parkinson's disease is an imbalance in the two neurotransmitters dopamine and acetylcholine (ACh) in the basal ganglia of the brain. This imbalance is caused by a failure of the nerve terminals in the substantia nigra to produce dopamine, which acts in the basal ganglia to control body movements. A correct balance between dopamine and ACh is needed for the proper regulation of posture, muscle tone, and voluntary movement. The deficiency of dopamine can also lead to excessive ACh activity because of the lack of dopamine's normal balancing effect. Symptoms of Parkinson's disease do not appear until approximately 80% of the dopamine store in the substantia nigra of the basal ganglia has been depleted.
2. Drug therapy is aimed at increasing the levels of dopamine at the remaining functioning nerve terminals. It is also aimed at blocking the effects of ACh and slowing the progression of the disease.
3. Amantadine causes the release of dopamine from nerve endings that are still intact. The result is higher levels of dopamine in the central nervous system.
4. It is most effective in the early stages of Parkinson's disease, but as the disease progresses and the number of functioning nerves diminishes, amantadine's effect is also reduced. The drug is usually effective for only 6 to 12 months.
5. Patients with Parkinson's disease often experience rapid swings in response to levodopa; this fluctuating response is known as the "on-off phenomenon."

This phenomenon is seen in patients who take levodopa for a long time. Such patients may experience periods when they have good control ("on" time) and periods when they have bad control or break-through Parkinson's disease ("off" time). Carbidopa is a peripheral decarboxylase inhibitor that does not cross the blood-brain barrier. As a result, carbidopa is able to prevent levodopa from breaking down in the periphery and allows more levodopa to reach and cross the blood-brain barrier. Levodopa-carbidopa combinations, such as Sinemet CR, may help decrease the "off" time.

CHAPTER 15
Psychotherapeutic Drugs

Chapter Review/Critical Thinking and Application

1. c
2. a
3. c
4. a, c, d
5. d
6. m
7. g
8. h
9. o
10. b
11. j
12. k
13. l
14. c
15. n
16. a
17. d
18. i
19. f
20. e
21. a. If Carl is taking a benzodiazepine for his anxiety and drinking alcohol, he is probably experiencing benzodiazepine toxicity or overdose.
    b. If ingestion is recent, Carl might be treated with gastric lavage. He might also be given flumazenil (Romazicon) to reverse the effect of the benzodiazepine overdose.
22. a. Mr. Delvini needs to be aware of the foods and drinks, including red wine, that he can no longer have because they contain tyramine.
    b. It appears that Mr. Delvini may have inadvertently ingested something containing tyramine, which has caused a hypertensive crisis.
23. Second-generation antidepressants offer an advantage over other antidepressants because they have fewer and less severe side effects.

24. If the antidepressant taken is a first-generation antidepressant, or tricyclic, excessive dosages could result in lethal cardiac dysrhythmias as well as seizures. These dysrhythmias are responsible for most of the deaths due to overdoses.

Case Study

1. See Table 15-3 for potential side effects and adverse effects of benzodiazepines. Most are related to their effects on the central nervous system. Patient teaching includes warning the patient to avoid driving or operating heavy equipment or machinery until he becomes accustomed to the side effects of the medication. In addition, measures should be taken to avoid orthostatic hypotension. Finally, he should avoid alcohol and other central nervous system depressants while taking this medication.
2. If he is experiencing life-altering anxiety, then he should also consider obtaining psychotherapy to assist him at this time.
3. Benzodiazepines are potentially habit forming and addictive, with possible withdrawal symptoms such as anxiety, panic attacks, convulsions, nausea, and vomiting. The medication should not be withdrawn abruptly. Patients should always be advised to take the medication as directed and never to stop taking the medicine abruptly. Benzodiazepines should be withdrawn gradually.
4. There is a potential for benzodiazepines to cause serious life-threatening toxicities, but when taken alone in normal dosages in otherwise healthy patients, they are very safe and effective anxiolytics. When they are taken with other sedating medications or with alcohol, however, life-threatening respiratory depression or arrest can occur. An overdose of benzodiazepines may result in one or more of the following symptoms: somnolence, confusion, coma, and respiratory depression. Overdose may be treated with gastric lavage and/or administration of activated charcoal and saline laxative. The benzodiazepine-specific antidote flumazenil may be used in severe cases.
5. Buspirone has the advantages of being both nonsedating and non–habit forming compared with the benzodiazepines.

CHAPTER 16
Central Nervous System Stimulants and Related Drugs

Chapter Review/Critical Thinking and Application

1. b
2. b, c, e
3. a
4. c

5. d
6. b
7. a. Stacey has narcolepsy.
   b. Methylphenidate, an amphetamine, or modanafil, a nonamphetamine, may be ordered.
   c. These drugs boost mental alertness, increase motor activity, and diminish the patient's sense of fatigue by stimulating the cerebral cortex and possibly the reticular activating system.
   d. (1) She should take her medication exactly as her physician prescribes, without skipping, omitting, or doubling up on her doses.
   (2) Stacey should avoid other central nervous system stimulants, in particular caffeine-containing products (e.g., coffee, tea, colas, and chocolate). She should check with her physician before taking any over-the-counter drug, and she should not consume any substance that contains alcohol.
8. Weight loss due to anorexia is associated with these drugs, and so it is important to monitor for weight gain or loss in children who are taking drugs for attention deficit hyperactivity disorder. Height and weight should be measured and recorded before therapy is initiated, and growth rate should be plotted during therapy. Nutritional status should be assessed, with attention to daily dietary intake as well as the amount eaten before drug therapy and after therapy is initiated.
9. With orlistat, patients need to watch dietary fat intake. Restricting the intake of fat to less than 30% of total caloric intake may help decrease the occurrence of gastrointestinal side effects. In addition, orlistat is to be taken with meals that contain fat. Supplementation with fat-soluble vitamins may be indicated.
10. These drugs work to reduce the severity of the headaches but do not prevent headaches.

Case Study

1. Serotonin agonists work by stimulating 5-HT1 receptors in the brain; this stimulation results in constriction of dilated blood vessels in the brain and decreased release of inflammatory neuropeptides.
2. Orally administered medications may not be tolerated because of the nausea and vomiting that often accompany the headaches. Alternative formulations such as subcutaneous self-injections and nasal sprays are advantageous. They also typically have a more rapid onset of action, producing relief in some patients in 10 to 15 minutes compared with 1 to 2 hours with tablets.
3. Use of sumatriptan is contraindicated in patients with ischemic heart disease, signs and symptoms consistent with ischemic heart disease, Prinzmetal's angina, and uncontrolled hypertension.

4. Foods containing tyramine should be avoided, because tyramine is known to precipitate severe headaches. Tyramine-containing foods include beer, wine, aged cheese, food additives, preservatives, artificial sweeteners, chocolate, and caffeine.
5. Keeping a journal of the occurrence of headaches, precipitating factors, and response to drug therapy is also encouraged so that the patient's progress and response to drug therapy can be followed.

CHAPTER 17
Adrenergic Drugs

Chapter Review/Critical Thinking and Application

1. d
2. b, d
3. a, b, d
4. a
5. c
6. a. The α-adrenergic activity of this drug causes vasoconstriction in the nasal mucosa. This produces shrinkage of the mucosa and promotes easier nasal breathing.
   b. Perhaps she administered the spray too often. Excessive use of nasal decongestants can lead to greater congestion because of a rebound phenomenon.
7. Use of the drug is contraindicated in patients who have a tumor that secretes catecholamines, such as a pheochromocytoma.
8. The action of dopamine depends on the dosage. At low dosages, it can dilate blood vessels in the brain, heart, kidneys, and mesentery, increasing blood flow to these areas. Increased renal flow may help remove excess fluid volume. At higher infusion rates, dopamine can improve contractility and cardiac output.
9. The toxic effects of adrenergic drugs are mainly an extension of their common adverse effects, such as seizures, hypotension or hypertension, dysrhythmias, and other effects, but the two most life-threatening toxic effects involve the central nervous system and cardiovascular system. Seizures can be managed effectively with diazepam. An extreme elevation in blood pressure poses the risk of hemorrhage in the brain and elsewhere in the body. To lower the blood pressure quickly, a rapid-acting α-adrenergic blocking drug can be used to reverse the adrenergic effects. Most of the adrenergic drugs have very short half-lives, and therefore their effects are relatively short-lived. Stopping the drug should quickly cause the toxic symptoms to subside. The treatment of overdoses often focuses on treating the symptoms and supporting the patient's respiratory and cardiac functions.

10. a. He is probably having an anaphylactic reaction to the antibiotic.
    b. First, stop the medication! Then notify the physician, but stay with the patient to monitor and support the ABC's (*a*irway, *b*reathing, and *c*irculation).
    c. Epinephrine is the drug of choice for anaphylactic reactions.

Case Study

1. Before giving this medication, the nurse should assess for hypersensitivity to albuterol and assess breath sounds and vital signs (blood pressure, pulse rate, respiratory rate) to obtain a baseline for comparative purposes. Because this medication may cause tachycardia and cardiac dysrhythmias, the patient's pulse rate and rhythm should be monitored during the treatment. Afterward, the nurse should assess the patient's vital signs and breath sounds again, and assess for therapeutic response to the medication.

2. Albuterol given orally has an onset of action of 30 minutes and peaks in 2.5 hours. Inhaled albuterol has an onset of action of 5 to 15 minutes and peaks in 1 to 1.5 hours. Therefore, the inhaled form will take effect faster than the oral form.

3. These are expected side effects of the albuterol and will soon wear off.

4. Salmeterol is indicated for asthma and prevention of bronchospasms in patients who may need long-term maintenance therapy for their asthma. Patients should be taught that salmeterol is not to be used for relief of acute symptoms, and education about its dosing is important. Dosing of salmeterol is usually at 2 puffs twice daily 12 hours apart for maintenance. For prevention of exercise-induced asthma, the recommendation is 2 puffs ½ to 1 hour before exercise and no additional dosing for 12 hours. If Maureen is still taking the inhaled steroid, then the bronchodilator should be taken first, and she should wait approximately 5 minutes before using the steroid inhaler. All equipment should be rinsed, and the patient should be encouraged to perform mouth care after the use of any inhaled forms of medication.

CHAPTER 18
Adrenergic-Blocking Drugs

Chapter Review/Critical Thinking and Application

1. a, b, d
2. a
3. c
4. b
5. d

6. Extravasation can cause vasoconstriction and ultimately tissue death (necrosis). If the vasoconstriction is not reversed quickly, the whole limb can be lost. Phentolamine, an α-blocker, can reverse this potent vasoconstriction and restore blood flow to the ischemic, vasoconstricted area. When phentolamine is injected subcutaneously in a circular fashion around the extravasation site, it causes α-adrenergic receptor blockade and vasodilation. This in turn increases blood flow to the ischemic tissue and thus prevents permanent damage.

7. Some β-blockers are considered cardioprotective because they inhibit stimulation by the circulating catecholamines released during muscle damage, such as that caused by a myocardial infarction. When a β-blocker occupies their receptors, the circulating catecholamines cannot bind to their receptors. Thus, the β-blockers "protect" the heart from being stimulated by these catecholamines, which would only further increase the heart rate and the contractile force, and thereby increase myocardial oxygen demand.

8. She should take her apical pulse for 1 full minute and monitor her blood pressure because cardiac depression can occur with these drugs. If her systolic blood pressure decreases to lower than 100 mm Hg or her pulse decreases to fewer than 60 beats/min, she should contact her physician. She should also report any weight gain, especially of more than 2 lb in a week, as well as any weakness, shortness of breath, or edema.

9. A common problem with the α_1-blockers such as prazosin is that when patients first start taking these drugs, they may experience lightheadedness and orthostatic hypotension. Patients should quickly develop a tolerance to this effect. He should be taught to take care when standing up to prevent falling if he gets lightheaded; taking the first dose at bedtime may help.

Case Study

1. Nonselective β-blockers (which block both β_1 and β_2 receptors) may precipitate bradycardia and hypotension; their use is contraindicated in asthma. Therefore, if the patient has heart disease as well as respiratory disease, a β_1-blocker, or "cardioselective" drug, would be very beneficial because it would not produce constriction or increased airway resistance as would β_2-blockers.

2. When a β-blocker is given, it occupies receptors and prevents circulating catecholamines (which are released when a myocardial infarction occurs) from binding to these receptors. The β-blocker thus prevents stimulation of the heart by these catecholamines, which would further increase

heart rate, contractile force, and myocardial oxygen demand. In addition, cardioselective β_1-blockers such as atenolol block the β_1-adrenergic receptors on the surface of the heart. This reduces myocardial stimulation, which in turn reduces heart rate, slows conduction through the atrioventricular node, prolongs sinoatrial node recovery, and decreases myocardial oxygen demand by decreasing myocardial contractile force (contractility).

3. Table 18-3 lists β-blocker–induced side effects and adverse effects. Patient teaching should include instructions to monitor the apical pulse for 1 full minute and monitor blood pressure because of the cardiac depression that can occur, and to notify the physician if systolic blood pressure decreases to lower than 100 mm Hg or pulse decreases to fewer than 60 beats/min. Patients should also report any weight gain, especially a gain of 2 lb or more in a 24-hour period or 5 lb or more in a week, as well as any weakness, shortness of breath, and edema. The patient should also be taught about orthostatic changes and cautioned to rise slowly when getting up to avoid syncope. For other teaching points, see Patient Teaching Tips in the text.

4. Make sure that patients are weaned off these medications slowly, if this is indicated, because of the possible rebound hypertension or chest pain that rapid withdrawal can precipitate.

CHAPTER 19
Cholinergic Drugs

Chapter Review/Critical Thinking and Application

1. h
2. g
3. f
4. b
5. j
6. e
7. i
8. a
9. c
10. b
11. b
12. d
13. c
14. b, c, d, f
15. a
16. SLUDGE stands for *S*alivation, *L*acrimation, *U*rinary incontinence, *D*iarrhea, *G*astrointestinal cramps, and *E*mesis.
17. a. Bethanechol is the drug of choice.
    b. None. Bethanechol use is contraindicated in patients with a genitourinary obstruction. The drug should be discontinued immediately.
18. a. Cholinergic crisis
    b. Ensure that atropine, the antidote, is readily available.
19. a. She should experience less eyelid drooping (ptosis), less double vision (diplopia), less difficulty swallowing and chewing, and/or less weakness.
    b. She should report any increased muscle weakness, abdominal cramps, diarrhea, or difficulty breathing.

Case Study

1. There are no "cures" for Alzheimer's disease, but there are several drugs available for management of symptoms. Their use can sometimes yield enough improvement in a patient's mental status to make a noticeable improvement in the quality of life for patients as well as caregivers and family members. However, individual response to these medications does vary from patient to patient. Available drugs include donepezil (Aricept), tacrine (Cognex), galantamine (Razadyne, Reminyl), rivastigmine (Exelon), and memantine (Namenda).
2. Because of his history of hepatitis A, caution should be exercised if galantamine is chosen; the dosage of this drug should be reduced for patients with moderately reduced renal or hepatic function. Results of liver function studies should be monitored if he is given this medication.
3. Direct-acting cholinergic agonists bind to cholinergic receptors and activate them. Indirect-acting cholinergic agonists act by making more acetylcholine (ACh) available at the receptor site. As a result, ACh binds to and stimulates the receptor. They do this by inhibiting the action of cholinesterase, the enzyme responsible for breaking down ACh.
4. Side effects of rivastigmine include dizziness, headache, nausea and vomiting, diarrhea, and anorexia (loss of appetite). Administering this drug with meals helps decrease the gastrointestinal side effects, although absorption may also be decreased. Patients who become dizzy with the therapy should be assisted with ambulation.

CHAPTER 20
Cholinergic-Blocking Drugs

Chapter Review/Critical Thinking and Application

1. a
2. a, c, d
3. b
4. c
5. b

6. Atropine sulfate is used preoperatively to reduce salivation and excessive secretions in the respiratory and gastrointestinal tracts. Glycopyrrolate (Robinul) is also used for this purpose.

7. a. Initially, Mr. Miller should be treated with hospitalization and close, continuous monitoring (including continuous electrocardiographic monitoring). The stomach should be emptied with gastric lavage. Fluid therapy and other standard measures used to treat shock should be instituted as needed. Activated charcoal may be effective in removing the drug that has already been absorbed.

   b. In the case of hallucinations, physostigmine has proved helpful, although its use is somewhat controversial because it causes severe adverse effects with routine use.

8. Antihistamines can have additive effects with cholinergic blockers, resulting in increased effects.

9. a. In the treatment of symptomatic bradycardia, higher dosages of atropine result in an increase in heart rate because of the cholinergic-blocking effects on the heart's conduction system. Atropine blocks the inhibitory vagal (cholinergic) effects on the pacemaker cells of the sinoatrial and atrioventricular nodes, which will hopefully lead to an increased heart rate due to unopposed sympathetic stimulation.

   b. Atropine has a therapeutic effect in cases of exposure to organophosphate insecticides because of its anticholinesterase effects.

Case Study

1. Tolterodine should not be used in patients with narrow-angle glaucoma or urinary retention. Mrs. Walsh's "eye problems" should be evaluated further.

2. Tolterodine appears to be associated with a much lower incidence of dry mouth. This may be due to tolterodine's specificity for the bladder as opposed to the salivary glands.

3. When these cholinergic-blocking drugs are used to treat urinary incontinence, the inability to sweat or perspire should be managed with an increase in fluids and avoidance of extreme heat. Mrs. Walsh needs to avoid overheating when working outside.

4. Although this drug may be associated with a lower incidence of dry mouth, it may still cause this unpleasant side effect because it is a cholinergic-blocking drug. Dry mouth may be managed best by drinking adequate fluids, chewing gum, performing frequent mouth care, sucking on sugar-free hard candy, and using saliva substitute products.

CHAPTER 21
Positive Inotropic Drugs

Chapter Review/Critical Thinking and Application

1. b
2. c
3. d
4. a
5. b
6. a, c, d, f
7. Vomiting, headache, fatigue, and dysrhythmia are adverse effects of cardiac glycosides. The presence of a serum potassium level of more than 5 mEq/L, along with these symptoms, means that administration of digoxin immune Fab is indicated for the treatment of severe digoxin toxicity.

8. Because of digoxin's fairly long duration of action and half-life, the physician has prescribed a loading, or "digitalizing," dose for Mr. Davis to bring the serum levels of the drug up to a therapeutic level more quickly. The usual loading dose is 1 to 1.5 mg/day, whereas the usual maintenance dose is 0.125 to 0.5 mg/day.

9. The therapeutic window is the range of drug levels in the blood that is considered therapeutic. Drug levels below this range would be subtherapeutic, and drug levels above this range may be toxic. Because digoxin has such a narrow therapeutic window, patients require constant monitoring for side effects, adverse effects, and toxic symptoms.

10. Increased urinary output and decreased dyspnea and fatigue are therapeutic effects of digoxin. The constipation needs to be assessed. Mr. Ferris should not be allowed to consume large amounts of bran or other foods high in fiber because the bran will bind to the digitalis and make less of the drug available for absorption.

11. a. Amrinone increases the force of contraction (inotropic effect) and relaxes the blood vessels, causing a reduction in afterload, or the force against which the heart must pump to eject its volume.

    b. Phosphodiesterase inhibitors do not stimulate receptors to cause an increase in the force of contraction as other inotropic drugs do, and therefore the drug maintains its effectiveness for a longer period of time. As a result, increased dosages are not needed to maintain positive results, and therefore unwanted cardiac side effects do not occur.

    c. Thrombocytopenia

Case Study

1. Positive inotropic effect: increases myocardial contractility

Negative chronotropic effect: decreases heart rate
Negative dromotropic effect: slows the conduction of electrical impulses in the heart

2. Effects on
   - Stroke volume: increased
   - Venous blood pressure and vein engorgement: decreased
   - Coronary circulation: increased
   - Diuresis: increased due to improved circulation

3. First you should complete your assessment by checking her apical pulse, heart and lung sounds, and blood pressure. In addition, check her potassium level, because low levels of potassium may lead to digoxin toxicity. If you have not yet given the digoxin dose, hold it and call the physician immediately. Monitor her for signs of digoxin toxicity, especially dangerous dysrhythmias. The digoxin level of 3.5 ng/mL is above the therapeutic range.

CHAPTER 22
Antidysrhythmic Drugs

Chapter Review/Critical Thinking and Application

1. d
2. c
3. a
4. d
5. a
6. b
7. a, (3); b, (1); c, (2)
8. a.   Class II antidysrhythmics, or β-blockers, are indicated because they have been shown to significantly reduce the incidence of sudden cardiac death after myocardial infarction.
   b.   If Mr. Killian had asthma, use of most of the class II drugs would be contraindicated. Noncardioselective β-blockers block not only the β_1-adrenergic receptors in the heart but also the β_2-adrenergic receptors in the lungs. As a result, preexisting asthma could be worsened.
9. Amiodarone is considered a drug of last resort. Although it is very effective, amiodarone can penetrate and concentrate in the adipose tissue of any organ in the body, where it may have unwanted effects. It may cause either hypothyroidism or hyperthyroidism, corneal microdeposits, pulmonary toxicity, and even dysrhythmias. Amiodarone has a very long half-life, and the side effects may take months to subside.
10. a.   Lidocaine must be injected intramuscularly or intravenously; when lidocaine is taken orally, the liver converts most of it to inactive metabolites.

b.   Lidocaine is extensively metabolized in the liver. For patients in liver failure or with a history of cirrhosis, a dosage reduction of 50% is recommended.

11. Mrs. Inez should *not* double up on her medication. The physician should be contacted about the missed dose and about Mrs. Inez's symptoms of chest pain and dizziness, which are adverse effects of the quinidine.

Case Study

1. As their name implies, they work by inhibiting the slow-channel pathways, or the calcium-dependent channels. As a result, they depress phase 4 depolarization, slow sinoatrial and atrioventricular nodal conduction rates, and thus reduce the incidence of paroxysmal supraventricular tachycardia (PSVT).
2. Prevention or reduction of supraventricular rhythms.
3. Taking phenytoin, an anticonvulsant, along with diltiazem may result in reduced effectiveness of the calcium channel blocker.
4. The physician may prescribe adenosine, which is useful for the treatment of PSVT that has failed to respond to verapamil.

CHAPTER 23
Antianginal Drugs

Chapter Review/Critical Thinking and Application

1. c
2. c
3. a, c, d, e
4. d
5. a
6. b
7. Call 911 and assist the patient until the ambulance arrives. At this time you do not know the man's condition, and you certainly cannot administer someone else's medication to him. Isordil is available in a sublingual form, but you cannot administer one person's medication to another person, especially to someone with an undetermined condition.
8. Ms. Vickers might be taking a β-blocker. Fatigue and lethargy are the most common patient complaints with the use of β-blockers, and mental depression can be exacerbated, particularly in the elderly. Also, one of the central nervous system adverse effects of β-blockers is the occurrence of unusual dreams.
9. Theresa should always include in her journal a description of the activity she was performing at the time her angina occurred and the number of

tablets she had to take before the pain subsided. Also, she must keep the tablets in an airtight, dark glass bottle away from sunlight, because the active ingredient in nitroglycerin is easily destroyed.

Case Study

1. Chronic stable angina, also known as classic or effort angina, can be triggered by either exertion or stress (cold temperature or emotions).
2. When experiencing an acute anginal attack, he should take 1 sublingual tablet as soon as possible after the pain begins, lie down immediately, remain calm, and rest. He can take up to 3 sublingual tablets every 5 minutes if relief is not experienced after the first tablet.
3. If he obtains no relief after 15 minutes (3 sublingual tablets), his handball partner should call 911 and have emergency response personnel take him to the hospital. The emergency response team would be better equipped to help him should further complications occur.
4. The β-blockers are most effective in the treatment of typical exertional angina.

CHAPTER 24
Antihypertensive Drugs

Critical Thinking Crossword

Across
1. Secondary
5. Idiopathic
7. Orthostatic
8. Vasodilators

Down
2. Essential
3. Primary
4. Diuretics
6. ACE

Chapter Review/Critical Thinking and Application

1. c
2. b, d, e
3. b
4. a
5. d
6. Because nitroprusside has a very short half-life (10 minutes), the nurse should first discontinue the infusion. Placing the patient in the Trendelenburg position will also be helpful. Treatment for the hypotension is supportive; pressor drugs can be given to raise the blood pressure quickly if necessary.

7. a. According to the most recent guidelines (see Table 24-1 in the textbook), this patient would be considered prehypertensive.
   b. He has "compelling indications," which are conditions that make his prehypertension potentially more dangerous. To prevent long-term effects, he will be placed on drug therapy for the compelling indications as needed, but will be given no antihypertensive drugs at this time. He will need to be monitored closely for changes in his blood pressure.
8. a. Captopril is probably best for Irene. In critically ill patients, a drug with a short half-life, such as captopril, is better, because if problems arise, they will be short-lived. Also, Irene has liver dysfunction, so captopril has an advantage because it is not a prodrug (a prodrug is inactive in its initial form and must be biotransformed in the liver to its active form to be effective).
   b. Because of his history of poor compliance, Kory would benefit from a drug with a long half-life and long duration of action, which he would need to take only once a day. Therefore, one of the newer ACE inhibitors—benazepril, fosinopril, lisinopril, quinapril, or ramipril—would be best.
9. There is a first-dose effect with prazosin. This means that the patient will experience a considerable drop in blood pressure after taking the first dose, so he should take it while lying down or before bedtime and arise slowly. This effect decreases with time or with a reduction in the dosage, as ordered by the physician.
10. a. β-Blockers and ACE inhibitors
    b. Calcium channel blockers and diuretics

Case Study

1. With these blood pressure readings, his hypertension would be classified as stage 1 hypertension.
2. If there are no "compelling indications," initial drug therapy would include thiazide-type diuretics. Other drugs that may also be started include ACE inhibitors, angiotensin II receptor blockers, β-blockers, calcium channel blockers, or a combination. Because John is African American, calcium channel blockers would be chosen over β-blockers and ACE inhibitors.
3. "Compelling indications" are conditions such as heart failure, previous myocardial infarction, high cardiovascular risk, diabetes mellitus, chronic kidney disease, and recurrent stroke prevention. These conditions, combined with hypertension, may result in eventual organ damage if the hypertension is not controlled. If John has diabetes,

then the blood pressure goal would be lower than 130/80 mm Hg.

4. He should be taught about the possibility of orthostatic hypotension and instructed to change positions slowly—especially after stooping or bending over or when rising from supine or sitting to standing.

CHAPTER 25
Diuretic Drugs

Chapter Review/Critical Thinking and Application

1. c
2. f
3. e
4. i
5. g
6. j
7. h
8. a
9. d
10. b
11. a, c, d, e
12. c
13. a
14. d
15. b
16. a. Ms. Andersen was probably prescribed a carbonic anhydrase inhibitor (CAI).
    b. An undesirable effect of the CAIs is that they elevate the blood glucose level, causing glycosuria in diabetic patients. They may also interact with some oral antidiabetic drugs.
17. a. For mannitol to be effective in treating acute renal failure, enough renal blood flow and glomerular filtration must exist to enable the drug to reach the tubules.
    b. Mannitol is always administered intravenously through a filter, because it can crystallize when exposed to low temperatures (which is more likely to occur when concentrations exceed 15%).
    c. Arthur's headache and chills are probably side effects of the mannitol therapy. At this time the therapy should be continued, but Arthur should be monitored for the development of more serious adverse effects.
18. a. Mr. Ferrara will be prescribed spironolactone in high doses; this drug is used often for the treatment of ascites associated with cirrhosis of the liver.
    b. His serum potassium level will need to be monitored frequently because he has impaired renal function.

19. a. Impotence and decreased libido are among the side effects of thiazide. Brendan is possibly experiencing these effects.
    b. He should stop eating licorice, because its consumption can lead to an additive hypokalemia in patients taking thiazide. Brendan's fatigue may be the result of drug toxicity and should be evaluated.
20. It is likely that Mrs. Hill's neighbor was prescribed one of the potassium-sparing diuretics and thus was not instructed to eat additional potassium-rich foods. Mrs. Hill should follow the dietary recommendations provided for her, not for her neighbor.

Case Study

1. These symptoms suggest hypokalemia. Furosemide is a kaliuretic diuretic, which means that potassium is excreted along with sodium and water.
2. Foods high in potassium include bananas, oranges, dates, raisins, plums, fresh vegetables, potatoes (white and sweet), meat, fish, apricots, whole grain cereals, and legumes.
3. Spironolactone is a potassium-sparing diuretic; it causes sodium and water to be excreted, but potassium is retained.
4. The use of ACE inhibitors or potassium supplements in combination with potassium-sparing diuretics can result in hyperkalemia. When taken together, lithium and potassium-sparing diuretics can result in lithium toxicity. The use of nonsteroidal antiinflammatory drugs with potassium-sparing diuretics can reduce the effectiveness of the diuretics.

CHAPTER 26
Fluids and Electrolytes

Chapter Review/Critical Thinking and Application

1. a, b, d, e
2. c
3. d
4. c
5. b
6. b
7. **Advantages**: Crystalloids are less expensive than colloids and blood products for replacing fluids and better for emergency short-term plasma volume expansion. They also promote urinary flow. They do not carry the risk of transmission of viral diseases or anaphylaxis and do not promote bleeding. **Disadvantages:** The fluids can leak out of the plasma into the tissues and cells, which results in edema (such as peripheral edema or

pulmonary edema). They may dilute plasma proteins, resulting in lower colloid oncotic pressure (COP), and dilute erythrocyte concentration, resulting in decreased oxygen tension. Large volumes are needed to be effective, but prolonged infusions and administration of large volumes may worsen acidosis or alkalosis. Lastly, their effects are relatively short-lived compared with those of colloids.

8. a. Blood products
   b. They are the only fluids that contain hemoglobin.
   c. They are natural products that require human donors, which means that they can be incompatible with a recipient's immune system; these products can also transmit pathogens from the donor to the recipient.

9. a. Tanya is exhibiting early symptoms of hypokalemia.
   b. She should eat foods high in potassium, such as bananas, orange juice, and apricots. She may be placed on oral potassium supplements for a short time.

10. a. Hyponatremia
    b. Mr. Sanchez can take in sodium by eating foods high in salt, such as catsup, mustard, cured meats, and potato chips.
    c. Vomiting a possible side effect of oral administration of sodium chloride; if vomiting occurs, he needs to be careful about monitoring for further fluid and electrolyte loss.

11. a. Signs of transfusion reaction include apprehension, restlessness, flushed skin, increased pulse and respiration rate, dyspnea, rash, joint or lower back pain, swelling, fever and chills, nausea, weakness, and jaundice.
    b. Although it is possible for pathogens such as that causing acquired immunodeficiency syndrome (AIDS) to be transmitted via blood products, Victor's wife should be reassured that techniques are now used that have drastically reduced the incidence of such problems.
    c. Every 15 minutes or more often if needed
    d. Victor's restlessness and increased pulse need to be reported to the physician immediately, because these are signs of a reaction to the blood product. Have another nurse notify the physician; should stop the transfusion immediately and change the infusion to normal saline at a slow rate. Follow the facility's protocol for transfusion reactions.

Case Study

1. The normal total protein level is 7.4 g/dL. If the level drops below 5.3 g/dL, the COP becomes less than the hydrostatic pressure, and fluid shifts into the tissues, which results in edema.

2. Colloids increase the COP and move fluid from outside the blood vessels to inside the blood vessels, thus reducing the edema.

3. Colloids are the choice for this patient. Crystalloids can leak out of the plasma into the tissues and cells, resulting in edema anywhere in the body. Crystalloids also dilute the proteins that are in the plasma, further reducing the COP. Finally, crystalloids are more likely to cause edema because of the larger volumes needed to achieve the desired clinical effect. Colloids reduce edema and expand plasma volume by pulling fluid from the extravascular space into the blood vessels.

4. Colloids can alter the coagulation system, which results in impaired coagulation and possibly bleeding. They have no oxygen-carrying ability and contain no clotting factors, and they may also dilute the plasma protein concentration, which may impair the function of platelets.

CHAPTER 27
Coagulation Modifier Drugs

Chapter Review/Critical Thinking and Application

1. k
2. n
3. j
4. l
5. m
6. b
7. a
8. c
9. i
10. h
11. e
12. g
13. a, c, d
14. b
15. a
16. c
17. b, c, d, e
18. d
19. Yes. The injection site should not be massaged or rubbed before or after the injection because this may cause hematoma formation.
20. a. The anticoagulant effects of heparin can be reversed with protamine sulfate.
    b. In general, 1 mg of protamine sulfate can reverse the effects of 100 units of heparin.

c. The activated partial thromboplastin time is the test most commonly used.

21. If the warfarin therapy needs to be resumed, warfarin resistance is likely to occur, because a large dose of vitamin K will maintain its warfarin reversal effects for up to 1 week.

22. The physician will probably prescribe one of the antifibrinolytic drugs, which are used to stop excessive oozing from surgical sites, such as chest tubes.

23. Desmopressin is used in patients with type I von Willebrand's disease; it increases the levels of clotting factor VIII.

24. a. No. Alteplase is present in the body in a natural state, so it does not induce an antigen-antibody reaction.
    b. The alteplase can be readministered because it has a very short half-life of 5 minutes. Because of its short half-life, it is given along with heparin to prevent reocclusion of the infarcted blood vessel.

25. a. They are possible indications of bleeding problems related to the anticoagulation therapy.
    b. Ursula might also be exhibiting a change in pulse rate or rhythm, blood pressure, or level of consciousness.
    c. Notify the physician immediately. Do not administer any other anticoagulants; if Ursula is receiving a continuous infusion, stop the infusion. Prepare to administer the appropriate antidote.

Case Study

1. Use of aspirin is contraindicated in the presence of peptic ulcer disease. Doug has been started on the clopidogrel therapy to reduce the risk of stroke.

2. He should be taught to watch for signs of abnormal bleeding and should immediately report any of the following signs and symptoms to the health care provider: respiratory difficulty, back pain, skin rash, evidence of gastrointestinal bleeding, any other bleeding abnormality, diarrhea, acute severe headache, and change in vision (blurred vision or loss of vision).

3. He needs to take measures to prevent bleeding, such as using a soft toothbrush and an electric razor, and should take great care when trimming his nails, gardening, and participating in rough or contact sports. He needs to take precautions to protect himself from injury and subsequent bleeding or bruising, which can be extremely dangerous while he is taking antiplatelet drugs.

4. Herbal products that contain garlic, ginger, ginseng, and ginkgo should be avoided because they have anticoagulant properties.

CHAPTER 28
Antilipemic Drugs

Chapter Review/Critical Thinking and Application

1. d
2. a, c, d, e
3. a
4. b
5. d
6. c
7. a. Fibric acid derivative—it is believed that these drugs work by activating the lipoprotein lipase, an enzyme responsible for the breakdown of cholesterol.
    b. Lipid-lowering drug and vitamin—exact mechanism unknown; beneficial effects are believed to be related to its ability to inhibit lipolysis in adipose tissue, decrease esterification of triglycerides in the liver, and increase the activity of lipase.
    c. HMG-CoA reductase inhibitor—reduces blood cholesterol by decreasing the rate of cholesterol production.
    d. Bile acid sequestrant—binds bile, preventing the resorption of the bile acids from the small intestine. The insoluble bile acid and resin (drug) complex that is formed is excreted in the feces.

8. Unless Mr. Harris has additional risk factors, his high level of low-density lipoprotein (LDL) cholesterol alone does not warrant drug therapy at this time. All reasonable nonpharmaceutical means of controlling Mr. Harris's LDL level need to be tried and found to fail before he is given drug therapy. Mr. Harris needs to find time in his busy schedule to exercise and eat more wisely.

9. Mr. Jahnke's age and smoking are risk factors, as is the fact that his father died suddenly of heart disease before 55 years of age. Mr. Jahnke's asthma and arthritis are not risk factors, nor is his blood pressure. Mr. Jahnke's level of high-density lipoprotein (HDL) cholesterol is above 60 mg/dL, so it is considered a negative risk factor and can be subtracted from the total number of positive risk factors.

10. Mrs. Kim is experiencing constipation and belching associated with cholestyramine use (she may also be experiencing heartburn, nausea, and bloating). Mrs. Kim requires extra patient teaching and support to help her maintain compliance with the drug therapy; she should be assured that these adverse effects will probably diminish over time.

11. No. Justus is not a candidate for niacin therapy for two reasons: (1) niacin is not recommended with lovastatin because it can lead to the development

of rhabdomyolysis, and (2) niacin use is contraindicated in patients with peptic ulcer.

12. Mrs. Nguyen must take her antihypertensive and cholestyramine (Questran) at different times of the day because the bile acid sequestrant may interfere significantly with the absorption of other drugs taken at the same time. All other drugs should be taken at least 1 hour before or 4 to 6 hours after the administration of antilipemics. Also, the powder form of cholestyramine should be allowed to dissolve slowly in at least 2 oz of fluid, without stirring, for at least 1 minute; stirring causes the powder to clump. The powder may not mix totally in the glass, and more fluid may need to be added to the glass. The powder may also be mixed thoroughly with food, such as crushed pineapple.

Case Study

1. No, he is not right. Dietary measures are a part of antilipemic therapy. Nonpharmacologic measures include consumption of a low-fat, low-cholesterol diet; supervised, moderate exercise; weight loss; cessation of smoking or drinking; and relaxation therapy.
2. This drug is used primarily to lower total and LDL cholesterol levels as well as triglyceride levels; it has been shown to raise the HDL level as well.
3. Elevations in liver enzyme levels may also occur, and the patient should be monitored for excessive elevations, which may indicate the need for alternative drug therapy. In addition, total cholesterol level, LDL/HDL ratio, and triglyceride levels need to be monitored to evaluate therapeutic effect.
4. Myopathy (muscle pain) is an uncommon but clinically important side effect that may occur in some patients taking statins. It may progress to a serious condition known as rhabdomyolysis in which the breakdown of muscle protein occurs, leading to myoglobinuria and possible renal damage. Patients receiving statin therapy should be taught to report unexplained muscle pain to their health care providers immediately.

CHAPTER 29
Pituitary Drugs

Chapter Review/Critical Thinking and Application

1. a. Glucocorticoids, mineralocorticoids, androgens
   b. corticotropin
   c. Regulates anabolic processes related to growth and adaptation to stressors; promotes skeletal and muscle growth; increases protein synthesis; increases liver glycogenolysis; increases fat mobilization

   d. somatropin and somatrem
   e. Antidiuretic hormone
   f. vasopressin and desmopressin
   g. Promotes uterine contractions
   h. oxytocin
2. b, e, f
3. d
4. b
5. d
6. c
7. a. Dose per week for this child (44 lb = 20 kg) is 6 mg
   b. Dose per injection (6 daily injections) = 1 mg per dose per day for 6 days
8. a. Alexis might very well benefit from administration of corticotropin, not only to treat the pain associated with inflammation.
   b. Cautions include checking to see whether Alexis may be pregnant or nursing. Contraindications to corticotropin use include scleroderma, osteoporosis, heart failure, peptic ulcer disease, hypertension, recent surgery, and dysfunction of the adrenocortex. Drug interactions of which you should be mindful are interactions with amphotericin B and drugs that lower potassium level, such as some diuretics.
   c. Other parameters to assess include baseline levels of vital signs, electrolyte values, blood glucose levels, chest radiographic findings, complete blood count results, intake and output, daily weight, and cortisol levels.
   d. Patient teaching plans should include elements listed at length in the Patient Teaching Tips box in this chapter.
9. In addition to information about proper subcutaneous injection techniques, the teaching plan should include a reminder of the dosage form and amount and the importance of compliance with therapy. Show the parents how to keep a journal of Patricia's growth measurements.
10. Contraindications to the use of growth hormone (somatotropin and somatrem) include closure of the epiphyseal plates of the long bones. Jack should not receive the medication simply to get taller but only when diagnosed with an appropriate medical condition, and then only if he has not stopped growing. Chances are that at age 25 he has stopped growing.

Case Study

1. Mr. Collins will probably be found to have diabetes insipidus; if so, he will benefit from treatment with vasopressin or desmopressin.
2. Assessment strategies should include evaluating pulse, vital signs, intake and output, daily weight,

and edema. Desmopressin should be given cautiously in patients with migraine headaches, seizures, and asthma.

3. Treatment will be via nasal spray, 1 to 2 sprays administered into each nostril three times daily. This should increase water resorption in the distal tubules and collecting ducts of the nephron, performing all the physiologic functions of antidiuretic hormone.

4. It should eliminate his severe thirst and decrease his urinary output.

CHAPTER 30
Thyroid and Antithyroid Drugs

Critical Thinking Crossword

Across
3. Secondary
6. Thyroxine
7. Primary

Down
1. Levothyroxine
2. Hyperthyroidism
4. Propylthiouracil
5. Tertiary
6. Thyrotropin

Chapter Review/Critical Thinking and Application

1. c
2. d
3. a
4. a, c, d
5. c
6. Mrs. Westin probably has hypothyroidism, which may result in the formation of a goiter, an enlargement of the thyroid gland resulting from its overstimulation by elevated levels of thyroid-stimulating hormone. She may benefit from one of the thyroid drugs, including thyroid, thyroglobulin, levothyroxine, liothyronine, or liotrix. Levothyroxine is generally preferred because, as a chemically pure formulation of 100% thyroxine, its hormonal content is standardized; therefore, its effect is predictable.
7. Even if it can be determined that the last several symptoms are due to menopause, the combination of the rest of the symptoms, plus her history, indicates the strong possibility that Ms. Hilton has hyperthyroidism. This is especially worth investigating because it is often caused by Graves' disease.
8. Surgery to remove all or part of the thyroid gland is an effective way to treat hyperthyroidism, but as a result lifelong hormone replacement is normally required.

Case Study

1. Her symptoms suggest hypothyroidism, and a thyroid replacement hormone, such as levothyroxine, would be indicated for this condition.
2. The thyroid preparations are given to replace what the thyroid gland cannot itself produce to achieve normal thyroid levels, known as a "euthyroid" condition.
3. Thyroid preparations should be taken at the same time every day to maintain constant blood levels. Taking the medication in the morning will help reduce problems with insomnia, which may result when the medication is taken later in the day or in the evening.

CHAPTER 31
Antidiabetic Drugs

Chapter Review/Critical Thinking and Application

1. b
2. d
3. a
4. c
5. c
6. b
7. Four units ($238 - 150 = 88.88 \div 20 = 4.4$. (Answer is 4, because 20 divides into 88 four whole times. The "left-over" 8.88 does not add up to 20, so it does not count toward the insulin dose.)
8. a. Pramlintide, given by subcutaneous injection, works by mimicking the action of the natural pancreatic hormone amylin. Amylin is secreted along with insulin in response to food intake and influences postmeal glucose levels by slowing gastric emptying, suppressing glucagon secretion (which reduces the liver's glucose output), and centrally modulating the senses of appetite and satiety. As a result, blood glucose levels are reduced.
   b. Exenatide is also an injectable medication, which comes in a prefilled pen-type device. It mimics the incretins, a class of hormones that normally enhance glucose-driven insulin secretion from the pancreatic beta cells. The incretins also suppress excessive glucagon secretion and delay gastric emptying. As a result, fasting and postmeal blood glucose levels should be reduced in patients with type 2 diabetes.
9. a. Alice's diet should include a high intake of protein and a low intake of carbohydrates.
   b. The brain needs a constant amount of glucose to function; thus the central nervous system manifestations of hypoglycemia (such as irritability) are often the first to appear.

c. In the conscious person, oral forms of glucose are used, such as rapidly dissolving buccal tablets or semisolid gel forms designed for rapid mucosal absorption. She could also try corn syrup, honey, fruit juice, a nondiet soft drink, or a small snack such as crackers or half a sandwich.

10. a. Bill should check the order at least three times and have another registered nurse check the prepared injection to be sure it is in accordance with the physician's order.
    b. You, of course. Novolin-R is regular insulin, and regular insulin is clear.
    c. If left at room temperature, the insulin in the vial should have been used within 1 month; otherwise, it should have been refrigerated.

11. a. Alec requires an intermediate-acting insulin.
    b. Alec's religious beliefs might prohibit him from using insulin made from pork. His cultural practices will need to be assessed before a type of insulin is selected for him.

12. a. Mrs. Franklin needs to make some significant lifestyle changes. She must stop smoking, lose weight, and exercise regularly, which will help with both the high blood glucose level and the hypertension.
    b. Mrs. Franklin should continue with her exercise and weight loss program; however, because her blood glucose level is still elevated, she also requires an oral antidiabetic drug.

13. a. Hypoglycemia
    b. Dennis may have been drinking alcohol. Sulfonylureas may interact with alcohol in a way that is similar to the interaction with disulfiram, which is used to deter alcohol ingestion in persons with chronic alcoholism. This *disulfiram-type* reaction includes vomiting and hypertension.

14. a. Twenty units of NPH insulin plus 4 units regular insulin
    b. No coverage
    c. Six units of regular insulin

Case Study

1. The second-generation sulfonylureas have many advantages over the older drugs, including much greater potency. Also, chlorpropamide is dependent on the kidneys for elimination and can cause toxicity in patients with decreased renal function. Glipizide use is not contraindicated in patients with severe renal failure.

2. Glipizide has a rapid onset of action; its effect is thus much like the body's normal response to meals, when greater levels of insulin are rapidly required to deal with the increased glucose in the blood.

3. Glipizide works best if given 30 minutes before meals.

4. Mr. Dressel should contact his physician immediately. He may require a change in his diabetic treatment while he is sick, because vomiting and inability to eat can cause a change in his blood glucose levels.

CHAPTER 32
Adrenal Drugs

Chapter Review/Critical Thinking and Application

1. a
2. c
3. a, b, c
4. b
5. d
6. c
7. Ms. Rivera's glucocorticoid can interact with aspirin and other nonsteroidal antiinflammatory drugs (NSAIDs), producing additive effects. Also, she should avoid persons with infections, because her own immune system is suppressed. The children in the hospital may have infections. In addition, she should report any fever, increased weakness and lethargy, or sore throat.

8. a. The use of systemic glucocorticoids with antidiabetic drugs may reduce the hypoglycemic effect of those drugs. A baseline blood glucose level should be determined, and Peter should be monitored for any problems.
   b. Oral dosage forms should be taken with milk, food, or nonsystemic antacids (such as aluminum-, calcium-, or magnesium-containing antacids), unless contraindicated, to minimize gastrointestinal upset. Another option is for the physician to order a histamine-2 receptor antagonist or proton pump inhibitors to prevent ulcer formation (glucocorticoids may cause gastric ulcers). Patients should be encouraged *not* to take the drug with alcohol, aspirin, or other NSAIDs to minimize gastric irritation and gastric bleeding.

9. Intervene. The student nurse should, while wearing gloves, apply the medication with a sterile tongue depressor or cotton-tipped applicator if the skin is intact. If the skin is not intact, a sterile technique should be used.

10. In addition to routine teaching about inhaler administration technique, Nina should be instructed to rinse out her mouth with lukewarm water after using the inhaler to prevent the development of an oral fungal infection.

Case Study

1. Administration of prednisone causes the body to stop producing hormones; tapering the dose allows the body time to start making it again. Sudden discontinuation of these drugs can precipitate an adrenal crisis caused by a sudden drop in the serum levels of cortisone. Also, a short term of therapy will reduce the effects that often occur with long-term therapy.

2. Short- or long-term therapy may cause steroid psychosis. In addition, long-term effects cause cushingoid symptoms, including moon face, weight gain, muscle wasting, and increased deposition of fat in the trunk area, leading to truncal obesity.

3. Glucocorticoid. Biologic functions of glucocorticoids include antiinflammatory actions, maintenance of normal blood pressure, carbohydrate and protein metabolism, fat metabolism, and stress effects. Biologic functions of mineralocorticoids include sodium and water resorption, blood pressure control, and regulation of potassium levels in and pH of blood.

4. The best time is early in the morning (6:00 AM to 9:00 AM) because this results in the least amount of adrenal suppression.

CHAPTER 33
Women's Health Drugs

Chapter Review/Critical Thinking and Application

1. b, c, d, e
2. a
3. a
4. b
5. b
6. c, e, f
7. a. Ask Isabelle if she is taking medication for her depression. Estrogen therapy is indicated for the symptoms of menopause, but the use of estrogen with a tricyclic antidepressant may result in toxicity of the latter drug.
   b. The smallest dose of estrogen that alleviates the symptoms is used for the shortest possible time.
8. a. The physician will probably prescribe medroxyprogesterone, which is indicated for treatment of secondary amenorrhea.
   b. Ms. Keller's dose of antidiabetic drug may need to be adjusted because of a possible decrease in glucose tolerance when progestins and antidiabetic drugs are taken together.
9. a. Perhaps Jacklyn's prescription could be switched to a 28-day form of Ortho-Novum, which is taken for all 28 days of the menstrual cycle rather than for 3 weeks with 1 week off.

   b. One of the benefits of oral contraceptive use is decreased blood loss during menstruation.
10. a. Choriogonadotropin alfa is often given in a carefully timed fashion after follicle-stimulating hormone–active therapy with a drug such as menotropin or clomiphene, when patient monitoring indicates sufficient maturation of ovarian follicles. Once the ovaries have been sufficiently stimulated (with 9 to 12 days of therapy), then a single large dose of choriogonadotropin alfa is given the next day.
    b. This course of drugs may be repeated a second and third time if needed.
11. Mrs. Ingalls needs to know that smoking can diminish the therapeutic effects of the estrogen she is taking and add to the risk of thrombosis. Also, she should be cautioned to wear sunscreen while in Aruba, because estrogen makes the skin more susceptible to sunburn.
12. a. Mrs. Simmons is assuming that the medication is estrogen therapy. Alendronate (Fosamax) is indicated to prevent osteoporosis in postmenopausal women. You will need to explain to her that it is a nonestrogen, nonhormonal medication used for prevention of bone loss in the early postmenopausal period. For women who experience early menopause, a dose of 5 mg daily is recommended.
    b. We know that she experienced early menopause; other risk factors associated with the development of postmenopausal osteoporosis include thin body build, white or Asian race, family history of osteoporosis, and moderately low bone mass. She would need to be assessed for these other risk factors.
13. Ibandronate is only given once a month, which reduces the dangerous gastrointestinal problems often associated with the other oral bisphosphonates.

Case Study

1. The physician will probably prescribe terbutaline or ritodrine. These drugs work by stimulating the β-adrenergic receptors located on the uterine smooth muscle. The muscle then relaxes and stops contracting.

2. Ms. O'Hara should be placed in the left lateral recumbent position to minimize hypotension and increase renal blood flow and blood flow to the fetus.

3. Hyperglycemia and hypokalemia are metabolic adverse effects of tocolytic therapy.

4. No, because tocolytic therapy is indicated for premature labor between the twentieth and thirty-seventh weeks of gestation. At this time, her labor would not be considered premature.

CHAPTER 34
Men's Health Drugs

Chapter Review/Critical Thinking and Application

1. b
2. b, d, f
3. a
4. d
5. c
6. a
7. a. Testosterone's poor performance in the oral dosage form is due to the fact that most of a dose is metabolized and destroyed by the liver before it can reach the circulation.
   b. Methyltestosterone and fluoxymesterone are both testosterone derivatives that are effective when given buccally or orally.
   c. With either drug, contraindications that could apply to Mr. Michaels include significant cardiac, hepatic, or renal dysfunction; breast carcinoma; or known or suspected prostate cancer.
8. a. No. The manufacturer's guidelines suggest that the patient not swallow, chew, or eat the buccal tablet but that it be completely absorbed in the mouth. The part of the drug that is swallowed will not reach the intended site of action because of heavy first-pass metabolism.
   b. Patients taking any hormone-related drug should never abruptly stop the drug. The physician may consider whether a transdermal form is suitable for Mr. Michaels.
9. a. Finasteride works by inhibiting the enzymatic process responsible for converting testosterone to 5α-dihydrotestosterone (DHT), which is the principal androgen responsible for stimulating prostatic growth. It can dramatically lower the prostatic DHT concentrations, thereby reducing testosterone concentrations and causing the hypertrophied prostate to decrease in size.
   b. The patient teaching plan should include the rationale for therapy and a full disclosure of side effects.
10. The Testoderm patch is applied only to the scrotal skin. The skin should be clean, dry scrotal skin that has been shaved for optimal skin contact. These patches are replaced every 22 to 24 hours. Androderm patches should be applied to clean, dry skin on the back, abdomen, upper arms, or thighs; the scrotum and bony areas (shoulder, hip) should be avoided. These patches are often ordered to be changed every 7 days. AndroGel is applied to the shoulders, arms, or abdominal skin daily.

Case Study

1. Sildenafil (Viagra) should be used cautiously in patients with renal disorders, hypertension, diabetes, and cardiovascular disease, and is contraindicated if the patient is taking nitrates because of the potential for severe hypotensive effects.
2. Headache, flushing, and dyspepsia are the most common adverse effects reported. In addition, sildenafil is highly protein bound and may interact with many drugs. Mr. Edward should check with the doctor before taking any other medication. In addition, he should report any visual changes immediately.
3. Older individuals experience declining liver function, so drugs may not be metabolized as effectively as when they were younger. In addition, there have been reports of vision loss in men who have been taking this class of drugs.
4. Sildenafil should be taken 1 hour before intercourse.

CHAPTER 35
Antihistamines, Decongestants, Antitussives, and Expectorants

Chapter Review/Critical Thinking and Application

1. a, b, c
2. a
3. b
4. c
5. b
6. d
7. The antihistamines cannot push off histamine that is already bound to its receptor. Because they compete with histamine for unoccupied receptors, they work best when given early in a histamine-mediated reaction, before all of the histamine binds to receptors.
8. Yes. The traditional antihistamines have anti-cholinergic effects, which may make them more effective in some cases. Patients respond to and tolerate these drugs quite well. Also, because many traditional antihistamines are generically available at this time, they are often much less expensive.
9. No. Mrs. Ling is likely experiencing rebound congestion caused by sustained use of the naphazoline for several days.
10. Keith is exhibiting symptoms of the cardiovascular effects that can occur when a topically applied adrenergic nasal decongestant is somewhat absorbed into the bloodstream.

11. Benzonatate's mechanism of action is entirely different from that of the other drugs. It suppresses the cough reflex by numbing the stretch receptors, which keeps the cough reflex from being stimulated in the medulla. It is associated with fewer drug interactions than the opioid antitussives and dextromethorphan.

12. Ask Irene whether she is taking any thyroid medication. A drug interaction (an additive hypothyroid effect) can occur if she takes an expectorant with an antithyroid drug. Irene should call her physician before she goes to the drugstore.

13. First, Lisa's brother received Robitussin A-C, an opioid antitussive containing codeine, for his cough. Lisa has been prescribed Robitussin, an expectorant, for her nonproductive cough associated with bronchitis. Second, even if the two children were prescribed the same drug, Lisa is only 5 years old and requires a smaller dosage than her brother.

14. Some decongestants have stimulating effects on the cardiac and central nervous systems that may result in palpitations, insomnia, restlessness, and nervousness. Patients taking these products should avoid caffeine and caffeine-containing products to avoid further excessive central nervous system stimulation.

Case Study

1. James's diabetes should not affect his treatment.
2. The topical diphenhydramine might come in combination with a drug such as calamine, camphor, or zinc oxide.
3. He should be informed that taking any of the sedating antihistamines may precipitate drowsiness, and so he should be instructed to avoid driving or operating heavy machinery should these side effects occur or until he knows how he responds to the medication.
4. James should also be informed not to consume alcohol or take other central nervous system depressants because they may interact with the diphenhydramine to exacerbate drowsiness and sedation.

CHAPTER 36
Bronchodilators and Other Respiratory Drugs

Chapter Review/Critical Thinking and Application

1. b, d, e, f
2. d
3. d
4. b
5. c
6. a

7. The cause of idiopathic (or intrinsic) asthma is unknown; allergic asthma is caused by hypersensitivity to an allergen in the environment. Idiopathic asthma is not mediated by immunoglobulin E, whereas allergic asthma is.

8. Tom is exhibiting some side effects of theophylline therapy, and the level in his blood is probably too high (the common therapeutic range for theophylline is a blood level of 10 to 20 mcg/dL). Tom may require a reduction in dosage.

9. You need to know how much Willie weighs. The pediatric dosage for intravenous epinephrine is 0.8 to 1.2 mg/kg/hour continuously.

10. Sylvia is exhibiting dose-related adverse effects of the albuterol, probably because she used it too frequently. Sylvia needs to be reminded to use her medication exactly as prescribed.

11. a. Anticholinergics, corticosteroids, and beta-agonists.
    b. Of concern is Mrs. Voss's glaucoma. Use of ipratropium bromide (an anticholinergic) is contraindicated in patients with glaucoma.

12. a. The disadvantage of administering the corticosteroids orally is that they can then lead to systemic effects, such as adrenocortical insufficiency, increased susceptibility to infection, fluid and electrolyte disturbances, endocrine effects, dermatologic effects, and nervous system effects. They can also interact with other systemically administered drugs. (The advantage to administering corticosteroids by inhalation is that their action is limited to the topical site of action—the lungs. Thus they have no systemic effects and cannot interact with other systemically administered drugs.)
    b. Yes. The use of an inhaled corticosteroid frequently allows for a reduction in the daily dose of the systemic corticosteroid. This reduction should be gradual.

13. a. The stimulating effects of the xanthines on the central nervous system and cardiovascular system may be enhanced in children.
    b. It depends. Theophylline tablets come in regular and extended-release forms. The extended-release form, of course, cannot be crushed.

14. The albuterol is a β-agonist that can be used to treat acute bronchospasms. The fluticasone is a corticosteroid and is not effective for acute bronchospasm. Fluticasone is useful for long-term management of asthma and works to reduce inflammation.

Case Study

1. These drugs are not direct bronchodilators; they work to reduce the inflammatory response in the lungs.

2. They are primarily used for oral prophylaxis and chronic treatment of asthma and are not recommended for treatment of acute asthma attacks.
3. There are no interactions between ibuprofen and montelukast; however, Jennie should continue to check with her physician before taking other over-the-counter medications.
4. These drugs should be taken every night on a continuous schedule, even if symptoms improve.

CHAPTER 37
Antibiotics Part 1

Critical Thinking Crossword

Across
3. Prophylactic
6. tetracycline
7. Penicillin
8. Bactericidal
9. cephalosporin

Down
1. Macrolide
2. Sulfonamide
4. Bacteriostatic
5. Superinfection

Chapter Review/Critical Thinking and Application

1. b, d, e
2. a
3. b
4. c
5. d
6. Cefoxitin (Mefoxin) is frequently used in patients undergoing abdominal or colorectal surgeries because it can effectively kill intestinal bacteria such as gram-positive, gram-negative, and anaerobic bacteria.
7. a. Sean should not take the doxycycline with milk because that can result in a significant reduction in the oral absorption of the drug. Sean should also be aware that tetracyclines can cause photosensitivity; he should stay out of the sun.
   b. The diarrhea is probably the result of alteration of the intestinal flora caused by the drug therapy.
8. She is experiencing a superinfection because the antibiotics she has been taking for her bronchitis have reduced the normal vaginal bacterial flora, and the yeast that is usually kept in balance by this normal flora has an opportunity to grow and cause an infection.

Case Study

1. He should be assessed for renal problems and blood dyscrasias. Also, the use of co-trimoxazole is contraindicated in cases of known drug allergy to sulfonamides or chemically related drugs such as sulfonylureas (used for diabetes), thiazide and loop diuretics, and carbonic anhydrase inhibitors.
2. If he is taking a sulfonylurea for his type 2 diabetes, close monitoring is needed, because sulfonamides can potentiate the hypoglycemic effects of sulfonylureas in patients with diabetes. In addition, although he is currently receiving intravenous heparin and not warfarin, he may be switched to oral anticoagulants soon, so you should keep in mind that sulfonamides can potentiate the anticoagulant effects of warfarin and lead to hemorrhage.
3. These antibiotics achieve very high concentrations in the kidneys, through which they are eliminated. Therefore, they are primarily used in the treatment of urinary tract infections.
4. Sulfonamides do not actually destroy bacteria but inhibit their growth. For this reason they are considered bacteriostatic antibiotics. Bactericidal antibiotics kill bacteria.

CHAPTER 38
Antibiotics Part 2

Chapter Review/Critical Thinking and Application

1. c
2. b
3. a
4. a, b, c, d
5. The current practice is once-a-day aminoglycoside dosing. You can tell her that studies have shown that once-daily dosing provides a sufficient plasma drug concentration to kill bacteria and also has either an equal or lower risk of toxicity compared with multiple daily dosing. Hopefully this type of dosing will be safer and more effective for her.
6. A blood sample for measurement of "trough" level is drawn at least 18 hours after a dose is given (24 hours if the patient has renal impairment). The therapeutic goal is a trough level at or below 1 mcg/mL. If the trough level is above 2 mcg/mL, then the patient is at greater risk for ototoxicity and nephrotoxicity. Trough levels should be monitored once every 3 days until the drug is stopped. In addition, renal function is monitored by measuring serum creatinine levels. A rising serum creatinine level suggests reduced creatinine clearance by the kidneys. Serum creatinine level should be measured at least twice weekly.

7. Yes. In patients who receive amiodarone therapy, dangerous cardiac dysrhythmias are more likely to occur when quinolones are taken. Hopefully another drug besides levofloxacin has shown effectiveness against the bacteria that is causing his infection.
8. Nitrofurantoin is used primarily to treat urinary tract infections because it is renally excreted and concentrates in the urine. It can cause significant renal impairment but is usually well tolerated if the patient is kept well hydrated. The "force fluids" order will facilitate urinary elimination of the drug. As a result, the drug will exert its desired effect and the patient will not be at risk for renal damage.

Case Study

1. Ototoxicity and nephrotoxicity. Symptoms of ototoxicity include dizziness, tinnitus, and hearing loss. Symptoms of nephrotoxicity include urinary casts, proteinuria, and increased blood urea nitrogen and serum creatinine levels. Keeping the drug blood levels (peak and trough) within a specific therapeutic range can help prevent those toxicities.
2. The aminoglycosides and penicillins are often used together because they have a synergistic effect; that is, the combined effect of the two drugs is greater than that of either drug alone.
3. *Yes,* there is a concern! The desired trough level is 1 mcg/mL, so a level of 3 mcg/mL could mean that he is receiving a dose that is too high. The increased serum creatinine level is also a concern because it could be an indication of impaired renal function. The physician should be notified immediately and doses of the aminoglycoside withheld until the physician responds.

CHAPTER 39
Antiviral Drugs

Chapter Review/Critical Thinking and Application

1. d
2. d
3. a
4. c
5. a, b
6. Any drug that kills a virus can also kill healthy cells. Viruses must enter cells to replicate. Therefore, antiviral drugs must also enter the host cells. Few drugs can kill only the virus and leave the body's cells unharmed. Viruses are also difficult to kill because often by the time they are discovered, they have finished replicating. At that point, it is too late for antiviral drugs, which interfere with viral replication, to work.

7. Yes. Zidovudine, one of the few anti–human immunodeficiency virus (HIV) drugs known to prolong patient survival, can be used for maternal and fetal treatment. During the pregnancy, Amy can receive the oral form of the drug. During labor she can receive the drug intravenously. Drug therapy for the infant can begin within 12 hours of delivery and continue for 6 weeks.
8. a. Acyclovir (Zovirax) is indicated for the herpes zoster (shingles).
   b. Bailey's daily fluid intake should be at least 2400 mL while she is taking the acyclovir. Also, acyclovir capsules may be taken with food.
   c. Bailey will be treated with acyclovir again; it is the drug of choice for treatment of both initial and recurrent episodes of shingles.
9. a. Ribavirin is used to treat infections caused by respiratory syncytial virus.
   b. Yes. Brenda's treatment will last at least 3 days but not longer than 7 days.
10. a. The patient may be experiencing zidovudine's major dose-limiting adverse effect, which is bone marrow suppression.
    b. Eduardo should mix the powder solution in at least 4 oz of water—not fruit juice or a juice containing acid—and drink it immediately. The drug should be taken on an empty stomach 1 hour before meals or 2 hours after meals.
    c. No. Antacids taken concurrently with didanosine can cause increased absorption of the didanosine, which is a positive effect.
11. No. Your co-worker is doing fine. Acyclovir administered by intravenous infusion is first diluted in the solution recommended by the manufacturer and is administered slowly over at least 1 hour to prevent renal damage.
12. No. Therapy with oseltamivir (Tamiflu) should begin within 2 days of the onset of influenza. It is probably too late for this medication to be effective for Stacy.

Case Study

1. Mr. C. should use a glove when applying topical acyclovir (Zovirax) to the affected area, which should be kept clean and dry. Also, he should not use any other creams or ointments on the area.
2. Mr. C.'s herpes infection cannot be "cured," although the acyclovir will help to manage the symptoms.
3. Stress the importance of treatment for Mr. C. and his sexual partner, and discuss with him how to prevent transmission of the virus.

4. There are several viruses in the Herpesviridae family, including herpes simplex type 1 (HSV-1), which causes mucocutaneous herpes—usually blisters around the mouth; varicella-zoster virus (herpes simplex type 3, or HSV-3), which causes both chickenpox and shingles; herpesvirus type 4 (also called Epstein-Barr virus or EBV); and herpesvirus type 8, which is believed by some to cause Kaposi's sarcoma, a cancer associated with acquired immunodeficiency syndrome (AIDS).

CHAPTER 40
Antitubercular Drugs

Chapter Review/Critical Thinking and Application

1. a
2. b
3. a, b, c
4. c
5. a
6. a. Liver function studies should be performed because isoniazid can cause hepatic impairment. A complete blood count, including hemoglobin level and hematocrit value, should be checked because of the hematologic disorders isoniazid can cause.
   b. Diane may be a slow acetylator. Acetylation, the process by which isoniazid is metabolized in the liver, requires certain enzymes to break down the isoniazid. In slow acetylators, who have a genetic deficiency of these enzymes, the isoniazid accumulates. The dosage of isoniazid may need to be adjusted downward in these patients.
7. a. Streptomycin is administered intramuscularly, deep into a large muscle mass, and the sites are rotated.
   b. The side effects and adverse effects of streptomycin are ototoxicity, nephrotoxicity, and blood dyscrasias.
   c. Although it may not be a concern in terms of Ms. Innes's streptomycin therapy, oral contraceptives become ineffective when given with rifampin. If rifampin is part of her therapy, Ms. Innes should switch to another form of birth control.
8. A thorough eye examination may be called for before therapy is initiated, because ethambutol can cause a decrease in visual acuity resulting from optic neuritis, which is also a contraindication to the use of ethambutol.
9. a. Mr. Fiore needs to know that his compliance with therapy is essential for achieving a cure. Although he is keeping his follow-up appointments, Mr. Fiore also needs to take his medication as ordered. He should be warned not to consume alcohol, and he should be encouraged to take care of himself by ensuring adequate nutrition, rest, and relaxation.
   b. The therapeutic response can be confirmed by results of laboratory studies (sputum culture and sensitivity tests) and chest radiographic findings.
10. a. Frannie, like all patients taking antitubercular drugs, needs to be compliant with the therapy regimen and keep her follow-up appointments. She should be reminded that she can spread the disease (during the initial period of the illness); she should wash her hands frequently and cover her mouth when coughing or sneezing. Frannie also needs adequate nutrition and rest.
    b. It is likely that Frannie is on rifampin therapy. She should be told that her urine, stool, saliva, sputum, sweat, and tears may become red-orange-brown and that this is an effect of rifampin therapy.

Case Study

1. George's gout is a consideration; pyrazinamide can cause hyperuricemia, so gout or flare-ups of gout can occur in susceptible patients. His diabetes is a concern too; ethambutol should be used cautiously in patients with diabetes. A baseline hearing test should be performed if streptomycin is considered, because this drug may cause ototoxicity.
2. An individual with a genetic deficiency of the liver enzymes that metabolize drugs can be classified as a "slow acetylator." When isoniazid is taken by slow acetylators, the drug accumulates because there are not enough of the enzymes to break down the isoniazid. As a result, the dosage of isoniazid may need to be reduced.
3. Results of liver function studies should be assessed carefully before therapy is initiated, because some drugs (isoniazid, pyrazinamide) are hepatotoxic. Liver function test results should be monitored closely during therapy as well.
4. Patients should take pyridoxine (vitamin B_6) as prescribed by the physician to prevent some of the neurologic side effects of isoniazid, such as numbness and tingling of the extremities (peripheral neuritis).

CHAPTER 41
Antifungal Drugs

Chapter Review/Critical Thinking and Application

1. j
2. e
3. f

4. g
5. a
6. c
7. h
8. i
9. d
10. b
11. c
12. b, c, e
13. d
14. b
15. a
16. Mycotic infections are very difficult to treat, and research into new drugs has occurred at a slow pace, in part because the necessary chemical concentrations of the experimental drugs cannot be tolerated by humans.
17. a. Fluconazole (Diflucan), unlike itraconazole, can pass into the cerebrospinal fluid, which makes it useful in the treatment of cryptococcal meningitis. It is considered to be the most effective of the imidazoles for treating several infections.
    b. Unfortunately, Mr. Kim will need to remain on the medication (at a reduced dosage) for 10 to 12 weeks after the negative results on his cerebrospinal fluid culture.
18. a. The amphotericin B should be diluted according to the manufacturer's guidelines and administered using an infusion pump. Do not use solutions that are cloudy or that have visible precipitates.
    b. Fever, chills, hypotension, tachycardia, malaise, muscle and joint pain, anorexia, nausea and vomiting, and headache are possible side effects.
    c. No. Almost all patients experience these effects. To decrease their severity, the patient may be pretreated with antipyretic (e.g., acetaminophen), antihistamines, and antiemetics.
19. Lewis should be aware that he will be taking the medication for 2 to 6 weeks, until the infection clears. During that time, he should avoid alcohol because of the increased risk for hepatoxicity, and he should take the medication with food to avoid gastrointestinal upset. Ketoconazole also causes photophobia, so Lewis should avoid the sun or use sunscreen and sunglasses with ultraviolet protection.
20. Nystatin oral troches or lozenges should be dissolved slowly and completely in the mouth for the best effects and should not be chewed or swallowed. Chrissie needs a review of how to use this medication.

Case Study

1. Voriconazole is used to treat major fungal infections in patients who do not tolerate or respond to other antifungal drugs.
2. Use of voriconazole is contraindicated in patients taking other drugs that are metabolized by cytochrome P-450 enzyme 3A4 (e.g., quinidine) because of the risk of inducing serious cardiac dysrhythmias.
3. Careful cardiac monitoring should be performed if Sally is also taking quinidine while taking this antifungal drug.

CHAPTER 42
Antimalarial, Antiprotozoal, and Anthelmintic Drugs

Chapter Review/Critical Thinking and Application

1. a
2. b
3. c
4. b, e
5. d
6. c
7. Malaria is caused by *Plasmodium* organisms. During the asexual stage of the *Plasmodium* life cycle, which occurs in the human host, the parasite resides for a while outside the erythrocyte; this is called the exoerythrocytic phase. The most effective drug for eradicating the parasite during this phase is primaquine.
8. Before primaquine is administered, Professor Henson should be given a pregnancy test. This is a pregnancy category C drug, so you will need to know if certain precautions are needed in Professor Henson's case. She should also be assessed for hypersensitivity, anemia, lupus erythematosus, methemoglobinemia, porphyria, rheumatoid arthritis, methemoglobin reductase deficiency, and glucose-6-phosphate dehydrogenase (G6PD) deficiency.
9. Mefloquine is indicated for the treatment of chloroquine-resistant malaria. Quinine, an older drug, may also be used.
10. Each of these three patients has a protozoal infection. The patient with the intestinal disorder has giardiasis. The patient with acquired immunodeficiency syndrome (AIDS) has pneumocystosis. The patient with the sexually transmitted disease has trichomoniasis. See the Dosages table for antiprotozoal drugs in Chapter 42 for specific drugs used to treat these diseases.

Case Study

1. Intestinal roundworms are diagnosed based on symptoms and examination of stool specimens.
2. Contraindications include allergy to the medication and pregnancy. Even though she is only 15 years of age, she should be assessed for possible pregnancy before this medication is given. In addition, her liver function test results should be assessed, because use of pyrantel is contraindicated in patients with liver disease.
3. Based on her weight of 57 kg, the dose for her would be 627 mg (11 mg × 57 kg).
4. Adverse effects of pyrantel therapy include headache, dizziness, insomnia, and skin rashes, but more common effects are anorexia, cramps, diarrhea, nausea, and vomiting.

CHAPTER 43
Antiseptic and Disinfectant Agents

Critical Thinking Crossword

Across
1. Zephiran
3. Nosocomial
4. Aldehyde
6. Betadine
7. Hibiclens
9. Dakin's

Down
2. Antiseptic
4. Acetic
5. Disinfectant
8. Lysol

Chapter Review

1. b, c, d
2. d
3. c
4. a
5. b
6. c

Case Study

1. The use of hydrogen peroxide as a solution to irrigate wounds is controversial. Its use may be detrimental to wounds because it can destroy newly forming cells as well as bacteria. In addition, tincture of iodine may stain the skin and cause irritation and pain at the site.
2. Dakin's solution is a sodium hypochlorite solution that may be used at 0.25% or 0.5% concentrations.
3. Dakin's solution is a very weak solution. The strength of most household bleach solutions is 5.25% sodium hypochlorite.

4. After the procedure, you should wash your hands, dispose of contaminated dressings, record the nature of the procedure and findings, and maintain asepsis (surgical asepsis if the wound is open in any way or if the skin is not intact).

CHAPTER 44
Antiinflammatory, Antirheumatic, and Related Drugs

Chapter Review/Critical Thinking and Application

1. b
2. b
3. a, b, d
4. c
5. d
6. a
7. Symptoms of both salicylism (chronic salicylate intoxication) and acute salicylate overdose are similar except that the effects are often more pronounced and occur more quickly in the acute form. Acute salicylate overdose results from the ingestion of a single toxic dose. Chronic salicylate intoxication occurs as a result of either high dosages or prolonged therapy with high dosages.
8. Treatment of acute salicylate overdose consists of removing the salicylate from the gastrointestinal tract and preventing its absorption; correcting fluid, electrolyte, and acid-base disturbances; and implementing measures to enhance salicylate elimination, including hemodialysis.
9. Mr. Chestnut has an acute overdose of a nonsalicylate nonsteroidal antiinflammatory drug (NSAID). If the condition progresses, symptoms can include intense headache, dizziness, cerebral edema, cardiac arrest, and even death.
10. His treatment will consist of removing the NSAID from the gastrointestinal tract, followed by administration of activated charcoal. Supportive and symptomatic treatment will be implemented. Hemodialysis, however, is not helpful with this type of overdose.
11. Mr. Henry needs to know that compliance with the entire medical regimen is important for the success of his treatment for gout. Allopurinol should be taken with meals to help prevent the occurrence of gastrointestinal symptoms such as nausea, vomiting, and anorexia. Fluids should be increased to 3 L per day, and hazardous activities should be avoided if dizziness or drowsiness occurs with the medication. Also, alcohol and caffeine should be avoided, because these drugs will increase uric acid levels and decrease the levels of allopurinol.

12. Ketorolac (Toradol) is indicated for the short-term management (up to 5 days) of moderate to severe acute pain that requires analgesia at the opioid level. It is not indicated for treatment of minor or chronic painful conditions.

13. The vinegary odor means that the aspirin has experienced some chemical breakdown, and she should *not* use it! She should discard it safely and purchase a new bottle.

Case Study

1. The specific COX-2 selectivity of these drugs allows them to control the inflammation and pain without producing some of the toxicity associated with NSAID therapy.

2. The most common adverse effects include fatigue, dizziness, lower extremity edema, hypertension, dyspepsia, nausea, heartburn, and epigastric discomfort. Any stomach pain, unusual bleeding, or blood in vomit or stool should be reported to the physician immediately. Chest pain, palpitations, and any gastrointestinal problems should be reported as well.

3. She should avoid alcohol and aspirin while taking this medication and should check with her physician before taking any over-the-counter medications.

CHAPTER 45
Immunosuppressant Drugs

Chapter Review/Critical Thinking and Application

1. b
2. c
3. c
4. a
5. a, c, d
6. a
7. a. Daclizumab can help prevent organ rejection. If her immune system cannot recognize the new kidney as foreign, it will not mount an immune response against it.
   b. Laboratory tests should include hemoglobin level, hematocrit, white blood cell count, and platelet count. These studies should be done before, during, and after therapy. If the leukocyte count should drop below $3000/mm^3$, the drug should be discontinued after the physician is notified.
   c. The antifungal drug is added several days before surgery as prophylaxis for *Candida* infections.
8. Encourage the patient to take the drug with meals or mixed with milk to prevent stomach upset.

9. Tess is experiencing symptoms consistent with side effects or adverse effects of muromonab-CD3.

10. Glatiramer acetate is the only immunosuppressant drug that is currently indicated for the treatment of relapsing-remitting multiple sclerosis. Hopefully it will help to reduce the frequency of his relapses.

Case Study

1. Yes, immunosuppressant therapy will be lifelong.
2. White patches on the tongue, mucous membranes, and oral pharynx would be indicative of candidiasis.
3. Mr. K. needs to be seen by a physician immediately. These symptoms could indicate that he has a severe infection.
4. If the leukocyte count drops below $3000/mm^3$, then the drug should be discontinued, because he is experiencing a severely immunosuppressed state.

CHAPTER 46
Immunizing Drugs and Biochemical Terrorism

Chapter Review/Critical Thinking and Application

1. a. Varicella vaccine
   b. Active
   c. Active
   d. *Haemophilus influenzae* type b prophylaxis
   e. Hepatitis B virus vaccine (recombinant)
   f. $Rh_0(D)$ immune globulin
   g. Passive
   h. Active
   i. Tuberculosis prophylaxis
   j. Active
   k. Diphtheria, tetanus, and pertussis prophylaxis, pediatric
   l. Passive
   m. Postexposure passive tetanus prophylaxis
   n. Active
   o. Diphtheria and tetanus prophylaxis (pediatric and adult)
2. b
3. d
4. a
5. a
6. c
7. Sometimes, after vaccination, the levels of antibodies against a particular pathogen decline over time and a second dose of the vaccine is given to restore the antibody titers to a level that can protect the person against the infection. This second dose is referred to as a *booster shot*.

8. Each year a new influenza vaccine is developed that contains three influenza virus strains that represent the strains most likely to circulate in the United States in the upcoming winter. The vaccination from the previous year may not be effective for the influenza virus strains occurring in the current year.

9. Carl may experience localized swelling, redness, discomfort, and warmth at the injection site. Acetaminophen and rest are recommended for the relief of these side effects, and application of warm compresses to the injection site may also help ease some of the discomfort.

10. There are three routes of inoculation (what the neighbor calls "types") of anthrax: cutaneous, inhalational, and gastrointestinal. Of the three, anthrax contracted by inhalation of the bacterial spores is the most deadly and has a mortality rate of more than 80%.

11. Paul is experiencing more than the expected side effects of his vaccinations. He is probably experiencing "serum sickness," which may occur after repeated injections of equine-derived immunizing drugs. Because his symptoms may indicate respiratory impairment, he needs to be taken to the hospital for evaluation and monitoring. He may receive analgesics, antihistamines, epinephrine, and/or corticosteroids to treat this reaction.

Case Study

1. Rabies is a very potent virus.
2. Those at high risk for rabies exposure, such as veterinarians, will receive the rabies virus vaccine (Imovax, RabAvert) as preexposure prophylaxis, followed by booster shots every 2 to 5 years based on blood titers. This is a type of active immunization.
3. You will receive drugs that give both active and passive immunization. Postexposure prophylaxis consists of injections of the rabies virus vaccine (see answer 2) and also rabies immune globulin (Imogam Rabies-HT). Because rabies can progress so rapidly, the body does not have time to mount an adequate immune defense—death occurs before it can do so. The passive immunization confers a temporary protection that is usually sufficient to keep the invading organism from causing death, even though it does not stimulate an antibody response. The active immunization you receive will stimulate an antibody response.
4. The rabies virus vaccine will be given intramuscularly on the day of exposure (day 0) and on days 3, 7, and 14, with 1 dose of rabies immune globulin given within 8 days of the first vaccine dose. The rabies immune globulin is given as a single dose (20 international unit/kg); as much of the dose

as possible is infiltrated into the bite wound area, and the remainder is given intramuscularly—but not in the same injection site as the rabies vaccine.

CHAPTER 47
Antineoplastic Drugs Part 1: Cancer Overview and Cell Cycle–Specific Drugs

Critical Thinking Crossword

Across
1. Bifunctional
6. Emetic
9. Folic
11. Malignancy
12. Extravasation
13. Nadir

Down
2. Leucovorin
3. Benign
4. Leukemia
5. Spread
7. Alkylation
8. Mitosis
10. Limiting

Chapter Review

1. a, b, c, e, f
2. d
3. a
4. b
5. c

Case Study

1. Methotrexate is an antimetabolite—specifically, a folic acid antagonist. It inhibits the action of an enzyme that is responsible for converting folic acid to a substance used by the cell to synthesize DNA for cell reproduction. As a result, the cell dies.
2. Laboratory test results should be checked for white blood cell and red blood cell counts, hemoglobin level and hematocrit, platelet counts, and renal and liver function studies.
3. The concurrent administration of nonsteroidal antiinflammatory drugs (NSAIDs) and methotrexate may lead to severe bleeding tendencies. Allen should be instructed to avoid all NSAIDs, including aspirin, while taking methotrexate.
4. Antiemetic therapy and antacids are often needed to decrease nausea, vomiting, and gastrointestinal upset. Because methotrexate may cause hyperuricemia (increased uric acid levels) associated with tumor lysis syndrome, allopurinol (Zyloprim)

may be given. Leucovorin may be used to protect the patient from potentially fatal bone marrow suppression, a toxic effect of methotrexate.

CHAPTER 48
Antineoplastic Drugs Part 2: Cell Cycle–Nonspecific and Miscellaneous Drugs

Chapter Review/Critical Thinking and Application

1. c
2. d
3. b
4. a, c, e, f
5. a
6. d
7. Cytoprotective drugs help to reduce the toxicity of various antineoplastics. As a result, the adverse effects may be reduced or increased dosages of the antineoplastic medication may be tolerated, which allows greater cancer cell kill. Examples include the following:
   Amifostine (Ethyol) used during therapy with cisplatin
   Dexrazoxane (Zinecard), used during therapy with doxorubicin
   Leucovorin (Wellcovorin) and allopurinol (Zyloprim), used during therapy with methotrexate
8. Patients receiving bleomycin must be monitored closely for the development of pulmonary fibrosis and pneumonitis. Mrs. Smythe needs to be assessed carefully for these possible problems.
9. During surgery to remove or reduce the size of (debulk) the brain tumor, the surgeon can place carmustine wafers. These wafers are implanted directly at the target site, in the area of the brain where the tumor is or was located.
10. *No!* In most facilities, institutional guidelines direct that the pharmacy department mix these drugs. Special requirements must be met for the safety of those working with these drugs, including the use of a laminar airflow hood and appropriate personal protection equipment (such as gown, mask, and gloves). It would not be safe for you or for those around you to mix the chemotherapy drug on the nursing unit.
11. You will stop the infusion immediately, but you won't pull out the intravenous catheter quite yet. The physician should be notified immediately, and you should expect to receive orders to treat this extravasation of mechlorethamine by injecting a solution of 10% sodium thiosulfate and sterile water (see Table 48-3) through the existing line into the extravasated site. The line can then be removed. Over the next few hours, the patient will

receive repeated subcutaneous injections into the area, and cold compresses should be applied to the site.

Case Study

1. Nephrotoxicity (possible damage to the kidneys), peripheral neuropathy (possible damage to peripheral nerves), and ototoxicity (possible damage to hearing).
2. Baseline renal studies should be performed, because this drug is highly nephrotoxic. If Dottie is receiving any other drugs that are potentially nephrotoxic (such as aminoglycoside therapy), dosage changes will need to be considered. If she has gout and is receiving treatment with probenecid or sulfinpyrazone, concurrent use of cisplatin may result in hyperuricemia or worsening of the gout. Baseline auditory studies should be performed, as well as baseline liver function studies and measurement of white blood cell count, hemoglobin level, hematocrit, and platelet level, because of the anticipated bone marrow suppression.
3. Because peripheral neuropathies may occur, numbness, tingling, or pain in the extremities should be reported to the physician immediately to prevent complications and enhance comfort.
4. Yes, this is a concern, because dehydration while taking cisplatin may lead to renal damage. Patients who are at home after treatment with this drug should be reminded of the importance of hydration and should be told to contact the physician if they experience dry mucous membranes, very dark amber urine, or little or no urinary output or vomiting of large amounts over a period of 8 hours or less. It may be a challenge, but she needs to try to take in 3000 mL of fluid per day to prevent dehydration.

CHAPTER 49
Biologic Response–Modifying Drugs

Chapter Review/Critical Thinking and Application

1. e
2. a
3. g
4. b
5. h
6. d
7. c
8. d
9. b
10. a, b, d, e
11. c

12. The major dose-limiting side effect of interferons is fatigue. Patients taking high dosages become so exhausted that they are often confined to bed. Sonja needs to know this before she starts the therapy.

13. Colony-stimulating factors (CSFs) such as filgrastim (Neupogen), pegfilgrastim (Neulasta), and sargramostim (Leukine) can be given for chemotherapy-induced leukopenia. These drugs should be administered 24 hours after the chemotherapy drugs have been given, because the myelosuppressive effects of the chemotherapy drugs tend to cancel out the therapeutic benefits of the CSFs.

14. She will receive oprelvekin (Neumega), which is given via subcutaneous injections daily for up to 21 days. Because she has severe thrombocytopenia, however, the nurse must be careful to prevent excessive bleeding and bruising at the injection sites and to teach Brittany measures to reduce bleeding risks.

Case Study

1. Epoetin alfa is a synthetic derivative of the human hormone erythropoietin, which is produced primarily by the kidneys. It promotes the synthesis of erythrocytes (red blood cells) by stimulating the production of red blood cell precursors.

2. Hemoglobin level and hematocrit should be monitored carefully. If therapy is not halted when the target hemoglobin level of 12 g/dL is reached or if the hemoglobin level and hematocrit rise too quickly, hypertension and seizures can result.

3. The drug is synthetically manufactured in mass quantities by means of recombinant DNA technology. This technology allows the drug to be essentially identical to its endogenously produced counterpart in the body.

4. Epoetin can be given either intravenously or subcutaneously; for administration at home, she will need to be taught subcutaneous administration.

5. Darbepoetin alfa (Aranesp) can be given weekly, so that the number of injections is reduced.

CHAPTER 50
Gene Therapy and Pharmacogenomics

Chapter Review/Critical Thinking and Application

1. g
2. f
3. b
4. c
5. d
6. DNA is deoxyribonucleic acid, located in the nucleus of all body cells as strands of chromosomes, collectively called *chromatin*. Protein synthesis is the primary function of DNA in the nuclei of human cells.

7. The goal of this scientific project was to map the entire DNA sequence (genome) of a human being.

8. The development of gene therapy and pharmacogenomics.

9. Recombinant DNA is DNA that has been artificially synthesized or modified in a laboratory setting. This technology is used to make recombinant forms of drugs such as hormones, vaccines, and antitoxins. The most common example of this technology is the alteration of the *Escherichia coli* genome so that these bacteria manufacture a recombinant form of human insulin.

10. The general goal of gene therapy is to transfer to the patient exogenous genes that will either provide a temporary substitute for or initiate permanent changes in the patient's own genetic functioning to treat a given disease. Gene therapy techniques are being studied for the treatment of acquired illnesses such as cancer, heart disease, and diabetes, but to date no gene therapy has received Food and Drug Administration approval for the routine treatment of disease.

CHAPTER 51
Acid-Controlling Drugs

Chapter Review/Critical Thinking and Application

1. h
2. e
3. i
4. k
5. c
6. a, b
7. f
8. d
9. b
10. g
11. b
12. c
13. d
14. b, d, e
15. You need to let him know that long-term self-medication with antacids may mask symptoms of serious underlying diseases. He needs to be evaluated for possible bleeding ulcer or even a malignancy, but you may not want to scare him with those possibilities! If his current self-treatment is no longer working, he needs a medical evaluation.

16. Omeprazole should be taken before meals, and the capsule should be taken whole, not crushed, opened, or chewed. Omeprazole may also be given with antacids, if ordered. Like omeprazole,

most of the other proton pump inhibitors are given short term, which should be emphasized to patients.

17. Patients with heart failure or hypertension should use antacids that are low in sodium. He should also be told to take the antacid alone, not at the same time as other medications (unless specifically instructed to do so), because the antacid will interfere with the absorption of the other medications. Antacids should be taken 1 hour before or 1 to 2 hours after other medications. If symptoms continue or worsen, he should consult his health care provider.

18. Antacids may promote premature dissolving of the enteric coating; if the coating is destroyed early in the stomach, gastrointestinal upset may occur. He should take the aspirin tablets with food, not with antacids.

19. Regimen 1 therapy is one of eight FDA-approved regimens for eradication of *Helicobacter pylori*. It consists of therapy with both the proton pump inhibitor omeprazole and the antibiotic clarithromycin in specific dosages for each.

Case Study

1. Although histamine-2 (H₂) antagonists are available over the counter, the dose of the over-the-counter preparation will not be the same strength as the usual dose of the prescription formulation.

2. The drug effects of the H₂ blockers are limited to specific blocking actions on the parietal cells of the gastric glands in the stomach. As a result, hydrogen ion production is decreased, which leads to an increase in the pH of the stomach (i.e., decreased stomach acid).

3. Use of H₂ receptor antagonists is contraindicated in patients with known drug allergy or impaired renal function or liver disease. Cautious use is recommended in patients who are confused, disoriented, or elderly. Interactions may occur with drugs that have a narrow therapeutic range. Caution should be used if she is taking theophylline for her asthma. Patients requiring these medications should avoid aspirin and other nonsteroidal antiinflammatory drugs, alcohol, and caffeine because of their ulcerogenic or gastrointestinal tract–irritating effects.

4. Smoking has been shown to decrease the effectiveness of H₂ blockers because the absorption of H₂ antagonists is impaired in individuals who smoke. Hopefully if she herself is not smoking, this will not be a problem for her, but spending several hours in a smoke-filled room may have an effect. Also, the beer and possibly spicy pizza may aggravate the underlying condition.

CHAPTER 52
Antidiarrheals and Laxatives

Critical Thinking Crossword

Across
1. Saline
4. Bulk forming
7. Hyperosmotic

Down
2. Adsorbent
3. Anticholinergic
5. Emollient
6. Stimulant
8. Opiates

Chapter Review/Critical Thinking and Application

1. d
2. a
3. d
4. c
5. a, d
6. Darkening of the tongue or stool is a temporary and harmless side effect associated with the use of bismuth subsalicylate (Pepto-Bismol).
7. Use of the belladonna alkaloid preparations, such as Donnatal, are contraindicated in patients with narrow-angle glaucoma. She should not use this drug.
8. Several factors may be causing Hillary's constipation: lack of proper exercise, poor diet (which might involve inadequate roughage and an excess of dairy products), use of aluminum-containing antacids, and stress.
9. a. The bulk-forming laxatives tend to produce normal stools, have few systemic effects, and are among the safest available.
   b. Ira should mix the medication with at least 6 to 8 oz of fluid and drink it immediately. He should never take it dry.
10. a. Because glycerin is very mild, it is often used in children.
    b. Abdominal bloating and rectal irritation
11. a. It will probably be determined based on Kyle's weight.
    b. She should not give Kyle any more medication, and she should contact the physician immediately.

Case Study

1. Antibiotic therapy destroys the balance of normal flora in the intestines, and diarrhea-causing bacteria proliferate.

2. *Lactobacillus acidophilus* is indicated for diarrhea caused by antibiotic treatment that has destroyed the normal intestinal flora.

3. Exogenously supplying these bacteria helps restore the balance of normal flora and suppress the growth of diarrhea-causing bacteria.

4. It is considered a dietary supplement. It is often used to treat uncomplicated diarrhea, although this is an off-label use (not approved by the Food and Drug Administration).

CHAPTER 53
Antiemetic and Antinausea Drugs

Chapter Review/Critical Thinking and Application

1. a
2. c, e
3. d
4. c
5. b
6. Neuroleptic antiemetics. If Norman is taking levodopa for his Parkinson's disease, the beneficial effects of the levodopa could be reduced or canceled because of a drug interaction with the neuroleptic drug.
7. a. Petra should take the metoclopramide 30 minutes before meals and at bedtime.
   b. Petra should be cautioned about taking her medication with alcohol because of the possible toxicity and central nervous system depression that can occur.
8. This drug comes in oral, intramuscular, intravenous, and rectal forms, but because she on "nothing-by-mouth" status and has no intravenous access, the intramuscular route was ordered. You can call her physician to get an order for an alternate route, but you cannot change the route without an order, because the dosage may also be different.
9. Dronabinol is a synthetic derivative of the major active substance in marijuana. You explain to him that it is used to stimulate appetite and weight gain in patients with acquired immunodeficiency syndrome (AIDS).

Case Study

1. There are no significant drug interactions associated with the serotonin blockers such as ondansetron.

2. Antiemetics are often administered before a chemotherapy drug is given, frequently ½ to 3 hours before treatment.

3. The headache is caused by the ondansetron and can be relieved with acetaminophen.

CHAPTER 54
Vitamins and Minerals

Chapter Review/Critical Thinking and Application

1. c
2. g
3. b
4. h
5. e
6. k
7. i
8. d
9. j
10. a
11. l
12. f
13. a, d, e
14. b
15. d
16. d
17. By "endogenous," the physician meant the form of vitamin D synthesized in the skin through exposure to ultraviolet radiation. Dietary sources of vitamin D include fish oils, salmon, sardines, and herring; fortified milk, bread, and cereals; and animal livers, tuna fish, eggs, and butter.
18. a. Pernicious anemia
    b. The oral absorption of cyanocobalamin (vitamin B_{12}, or extrinsic factor) requires the presence of intrinsic factor, which is a glycoprotein secreted by gastric parietal cells. Damage to the gastrointestinal tract may reduce the amount of intrinsic factor available.
    c. The patient education card for Ms. Evans should focus on foods containing cyanocobalamin; these include foods of animal origin such as liver, kidney, fish, shellfish, meat, and dairy products.
19. To avoid venous irritation, calcium should be given via an infusion pump when given intravenously. It should be infused slowly (less than 1 mL/min for adults) to avoid cardiac dysrhythmias and cardiac arrest. The physician is correct in ordering infusion with 1% procaine. This will reduce vasospasm and dilute the effects of calcium on surrounding tissues. In either case, monitor for extravasation; if it occurs, you should discontinue administration immediately.
20. The orange juice contains ascorbic acid (vitamin C), which enhances the absorption of iron.

Case Study

1. Broad-spectrum antibiotics can inhibit the intestinal flora, which provide the body with vitamin K_2

As a result, a deficiency may occur. Vitamin K can be given either orally or by injection in adults.

2. Vitamin K is essential for the synthesis of blood coagulation factors, which takes place in the liver.

3. Deficiency states can also be seen in newborns because of malabsorption attributable to inadequate amounts of bile. The deficiency may also be seen in patients receiving specific anticoagulants that inhibit hepatic vitamin K activity.

4. Dietary sources of vitamin K are green leafy vegetables (cabbage, spinach, etc.), meats, and milk.

CHAPTER 55
Nutrition Supplements

Critical Thinking Crossword

Across
1. Erythromycin
4. Anabolism
5. Gastrostomy
8. Absorptive
10. Fatty acid
11. Essential
12. Nitrogen

Down
2. Catabolism
3. Enteral
6. Semiessential
7. Metabolism
8. Arginine
9. Phlebitis

Chapter Review/Critical Thinking and Application

1. a
2. c
3. a, c, d, e
4. c
5. a
6. d
7. a. Advantages of the newer tubes are that they are thinner, have a smaller diameter, and are more pliable for better patient tolerance. However, they also make checking for gastric aspiration more difficult.
   b. Patients who suffer from this condition experience cramping, diarrhea, abdominal bloating, and flatulence with the ingestion of lactose. In this case, lactose-free solutions should be used.
   c. The residual should not be more than 2 hours' worth of feeding—in this case, no more than 100 mL. You should return the aspirate, withhold the feeding, elevate the head of the bed, and notify the physician.

8. Mr. Robbins shows signs of fluid overload. The first thing you should do is slow his infusion rate, then remain with him and contact the physician immediately. Continually assess his vital signs. Next time you can prevent this by maintaining intravenous rates, assessing the intravenous infusion every hour, and monitoring the patient's fluid status.

Case Study

1. If total parenteral nutrition is discontinued abruptly, rebound hypoglycemia may occur because the pancreas has not had time to adjust to the reduced blood glucose levels. Hypoglycemia is manifested by cold, clammy skin, dizziness, tachycardia, and tingling of the extremities.

2. To prevent hypoglycemia, hang a solution of 5% to 10% glucose to infuse until bag No. 4 is ready. You should also call to make sure the pharmacy is preparing the infusion bag.

3. During this infusion, her blood glucose levels should be monitored on a regular basis. You should assess for signs of both hyperglycemia and hypoglycemia, signs of infection, and signs of fluid overload.

CHAPTER 56
Blood-Forming Drugs

Chapter Review/Critical Thinking and Application

1. d
2. b
3. c
4. a, b, c
5. b, c, d
6. d
7. Anyone who is about to receive his first dose of iron dextran is at risk for fatal anaphylaxis. Because of this, a test dose of 25 mg of iron dextran should be administered by the chosen route and appropriate method. An anaphylactic reaction should occur within a few moments, although waiting at least 1 hour before giving the rest of the initial dose is recommended. Intramuscular iron should be administered deep in a large muscle mass using a Z-track method and a 23-gauge 1½-inch needle.

8. Dietary sources of iron include meats and certain vegetables and grains. These forms of iron must be converted by gastric juices before they can be absorbed. Other foods such as orange juice, veal, fish, and ascorbic acid may help with iron absorption. Conversely, eggs, corn, beans, and many cereal products containing chemicals known as *phytates* may impair absorption of iron from

other iron-containing foods or iron supplements. However, it should also be noted that both beans and eggs are themselves common dietary sources of iron. Antacids and milk products decrease the absorption of iron.

9. Treatment should include suction and maintenance of the airway, correction of acidosis, and control of shock and dehydration with intravenous fluids or blood, oxygen, and a vasopressor. Abdominal radiographs can allow visualization of the tablet. A serum concentration of more than 300 mcg/dL will place David at serious risk for toxicity. His stomach should be emptied immediately. Because many of the iron products are extended-release formulations that liberate their contents in the intestines rather than in the stomach, whole-gut lavage is generally believed to be superior to and more effective than gastric lavage. This is followed by a saline cathartic or possible surgical removal of ingested iron tablets.

10. Patients with severe symptoms will exhibit coma, shock, or seizures. Chelation therapy with deferoxamine should be initiated.

Case Study

1. Oral forms should be given with juice (but not antacids or milk) between meals for maximal absorption. Should gastrointestinal distress occur, however, the iron can be taken with meals.

2. She should be reminded that use of any iron product will cause the stools to turn tarry and black.

3. She should be told that one iron product cannot be substituted for another because each product contains different forms of the iron salt in different amounts.

4. Liquid oral forms of iron should be diluted per the manufacturer's instructions and taken through a plastic straw to avoid discoloration of tooth enamel.

CHAPTER 57
Dermatologic Drugs

Chapter Review/Critical Thinking and Application

1. a
2. b
3. a
4. b
5. a, b, d
6. d
7. You may first ask Mr. Mugler about any allergies to other forms of drugs. If he has an allergy to a particular antibacterial drug, that drug should not be used topically either. If culture and sensitivity

testing is to be carried out, be sure to collect the specimen before the first application of the antibacterial drug. In this case, you can simply apply a thin film of clindamycin and monitor for signs of allergy to clindamycin.

8. Gloves are used not only to prevent contamination from secretions but also to prevent absorption of the medication through the skin of the person applying the medication.

9. Mr. Lacroix and his children are being treated for head lice. Tell him the following: "Leave the shampoo on for 4 minutes, then rinse and dry the hair. Then use a nit comb to remove nits (eggs) from the hair shafts." Other measures he should take include decontaminating the clothing and personal articles of the infested persons. All clothing, linens, stuffed toys, and so on should be washed in hot, soapy water or dry-cleaned.

10. A patient taking any anti-acne drug should avoid ultraviolet light, weather extremes, sunlight, abrasive cleansers, and other keratolytic products. Sunscreen should be worn during therapy. Tretinoin is available in many topical formulations, including creams, gels, and a liquid. Because of its potential to cause severe irritation and peeling, it may initially be applied once every 2 or 3 days, often starting with a lower-strength product. Benzoyl peroxide generally produces signs of improvement in 4 to 6 weeks, and side effects are infrequent and rarely a problem. Most are confined to the skin and involve peeling of the skin, redness, or a sensation of warmth. Benzoyl peroxide is applied sparingly one to four times daily and is available as a cleansing bar, liquid, lotion, mask, cream, gel, and cleanser.

11. The patient should be assessed for allergy to iodine. Cadexomer iodine (Iodosorb) is used to chemically débride the wound by absorbing exudates. It is not harmful to viable cells, but it does stain tissue.

12. It is possible that the patient is not a candidate for surgery at this time or is taking anticoagulants, which could cause the area to bleed excessively if surgical débridement is performed. The prescribed medication selectively removes necrotic tissue without harming normal tissue and can be used on infected wounds.

Case Study

1. Judy's allergies, especially any allergies to sulfonamide drugs, should be assessed. This cream should be applied only to areas that have been cleansed and débrided. The wound bed may need to be débrided before the cream can be applied.

2. The dressing helps keep the medication at the intended site and provides protection to the wound. In addition, it keeps the cream from soiling the clothing.

3. No! He should prevent contamination of the medication and avoid exposure to Judy's wound secretions. He should apply the cream with a sterile, gloved hand.

4. The side effects of silver sulfadiazine are similar to those of other topical drugs and include pain, burning, and itching.

CHAPTER 58
Ophthalmic Drugs

Chapter Review/Critical Thinking and Application

1. c
2. h
3. j
4. k
5. a
6. d
7. b
8. f
9. g
10. e
11. c
12. b
13. b
14. d
15. b, c, d
16. c
17. The effect is less pronounced in individuals with dark eyes (brown or hazel), because pigment absorbs the drugs and dark eyes have more pigment than light eyes (blue).
18. a. Dipivefrin (Propine), a prodrug of epinephrine, has better lipophilicity than epinephrine and can penetrate into the anterior chamber of the eye. It is 4 to 11 times more potent than epinephrine in reducing intraocular pressure.
    b. Mrs. Ngo should report any stinging, burning, itching, lacrimation, or puffiness of the eye.
    c. No. Systemic effects are rare; they include cardiovascular effects and possibly headaches and faintness.
19. Ned may have had an allergic reaction to a preservative, such as benzalkonium chloride, in the first drug that was tried. Timolol is available in a preservative-free product.
20. a. Oral glycerin is indicated before iridectomy to reduce intraocular pressure in individuals with acute narrow-angle glaucoma.
    b. Mrs. O'Rourke should lie flat during and after oral administration of glycerin to diminish any headache caused by cerebral dehydration.

When they are tolerated, she should also take in sufficient fluids.

21. a. Purulent drainage or exudate would inhibit the product's effectiveness.
    b. The solution must have been cloudy; in that case, it should be discarded—only clear solutions should be administered.
22. The nonsteroidal antiinflammatory drugs are considered less toxic, and they are preferred over the corticosteroids as initial topical therapy for injuries.
23. Stinging is normal after instillation of the drops. Ms. Luna should not wear her contact lenses while taking this medication.

Case Study

1. Ocular cytomegalovirus (CMV) infection is one of the many potential opportunistic infections that is associated with acquired immunodeficiency syndrome (AIDS). He did not contract the infection because he had poor hygiene; his immunosuppressed condition made him more susceptible to this infection.
2. Ophthalmic viral infections can be treated by implanting a medicated disk or administering an intravitreal (into the vitreous humor) injection of the appropriate drug.
3. The ganciclovir will be in the form of an implant (disk) that is surgically placed in the posterior of the eye. Implantation normally takes less than 1 hour and is an outpatient procedure performed under local anesthesia.
4. The medication in this implant will be released over a period of 5 to 8 months.

CHAPTER 59
Otic Drugs

Chapter Review/Critical Thinking and Application

1. a, b, d, e
2. d
3. b
4. a
5. c
6. The patient needs medical care immediately. His symptoms may be indicative of head trauma.
7. To take advantage of the steroidal antiinflammatory, antipruritic, and antiallergic drug effects.
8. a. Clean the ear, remove all cerumen by irrigation, and clean the dropper with alcohol. The drops also need to be at room temperature.
    b. He might become dizzy, so he should be supine when the drops are instilled.

9. a. The hydrocortisone will help reduce the inflammation and itching associated with the infection.
    b. A drug hypersensitivity or a perforated eardrum.
10. Many ear disorders involve pain and inflammation; the anesthetic effect of the local anesthetic drugs makes them beneficial in treating these conditions.
11. a. The instructions are different for each boy. The pinna should be held up and back during instillation of eardrops in children older than 3 years of age, like Drew. For children 3 years of age or younger, like Ben, the pinna should be gently pulled down and back.
    b. Reduced pain, redness, and swelling are therapeutic effects of the medication.
12. a. Esther's husband should warm the eardrops to body temperature by holding the bottle under warm running water, not by soaking it in hot water—especially because he should be careful not to let water get into the bottle or damage the label.
    b. Esther should not sit up right away. She should lie down on the side opposite the side of the affected ear for about 5 minutes after the drug is instilled. As an alternative, she can gently insert a small cotton ball into the ear canal to keep the drug in place, but the cotton ball should not be forced into the ear canal.

Case Study

1. Mark probably has an impaction of earwax in his ear canal. Such a buildup can cause pain and temporary deafness.
2. He should be taught that he should *not* insert anything into his ear canal. He will need to know how to clean his ears properly and how to use cerumen removal drugs. You may need to irrigate his ear canals before medication therapy is started.
3. This medication is given as otic (ear) drops. He will need to follow the manufacturer's recommendations for administration. He should lie on the side opposite the side of the affected ear for about 5 minutes after instillation of the drug. A small cotton ball may be inserted gently into the ear canal to keep the drug there, but it should not be forced or jammed down into the ear canal. When administering the drops, he should pull the pinna of his ear up and back.
4. The carbamide peroxide will slowly release hydrogen peroxide and oxygen, and this effervescent effect will mechanically act to loosen the cerumen. In addition, the glycerin will soften the cerumen, making it easier to remove.

OVERVIEW OF DOSAGE CALCULATIONS

Introduction

Interpreting Medication Labels

1. Generic name: rifampin
    Trade name: Rifadin
    Unit dose: 300-mg capsule
    Total in container: 30 capsules
    Route: oral
2. Generic name: loracarbef
    Trade name: Lorabid
    Unit dose: 200 mg per 5 mL
    Total in container: 75 mL (when mixed)
    Route: oral
3. Generic name: medroxyprogesterone acetate suspension
    Trade name: Depo-Provera
    Unit dose: 400 mg per mL
    Total in container: 2.5 mL
    Route: Intramuscular use only

Section I

Basic Conversions Using Ratio and Proportion

1. 600,000 mcg
2. 1,500,000 mcg
3. 5 mg
4. 5000 mg
5. 2500 mg
6. 0.9 g *(Don't forget the leading zero.)*
7. 8000 g
8. 0.75 L *(Don't forget the leading zero.)*
9. 975,000 mL
10. 0.5 L *(Don't forget the leading zero.)*
11. 960 mg
12. 1.5 gr
13. 20 mL
14. 12 tsp
15. 6 tbsp
16. 90 mL
17. 0.2 oz *(Don't forget the leading zero.)*
18. 198 lb
19. 68.2 kg *(rounded to tenths)*
20. 24.2 lb

Section II

Calculating Oral Doses

1. 1 tablet
    0.5 g = 500 mg; each tablet is 500 mg; therefore 1 tablet is needed

2. 2 tablets
0.5 mg = 500 mcg;
250 mcg : 1 tablet :: 500 mcg : x tablet
Proof: $250 \times 2 = 500; 1 \times 500 = 500$

3. 0.5 tablet
0.25 g = 250 mg;
500 mg : 1 tablet :: 250 mg : x tablet
Proof: $500 \times 0.5 = 250; 1 \times 250 = 250$

4. 20 mL
12.5 mg : 5 mL :: 50 mg : x mL
Proof: $12.5 \times 20 = 250; 5 \times 50 = 250$

5. 2 tablets
600 mg = gr x; gr v : 1 tablet :: gr x : x tablet
Proof: gr v $\times 2$ = gr x; $1 \times$ gr x = gr x
NOTE: With this problem, since most are more familiar with metric doses, you may convert the dose on hand, gr v, to 300 mg. Then set up your problem:
300 mg : 1 tab :: 600 mg : x

6. 4 mL
0.1 g = 100 mg; 125 mg : 5 mL :: 100 mg : x mL
Proof: $125 \times 4 = 500; 5 \times 100 = 500$

7. 3 tablets
0.3 g = 300 mg;
100 mg : 1 tablet :: 300 mg : x
Proof: $100 \times 3 = 300; 1 \times 300 = 300$

8. 22.5 mL
20 mEq : 15 mL :: 30 mEq : x
Proof: $20 \times 22.5 = 450; 15 \times 30 = 450$

9. 3 capsules
0.15 g = 150 mg;
50 mg : 1 capsule :: 150 mg : x
Proof: $50 \times 3 = 150; 1 \times 150 = 150$

10. 4 tablets
2 g = 2000 mg;
500 mg : 1 tablet :: 2000 mg : x
Proof: $500 \times 4 = 2000; 1 \times 2000 = 2000$

Section III

Reconstituting Medications

1. 2 mL
100 mg : 1 mL :: 200 mg : x
Proof: $100 \times 2 = 200; 1 \times 200 = 200$

2. 1.5 mL
40 mg : 1 mL :: 60 mg : x
Proof: $40 \times 1.5 = 60; 1 \times 60 = 60$

3. 0.8 mL
10,000 units : 1 mL :: 8000 units : x
Proof: $10,000 \times 0.8 = 8000; 1 \times 8000 = 8000$

4. 1.5 mL
500 mg : 1 mL :: 750 mg : x
Proof: $500 \times 1.5 = 750; 1 \times 750 = 750$

5. 20 mL
125 mg : 5 mL :: 500 mg : x
Proof: $125 \times 20 = 2500; 5 \times 500 = 2500$

6. Choose the concentration using 4.6-mL diluent. Using the 9.6-mL diluent would necessitate giving 3 mL intramuscularly versus 1.5 mL using the 4.6-mL diluent.
1.5 mL
200,000 units : 1 mL :: 300,000 units : x mL
Proof: $200,000 \times 1.5 = 300,000;$
$1 \times 300,000 = 300,000$

7. 0.75 mL
First: Convert mcg to mg : 750 mcg = 0.75 mg
1:1000 indicates 1 g in 1000 mL, or 1000 mg in 1000 mL, or 1 mg/mL.
1 mg : 1 mL :: 0.75 mg : x
Proof: $1 \times 0.75 = 0.75; 1 \times 0.75 = 0.75$

8. 1 mL
NOTE: 1:5000 indicates 1 g in 5000 mL, or 1000 mg in 5000 mL, or 0.2 mg/mL.
0.2 mg : 1 mL :: 0.2 mg : x
Proof: $0.2 \times 1 = 0.2; 1 \times 0.2 = 0.2$

9. 9 mL
NOTE: 10% indicates 10 g per 100 mL, or 0.1 g/mL.
Need to ensure units that are alike: 900 mg = 0.9 g
0.1 g : 1 mL :: 0.9 g : x
Proof: $0.1 \times 9 = 0.9; 1 \times 0.9 = 0.9$

10. 8 mL
NOTE: 50% indicates 50 g per 100 mL, or 0.5 g/mL.
0.5 g $\times$ 1 mL :: 4 g : x
Proof: $0.5 \times 8 = 4; 1 \times 4 = 4$

Section IV

Pediatric Calculations

1. a. 0.46 to 47.3 mg/hr
40 lb = 18.2 kg
Low dose: 0.025 mg/kg/hr $\times$ 18.2 kg = 0.455, rounded to 0.46 mg/hr
High dose: 2.6 mg/kg/hr $\times$ 18.2 kg = 47.32, rounded to 47.3 mg/hr
b. Yes, the ordered dose of 1 mg/hr falls within the safe range for this child.

2. a. 75 to 150 mg/dose
33 lb = 15 kg
Low dose: 5 mg/kg/dose $\times$ 15 kg = 75 mg/dose
High dose: 10 mg/kg/dose $\times$ 15 kg = 150 mg/dose
b. 600 mg (40 mg $\times$ 15 kg = 600 mg/kg/24 hr)
c. Yes, the ordered dose of 120 mg falls within the safe and therapeutic range for this child.

3. a. 3180 to 4770 mg/24 hr
70 lb = 31.8 kg
Low dose: 100 mg/kg/24 hr $\times$ 31.8 kg = 3180 mg/24 hr
High dose: 150 mg/kg/24 hr $\times$ 31.8 kg = 4770 mg/24 hr

b. 1060 to 1590 mg/dose

Three doses in 24 hours; 3180 ÷ 3 = 1060 mg/dose; 4770 ÷ 3 = 1590 mg/dose

c. No. 1.7 g = 1700 mg, which exceeds the safe dosage range for this drug for this child. (Did you remember to convert g to mg?)

4. a. 0.14 to 0.34 mg/day

15 lb = 6.8 kg

Low dose: 0.02 mg/kg/day × 6.8 kg = 0.136 rounded to 0.14 mg/day

High dose: 0.05 mg/kg/day × 6.8 kg = 0.34 mg/day

b. 0.07 to 0.17 mg/dose

"bid" doses are given twice in 24 hours. 0.14 ÷ 2 = 0.07 mg/dose; 0.36 ÷ 2 = 0.17 mg/dose

c. Yes, 150 mcg = 0.15 mg, which falls within the safe and therapeutic dosage range for this child. (Did you remember to convert mcg to mg?)

5. a. 15.5 to 34.1 mg/kg/dose

34 lb = 15.5 kg

Low dose: 1 mg/kg/dose × 15.5 kg = 15.5 mg/dose

High dose: 2.2 mg/kg/dose × 15.5 kg = 34.1 mg/dose

b. Yes, the ordered dose of 30 mg is within the safe and therapeutic dose range for this child.

6. a. 90.8 to 113.5 mcg/kg/day

50 lb = 22.7 kg

Low dose: 4 mcg/kg/day × 22.7 kg = 90.8 mcg/day

High dose: 5 mcg/kg/day × 22.7 kg = 113.5 mcg/day

b. No. The ordered dose, 0.2 mg = 200 mcg, which exceeds the safe and therapeutic dosage range for this child. (Did you remember to convert mcg to mg?)

Section V

Basic Intravenous Calculations

1. Start at STEP 1. You need to calculate the hourly rate.

a. 167 mL/hr

1000 mL :: 6 hr :: x : 1 hr

$(1000 \times 1) = (6 \times x)$; $1000 = 6x$;

$x = 1000/6 = 166.66$ (Round to nearest whole number.)

Proof: $1000 \times 1 = 1000$; $6 \times 167 = 1002$ (slight difference due to previous rounding)

(Alternate method: 1000 mL ÷ 6 hr = 166.67 or 167 mL/hr)

b. 42 gtt/min (Round to nearest whole number.)

STEP 2:

$$\frac{\text{drop factor}}{\text{time (min)}} \times \text{hourly rate} = 15/60 \times 167 =$$
$$1/4 \times 200 = 41.75 \text{ (rounded to nearest whole number)}$$

2. Start at STEP 1. You need to calculate the hourly rate.

a. 200 mL/hr

600 mL : 3 hr :: x : 1 hr

$(600 \times 1) = (3 \times x)$; $600 = 3x$;

$x = 600/3 = 200$

Proof: $600 \times 1 = 600$; $3 \times 200 = 600$

(Alternate method: 600 mL ÷ 3 hr = 200 mL/hr)

b. 33 gtt/min (Round to nearest whole number.)

STEP 2:

$$\frac{\text{drop factor}}{\text{time (min)}} \times \text{hourly rate} = 10/60 \times 200 =$$
$$1/6 \times 200 = 33.33 \text{ (rounded to nearest whole number)}$$

3. Start at STEP 1. You need to calculate the hourly rate.

a. 83 mL/hr

1000 mL : 12 hr :: x : 1 hr

$(1000 \times 1) = (12 \times x)$; $1000 = 12x$; $x = 1000/12 = 83.33$ (Round to nearest whole number.)

Proof: $1000 \times 1 = 1000$; $12 \times 83 = 996$ (slight difference due to previous rounding)

(Alternate method: 1000 mL ÷ 12 hr = 83.33 or 83 mL/hr)

b. 21 gtt/min (Round to nearest whole number.)

STEP 2:

$$\frac{\text{drop factor}}{\text{time (min)}} \times \text{hourly rate} = 15/60 \times 83 =$$
$$1/4 \times 83 = 20.75 \text{ (rounded to nearest whole number)}$$

4. Start at STEP 1. You need to calculate the hourly rate.

a. 100 mL/hr

200 mL : 2 hr :: x : 1 hr

$(200 \times 1) = (2 \times x)$; $200 = 2x$;

$x = 200/2 = 100$

Proof: $200 \times 1 = 200$; $2 \times 100 = 200$

(Alternate method: 200 mL ÷ 2 hr = 100 mL/hr)

b. 100 gtt/min

STEP 2:

$$\frac{\text{drop factor}}{\text{time (min)}} \times \text{hourly rate} = 60/60 \times 100 =$$
$$1 \times 100 = 100$$

c. The drop factor for microdrip tubing is 60 gtt/mL.

5. Start at STEP 2. The hourly rate has been provided (75 mL/hr).

13 gtt/min (Round to nearest whole number.)

STEP 2:

$$\frac{\text{drop factor}}{\text{time (min)}} \times \text{hourly rate} = 10/60 \times 75 = 1/4 \times 75 = 12.75 \text{ (rounded to nearest whole number)}$$

6. Start at STEP 2. The hourly rate has been provided (75 mL/hr).

19 gtt/min (Round to nearest whole number.)

STEP 2:

$$\frac{\text{drop factor}}{\text{time (min)}} \times \text{hourly rate} = 15/60 \times 75 = 1/4 \times 75 = 18.75$$

7. Start at STEP 2. The hourly rate has been provided (75 mL/hr).

25 gtt/min

STEP 2:

$$\frac{\text{drop factor}}{\text{time (min)}} \times \text{hourly rate} = 20/60 \times 75 = 1/3 \times 75 = 25$$

8. As the drop factor increases, the gtt/min also increases.

9. a. 100 mL/hr

b. and c. Since the infusion pump delivers in mL/hr, it is unnecessary to calculate gtt/min.

Start at STEP 1. You need to calculate the hourly rate. Remember, 30 min = 0.5 hr.

50 mL : 0.5 hr :: x mL : 1 hr

$(50 \times 1) = (0.5 \times x)$; 50 = 0.5$x$;

x = 50/0.5 = 100

Proof: $50 \times 1 = 50$; $0.5 \times 100 = 50$

(Alternate method: 50 mL ÷ 0.5 hr = 100 mL/hr)

10. Start at STEP 1. You need to calculate the hourly rate.

a. 125 mL/hr

500 mL : 4 hr :: x : 1 hr

$(500 \times 1) = (4 \times x)$; 500 = 4$x$;

x = 500/4 = 125

Proof: $500 \times 1 = 500$; $4 \times 125 = 500$

(Alternate method: 500 mL ÷ 4 hr = 125 mL/hr)

b. 125 gtt/min

STEP 2:

$$\frac{\text{drop factor}}{\text{time (min)}} \times \text{hourly rate} = 60/60 \times 125 = 1 \times 125 = 125$$

PRACTICE QUIZ

1. 0.75 mg

1000 mcg : 1 mg :: 750 mcg : x mg

Proof: $1000 \times 0.75 = 750$; $1 \times 750 = 750$

2. 8000 mg

1 g : 1000 mg :: 8 g : x mg

Proof: $1 \times 8000 = 8000$; $1000 \times 8 = 8000$

3. 113.6 kg

1 kg : 2.2 lb :: x kg : 250 lb

Proof: $1 \times 250 = 250$; $2.2 \times 113.6 = 249.92$ (rounds to 250)

4. 165 lb

1 kg : 2.2 lb :: 75 kg : x lb

Proof: $1 \times 165 = 165$; $2.2 \times 75 = 165$

5. 15 mL

1 tsp : 5 mL :: 3 tsp : x mL

Proof: $1 \times 15 = 15$; $5 \times 3 = 15$

6. 600 mg

gr i (1) : 60 mg :: gr x (10) : x mg

Proof: 1 (gr i) $\times 600 = 600$; 60×10 (gr x) = 600

7. 10 mL

25 mg : 5 mL :: 50 mg : x mL

Proof: $25 \times 10 = 250$; $5 \times 50 = 250$

8. 1 tablet

STEP 1: Convert g to mg : 0.5 g = 500 mg

500 mg : 1 tablet :: 500 mg : x tablet

Proof: $500 \times 1 = 500$; $1 \times 500 = 500$

9. 2 mL

50 mg : 1 mL :: 100 mg : x mL

Proof: $50 \times 2 = 100$; $1 \times 100 = 100$

10. 5 mL

1% indicates 1 g in 100 mL, which equals 1000 mg/100 mL, or 10 mg/1 mL.

10 mg : 1 mL :: 50 mg : x mL

Proof: $10 \times 5 = 50$; $1 \times 50 = 50$

11. 0.25 mL

1:1000 indicates 1 g in 1000 mL, which equals 1000 mg/1000 mL, or 1 mg/mL.

1 mg : 1 mL :: 0.25 mg : x mL

Proof: $1 \times 0.25 = 0.25$; $1 \times 0.25 = 0.25$

12. 1.5 mL

10,000 units : 1 mL :: 15,000 units : x mL

Proof: $10,000 \times 1.5 = 15,000$; $1 \times 15,000 = 15,000$

13. a. 0.2 to 0.8 mg/dose

b. No, the dose of 1 mg exceeds the safe and therapeutic dosage range for this child.

22 lb = 10 kg

Low range: 0.02 mg/kg/dose $\times$ 10 kg = 0.2 mg/dose

High range: 0.08 mg/kg/dose $\times$ 10 kg = 0.8 mg/dose

14. a. 63 mL/hr

500 mL ÷ 8 hr = 62.5 (rounded to 63 mL/hr)

b. 16 gtt/min

$$\frac{\text{drop factor}}{\text{time (min)}} \times \text{hourly rate} = 15/60 \times 63 = 1/4 \times 63 = 15.75 \text{ (rounded to nearest whole number)}$$

15. a. Infusion pumps deliver mL/hr.

b. 50 mL/hr (as stated in the question)

16. a. 42 mL/hr
    1000 mL ÷ 24 hr = 41.67 (rounded to
        42 mL/hr)

    b. 42 gtt/min (Remember that if the drop factor is
    60, the rate is the same as the gtt/min.)

    $$\frac{\text{drop factor}}{\text{time (min)}} \times \text{hourly rate} = 60/60 \times 42 = 1 \times 42 \text{ gtt/min}$$

17. a. 1 g

    b. 2.5 mL
    200 mg : 1 mL :: 500 mg : x mL
    Proof: 200 × 2.5 = 500; 1 × 500 = 500

18. a. 200,000 units/mL

    b. 23 mL

    c. 1 mL (concentration is 200,000 units per
    1 mL)

    d. Label the multidose vial with the date, time,
    amount of diluent used, and user's initials.

19. a. 6 mL
    100 mg : 1 mL :: 600 mg : x mL
    Proof: 100 × 6 = 600; 1 × 600 = 600

    b. Up to 1410 mg/24 hr
    31 lb = 14.1 kg; 14.1 kg × 100 mg/kg/day =
        1410 mg/24 hr (safe dose)

    c. 705 mg/dose
    There are two doses per day; 1410 mg ÷ 2 =
        705 mg/dose

    d. Yes
    The ordered dose of 600 mg does not exceed
        the 705 maximum dose.

20. 2.5 mL
    125 mcg = 0.125 mg
    0.05 mg : 1 mL :: 0.125 mg : x mg
    Proof: 0.05 × 2.5 = 0.125 × 0.125 = 0.125

BARRON'S

CLEP*

12TH EDITION

College Composition
John Bechtle, D.Min.
Director, The Telos Institute International
William C. Doster

Humanities
Ruth S. Ward
Philip Geer, Ed.M.

Mathematics
Shirley O. Hockett, M.A.
Ithaca College (retired)
David Bock, M.S.
Author, Consultant
Benjamin Kirk, M.A.
Ithaca High School

Natural Sciences
Adrian W. Poitras
Louis Gotlib, M.A.T.
Wissahickon Sr. High School

Social Sciences—History
Robert Bjork
Philip Geer, Ed.M.

Introductions
John Bechtle, D.Min.

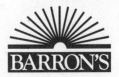
BARRON'S

All inquiries should be addressed to:
Barron's Educational Series, Inc.
250 Wireless Boulevard
Hauppauge, New York 11788
www.barronseduc.com

ISBN: 978-1-4380-0628-4

ISSN: 2380-7156

PRINTED IN THE UNITED STATES OF AMERICA
9 8 7 6 5 4 3 2 1

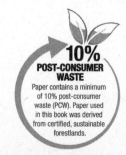

10%
POST-CONSUMER
WASTE
Paper contains a minimum
of 10% post-consumer
waste (PCW). Paper used
in this book was derived
from certified, sustainable
forestlands.

Contents

THE COLLEGE MATHEMATICS EXAMINATION

THE SOCIAL SCIENCES–HISTORY EXAMINATION

THE NATURAL SCIENCES EXAMINATION

Introduction to the College-Level Examination Program

1

WHAT IS THE CLEP EXAM PROGRAM?

The College-Level Examination Program (CLEP) is a nation-wide testing program developed by the College Board, in cooperation with the Educational Testing Service (ETS). It began in 1965 and is now administered at 1,800 colleges. Nearly 3,000 colleges award credit to students who perform well on the exams.

WHO TAKES CLEP EXAMS?

Most students who take the CLEP Exams are people who have acquired significant amounts of knowledge outside the college classroom. By taking CLEP Exams, they can demonstrate that they have achieved college-level learning so that they are not required to enroll in certain courses when they pursue a college degree.

CLEP Exams have proven valuable for:

- Adult learners who have engaged in self-study and achieved significant learning on the job.
- Home-educated students who have undertaken advanced studies during their high school years.
- High school students who have taken advanced courses during their high school years.
- Students from nonaccredited institutions who need to have their records validated so they can pursue a degree at an accredited institution.
- Applicants for employment with government agencies who value a standardized evaluation of skills.
- Individuals who desire to evaluate their level of learning for the purpose of personal growth, rather than pursuit of a college degree.

CLEP SUBJECT EXAMS

This book will help you prepare for five of the CLEP Exams that cover the material typically taught in introductory courses during the first two years of college: College Composition, Humanities, Mathematics, Natural Sciences, and Social Sciences and History.

Overview of Exams

Test	Content
College Composition	Part 1—Conventions of standard written English, revision skills, ability to use source materials, rhetorical analysis
	Part 2—Two essays, one of which involves analysis and citation of sources
College Composition Modular	Part 1—Conventions of standard written English, revision skills, ability to use source materials, rhetorical analysis
	Part 2—To be determined by the credit-granting institution
Humanities	Literature (drama, poetry, fiction, nonfiction, including philosophy)
	The Arts (visual arts, music, performing arts, architecture)
Mathematics	Sets, logic, real number system, functions and graphs, probability and statistics
Natural Sciences	Biological science, physical science
Social Sciences and History	History, political science, sociology, economics, psychology, geology, anthropology

GENERAL INFORMATION ABOUT THE EXAMS COVERED IN THIS BOOK

Each of the CLEP Exams covered in this book emphasizes the general principles of the subject area being tested, not the mere facts anyone might remember from a specific course. More specific information about the areas covered is given in each of the sections of this book dealing with the five exams. In general, however, the entire battery of five tests covers what anyone might be expected to know from the first two years of college work or the equivalent.

Most colleges have a required series of courses that provide the type of general information and educational experience that every person should have as he or she goes into a specialized area; these CLEP Examinations do not go beyond the content of these "general education" courses, as they are often called. Obviously, different schools provide varied content in each of these courses, and some schools have no such general education requirements. Students with different backgrounds may find that they are deficient in one area but very good in another. However, it is normally the overall score that matters.

You do not have to take all five Examinations. You may choose any one or more of the exams, scheduling the test dates at your convenience.

HOW THE SYSTEM WORKS

The CLEP examination process requires you to interact with three different institutions.

> 1. The College Board
> 2. A local test center connected to the Educational Testing Service
> 3. A college (if you wish to receive college credit)

The **College Board** develops the CLEP Exams, keeps and reports the scores, and oversees the process. A network of 1,800 **test centers**, located at colleges and universities, administer the exams. Over 2,900 **colleges** grant credit for satisfactory scores.

Understanding how the process is organized will help you achieve your educational objectives most effectively. To earn college credit through CLEP Exams, you should take the following steps:

1. Become familiar with the exams and decide which one(s) you wish to take.
2. Make contact with the college where you intend to receive credit. Obtain information on their policies to learn how much credit is possible, what scores are required, and how your results will be handled.
3. Develop a plan to prepare for the exam, using materials like this handbook.
4. Visit *www.clep.collegeboard.org* and register to take the test (see below for more information on registering)
5. Report to the test center at your scheduled time.
6. After you log into the computer, but before the test begins, you will be asked to indicate your "Score Recipient." Here you will select the college of your choice, and your score report will automatically be sent to it.
7. You will receive an unofficial score report as soon as you complete the test, except for College Composition. Keep this in your records. You will receive your official score report for College Composition in 2 to 4 weeks because your essays must be graded and included in the scoring.
8. Check with the college you selected to receive your score to see if there is anything you need to do to have the credit added to your transcript.

HOW TO ARRANGE TO TAKE THE CLEP EXAMINATIONS

Educational Testing Service has established test centers at major colleges in all parts of the United States. Some test centers are open only to their own students; others are open to the public. You can locate the nearest test center by consulting the College Board website at *www.clep.collegeboard.org/search/test-centers*. You can also contact them by phone at (800) 257-9558.

There are three easy steps to taking CLEP exams:

STEP 1 When you are ready to take your CLEP exam, go to *www.clep.collegeboard.org* and pay for the exam by creating a My Account. The CLEP fee is $80. **After you pay, you will need to print your Registration Ticket and bring it with you on the day of your exam.**

STEP 2 Fill out the REGISTRATION FORM to make an appointment to take your test.

STEP 3 **On your test day**, come to the Testing Center with two forms of ID (primary ID must have a photo AND a signature—a driver's license works great; secondary ID can have either a picture OR a signature—Student ID, passport, and birth certificate are some examples). Also, each Test Center will have a fee for proctoring the test. Please check with the Center about this fee and bring money to cover the fee, usually payable with cash, check, or card.

Please also review the test center's *Check-In Policies* before you come to take your exam.

Each test center will provide detailed information on their procedures and fees. In addition, the College Board maintains regional offices in each section of the country, which can provide additional information.

HOW SCORES ARE HANDLED

All CLEP Exams are now administered on computers. Most of them are scored immediately, so that you will know your score before you leave the exam session. Exceptions include the College Composition and the College Composition Modular. Unlike exams in multiple-choice format, the College Composition essays are scored by college professors, rather than computers. Essays are scored twice a month, and scores are combined with the scores on the multiple-choice section of the exam. The combined score is then reported to the student. Some colleges provide and score their own essay section for the College Composition Modular exam.

Because the exams are computer-based, you must be careful to follow instructions exactly. We suggest that you visit the College Board's website at *www.clep.collegeboard.org/test-preparation*. From this page you can click on CLEP Tutorial Testing Platform so that you can become familiar with the process of completing the exam on a computer.

The total number of questions you have answered correctly will be converted to a "scaled score" between 20 and 80. The scaled score will be reported to any college you designate. When you take the exam, you have the option to have the score sent to a college or employer at no charge. If you request a score report at a later date, there is a nominal fee.

FINAL CAUTION

Before you register for a CLEP Exam, consult the staff at the institution where you plan to have your scores sent. You should find out exactly how the scores will be interpreted, what uses will be made of the scores, and what specific scores are required by that college to receive credit.

> The format and content of the CLEP Examinations are changed periodically. You should check the CLEP website or contact the nearest College Board regional office to obtain the latest information on each exam.

Neither the College Board nor Educational Testing Service sets a passing or failing score. Evaluating your scores and granting credit is solely the responsibility of the college to which your scores are submitted. Since most institutions have different policies on these matters, you should have that information before you take the examinations.

How to Use This Book in Preparing for the CLEP Examinations

2

HOW TO STUDY FOR THE CLEP EXAMINATIONS

The CLEP Examinations represent a survey of basic subjects. This book covers five basic subjects. When the test is constructed, each subject is outlined or divided up into a number of main topics. Questions are written that fall under the main headings. Because the test has only a limited number of questions, these questions will, for the most part, cover only the main points of any one category. Therefore, in studying for the examination the student should survey the entire subject, draw up an outline of the subject, review the main points in familiar areas, and study those topics with which he or she is less familiar.

This book helps you get used to the actual process of taking multiple-choice tests. At the same time each sample question reveals a topic or subject area that may be on the actual test. Because these questions and those presented on the actual test are not identical, it is best not to simply memorize answers to the questions in this book. Instead, when you encounter questions you can't answer, look at the answer key to determine the correct answer. When you find the answer, try to understand the concept or idea involved. You might keep track of the questions you miss and see if they fall in the same category. In this way you can direct your review toward those areas in which you are least proficient. You may have difficulty with a question because the question contains words you do not know. In this case, write the words down as you confront them and find out what they mean by consulting a dictionary or other reference book.

Because the CLEP Examinations cover a wide area of general knowledge, it would be difficult to start from scratch, learning everything that might be included in the test. However, you should realize that you are not starting from scratch. If you are a recent high school graduate, you will discover that most of the material on the tests is material with which you are already familiar from high school and elementary school courses. If you have been out of school for some time, you will find that much of the material on the actual examination is familiar to you from newspapers, magazines, websites, and your general experience.

In preparing for the test it is best to use books that outline the material to be covered in a brief but concise way. You need to know the main points of a subject. If you do not already have extensive knowledge in a field, it is unreasonable to expect to acquire it now and for the most part it will be unnecessary in terms of this particular examination. The questions on a CLEP Exam are designed to do more than merely test your memory of an endless list of facts; they call on you to use your knowledge of broad features and key principles to determine the most likely answers to the questions. Main points you should know include the major persons in a field, the main events, principles involved, and the vocabulary of each field.

The Examination in College Mathematics covers material that is generally taught in a college course for nonmathematics majors. Some of the topics are sets, logic, the real number system, functions and graphs, probability and statistics, and additional topics from algebra and geometry. The bibliography given in Chapter 10 will be helpful if you feel the need for a general review of mathematics.

It is important to remember that survey courses for freshmen and sophomores in college, for the most part, repeat a good deal of material that the student should have learned in high school. To be sure, college courses are more compact or concise and may go into the subject in greater depth. Nevertheless, many of the main topics covered are the same as those covered in high school. Do not be overwhelmed by the idea that these are "college" examinations. They are designed for the person who has acquired a basic education on his or her own. Working out the items offered in this book and answering the questions will be one way in which you can review what you have already learned, either in a classroom or on your own.

STRATEGIES FOR PREPARING FOR THE CLEP EXAMS

How the Book Is Organized

This book is arranged in five major parts, one part for each of the five CLEP Exams. Each part opens with a Trial Test, which gives you an idea of what the examination is like. It also lets you determine how you would score on the examination without any specific preparation or practice. Then there is a chapter that provides general information about the examination and a number of items illustrating the basic principles of the subject area as well as the different kinds of information you will need to have or the different responses you might be called upon to make. You will find these sample items arranged in small groups, and we have provided answers and explanations for these answers immediately following each group of questions. You may work through these groups of items at your own pace. The specific questions we give you will help you become familiar with the basic principles of the subject area. Each of these chapters includes a brief bibliography of reference works and textbooks that you may want to review if you find that you are weak in one of the subject areas. Most of these books are available in a good public library.

The remainder of each section consists of a chapter containing two sample examinations. You may take these exams to track your progress as you prepare to take the CLEP Exam of your choice. An answer key is included at the end of each test so you can check yourself immediately. Answer explanations are also provided; these explanations will help you learn how to read each question carefully and answer exactly what is asked. They will also help you recognize your weak spots so you can plan your studies. When taking the sample tests, we suggest that you follow the time limit that will be imposed during an actual CLEP Examination, so you get into the habit of having that limitation as part of the test procedure.

Planning Your Study Strategy

1. DECIDE WHICH EXAMS TO TAKE

You can't take all the exams on the same day, and most people will want to study for one or two exams at a time. If you do prepare for more than one test at a time, plan a schedule that allows you to skip back and forth between the two exam sections. This variety will give you a needed break.

Start with the subject you know best, so that you will have a quick initial success.

It is important to understand what kind of knowledge the CLEP Exams are designed to measure. The Exams represent a survey of five basic subjects. When the test is constructed, each subject is outlined or divided up into a number of main topics.

Questions are written to evaluate mastery of the main headings. Because the test has only a limited number of questions, these questions will, for the most part, cover only the main points of any one category. When you study, therefore, you should survey the entire subject, reviewing the main points in familiar areas and studying more intensively in the areas which are less familiar. Even though the test questions may refer to facts you have not mastered, you can often determine the correct answer by using your knowledge of basic principles to eliminate unlikely choices and focus on the most likely options.

2. TAKE THE TRIAL TEST

You probably have a fairly accurate idea of which subjects are your strongest areas and which will require more intensive preparation.

By taking the Trial Test, you can confirm your self-evaluation and gain a more precise idea of how much preparation you should plan.

- If you have strong knowledge of the subject, you can simply use the material in this handbook to review. A score of 60 or above normally represents a fairly strong grasp of the material.
- If your knowledge of the subject is moderate, you should probably use one of the texts listed in the bibliography of each chapter to do a more extensive review of the subject. In preparing for the tests, it is best to use books that outline the material to be covered in a brief but systematic way. You may wish to obtain a textbook used by a local college. You need to know the main points of the subject, such as the major persons, the main events, the principles involved, and the vocabulary of each field.
- If you have a particularly weak background in one particular area, it may be more reasonable for you to take a college-level course in the subject. CLEP Examinations are designed to help you receive credit for what you have already learned, and if you do not already have adequate knowledge in a field, it is unreasonable to expect that you can master it without extensive study.

3. SET UP A PERSONAL STUDY PLAN

Determine your study goals and decide how much time you can devote to preparation. Set aside a time and place to work on the exam so that you can make steady progress.

4. WORK THROUGH THE CHAPTER ON BACKGROUND AND PRACTICE QUESTIONS

Do not attempt to take any of the complete Sample Examinations until you have worked through all the sample items in this chapter. As you try the small groups of questions, you will see that each of these groups deals with just one part of the subject area. In the complete examinations, on the other hand, questions are arranged in a more random order to cover the whole subject area.

5. TAKE THE SAMPLE EXAMS

If you complete this entire book with the illustrative and sample test items we have prepared for you, you will have worked through almost 3,000 different test items.

Why so many? We believe that this much practice is necessary for you to do well on the CLEP exam battery. We do not, of course, expect that anyone will attempt to finish the whole book in just a few days. Take your time, and you will be better off.

Observe the time limits when you take each Sample Examination, so that you will become accustomed to the discipline of working within time limits. Do not be disappointed if you do not finish each Sample Examination within the prescribed time limit. Test experts tell us that many people do not finish the tests for various reasons. Simply do the best you can. If you can get about 50 percent of each test correct, your score will be above the average score of all college sophomores in the United States.

The vocabulary level of the test items is about Grade 14, which means that the words used are those that any college sophomore should recognize and understand from his or her reading. Sentence structure and syntax are at the same level. You should not use a dictionary or any other reference tool while you are taking a sample exam because you will not have access to such tools during the actual examination period. After completing the Sample Exam, however, you may find it helpful to consult a good dictionary to learn the meaning of any words you did not understand.

You will take the actual CLEP Exams on a computer, but we have provided answer sheets for the Trial Tests and Sample Examinations.

This book helps you get used to the actual process of taking multiple-choice tests. In addition, each sample question reveals a topic or subject area that may be represented on the actual test. None of the questions in the book appears in an actual CLEP Exam, so it is best not to simply memorize answers to the questions in this book. Instead, you should use the following procedure:

- ✔ Mark each question that you cannot answer.
- ✔ Read the explanation of the question in the section following the test, and try to understand the concept you missed.
- ✔ Look for patterns of weakness or blind spots. If several of the questions you missed fall into the same category, you can focus extra effort on study in that area.

6. BE SURE THAT YOU ARE COMFORTABLE WITH COMPUTER-BASED TESTING

You will take your CLEP Exam on a computer, so it is important to become comfortable with that format so that you will not be distracted during the test. You can download the *CLEP Tutorial-Testing Platform* from the CLEP website to recreate the experience of taking a CLEP Exam on your computer. Go to *www.clep.collegeboard.org/test-preparation*, then click on *CLEP Tutorial-Testing Platform*. If you have a learning disability or physical disability that would make it difficult for you to take a CLEP Exam in the standard format, you may request special testing accommodations. You should contact the test center that you plan to use well in advance to find out how they can help you.

Strategies for Taking the CLEP Examinations

1. BEFORE THE TEST DAY

✔ Get plenty of sleep. An important aid in taking an examination is to rest the night before. Fatigue can lower your self-confidence and your ability to concentrate. It can also slow you down when taking the examination and can ultimately lower your score.

✔ Eat normally. Do not take any tranquilizers or stimulants that might interfere with your performance. Do not drink too many liquids so that you can avoid the necessity of interrupting the exam for a visit to the restroom.

✔ Be sure that you know the location of the test center, including parking, so that you will not be delayed.

✔ Contact the test center to be sure that you know what ID to bring and what form of payment is acceptable.

2. ON THE TEST DAY

✔ Arrive early so that you will not feel rushed and will have time to adjust to the surroundings. This will give you time to ask questions and arrange your personal belongings before the exam begins.

✔ Be sure you have remembered to bring the required personal identification and payment. Bring any registration forms required by the test center. Your personal identification should include a driver's license, passport, or other government-issued identification that includes your photograph and signature. You may also need secondary identification such as a social security card or student ID that includes your photo or signature.

✔ Wear comfortable clothes. Since you do not know whether the examination room will be warm or cold, wear layers of clothing that can removed or added as needed.

✔ Bring two pencils with good erasers, to write ideas for an essay or to do math calculations. You may not bring a mechanical pencil. Do not bring scratch paper; it will be provided by the test center. If you take the Mathematics Exam, you will not need a calculator; the test software includes a calculator.

A credit card is the most common method of payment, but you may also pay by check or money order.

3. DURING THE EXAM

Different strategies work for different people in taking exams. You should follow whatever procedure works best for you. Because each test is timed, however, it is crucial that you do not linger too long on any single question. As soon as it becomes obvious to you that you do not know the answer, you should move on to the next question. Many poor test takers get bogged down on one or two questions and don't have time to complete all the questions they could have answered.

Here is a strategy that seems to work for many people:

STRATEGY

The Process of Elimination

The scientist who invented the first usable electric light was

(A) Benjamin Franklin
(B) George Washington
(C) Thomas Edison
(D) Henry Ford
(E) Marie Curie

You may not know a thing about electricity but certainly you can eliminate the names of George Washington and Henry Ford. You have bettered your odds; your chances are now one-in-three instead of one-in-five. If you are still not sure which is correct, but have a hunch, then play that hunch.

✔ Read the question and try to *recall* or determine the right answer.

✔ If you cannot recall or determine the right answer, read the question again and see if you *recognize* the correct answer. Be sure to read all the choices before answering, then choose the best answer.

✔ If you do not recognize the right answer, use the "Mark" tool on the screen to identify that question so you can return to it later. Then immediately go on to the next question. In this way you will spend your time on what you know. The secret of taking this type of test is to decide immediately whether or not you know the answer. If you cannot decide quickly, mark the questions and go on to the next item so that no time is wasted.

✔ When you have completed all the answers that you were sure of, you will probably have time to go back and look more closely at the questions you marked the first time around. When you come back to take a second look, you will find that you immediately recognize some of the answers.

✔ For any items that still give you difficulty, you should use the process of elimination to weed out any obviously incorrect answers.

✔ Make your best guess. **There is no penalty for wrong answers, so it is better to guess than to leave an item blank.**

Often, you will have heard or read the correct answer, even though you do not consciously remember it. So you will often be correct if you follow your instincts. If you have chosen an answer and still aren't sure about it, it is usually best to stick with your first answer. Research studies have demonstrated that the first guess is more likely to be correct than a revised guess later on.

OTHER HINTS

- **DON'T ASSUME ANYTHING ABOUT THE TEST INSTRUCTIONS.** You will be given time to read the test directions before the test begins. Even if you feel completely familiar with the directions from other experiences, take time to read them on this particular test, so that you know exactly what to expect.
- **RELAX.** Don't let last minute nervousness get the better of you. Almost everyone is a little tense before an examination, and being a little keyed up can help you focus on the task at hand. But too much tension can interfere with your performance. If you freeze or clutch during the examination, then forget the questions for a few moments and concentrate on something else. Don't worry about the few minutes you lose. You'll waste more time and will be less efficient if you try to struggle through the test with that "locked up" feeling. Relax and be calm. Remind yourself that you're pretty smart and you have what it takes. Then, when you are calmer, go back to the exam.
- **PACE YOURSELF.** Check the time fairly often to make sure you're not going too slowly. You should have finished one quarter of the questions when one quarter of the time is up, half of the questions when half the time is up. If you find you have been taking too long, try to speed up a bit for the rest of the test. And remember not to spend too long on any one question.
- **READ ALL OF THE ANSWER CHOICES BEFORE CHOOSING YOUR ANSWER.** The first or second answer might seem correct, but the fourth or fifth one might be even better—and usually the directions instruct you to pick the *best* answer choice.
- **DO NOT TRY TO FIGURE OUT A CERTAIN PATTERN OF ANSWERS.** Some students think that if the answer to one question is (A), the answer to the next question will probably be (D), and the correct response to the following question might be (B). The CLEP Exams are designed so that no such patterns exist.
- **DO NOT LOOK FOR "TRICK QUESTIONS."** CLEP Exams are written to ask straightforward questions to find out what you know. They do not build in traps or surprises.

> **NOTE**
>
> **You should use a slightly different approach when taking the College Mathematics Exam. See the section on the Math Exam for details.**

When you finish this book, look back through the questions, and check to see just how much factual information you can recall from your experiences with the sample items. We think that you will be pleasantly surprised.

Good luck!

NOTE

No sample question in this book has ever appeared on an actual CLEP examination. The examinations are security tests, and all material on those tests is protected by copyright in the name of the Educational Testing Service. The test items in this book are meant to be similar in format to an actual CLEP examination, not actual items that you might find when you take one or more of the examinations.

Progress Chart

	Trial Test	Exam 1	Exam 2
College Composition 50 minutes for multiple choice, 70 minutes for essays			
College Composition Modular 90 minutes for multiple choice, 70 minutes for the optional essay			
Humanities 90 minutes			
Mathematics 90 minutes			
Natural Sciences 90 minutes			
Social Sciences–History 90 minutes			

The College Composition Examination

ANSWER SHEET
Trial Test

COLLEGE COMPOSITION

1. Ⓐ Ⓑ Ⓒ Ⓓ Ⓔ
2. Ⓐ Ⓑ Ⓒ Ⓓ Ⓔ
3. Ⓐ Ⓑ Ⓒ Ⓓ Ⓔ
4. Ⓐ Ⓑ Ⓒ Ⓓ Ⓔ
5. Ⓐ Ⓑ Ⓒ Ⓓ Ⓔ
6. Ⓐ Ⓑ Ⓒ Ⓓ Ⓔ
7. Ⓐ Ⓑ Ⓒ Ⓓ Ⓔ
8. Ⓐ Ⓑ Ⓒ Ⓓ Ⓔ
9. Ⓐ Ⓑ Ⓒ Ⓓ Ⓔ
10. Ⓐ Ⓑ Ⓒ Ⓓ Ⓔ
11. Ⓐ Ⓑ Ⓒ Ⓓ Ⓔ
12. Ⓐ Ⓑ Ⓒ Ⓓ Ⓔ
13. Ⓐ Ⓑ Ⓒ Ⓓ Ⓔ
14. Ⓐ Ⓑ Ⓒ Ⓓ Ⓔ
15. Ⓐ Ⓑ Ⓒ Ⓓ Ⓔ
16. Ⓐ Ⓑ Ⓒ Ⓓ Ⓔ
17. Ⓐ Ⓑ Ⓒ Ⓓ Ⓔ
18. Ⓐ Ⓑ Ⓒ Ⓓ Ⓔ
19. Ⓐ Ⓑ Ⓒ Ⓓ Ⓔ
20. Ⓐ Ⓑ Ⓒ Ⓓ Ⓔ
21. Ⓐ Ⓑ Ⓒ Ⓓ Ⓔ
22. Ⓐ Ⓑ Ⓒ Ⓓ Ⓔ
23. Ⓐ Ⓑ Ⓒ Ⓓ Ⓔ

24. Ⓐ Ⓑ Ⓒ Ⓓ Ⓔ
25. Ⓐ Ⓑ Ⓒ Ⓓ Ⓔ
26. Ⓐ Ⓑ Ⓒ Ⓓ Ⓔ
27. Ⓐ Ⓑ Ⓒ Ⓓ Ⓔ
28. Ⓐ Ⓑ Ⓒ Ⓓ Ⓔ
29. Ⓐ Ⓑ Ⓒ Ⓓ Ⓔ
30. Ⓐ Ⓑ Ⓒ Ⓓ Ⓔ
31. Ⓐ Ⓑ Ⓒ Ⓓ Ⓔ
32. Ⓐ Ⓑ Ⓒ Ⓓ Ⓔ
33. Ⓐ Ⓑ Ⓒ Ⓓ Ⓔ
34. Ⓐ Ⓑ Ⓒ Ⓓ Ⓔ
35. Ⓐ Ⓑ Ⓒ Ⓓ Ⓔ
36. Ⓐ Ⓑ Ⓒ Ⓓ Ⓔ
37. Ⓐ Ⓑ Ⓒ Ⓓ Ⓔ
38. Ⓐ Ⓑ Ⓒ Ⓓ Ⓔ
39. Ⓐ Ⓑ Ⓒ Ⓓ Ⓔ
40. Ⓐ Ⓑ Ⓒ Ⓓ Ⓔ
41. Ⓐ Ⓑ Ⓒ Ⓓ Ⓔ
42. Ⓐ Ⓑ Ⓒ Ⓓ Ⓔ
43. Ⓐ Ⓑ Ⓒ Ⓓ Ⓔ
44. Ⓐ Ⓑ Ⓒ Ⓓ Ⓔ
45. Ⓐ Ⓑ Ⓒ Ⓓ Ⓔ
46. Ⓐ Ⓑ Ⓒ Ⓓ Ⓔ

47. Ⓐ Ⓑ Ⓒ Ⓓ Ⓔ
48. Ⓐ Ⓑ Ⓒ Ⓓ Ⓔ
49. Ⓐ Ⓑ Ⓒ Ⓓ Ⓔ
50. Ⓐ Ⓑ Ⓒ Ⓓ Ⓔ
51. Ⓐ Ⓑ Ⓒ Ⓓ Ⓔ
52. Ⓐ Ⓑ Ⓒ Ⓓ Ⓔ
53. Ⓐ Ⓑ Ⓒ Ⓓ Ⓔ
54. Ⓐ Ⓑ Ⓒ Ⓓ Ⓔ
55. Ⓐ Ⓑ Ⓒ Ⓓ Ⓔ
56. Ⓐ Ⓑ Ⓒ Ⓓ Ⓔ
57. Ⓐ Ⓑ Ⓒ Ⓓ Ⓔ
58. Ⓐ Ⓑ Ⓒ Ⓓ Ⓔ
59. Ⓐ Ⓑ Ⓒ Ⓓ Ⓔ
60. Ⓐ Ⓑ Ⓒ Ⓓ Ⓔ
61. Ⓐ Ⓑ Ⓒ Ⓓ Ⓔ
62. Ⓐ Ⓑ Ⓒ Ⓓ Ⓔ
63. Ⓐ Ⓑ Ⓒ Ⓓ Ⓔ
64. Ⓐ Ⓑ Ⓒ Ⓓ Ⓔ
65. Ⓐ Ⓑ Ⓒ Ⓓ Ⓔ
66. Ⓐ Ⓑ Ⓒ Ⓓ Ⓔ
67. Ⓐ Ⓑ Ⓒ Ⓓ Ⓔ
68. Ⓐ Ⓑ Ⓒ Ⓓ Ⓔ
69. Ⓐ Ⓑ Ⓒ Ⓓ Ⓔ

70. Ⓐ Ⓑ Ⓒ Ⓓ Ⓔ
71. Ⓐ Ⓑ Ⓒ Ⓓ Ⓔ
72. Ⓐ Ⓑ Ⓒ Ⓓ Ⓔ
73. Ⓐ Ⓑ Ⓒ Ⓓ Ⓔ
74. Ⓐ Ⓑ Ⓒ Ⓓ Ⓔ
75. Ⓐ Ⓑ Ⓒ Ⓓ Ⓔ
76. Ⓐ Ⓑ Ⓒ Ⓓ Ⓔ
77. Ⓐ Ⓑ Ⓒ Ⓓ Ⓔ
78. Ⓐ Ⓑ Ⓒ Ⓓ Ⓔ
79. Ⓐ Ⓑ Ⓒ Ⓓ Ⓔ
80. Ⓐ Ⓑ Ⓒ Ⓓ Ⓔ
81. Ⓐ Ⓑ Ⓒ Ⓓ Ⓔ
82. Ⓐ Ⓑ Ⓒ Ⓓ Ⓔ
83. Ⓐ Ⓑ Ⓒ Ⓓ Ⓔ
84. Ⓐ Ⓑ Ⓒ Ⓓ Ⓔ
85. Ⓐ Ⓑ Ⓒ Ⓓ Ⓔ
86. Ⓐ Ⓑ Ⓒ Ⓓ Ⓔ
87. Ⓐ Ⓑ Ⓒ Ⓓ Ⓔ
88. Ⓐ Ⓑ Ⓒ Ⓓ Ⓔ
89. Ⓐ Ⓑ Ⓒ Ⓓ Ⓔ
90. Ⓐ Ⓑ Ⓒ Ⓓ Ⓔ

Trial Test

3

This chapter contains a Trial Test in College Composition. Take this Trial Test to learn what the actual exam is like and to determine how you might score on the exam before any practice or review.

The CLEP Exam in College Composition measures your knowledge of English, including usage, sentence correction, paragraph revising, analysis, and construction shift.

There are two CLEP Exams in College Composition

- **COLLEGE COMPOSITION EXAM.** The College Composition Exam consists of two parts: the first part involves 50 multiple-choice questions, and the second part involves two essays.
- **COLLEGE COMPOSITION MODULAR EXAM.** The College Composition Modular Exam normally consists of two parts: the first part involves 90 multiple-choice questions, and the second part generally involves one or two essays, determined by the policies of the college granting credit.

NUMBER OF QUESTIONS ON THE TRIAL TEST

Part One: 50 questions
Part Two: 40 questions

PART ONE TIME LIMIT: 50 MINUTES
PART ONE AND PART TWO TIME LIMIT: 90 MINUTES

The Trial Exam is divided into two parts. Part One includes 50 questions that represent the types of questions found on the College Composition Exam. Part Two contains an additional 40 questions. The combination of Part One and Part Two matches the number and types of questions found on the College Composition Modular Exam.

If you intend to take the College Composition Exam, you may complete Part One and ignore Part Two.

If you intend to take the College Composition Modular Exam, you should complete both Part One and Part Two.

Part One

This part of the Trial Test consists of 50 questions, and you have 50 minutes to complete it. If you plan to take the College Composition Exam, you should complete only Part One of this test. If you plan to take the College Composition Modular Exam, you should complete Part One, then go on to complete Part Two. You may also proceed to Part Two if you simply wish to get extra practice in answering the questions.

> **DIRECTIONS:** Read each sentence carefully, paying attention to the underlined portions. Assume that elements of the sentence that are not underlined are correct and cannot be changed. In choosing answers, follow the requirements of Standard Written English.
>
> If there is an error, select the one underlined part that must be changed to make the sentence correct.
>
> If there is no error, select "No error," answer (E).

1. Looking out of the window was my pleasure for many
       A
    hours, for I could not understand the countryside until I had concentrated
         B   C
    on the different effects of it's beautiful scenes. No error.
                   D   E

2. Chinese art with its subtle shadings and almost suggestive
                A
    curving lines demonstrates those characteristics that set them apart
            B   C
    from all other people of the world. No error.
         D   E

3. Brazil is larger than any country in the world; if you argue with this bold
         A   B   C
    statement, look at the map of the world, either an atlas or any projection
                                  D
    of the world on a flat surface. No error.
                    E

4. <u>Most of the evidence</u> the prosecutor so carefully presented in his
       A

summation was ignored <u>by the jury</u> because <u>the defense attorney made</u>
             B   C

such an emotional speech <u>explaining his client's actions.</u> <u>No error.</u>
                          D   E

5. <u>As Joel reflected</u> on his experience at his <u>last job, he has realized</u> that he
     A   B

learned <u>some valuable life lessons</u> that would help him <u>at his current job.</u>
              C   D

<u>No error.</u>
  E

DIRECTIONS: The following passages are early drafts of essays.

Read each passage and then answer the questions that follow. Some questions refer to particular sentences or parts of sentences and ask you to improve sentence structure or diction (word choice). Other questions refer to the entire essay or parts of the essay and ask you to consider the essay's organization, development, or effectiveness of language. In selecting your answers, follow the conventions of Standard Written English.

<u>Questions 6–12</u> are based on the following draft of an essay.

(1) Some people like to relax by engaging in sports like tennis or softball. (2) Others go in for yoga exercises or read spy stories or they like to work in the garden. (3) One woman I know works on her car whenever she feels tense and nervous. (4) Her car is always in tip-top shape, and she keeps up on the latest automotive technology, too. (5) Me, I play computer games.

(6) A lot of people claim computer games are a waste of time. (7) They say that teenagers are flipping shapes around on Tetris when they should be doing their homework while young children are zapping digitized monsters instead of getting some physical exercise. (8) But there is a place for computer games. (9) All you have to do is remember that they are games, and belong in relaxation time, so you shouldn't be doing them in work time.

(10) Sometimes computer games serve a very useful purpose. (11) A spy was discovered when his boss borrowed his computer to play a computer game and found a file with all the information the spy had collected to pass to the enemy.

(12) The great advantage of computer games is that they are always there. (13) If you need a break from the research paper you're working on or the calculus problem you're having trouble with, just hit a few keys and you're off on a game that may require some concentrated eye-hand coordination, but will give your brain a much-needed rest.

6. Which is the best version of the underlined portion of sentence 2 (reproduced below)?

Others go in for yoga exercises or read spy stories or they like to work in the garden.

(A) (as it is now)
(B) and they like to work
(C) and work
(D) or work
(E) or they work

7. What should be done with sentence 4?

(A) Leave it as it is.
(B) Delete it.
(C) Combine it with sentence 3, using a colon.
(D) Put it after sentence 5.
(E) Combine it with sentence 3, using a comma.

8. What is the best version of the underlined portion of sentence 6 (reproduced below)?

A lot of people claim computer games are a waste of time.

(A) (as it is now)
(B) Most people say
(C) Many people claim that
(D) They say
(E) Although people claim that

9. What should be done with "while" in sentence 7?

(A) It should be left as it is.
(B) It should be deleted.
(C) It should be replaced with a semicolon.
(D) It should be replaced by "and that."
(E) It should be replaced by "so that."

10. What should be done with paragraph 3?

(A) It should be left as it is.
(B) It should be deleted.
(C) It should be placed before paragraph 1, so that it begins the essay.
(D) It should be placed after paragraph 4, so that it ends the essay.
(E) It should be combined with paragraph 2.

11. Which is the best version of the underlined portion of sentence 9 (reproduced below)?

All you have to do is remember that they are games, and belong in relaxation time, so you shouldn't be doing them in work time.

(A) (as it is now).

(B) so you shouldn't do them in work time.

(C) so you shouldn't do them when you should be working instead.

(D) not in work time.

(E) not when you should be working.

12. Which is the best version of sentence 12 (reproduced below)?

The great advantage of computer games is that they are always there.

(A) (as it is now)

(B) The great advantage of computer games is their constant availability.

(C) For those of us who use them, the great advantage of computer games is that they are always there on the computer.

(D) Computer games are always there.

(E) If you spend long hours working at a computer, the great advantage of computer games is that they are always there.

Questions 13–18 are based on the following passage:

(1) There used to be an old ad that said, "They laughed when I sat down at the piano." (2) Well, all through my childhood, they just left when I sat down at the piano.

(3) Mother was determined that I should be a musician, and she started me on piano lessons when I was seven. (4) Little girls who take piano lessons also have to practice. (5) There's no point in taking piano lessons if you don't practice. (6) This is what she kept pointing out to my father and my two brothers. (7) "There's no point in having her take piano lessons if she doesn't practice," Mother told my father and my two brothers every evening at six o'clock, half an hour before dinner, when I did my practicing. (8) That's when my father went out to the garage. (9) That's when my brothers went up to their room. (10) That's when the dog started scratching the door to be let out. (11) Even my mother, who was the one who said I had to practice, headed for the kitchen and started banging pots and pans.

(12) It wasn't that my family didn't love me. (13) I was the baby of the family, and most of the time they were willing to spoil me rotten. (14) The problem was that they weren't deaf— not even tone-deaf. (15) They just couldn't bear to listen.

(16) Then I began to practice. (17) My fingers stumbled over even the easiest scales sitting at the piano. (18) I couldn't play anything without hitting the wrong notes. (19) And what is more, I therefore had no sense of rhythm.

13. What is the best position in the essay for paragraph 4?

    (A) (where it is now)
    (B) following paragraph 1
    (C) following paragraph 2
    (D) at the start of the essay
    (E) omitted from the essay

14. Which is the best word to replace "and" in sentence 3?

    (A) None. A semicolon should be used.
    (B) but
    (C) yet
    (D) because
    (E) so

15. What is the best way to treat sentences 5 and 6?

    (A) Combine them into a single sentence, joining them with "and."
    (B) Delete them.
    (C) Move them to the end of the paragraph.
    (D) Put them after sentence 7.
    (E) Put them at the beginning of the paragraph.

16. Keeping in mind the sense of the passage as a whole, which of the following would be the best transition word to introduce sentence 4?

    (A) However,
    (B) Therefore,
    (C) Consequently,
    (D) Thus,
    (E) Besides,

17. Which of the following is the best version of the underlined portion of sentence 17 (reproduced below)?

My fingers stumbled over even the easiest scales sitting at the piano.

    (A) It should be left as it is.
    (B) It should be deleted.
    (C) while sitting at the piano.
    (D) seated at the piano.
    (E) when on the piano bench.

18. Which of the following is the best version of the underlined portion of sentence 19 (reproduced below)?

And what is more, I therefore had no sense of rhythm.

(A) (as it is now)
(B) I had
(C) Therefore, I had
(D) And I thus had
(E) What is more, I thus had

Questions 19–25 are based on the following passage:

(1) In 1869, Antonio Lopez de Santa Anna, the brave Mexican leader of the Alamo attack, moved to Staten Island, New York. (2) He had been exiled from Mexico because his forces slaughtered the Texas insurgents in their battle for independence. (3) Santa Anna had brought with him several objects from home, including a large lump of chicle, the elastic sap of the Sapodilla tree. (4) The Mayan Indians had been chewing this substance for hundreds of years. (5) Today, many people like breath mints as well as gum, although both products sell very well. (6) Santa Anna wasn't interested in chewing the chicle, he hoped that the inventor Thomas Adams could refine the substance into a substitute for rubber and Adams did his best, but he could not transform chicle into rubber.

(7) Adams was walking down the street one day he saw a small child buying a wax called "paraffin" at a pharmacy. (8) This gave Adams a great idea. (9) He asked the pharmacy manager if he would sell a brand new kind of gum. (10) The pharmacist agreed. (11) Dashing home, Adams immersed the chicle in water until it was soft. (12) Then he squeezed and was pressing the chicle into little round shapes. (13) They were a drab gray color, but every single ball of "gum" was sold the very next day. (14) With his profits, Adams went into business producing Adams New York Gum No. 1.

(15) The process of making chewing gum is surprisingly similar today. (16) Now, small pieces of latex—still obtained from the Sapodilla trees of Central and South America—are kneaded until soft. (17) Today, however, the chicle is added to a hot sugar-corn syrup mixture. (18) When the mixture is smooth, it is flavored, usually with mint (a great flavor), and rolled into thin strips or squares.

19. Which is the relationship between sentences 1 and 2?

(A) cause-effect
(B) chronological order
(C) problem-solution
(D) compare-contrast
(E) no connection

20. A reasonable criticism of sentence 5 would be that it

    (A) does not serve as an example of the Alamo attack.

    (B) endorses commercial products.

    (C) is off the topic.

    (D) lacks specific details to support the generalization.

    (E) is not a complete sentence, since it lacks a verb.

21. Which is the best version of sentence 6 (reproduced below)?

Santa Anna wasn't interested in chewing the chicle, he hoped that the inventor Thomas Adams could refine the substance into a substitute for rubber and Adams did his best, but he could not transform chicle into rubber.

    (A) (as it is now)

    (B) Santa Anna wasn't interested in chewing the chicle but he hoped that the inventor Thomas Adams could refine the substance into a substitute for rubber and even though Adams did his best, but he could not transform chicle into rubber.

    (C) Santa Anna wasn't interested in chewing the chicle. He hoped that the inventor Thomas Adams could refine the substance into a substitute for rubber. Adams did his best, but he could not transform chicle into rubber.

    (D) Santa Anna wasn't interested in chewing the chicle; instead, he hoped that the inventor Thomas Adams could refine the substance into a substitute for rubber. Adams did his best, but he could not transform chicle into rubber.

    (E) Santa Anna hoped that the inventor Thomas Adams could refine the substance into a substitute for rubber because he wasn't interested in chewing the chicle and Adams could not transform chicle into rubber but he did his best.

22. Which is the best version of sentence 7 (reproduced below)?

Adams was walking down the street one day he saw a small child buying a wax called "paraffin" at a pharmacy.

    (A) (as it is now)

    (B) Adams was walking down the street one day, he saw a small child buying a wax called "paraffin" at a pharmacy.

    (C) Adams was walking down the street one day when he saw a small child buying a wax called "paraffin" at a pharmacy.

    (D) At a pharmacy, a small child buying a wax called "paraffin" was seen by Adams as one day he was walking down the street.

    (E) A small child buying a wax called "paraffin" at a pharmacy was seen by Adams as he was walking down the street one day.

23. Sentence 12 is weak because

    (A) it is vague and unclear.

    (B) it is lacking a subject.

    (C) it has a misplaced modifier.

    (D) it has a dangling participle.

    (E) the verbs are not parallel.

24. Which is the best version of sentence 13 (reproduced below)?

They were a drab gray color, but every single ball of "gum" was sold the very next day.

(A) (as it is now)
(B) They were a drab gray color, but every single ball of "gum" were sold the very next day.
(C) Every single ball of "gum" was sold the very next day; they were a drab gray color.
(D) Every single ball of a drab gray colored "gum" were sold the very next day.
(E) A drab gray color, every single ball of "gum" was sold the very next day.

25. The apparent purpose of this passage is to

(A) persuade the reader that gum is an important product, in the past as well as the present.
(B) explain the history of chewing gum.
(C) compare and contrast marketing in the past and present.
(D) describe how chewing gum is made.
(E) highlight the contributions of people from other cultures.

DIRECTIONS: The following questions test your familiarity with basic research, reference, and composition skills. Some questions refer to passages, whereas other questions are self-contained. For each question, choose the best answer.

26. What is the best source to use in discovering the current world chess champion?

(A) An almanac
(B) An encyclopedia
(C) A book on the history of chess
(D) A copy of the most recent issue of a chess magazine
(E) A Web search

27. Wheeler, Sarah. "The Magnetic North: Notes from the Arctic Circle." *Slate* 24 February 2011. 25 February 2011. *http://ww.slate.com/id/2285394/entry/0/.*

In the above entry, 24 February 2011 provides what information?

(A) The date when the research paper was due
(B) The date when it was accessed by the writer
(C) The date when it was last revised
(D) The date when it was published
(E) The date when it was removed from the website

Questions 28–30 are based on the following passage:

Balkanization, division of a multinational state into smaller, ethnically homogeneous entities. It also is used to refer to ethnic conflict within multiethnic states. The term was coined at the end of World War I to describe the ethnic and political fragmentation that followed the breakup of the Ottoman Empire, particularly in the Balkans. The term is today invoked to explain the disintegration of some multiethnic states and their devolution into dictatorship, ethnic cleansing (q.v.), and civil war.

Balkanization has occurred in places other than the Balkans, including Africa in the 1950s and 1960s following the dissolution of the British and French colonial empires there. In the early 1990s the disintegration of Yugoslavia and the collapse of the Soviet Union led to the emergence of several new states—many of which were unstable and ethnically mixed—and then to violence between them. Many of the successor states contained seemingly intractable ethnic and religious divisions, and some made irredentist territorial claims against their neighbours. Armenia and Azerbaijan, for example, suffered from intermittent violence over ethnic enclaves and borders. In the 1990s in Bosnia and Herzegovina, ethnic divisions and intervention by Yugoslavia and Croatia led to widespread fighting among Serbs, Croatians, and Bosnians (Muslims) that resulted in the deaths of more than 10,000 people.

(R.W.P.)

Source: *The New Encyclopedia Britannica*, Vol. 1, Micropaedia. 15th ed. Chicago: Encyclopedia Britannica, 2005, p. 833.

28. Which of the following statements is NOT supported by the above entry?

    (A) Balkanization is often connected to ethnic divisions.
    (B) Balkanization is a term that originated in the aftermath of World War I.
    (C) Balkanization is the name of a portion of the territory originally included inthe Ottoman Empire.
    (D) Balkanization is a term used to describe the breakup of a state into smaller divisions along ethnic lines.
    (E) Africa was the scene of ethnic divisions in the mid-twentieth century.

29. In this entry, the abbreviation *q.v.* means that the student should

    (A) see the previous article for a fuller explanation of the term.
    (B) consult a dictionary for a definition of ethnic cleansing.
    (C) recognize that a non-standard meaning of the term is used.
    (D) notice that ethnic cleansing is given special emphasis.
    (E) refer to the article on "ethnic cleansing" for more information.

30. This passage points out that Balkanization in Africa

   (A) resulted from the dissolving of the British and French colonial system.
   (B) is not an accurate description of the historical facts.
   (C) was a direct result of conflict in the Balkan region.
   (D) resulted in the dismantling of the British presence in the region.
   (E) caused widespread conflict that resulted in thousands of deaths.

Questions 31–34 are based on the following passage:

[1]**plot** \ plät\ *n* [ME, fr. OE] (bef. 12c) **1 a :** a small area of planted ground < a vegetable ~ > **b :** a small piece of land in a cemetery **c :** a measured piece of land : LOT **2 :** GROUND PLAN, PLAT **3 :** the plan or main story (as of a movie or literary work) **4** [perh. back-formation fr. *complot*] **:** a secret plan for accomplishing a usu. evil or unlawful end INTRIGUE **5 :** a graphic representation (as a chart)— **plot·less** \-ləs\ *adj* — **plot·less·ness** *n*

   syn PLOT, INTRIGUE, MACHINATION, CONSPIRACY, CABAL means a plan secretly devised to accomplish an evil or treacherous end. PLOT implies careful foresight in planning a complex scheme < an assassination *plot* >. INTRIGUE suggests secret underhanded maneuvering in an atmosphere of duplicity < backstairs *intrigue* >. MACHINATION implies a contriving of annoyances, injuries, or evils by indirect means < the *machinations* of a party boss >. CONSPIRACY implies a secret agreement among several people usu. involving treason or great treachery < a *conspiracy* to fix prices >. CABAL typically applies to political intrigues involving persons of some eminence < a *cabal* among powerful senators >. ***syn*** see in addition PLAN

[2]**plot** *vb* **plot·ted; plot·ting** *vt* (1588) **1 a :** to make a plot, map, or plan of **b :** to mark or note on or as if on a map or chart **2 :** to lay out in plots **3 a :** to locate (a point) by means of coordinates **b :** to locate (a curve) by plotted points **c :** to represent (an equation) by means of a curve so constructed **4 :** to plan or contrive esp. secretly **5 :** to invent or devise the plot of (as a movie or a literary work) ~ *vi* **1 :** to form a plot : SCHEME **2 :** to be located by means of coordinates (the data ~ at a single point)

Source: *Merriam-Webster's Collegiate Dictionary.* 11th ed.
Springfield, MA: Merriam-Webster, 2003.

31. This dictionary lists two entries for the word *plot* because

   (A) the first entry gives literal meanings, whereas the second gives figurative meanings.
   (B) the word can be spelled in more than one way.
   (C) the first entry gives the more common meanings, whereas the second gives less common meanings.
   (D) the word developed historically from two different words.
   (E) the word occurs both as a noun and as a verb.

32. What is the purpose of the paragraph that begins with *syn*?

   (A) To show the importance of the word *plot* in scholarly discussion
   (B) To demonstrate how the word *plot* is used in various contexts
   (C) To compare the meanings of several synonyms for *plot*
   (D) To explain the history of the word *plot*
   (E) To compare the most common meanings of *plot*

33. What information is provided by the material between < and >?

   (A) Explanations of other words with similar meanings
   (B) Historical information on the origin of the word
   (C) Examples of the word as used in a phrase
   (D) Grammatical information about the usage of the word
   (E) Alternate spellings of the word

34. Which of the following statements is best supported by the definition above?

   (A) When *plot* is used to describe a secret plan, the aim of the plan is usually evil.
   (B) *Plot* is almost always used as a noun.
   (C) *Plot* is normally used to describe political schemes.
   (D) The *plot* of a movie or literary work involves careful plotting to achieve a complex scheme.
   (E) When used of land, *plot* refers to a garden or cemetery.

   _____

35. What is the difference between a footnote and an endnote?

   (A) A footnote provides more complete information than an endnote.
   (B) They differ both in the information they provide and in their location in the paper.
   (C) Both appear in the same location in the paper, but they provide different information.
   (D) An endnote provides more complete information than a footnote.
   (E) Both contain the same information, but are found in different locations in the paper.

36. A parenthetical reference such as (Crowe 235) gives only partial information on the source of information. Where can a reader find complete information on the source?

   (A) A footnote at the end of the paper
   (B) An Endnotes page
   (C) A footnote at the bottom of the page
   (D) A Works Cited page
   (E) A separate document

37. Which type of information are you most likely to find in a glossary?

    (A) A list of geographical locations mentioned in a source

    (B) A list providing definitions of terms used in a specific area of study

    (C) A list of the topics discussed in a book

    (D) A collection of quotations from noted authors

    (E) A brief summary of the arguments presented in a larger work

---

DIRECTIONS: The following questions test your ability to analyze writing. Some questions refer to passages, whereas other questions are self-contained. For each question, choose the best answer.

Questions 38–44 are based on the following passage:

(1) People often find excuses for not getting a flu vaccine each year. (2) Sometimes they get busy or do not understand the serious consequences of this respiratory infection. (3) In addition, people often confuse it with other milder infections. (4) The flu can cause prolonged stress on a body. (5) People with heart problems are especially vulnerable as are children and the elderly. (6) Even healthy people should get the shot each October or November. (7) For those squeamish of shots, there is even a nasal-spray vaccine. (8) On the other hand, people allergic to chicken eggs should first consult their physicians before getting the shot. (9) Eggs are used in several vaccines. (10) If people got their annual flu vaccines, tens of thousands of people would not become hospitalized or possibly even die from this dangerous illness.

38. What should be done with sentence 9?

    (A) It should be placed before sentence 8.

    (B) It should be omitted.

    (C) It should end the paragraph.

    (D) It should begin with the word <u>however</u>.

    (E) It should be placed just after sentence 6.

39. From the tone of the passage, a reader might conclude

    (A) that it was written for a scientific journal

    (B) that this was an excerpt from a high school social studies assignment

    (C) that the author intended to persuade the readers to get a flu shot

    (D) that the author believes the formality of the passage will convey intellectual curiosity

    (E) that the author believes people overreact to insignificant illnesses

40. The paragraph is an example of

   (A) satire
   (B) argumentative writing
   (C) narration
   (D) a process paper
   (E) an informative paper

41. The function of sentence 5 is to

   (A) provide a contrast for sentence 4
   (B) exclude some people who don't need vaccines
   (C) imply that there is an alternative to vaccines
   (D) develop an argument against using eggs in vaccines
   (E) provide an example of whom the author feels most needs to take action

42. What is the best transition to begin sentence 6?

   (A) However,
   (B) Therefore,
   (C) In addition,
   (D) Furthermore,
   (E) Hence,

43. What tone does the author take in sentence 10?

   (A) Accusatory
   (B) Tense
   (C) Conciliatory
   (D) Advisory
   (E) Prophetic

44. Which of the following pairs of sentences could most logically be combined?

   (A) sentences 3 and 4
   (B) sentences 4 and 5
   (C) sentences 6 and 7
   (D) sentences 7 and 8
   (E) sentences 8 and 9

Questions 45–50 are based on the following passage:

(1) Language can convey pleasant or unpleasant thoughts; language can be used to speak tender thoughts of love and admiration or to declare unending hostility—the expressed ideas, themselves, are beside the point, however. (2) Can you imagine how thwarted a loving couple would be if they could not exchange outpourings of the affection they feel? (3) Suzanne Langer, a philosopher, in an essay called "The Language Line" says that it is not a collection of physical characteristics that separate people from the lower animals but very simply the ability to use language as a vehicle of communication. (4) Since almost all language is used in a social context, we must include this characteristic as one of those essential to a definition of language.

45. What is the purpose of sentence 2?

   (A) To illustrate the point of sentence 1
   (B) To intrude a new idea into the discussion
   (C) To limit the uses of language to lovers' conversations
   (D) To ask an unanswerable question
   (E) To contradict the idea of sentence 1

46. The author uses material from a Suzanne Langer essay in which of the following forms?

   (A) A direct quotation
   (B) A paraphrase
   (C) A summary
   (D) A qualified quotation
   (E) The reader cannot tell because the whole selection is not given.

47. In sentence 4, the phrase *social context*

   (A) should have been more clearly defined
   (B) may have several different meanings
   (C) is sociological jargon
   (D) indicates social aspects of communication implied in earlier sentences
   (E) refers to a radical political belief

48. The author identifies Ms. Langer as a philosopher

   (A) to explain the use of big words in the sentence
   (B) to lend intellectual support to his idea
   (C) to appeal to intellectual snobs among the readers
   (D) to limit the application of the remark to philosophy
   (E) to demonstrate his respect for Ms. Langer as a scholar

49. In sentence 1, the author uses

    (A) several positive and negative characteristics of language.

    (B) an unnecessarily complex system of punctuation—a semicolon, dashes, commas.

    (C) techniques of balancing complete opposite notions that language can express.

    (D) the group of words after the dash to contradict the ideas expressed in the first part of the sentence.

    (E) too much information for even a long sentence.

50. That this passage was taken from a longer essay is shown most clearly in

    (A) sentence 1

    (B) sentence 4

    (C) sentence 2

    (D) sentence 3

    (E) sentences 1 and 3

Part Two

This part of the Trial Test consists of 40 questions, and you have 40 minutes to complete it. If you plan to take the College Composition Exam, you need to complete only Part One of this test. However, if you plan to take the College Composition Modular Exam, you should go on to complete Part Two. The combination of Parts One and Two is equivalent to the College Composition Modular Examination. You may also complete Part Two if you simply wish to get extra practice in answering the questions.

DIRECTIONS: The following sentences test your knowledge of grammar, usage, diction (choice of words), and idioms. Some sentences are correct. No sentence contains more than one error.

Read each sentence carefully, paying attention to the underlined portions. You will find that the error, if there is one, is underlined. Assume that elements of the sentence that are not underlined are correct and cannot be changed. In choosing answers, follow the requirements of standard written English.

If there is an error, select the <u>one underlined part</u> that must be changed to make the sentence correct.

If there is no error, select "No error," answer (E).

---

51. In his speech, <u>George Bush made many illusions</u> to the United States,
                                    A

    <u>its government</u> and its citizens, <u>its almost overwhelming diversity</u> and
         B   C

    immensity, and <u>its great past and future potential.</u> <u>No error.</u>
                              D   E

52. Many current officeholders <u>must of been</u> aware that <u>their continuing effort</u>
                                          A   B

    to waste money while <u>refusing to increase taxes</u> can only
                                    C

    <u>make budget deficits larger.</u> <u>No error.</u>
                D   E

53. Frank Sinatra and <u>Barbra Streisand have had</u>
                              A

    <u>more influence upon contemporary</u> music <u>as any other singers</u>
                   B   C

    <u>recording songs</u> by the thousands each week. <u>No error.</u>
          D   E

54. Some users of deadly <u>drugs have excused</u> <u>their fatal addiction</u> as their
                                A   B

    wanting to escape <u>the many problems</u> <u>that may afflict</u> those who have
                             C   D

    been searching for happiness. <u>No error.</u>
                                   E

DIRECTIONS: In each of the following sentences, part of the sentence or the entire sentence is underlined. Below each sentence you will find five ways of phrasing the underlined part. Select the answer that produces the most effective sentence, one that is clear and exact, without awkwardness or ambiguity. In choosing answers, follow the requirements of standard written English. Choose the answer that best expresses the meaning of the original sentence.

Answer (A) is always the same as the underlined part. Choose answer (A) if you think the original sentence needs no revision.

---

55. In these times of overwhelming social upheaval, we can understand that our past <u>was not as productive as we thought it was.</u>

    (A) was not as productive as we thought it was
    (B) was not so productive as we thought it was
    (C) was not as productive so that we thought about it
    (D) is not what we hoped it would be
    (E) was not as productive as we thought they were

56. The minister made the congregation a little upset <u>in the course of the initial</u> sermon by demanding money in the collection plates.

    (A) in the course of the initial
    (B) during his first
    (C) during the exciting
    (D) in the course of the foremost
    (E) in the coarse of the initial

57. It is an amazing observation <u>of today's modern world</u> that no one seems to have the ability of laughing at his or her mistakes.

    (A) of today's modern world
    (B) of the world of today
    (C) of today's world
    (D) with today's modern world
    (E) from all that I see around me today

58. <u>Americans has the responsibility of changing their government form if they</u> <u>believe it no longer responds to their needs.</u>

   (A) Americans has the responsibility of changing their government form if they believe it no longer responds to their needs.

   (B) When Americans find it no longer responds to their needs, they can change their form of government.

   (C) Americans can change their form of government if it no longer responds to their needs.

   (D) Americans who are unhappy with their government has the right to change its form.

   (E) Americans has the right to change their form of government; when they are unhappy with it.

59. The city council member introduced <u>an ordinance prohibiting rock concerts</u> within the city limits.

   (A) an ordinance prohibiting rock concerts

   (B) an ordinance that discouraged rock concerts

   (C) an ordinance that makes it possible for rock concerts

   (D) an ordinance for making illegal rock concerts

   (E) an ordinance permitting rock concerts

60. <u>The candidate for president worked hard for voters, dashing from precinct</u> <u>to precinct on a motor scooter.</u>

   (A) The candidate running for president worked hard for voters, dashing from precinct to precinct on a motor scooter.

   (B) On a motor scooter, the candidate rushed from place to place as they campaigned for election.

   (C) Rushing from place to place, the motor scooter was campaigning for voters.

   (D) The candidate campaigned hard for voters; rushing from place to place on a motor scooter.

   (E) The candidate having been campaigning hard for voters; rushing from place to place on a motor scooter.

61. <u>Suburbanites who are accustomed to riding trains on the daily round-trip do</u> <u>not get disturbed if exact schedules are not maintained.</u>

   (A) Suburbanites who are accustomed to riding trains on the daily round-trip do not get disturbed if exact schedules are not maintained.

   (B) Some of the suburbanites commuting into a city by train is not upset if a train is late once in a while.

   (C) A train being late once in a while does not upset those suburbanites whom expect such delays.

   (D) Schedules not being maintained as published do not disturb many suburbanites who commuted to a city for a job.

   (E) Those suburbanites who commute to the city by train doesn't get bothered if trains are sometimes late.

62. Jonathan's father, <u>the male child of</u> a native prince and a foreign sugarcane worker, was born in Grenada.

   (A) the male child of
   (B) being the male child of
   (C) having been sired by
   (D)   the only male son of
   (E)   the son of

63. <u>Jessica wanted to succeed as a doctor or a lawyer, which is one of the highest ambitions anyone can have.</u>

   (A) Jessica wanted to succeed as a doctor or a lawyer, which is one of the highest ambitions anyone can have.
   (B) Jessica wanted to succeed as a doctor or to be a lawyer, two of the highest ambitions anyone can have.
   (C) Jessica wanted to succeed in medicine or law, two professions in which people with high ambitions have been successful.
   (D) Among her other ambitions, Jessica wanted to study doctor and lawyer.
   (E) More than anything else, Jessica wanted to achieve eminence as a doctor or to be a lawyer.

64. Motorists who cross Death Valley <u>is often told to take</u> plenty of water for car radiators.

   (A) is often told to take
   (B) cannot but be warned
   (C) are advised to
   (D) is told to beware the dangers of dryness
   (E) could be constantly advised to

65. <u>Because George Washington knew how to submit an accurate expense account was the only reason he had so little trouble collecting money due him.</u>

   (A) Because George Washington knew how to submit an accurate expense account was the only reason he had so little trouble collecting money due him.
   (B) George Washington knew how to submit an accurate expense account; therefore, he had little trouble collecting money due him.
   (C) The reason that George Washington had so little trouble collecting money due him was because he knew how to submit an accurate expense account.
   (D) George Washington had little trouble collecting money due him, he knew how to submit an accurate expense account.
   (E) George Washington's expense account, having been so carefully submitted that the cost was paid almost immediately.

66. Since the package was actually addressed to both of us, you <u>should not of been so startled</u> when I opened it.

    (A) should not of been so startled
    (B) could not have been so startled
    (C) should of been so startled
    (D) would not have been so startled
    (E) should not have been so startled

67. Without being asked, <u>the woman took</u> a seat at one of the cocktail tables and ordered white wine.

    (A) the woman took
    (B) the woman should have taken
    (C) the woman has taken
    (D) the woman should of taken
    (E) the woman had took

68. In the South, dogwood and azaleas announce the arrival of spring <u>by bursting into bloom in many gardens.</u>

    (A) by bursting into bloom in many gardens
    (B) after they explode into bloom in every garden
    (C) even though they force their buds into bloom
    (D) since they have burst into bloom
    (E) while they bloom in every garden

69. Luggage inspectors at airports must confiscate food and exotic pets, not necessarily because they might contain weapons, <u>but diseases could be spread</u>.

    (A) but diseases could be spread
    (B) but the fact that they might cause diseases is terrifying
    (C) but what would we do if anyone got sick?
    (D) but because they might carry diseases
    (E) but they might could have diseases

70. Ms. Cruz is <u>one of the commuters who takes</u> the train from Hunter's Point every evening.

    (A) one of the commuters who takes
    (B) one of the commuters that takes
    (C) one of the commuters and they take
    (D) one of the commuters who take
    (E) one of the commuters, they take

Questions 71–72 are based on the following excerpt from a research paper using the APA format:

John Adams believed that "the greatest happiness in Britain had occurred during Elizabeth's reign, during the years of the Commonwealth, and after 1688, the periods when the Commons were dominant." (Cowing, 1971, p. 161).

71. The number 1971 in this parenthetical citation refers to:

   (A) the page number of the original quotation
   (B) the date of publication
   (C) the page number of a secondary source
   (D) the date when Adams made the statement
   (E) the call number in the Dewey Decimal System

72. Which of the following in-text citations would be the correct form if the paper had been written using the MLA format?

   (A) (Cowing, p. 161)
   (B) (Cowing 161)
   (C) (Cowing, 1971, p. 161)
   (D) (Cowing, Adams 161)
   (E) (161)

Questions 73–76 are based on the following passage:

(1) Obesity affects all ages, sexes, racial/ethnic groups, and educational levels. (2) However, the highest percentage of obese people can be found in the lower class. (3) It is because the lower class typically eats cheaper, highly processed, high-calorie foods and is ignorant about healthy diet and living. (4) The country most greatly affected by obesity is the United States. (5) At least 84% of Americans eat unhealthily, and 86% do not get enough physical exercise. (6) It is recorded that more than two-thirds of American adults are obese (Lemonick 14). (7) Not surprisingly, obesity is the second largest cause of death in America ("Obesity").

(8) Obesity is, in fact, growing exponentially. (9) There are now approximately 1.6 billion obese people in the world. (10) Moreover, in the past 20 years, the rates of obesity have tripled in developing countries. (11) While the number of overweight people has surged to 1.6 billion, the world's underfed population has declined slightly since 1980 to 1.1 billion (World Watch Institute). (12) Obesity contributes to around 18 million deaths each year. (13) Heart disease, diabetes, and certain types of cancer are factors that result from obesity. (14) Obesity causes an additional 4 million deaths due to other conditions, such as stroke. (15) The World Health Organization also predicted that by 2015, more than 2.3 billion people will be obese. (16) Obesity is also now rampant in children. (17) Twenty million children under the age of five are overweight as of 2005. (18) One out of four children in America is recorded to be affected by the disorder (Nedley 283). (19) According to the International Obesity Task Force, a total of 155 million children worldwide are overweight or obese (IASO). (20) Unfortunately, childhood obesity is now becoming the norm and not many people care to correct it.

73. What part of sentence 20 is supported by the statistics given?

   (A) The entire sentence
   (B) Not many people care to correct it.
   (C) Childhood obesity is now becoming the norm
   (D) None of the sentence
   (E) Unfortunately

74. Which of the following sentences does NOT directly support the statement in sentence 8?

   (A) Sentence 10
   (B) Sentence 11
   (C) Sentences 12–14
   (D) Sentence 15
   (E) Sentence 17

75. Which statistic is repeated unnecessarily?

   (A) The number of obese people in the world is 1.6 billion.
   (B) The obese population will reach 2.3 billion in 2015.
   (C) Twenty million children under age five were obese in 2005.
   (D) 155 million children in the world are overweight.
   (E) Obesity contributes to 18 million deaths annually.

76. Which of the following sentences does not provide documentation for the statistic that it gives?

    (A) Sentence 6
    (B) Sentence 7
    (C) Sentence 11
    (D) Sentence 15
    (E) Sentence 18

    _____

77. When is it unnecessary to provide documentation?

    (A) When the information is paraphrased from a source
    (B) When the information is common knowledge
    (C) When the information is a direct quotation
    (D) When the information is a summary of the source
    (E) When the information is an indirect quotation

78. When a library lists the call number of a book as BR 118.D625, what system of cataloging is it using?

    (A) Modern Language Association system
    (B) Dewey Decimal system
    (C) Library of Congress system
    (D) University of Chicago system
    (E) Universal Library system

79. Blackwood, Cecil. "Undaunted Courage: Shackleton's Antarctica."
    Historical Digest 27 (2005) 37-42.

    What type of source is described in this Works Cited entry?

    (A) Encyclopedia article
    (B) Article in a journal
    (C) Article on a website
    (D) Book by one author
    (E) Multi-volume set of books

80. Which of these abbreviations means "cited from the same source listed in the footnote immediately preceding this one"?

    (A) et al.
    (B) op. cit.
    (C) loc. cit.
    (D) Ibid.
    (E) sic

DIRECTIONS: The following questions test your ability to analyze writing. Some questions refer to passages, whereas other questions are self-contained. For each question, choose the best answer.

Questions 81–85 are based on the following passage:

(1) In the early days, the streets of Etowah were extremely muddy, and women wore high top shoes, some women losing them in the mud. (2) This continued until 1921, when Etowah's main street, Tennessee Avenue, was paved. (3) Many wagons and teams became stuck in the mud and had to be pulled loose.

(4) With the incorporation of Etowah in 1909 as a "town," it became a municipality with a commission form of government. Five commissioners served two-year terms, and the chairman was responsible to carry out the duties of "mayor." (5) The first chairman was A. J. McKinney, a drygoods merchant, and the first recorder was E. F. Vandivere, a railroad employee. (6) The first Board of Education consisted of Dr. J. O. Nichols, C. A. Clayton, and P. A. Kinser; and their terms were staggered at two, four, and six years. (7) This policy still remains, although attempts to change it to a five member board failed in 1964 and again in 1966 when new charter changes were requested. (8) At the present a movement is on foot to ask for an amendment to adopt a five-member school board in August 1988.

(9) The commission form of government continued to be in effect until December 1950, when it was changed to a Mayor-Commission form, with the Mayor and Commissioner of Finance, Commissioner of Streets and Sanitation, Commissioner of Education and Recreation, Commissioner of Fire and Police, and City Recorder. (10) These charter changes designated Etowah as a "city." (11) George Woods was the first elected mayor under the first charter since 1938 and was re-elected in December of 1950. (12) He continued as recorder until his death on September 15, 1983, a period of 49 years, and was perhaps the longest-termed official ever in the state.

81. What should be done with sentences 6–8?

   (A) Leave them unchanged
   (B) Omit them
   (C) Make them a separate paragraph and move them to the end.
   (D) Combine them into a single sentence
   (E) Omit sentence 8

82. What should you do with sentence 3?

    (A) Leave the sentence unchanged.
    (B) Use it to begin the paragraph.
    (C) Put it after sentence 1.
    (D) Omit the sentence.
    (E) Move the sentence to begin the next paragraph.

83. Which of these is the best way to begin sentence 11?

    (A) George Woods was the first elected mayor under the first charter since 1938
    (B) George Woods was the first elected mayor since 1938
    (C) George Woods was the first mayor since 1938
    (D) George Woods was elected as mayor under the first charter in 1938
    (E) The first charter elected George Woods as mayor in 1938

84. What logical connection exists between the first paragraph and the rest of the passage?

    (A) The first paragraph demonstrates the need for strong civic government.
    (B) The first paragraph describes some of the problems faced by early governments.
    (C) Both paragraphs refer to the history of Etowah in the early 1900s.
    (D) The first paragraph shows that the town was very small.
    (E) The first paragraph describes one of the first accomplishments of the town government.

85. Which of these versions of sentence 9 is most effective in making clear that the Mayor and the Commissioner of Finance are two separate offices?

    (A) with offices for the Mayor and Commissioner of Finance
    (B) with the Mayor and Commissioner of Finance
    (C) with a Mayor and Commissioner of Finance
    (D) with the offices of Mayor, Commissioner of Finance,
    (E) led by a Mayor and Commissioner

Questions 86–90 are based on the following passage:

(1) Although numerous studies have been done to establish exactly how alcohol affects drivers and how many crashes can be blamed on drinks, similar data do not exist about legal drugs and driving. (2) The Food and Drug Administration requires warnings to drivers on all sedatives, but the requirement is based on an assumption that such drugs as tranquilizers, painkillers, and antihistamines affect driving skills, not on actual tests.

(3) The information that does exist indicates that the problem of legal drugs and driving is far-reaching. (4) Simulated road tests at the Southern California Research Institute showed that the drug diazepam, more commonly known as Valium, impaired drivers' abilities to stay in their lane, maintain an even speed, and determine exits, and increased the time and distance needed to stop the car.

(5) One study found that psychiatric patients taking one or more medications have two or three times as many accidents as psychiatric patients who are not taking drugs. (6) Another determined that allergy sufferers have 50 to 100 percent more accidents and time lost from work because of accidents than nonallergy sufferers.

(7) A study of accident victims admitted to Oslo hospitals indicated that 20 percent showed Valium in their blood. (8) Eleven percent of those showed evidence of Valium alone; the rest showed a mixture of Valium and alcohol. (9) A similar study in Dallas found Valium in the blood of 10 percent of drivers killed in car crashes.

(10) "The weight of the circumstantial evidence in this case builds to an irrefutable conclusion," said J. F. O'Hanlon, a professor at the Traffic Research Center in the Netherlands.

86. What is the "irrefutable conclusion" described by the professor in sentence 10?

   (A) The passage does not give his conclusion.
   (B) Valium increases the probability of accidents.
   (C) Allergy drugs are as dangerous as alcohol for a driver.
   (D) Psychiatric patients should not drive.
   (E) Driving under the influence of legal drugs should be restricted.

87. In sentence 6, what logical conclusion does the writer want readers to draw?

   (A) Allergy sufferers are prone to accidents.
   (B) Allergy sufferers have more accidents because of their medications.
   (C) Allergies are a major cause of accidents.
   (D) Allergy medications are the major cause of accidents.
   (E) Allergy sufferers have the same number of accidents as psychiatric patients.

88. In sentence 3, the writer claims that the problem of legal drugs and driving is far-reaching. Which portion of the passage provides evidence that the problem affects a significant proportion of the population?

(A) Sentences 7–9
(B) Sentence 4
(C) Sentences 5
(D) Sentence 10
(E) Sentence 6

89. What form of argument is used in this selection?

(A) Circular
(B) Inductive
(C) Analogy
(D) Ad hominem
(E) Deductive

90. In sentence 2, why does the writer mention sedatives in the first clause, but change in the second clause to refer to tranquilizers, painkillers, and antihistamines?

(A) To argue that the FDA should require warning labels on additional drugs
(B) To show that several categories of medication can be dangerous
(C) To provide more detailed information for physicians
(D) To give specific examples of a broader term
(E) To make it clear that the restriction on sedatives is based on actual tests, unlike restrictions on the other drugs

STOP

If there is still time remaining, you may review your answers.

ANSWER KEY
Trial Test

COLLEGE COMPOSITION

1. **D**	24. **A**	47. **D**	70. **D**
2. **C**	25. **B**	48. **B**	71. **B**
3. **B**	26. **E**	49. **C**	72. **B**
4. **E**	27. **D**	50. **B**	73. **C**
5. **B**	28. **C**	51. **A**	74. **C**
6. **D**	29. **E**	52. **A**	75. **A**
7. **B**	30. **A**	53. **C**	76. **D**
8. **C**	31. **E**	54. **E**	77. **B**
9. **D**	32. **C**	55. **A**	78. **C**
10. **B**	33. **C**	56. **B**	79. **B**
11. **D**	34. **A**	57. **C**	80. **D**
12. **E**	35. **E**	58. **C**	81. **C**
13. **C**	36. **D**	59. **A**	82. **C**
14. **E**	37. **B**	60. **A**	83. **D**
15. **B**	38. **B**	61. **A**	84. **C**
16. **A**	39. **C**	62. **E**	85. **D**
17. **B**	40. **E**	63. **C**	86. **A**
18. **B**	41. **E**	64. **C**	87. **B**
19. **A**	42. **A**	65. **B**	88. **A**
20. **C**	43. **D**	66. **E**	89. **B**
21. **D**	44. **B**	67. **A**	90. **D**
22. **C**	45. **A**	68. **A**	
23. **E**	46. **E**	69. **D**	

SCORING CHART

After you have scored your Trial Test, enter the results in the chart below, then transfer your score to the Progress Chart on page 12. As you complete the Sample Examinations later in this part, you should be able to achieve increasingly higher scores.

Total Test	Number Right	Number Wrong	Number Omitted
90			

ANSWER EXPLANATIONS

1. **(D)** It's is incorrect. Its (no apostrophe) is the correct form.

2. **(C)** Them is vague. It refers to Chinese people, and Chinese people are not mentioned.

3. **(B)** Any country should be any other country to make the comparison accurate.

4. **(E)** The sentence is correct.

5. **(B)** Has realized is the present perfect tense. The simple past, realized, is needed.

6. **(D)** This is the only choice that maintains the parallel construction, go . . . or read . . . or work.

7. **(B)** This sentence has nothing to do with the topic of the passage, the value of computer games for relaxation, and so should be taken out.

8. **(C)** This choice corrects the original a lot, which is not acceptable in standard English. Most (B) is not justified by anything in the passage; they say (D) is vague and should be avoided whenever possible; and (E) begins a contrast the sentence does not complete.

9. **(D)** The two clauses are of comparable importance and are best joined with *and*.

10. **(B)** Again, the information contained here, though interesting, has nothing to do with the topic of the passage.

11. **(D)** This choice makes the contrasting phrase parallel to in relaxation time.

12. **(E)** This choice provides a logical justification for the claim made in sentence 12. Obviously, computer games are not "always there" for people who do not normally use a computer.

13. **(C)** Paragraph 3 is a far better conclusion for the passage than paragraph 4 is. Putting paragraph 4 after paragraph 2 makes the sequence of events logical.

14. **(E)** So makes the cause-and-effect relationship clear.

15. **(B)** These sentences simply say what is said more effectively in sentence 7, so they should be removed.

16. **(A)** However, makes clear the problem created by sentence 3. The other choices make no sense in terms of the passage as a whole.

17. **(B)** Because the scales were not sitting at the piano, the simplest way to deal with this dangling modifier is to remove it from the sentence.

18. **(B)** This choice keeps the sentence parallel with the other sentences in the paragraph and avoids unnecessary verbiage.

19. **(A)** There is a cause-and-effect relationship between these two sentences. The *cause* is *why* something happens; the *effect* is *what* happens, the result. Sentence 1 is the effect; sentence 2 is the cause. None of the other relationships is valid.

20. **(C)** The sentence is off the topic. (B) and (D) are incorrect. (A) and (E) are illogical.

21. **(D)** Eliminate (A) because it is a run-on sentence. (B) is stringy, with too many independent clauses strung together. (C) is choppy because it does not show the relationship between ideas. (E) does not make sense, largely because of the word "and" in the final clause. (D) correctly links ideas by using coordination.

22. **(C)** The original sentence is a run-on, where two independent clauses are incorrectly joined. (B) does not correct the error; rather, it creates a comma splice. Only a semicolon, colon, dash, or subordinating conjunction can join two independent clauses. (D) and (E) are in the passive voice, which should be used only when the doer of the action is unknown or the writer does not want to identify the doer to save embarrassment ("A mistake was made" rather than "You made a mistake"). (C) provides the best subordinating conjunction ("when") to show the relationship between clauses.

23. **(E)** The verbs are not parallel. The sentence should read: Then he *squeezed* and *pressed* the chicle into little round shapes.

24. **(A)** The sentence is correct as written. It is both grammatical and elegant.

25. **(B)** Choice (A) and (C) are not supported in the passage. (D) is incorrect because it is the subject of only the final paragraph. (E) is too limited for the same reason. (B) correctly states the author's purpose.

26. **(E)** Changes in the status of chess players can be posted immediately on Web sites, making it possible to access the most recent information.

27. **(D)** The entry for an article from a Web site normally lists the date of publication first. The date when it was accessed by the researcher is listed later.

28. **(C)** All of the other choices are mentioned in the article.

29. **(E)** The abbreviation *q.v.* comes from a Latin phrase meaning "which see," and informs the student that additional information is available in the article on ethnic cleansing found elsewhere in the encyclopedia.

30. **(A)** The entry states that Balkanization in Africa was part of the aftermath of the dissolution of the European colonial empires there. (D) reverses the cause-and-effect sequence, making Balkanization the cause, rather than the effect, of colonialism's collapse. (E) may be true, but the article did not state it.

31. **(E)** When a word is used as either a noun or a verb, the two sets of definitions are given separately.

32. **(C)** Dictionaries often provide comparisons between the usage of closely related synonyms.

33. **(C)** This dictionary entry provides examples of word usage in a phrase, to clarify the definitions given.

34. **(A)** None of the other choices are justified by the entry.

35. **(E)** Footnotes and endnotes generally contain the same information; however, their placement in the paper is different. Footnotes appear at the bottom of the page where the information is cited; endnotes are listed in a separate page at the end of the paper.

36. **(D)** Complete information on sources is given in a Works Cited page (MLA format) or Reference page (APA format) at the end of the paper.

37. **(B)** A glossary is a list of terms used in a specific field. It often appears at the end of a book, explaining and defining unusual or difficult terms used.

38. **(B)** This sentence does not advance the paragraph. It hurts the unity of the paragraph.

39. **(C)** Each of the other choices is inaccurate: (A) This paragraph does not contain scientific jargon or research. (B) This paper does not reflect social studies issues. (D) This paper is not formal. (E) The author does not mention overreacting. This paper contains a call to action, so (C) is the best choice.

40. **(E)** The paper does not have the characteristics of satire, argumentation, narration, or process work.

41. **(E)** (A) There is no contrast to sentence 4. (B) The author advocates vaccines for these people. (C) There is no mention of an alternative to getting a vaccine. (D) This paragraph advises people to stay healthy by getting vaccinated.

42. **(A)** However shows a contrast between the most vulnerable and the healthy. Both groups are encouraged to get a vaccine.

43. **(D)** This paragraph advises people to stay healthy by getting a flu vaccine.

44. **(B)** There is a connection between the damage the flu can cause and who is most likely to suffer greater consequences from contracting the flu.

45. **(A)** Sentence 2 serves as a concrete example of the importance of language.

46. **(E)** Since the whole selection is not given, the reader cannot tell whether this is (B) a paraphrase, (C) a summary, or (D) a qualified quotation. The reader can tell, however, that it is not (A) a direct quotation.

47. **(D)** In sentences 1, 2, and 3, language as a means of communication is discussed. In each case, the examples used have to do with language in a social context.

48. **(B)** Writers often support their ideas with confirming statements from an authority in the field.

49. **(C)** The author makes effective use of the technique of balancing opposites in this sentence.

50. **(B)** Sentence 4, the last sentence of the passage, mentions that this is one characteristic of a definition of language. We can assume that other characteristics will be discussed in following paragraphs.

51. **(A)** Illusions and allusions refer to two different ideas. The correct term is allusions.

52. **(A)** Must of should be must have, the correct verb form.

53. **(C)** As should be than. We say more than, not more as.

54. **(E)** The sentence is correct.

55. **(A)** Choice (B) contains a poor idiom (so-as). (C) is wordy. (D) It is is a vague usage. (E) they, a plural word, does not fit with the singular words.

56. **(B)** Choice (A) has too many words. (C) exciting changes the meaning of the sentence too much. (D) contains excess verbiage. (E) coarse is an incorrect word choice.

57. **(C)** Choice (A) Today's modern is redundant. (B) contains too many words. (D) with is an incorrect preposition. (E) is too wordy.

58. **(C)** Has in (A), (D), and (E) is a singular form when the sense of the idea is plural. (B) has it, their, and they as vague pronouns. The semicolon in (E) is also incorrect.

59. **(A)** Choice (B) and (E) change the meaning of the sentence too much. (C) is too wordy. (D) distorts the meaning of the sentence too much.

60. **(A)** Choice (B) they is a vague pronoun. (C) the sentence says the motor scooter was trying to get voters. (D) Use a semicolon to connect to independent clauses. "Rushing from place to place..." is a fragment. (E) is a vague sentence.

61. **(A)** Choice (B) has an error in agreement—is is singular, some is plural. (C) Whom is the wrong case for a subject. (D) do not disturb is present tense, commuted is past tense. (E) doesn't is singular, not plural.

62. **(E)** Choice (A) male child is redundant. (B) being is unnecessarily wordy. (C) having been sired by does not really make sense. (D) male son is repetitious.

63. **(C)** Choice (A) implies that medicine or law are one job; note the singular is. (B) A doctor or to be a lawyer are distorted comparisons. (D) Doctor and lawyer are not parallel with ambitions. (E) has incorrect parallelism in the last part of the sentence.

64. **(C)** Choice (A) and (D) contain an error in agreement of subject and verb. (B) contains a vague phrase cannot but be. (E) could is not a strong enough word for the sentence.

65. **(B)** Choice (A) Because . . . the reason is redundant. (C) reason . . . was because is repetitious. (D) the comma creates a comma splice. (E) the response to the sentence is a sentence fragment.

66. **(E)** Choices (A) and (C) Should of is not a verb form. (B) could changes the tense relationship. (D) also changes the tense relationship.

67. **(A)** Choices (B) and (C) change the tense relationship. (D) Should of is not a verb form. (E) had took is an incorrect verb form.

68. **(A)** Choice (B) <u>After</u> is the wrong verb form because it involves a tense sequence that is not correct. (C) <u>Even though</u> makes no sense. (D) <u>since</u> also implies a past event. (E) <u>while</u> is an ambiguous word.

69. **(D)** Choice (A) This is a shift from active to passive voice. (B) This is wordy and not parallel. (C) This is a shift in tone and not parallel. (E) This is not standard English.

70. **(D)** The <u>who</u> refers to the commuters, plural, so the verb must be the plural form, <u>take</u>.

71. **(B)** In the APA format, the date of publication is listed after the author's last name in the parenthetical note.

72. **(B)** Parenthetical citations in the MLA format include only the last name of the author and the page number, with no additional punctuation.

73. **(C)** Sentences 16–19 present statistics on the prevalence of child obesity, but there are no statistics to show that there is a lack of concern about the problem.

74. **(C)** Sentences 12–14 show that obesity contributes to disease, but they do not show that it is growing exponentially.

75. **(A)** The number of obese people in the world is given in both sentence 9 and sentence 11.

76. **(D)** Although sentence 15 mentions the World Health Organization, it does not include a parenthetical citation to specify the source document.

77. **(B)** Documentation is not required for information that is common knowledge. If the information is not common knowledge, documentation may be necessary whether it is a direct quotation or it is in a more indirect format.

78. **(C)** Library of Congress call numbers follow this format.

79. **(B)** The entry represents an article in a journal.

80. **(D)** *Ibid.* is the abbreviation normally used in a set of footnotes or endnotes to indicate that the source is the same as that given in the previous footnote.

81. **(C)** These sentences describing the Board of Education are located between two sections on the overall form of city government. The flow of the discussion would be more logical if this section were moved to the end.

82. **(C)** Sentences 1 and 3 both describe the condition of the muddy streets before the repairs in sentence 2 were completed.

83. **(D)** The other choices are either awkwardly worded or unclear in expressing the idea.

84. **(C)** The first paragraph is only loosely related to the rest of the discussion. The primary connection is its reference to the early era of the town's history; the second paragraph deals with the early forms of municipal government.

85. **(D)** All other choices use the description "Mayor and Commissioner," which does not make it clear that the two offices are separate.

86. **(A)** The passage does not actually specify which conclusion the professor intended. The reader must infer a conclusion with a direct statement.

87. **(B)** The writer wants readers to conclude that allergy sufferers have a higher rate of accidents because of their allergy medications. Such a conclusion would support the main argument of the article.

88. **(A)** Only sentences 7–9 contain statistical analysis about the percentage of a population affected by the problem. All the other studies support the proposition that there is a problem, but they do not show how widespread it is. Legal drugs can have effects on driving and accident rate.

89. **(B)** The author uses an inductive argument, citing several specific instances as the basis for a generalization about the effect of legal drugs on driving.

90. **(D)** Sedatives are a broader category of medications, and the other drugs mentioned are specific examples of medications in that category.

Background and Practice Questions

4

DESCRIPTION OF THE COLLEGE COMPOSITION EXAMINATION

Note: The College-Level Exam Program (CLEP) has two different examinations that cover the material a student is expected to learn in most first-year courses in college composition:

1. The College Composition Exam
2. The College Composition Modular Exam

This chapter is designed to help you prepare for either of these exams.

The College Composition Exam requires you to complete a section of multiple-choice items and write two essays. The first essay is based on your own reading and experience, while the second essay requires you to build an argument using two sources that will be provided. You will have 50 minutes to answer approximately 50 multiple-choice questions, followed by 70 minutes to write the two essays.

The College Composition Modular Exam also involves a multiple-choice section and an essay section. You will have 90 minutes to answer approximately 90 multiple-choice questions. The essay portion of the exam may vary, depending on the policies of the college granting credit. It could involve the same type of essay assignments found in the College Composition Exam, or it could involve an alternate essay or writing project developed and scored by the college.

See the following chart for a summary of the content in the two exams:

TIP

Be sure you know which exam will be accepted by the institution to which you will send your score, so that you will take the appropriate examination.

College Composition

Content and Item Types	Time/Number of Questions

Part 1 Multiple-Choice Questions
   Conventions of Standard Written
      English (10%)
   Revision Skills (40%)
   Ability to Use Source Materials (25%)
   Rhetorical Analysis (25%)
	Part 1
	   50 questions—50 minutes

Part 2 Essays
   First Essay
   Second Essay using sources
	Part 2
	   Essay 1—30 minutes
	   Essay 2—40 minutes

College Composition Modular

Content and Item Types	Time/Number of Questions

Part 1 Multiple-Choice Questions
  Conventions of Standard Written English (10%)
  Revision Skills including Sentence-Level Skills (40%)
  Ability to Use Source Materials (25%)
  Rhetorical Analysis (25%)
	Part 1
	90 questions—90 minutes

Part 2 Essays
  Varies, depending on college policy
	Part 2
	  Varies depending on college policy

KINDS OF QUESTIONS THAT APPEAR ON THE EXAM

Both the College Composition Exam and the College Composition Modular Exam contain the following types of questions:

1. **CONVENTIONS OF STANDARD WRITTEN ENGLISH.** You will be asked to identify grammatical errors in sample sentences. The questions will test your awareness of a variety of logical, structural, and grammatical relationships within sentences and acceptable usage in areas such as those listed below:

   - Syntax (parallelism, coordination, subordination)
   - Sentence boundaries (comma splice, run-ons, sentence fragments)
   - Recognition of correct sentences
   - Concord/agreement (pronoun reference, case shift, and number; subject-verb; verb tense)
   - Diction
   - Modifiers
   - Idiom
   - Active/passive voice
   - Lack of subject in modifying word group
   - Logical comparison
   - Logical agreement
   - Punctuation

2. **REVISION SKILLS.** You will identify ways to improve an early draft of an essay. This type of question is used to measure your grasp of a number of skills, including:

   - Organization
   - Evaluation of evidence
   - Awareness of audience, tone, and purpose
   - Level of detail
   - Coherence between sentences and paragraphs
   - Sentence structure and variety
   - Main idea, thesis statement, and topic sentences
   - Rhetorical effects

- Use of language
- Evaluation of author's authority and appeal
- Evaluation of reasoning
- Consistency of point of view
- Transitions
- Sentence-level errors primarily relating to the conventions of Standard Written English

3. **ABILITY TO USE SOURCE MATERIALS.** You will have the opportunity to demonstrate your familiarity with basic reference and research skills:

- Use of reference materials
- Evaluation of sources
- Integration of resource material
- Documentation of sources, including, but not limited to, MLA, APA, and Chicago manuals of style

4. **RHETORICAL ANALYSIS.** You will be asked to read passages in different styles and answer questions about the content and organization of each passage, as well as the strategies used by each writer:

- Appeals
- Tone
- Organization and structure
- Rhetorical effects
- Use of language
- Evaluation of evidence

STUDY SOURCES

For review, you might consult the following books.

Cazort, Douglas. *Under the Grammar Hammer: The 25 Most Important Grammar Mistakes and How to Avoid Them.* New York: Lowell House, 1997.

Choy, Penelope, Dorothy Goldbart Clark, and James R. McCormick. *Basic Grammar and Usage,* 5th ed. New York: Harcourt, 1997.

Feierman, Joanne. *Actiongrammar: Fast, No-Hassle Answers on Everyday Usage and Punctuation.* New York: Fireside, 1995.

Glenn, Cheryl and Loretta Gray. *Hodges' Harbrace Handbook.* 16th ed. Boston: Thomson Wadsworth, 2007.

Kipfer, Barbara Ann. *Twenty-First Century Manual of Style.* New York: Dell, 1995.

Partridge, Eric. *Usage and Abusage: A Guide to Good English.* New York: W. W. Norton & Company, 1995.

Princeton Language Institute. Holland, Joseph (ed.). *21st Century Grammar Handbook.* New York: Dell, 1993.

Rozakis, Laurie. *Random House Webster's Pocket Grammar, Usage and Punctuation.* New York: Random House Reference, 1998.

Shertzer, Margaret D. *The Elements of Grammar.* New York: MacMillan General Reference, 1996.

Strunk, W. and E. B. White. *The Elements of Style.* Prentice Hall, May 1999.

Sutcliffe, Andrea (ed.). *New York Public Library Writer's Guide to Style and Usage.* New York: HarperCollins, 1994.

Zahler, Diane, Ellen Lichtenstein, and Claudia H. C. Q. Sorsby. *21st Century Guide to Improving Your Writing.* New York: Dell, 1995.

PRACTICE QUESTIONS FOR CONVENTIONS OF STANDARD WRITTEN ENGLISH

The directions and practice questions that follow will give you a good idea of what questions on conventions of standard written English are like. The directions, reprinted here by permission of Educational Testing Service, are the actual directions you will find in the test on the day of the exam.

> **DIRECTIONS:** Read each sentence carefully, paying attention to the underlined portions. Assume that elements of the sentence that are not underlined are correct and cannot be changed. In choosing answers, follow the requirements of Standard Written English.
>
> If there is an error, select the <u>one underlined part</u> that must be changed to make the sentence correct.
>
> If there is no error, select "<u>No error</u>," answer (E).

To help you review some of the basics of grammar and usage on which you will be tested, the practice questions for identifying sentence errors are grouped by type of grammatical error.

Errors in Pronoun Case

The spelling of a noun or pronoun may change, depending on its use in the sentence; this is called its *case*. For example, we usually show that a noun is possessive by adding *'s*.

Example: The cat's whiskers = the whiskers belonging to the cat.

Personal pronouns have one form when used as the subject of a sentence but often have a different form when used as the direct or indirect object of the sentence. They may also have a different spelling to show possession.

Examples: *I* rode in the car. The child saw *me*. Here is *my* book.

Here is a chart of the most common forms:

Nominative case (subject)	Objective case (object)	Possessive case
I	me	my (mine)
you	you	your (yours)
he	him	his
she	her	her (hers)
it	it	its
we	us	our (ours)
they	them	their (theirs)

Hint: When two pronouns appear in combination, try them one at a time to pick the right case.

Example: My mother called Sam and me.

EXAMPLES

1. Between <u>you and I</u>, that whole celebration was <u>really</u> an <u>elegant affair</u>,
             A   B   C
   <u>I thought</u>. <u>No error</u>.
   D   E

   Explanation: The underlined error is choice (A); I should be <u>me</u>, objective case, object of preposition <u>between</u>.

2. The history teacher, <u>whom</u> I think was the <u>best teacher</u> <u>I ever had</u>,
                       A   B   C
   <u>told us</u> that he had served overseas during World War II. <u>No error</u>.
   D   E

   Explanation: The underlined error is choice (A); <u>whom</u> should be <u>who</u>, subjective case, subject of the verb <u>was</u>.

Now, try your hand with the following twelve sentences. You will find the answers and the explanations immediately following the group of sentences:

1. My aunt, <u>whom we admire</u>, has <u>given we</u> <u>boys ten</u> dollars each to spend
                  A   B   C
   <u>at the fair</u> tomorrow. <u>No error</u>.
     D   E

2. When <u>I showed my</u> mother the suit <u>I had selected</u>, she <u>objected to me</u>
            A   B   C
   buying it; <u>she said it</u> was too expensive. <u>No error</u>.
            D   E

3. <u>Whomever is</u> going to the <u>meeting needs</u> to bring the <u>minutes from the last</u>
     A   B   C
   meeting <u>with him or her</u>. <u>No error</u>.
              D   E

4. <u>New York City</u> <u>with it's many</u> suburbs has been called America's fabulous
        A   B
   metropolis, <u>its dirtiest city</u>, and its most exciting <u>place for a</u> brief
                 C   D
   vacation. <u>No error</u>.
          E

5. Abraham Lincolns Gettysburg Address has been called a model of brevity,
    _____   A   _____ B
    the greatest short speech that anyone has ever delivered, and a speech
    _____ C _____ _____ D
    worth more than a longer one would have been. No error.
    _____
    E

6. Please ask whoever you wish to serve as a fourth member of the
    _____ _____ B
    A
    board I am appointing to study the pollution situation in your county.
    _____ C _____ D
    No error.
    _____
    E

7. The United Nations has performed many useful tasks through its various
    _____ A _____ B
    commissions although there are representatives on these commissions
    _____ C
    whom everyone knows are slow-moving. No error.
    _____ D _____ E

8. The Nobel Prize for Literature has been awarded to Toni Morrison, who's
    _____ A _____ B
    novels are now considered among the greatest that have been written in the
    _____ C _____ D
    United States in the twentieth century. No error.
    _____
    E

9. Even though we know that we are exercising our rights under the
    _____ A _____ B
    United States Constitution, Ashley and myself are arrested every
    _____ C
    time we picket the animal shelter. No error.
    _____ D _____ E

10. After the bell rang and signaled the end of classes for that day, the
    _____ A
    teacher told Sandeep and I that we would have to remain thirty
    _____ B _____ C
    minutes longer for whispering in the back of the room. No error.
    _____ D _____ E

Answer Explanations

1. **(B)** We should be us; it is the indirect object of the verb has given.

2. **(C)** Me should be my; the possessive case is used with the gerund; the object of the preposition is buying and not me.

3. **(A)** Whomever should be whoever; it is the subject of is and needs.

4. **(B)** It's should be its; the possessive case of it never has an apostrophe.

5. **(A)** Lincolns should be Lincoln's; this is a possessive, not a plural.

6. **(B)** Whoever should be whomever; objective case needed; object of wish.

7. **(D)** Whom should be who; subject of verb are.

8. **(B)** Who's should be whose; who's is a contraction of who is.

9. **(C)** Myself should be I; I, subject of are arrested; myself is a reflexive pronoun.

10. **(B)** I should be me; object of the verb told.

Errors in Agreement of Subject and Verb

The subject of each sentence should agree with its verb in number: singular subjects go with singular verbs, and plural subjects go with plural verbs.

> **Examples:** My brother drives to work every day.
>   My brothers drive to work every day.

A compound subject with two singular subjects joined by *and* is considered plural.

> **Example:** Jack and Jill are my friends.

Pay special attention to words like *each, either, everyone, someone* (singular) and *both, few* (plural).

EXAMPLES

1. The top three winners in the state competition. goes to the national finals to be
         A   B   C   D
   held this year in San Francisco, California. No error.
                                         E

   Explanation: The underlined error is choice (C); goes should be go, since the plural subject winners requires the plural verb go.

2. Either John or his two friends is going to find that passing a test on that
                                       A   B   C
   material is not the easiest thing they have ever done in school. No error.
                               D   E

   Explanation: The underlined error is choice (A); is going should be are going, to agree with the plural word friends.

---

1. The committee is deciding now which of the many applicants for the
                  A   B   C
   teaching position are going to be hired. No error.
                     D   E

2. Despite what each of the experts tell us about how to avoid bankruptcy,
                           A   B
   some people insist on spending more money each year than they make.
                 C   D
   No error.
    E

3. Each of the critics were assigned a book to read, to discuss within twenty
            A   B   C
   minutes, and to offer an opinion about. No error.
               D   E

4. Although the influence of television on America's buying proclivities
            A   B
   have been studied by many psychologists, no one has found exactly what
   C
   the influence has been. No error.
         D   E

5. No member of a circus troop have the right to play strictly to the
                    A   B
   audience so that other members of the team do not get their fair share
                         C   D
   of the applause. No error.
            E

6. No matter what statisticians report to the American Automobile
                  A
   Association, accidents just does not happen on today's superhighways
                     B   C
   unless some driver has been too careless at the wheel of his or her car.
              D
   No error.
    E

Answer Explanations

1. **(D)** <u>Are</u> should be <u>is</u>; subject <u>which</u> is singular.

2. **(A)** <u>Tell</u> should be <u>tells</u>; subject <u>each</u> is singular.

3. **(A)** <u>Were</u> should be <u>was</u>; subject <u>each</u> is singular.

4. **(C)** <u>Have</u> should be <u>has</u>; subject <u>influence</u> is singular.

5. **(A)** <u>Have</u> should be <u>has</u>; subject <u>member</u> is singular.

6. **(B)** <u>Does</u> should be <u>do</u>; subject <u>accidents</u> is plural.

Errors in Agreement Between a Pronoun and Its Antecedent

A pronoun usually refers to a noun or another pronoun elsewhere in the sentence, called the *antecedent*. The pronoun should agree with its antecedent in number and gender.

> **Example:** My sister asked me to wait for her.
> My friends asked me to wait for them.

The following words are considered singular, and you should use a singular pronoun to refer to them: *each, either, neither, one, everyone, nobody, anyone.*

These words are considered plural, and you should use plural pronouns when you refer to them: *both, few, several, many.*

These words may be either singular or plural, depending on how they are used: *some, any, none, all, most.*

EXAMPLES

1. The audience <u>was cheering</u> Kevin Kline's performance as Hamlet; <u>they refused</u>
               A   B   C
 to leave the theater <u>until he</u> took four curtain calls. <u>No error.</u>
                    D   E

 Explanation: The underlined error is choice (C); <u>they</u> should be <u>it</u> to match the singular subject <u>audience</u>.

2. No one is able to find <u>their seats</u> in a <u>darkened theater</u> so <u>it is necessary</u> to
                           A   B   C
 bring <u>a flashlight.</u> <u>No error.</u>
      D   E

 Explanation: The underlined error is choice (A); <u>their seats</u> should be <u>his seat</u>.

---

1. When anyone expresses <u>a desire</u> to <u>get married</u> <u>as quickly</u> as possible,
                  A   B   C

   <u>they always set</u> off gossiping tongues in the community. <u>No error.</u>
       D   E

2. When anyone <u>seeks employment</u> with a large corporation, <u>he or she should</u>
                    A   B

   always be sure <u>that his or her</u> qualifications fit <u>their needs.</u> <u>No error.</u>
                     C   D   E

3. Everyone always wants <u>their achievements</u> at work to be
                          A

   <u>rewarded by management</u> in the form of raises, promotions, and
               B

   <u>other tangible signs of appreciation</u>, even though the ability to get
                   C

   along with <u>others</u> is often as important to success as accomplishment
                 D

   itself. <u>No error.</u>
          E

4. When anyone <u>looks up a word</u> in any of the desk dictionaries <u>to check its</u>
                  A   B

   spelling, <u>you must make</u> sure that the word cannot be spelled
                 C

   <u>in more than</u> one acceptable way. <u>No error.</u>
       D   E

5. The congregation was <u>sitting reverently</u> <u>in their pews</u> when the organ
                         A   B

   <u>broke the silence</u> with the first <u>chords of a traditional</u> hymn. <u>No error.</u>
           C   D   E

6. The television industry <u>was</u> jolted when the Federal Communications
                       A

   Commission announced that cigarette advertising would not <u>be permitted</u>
                                                     B

   on television after <u>January 1, 1971</u>, a move that took away one <u>of their</u>
                   C   D

   prime sources of revenues. <u>No error.</u>
                     E

7. When you <u>finally decide upon</u> the career you will follow for the rest of
                    A

your life, <u>a person should</u> be sure that you have made <u>a choice that</u> will
                    B   C

bring you as much <u>personal gratification</u> as possible. <u>No error.</u>
                           D   E

Answer Explanations

1. **(D)** <u>They always set</u> should be <u>he or she always sets</u>; antecedent <u>anyone</u> is singular.

2. **(D)** <u>Their</u> should be <u>its</u>; antecedent <u>corporation</u> is singular.

3. **(A)** <u>Their</u> should be <u>his</u> or <u>her</u>; antecedent <u>everyone</u> is singular.

4. **(C)** <u>You</u> should be <u>he</u> or <u>she</u>; antecedent <u>anyone</u> is third person.

5. **(B)** <u>Their</u> should be <u>its</u>; antecedent <u>congregation</u> is singular here.

6. **(D)** <u>Their</u> should be <u>its</u>; antecedent <u>industry</u> is singular.

7. **(B)** <u>A person</u> should be <u>you</u>; antecedent <u>you</u> is second person.

Errors in Tense Sequence

A writer should normally choose one tense and maintain it throughout the entire sentence or paragraph. One should only switch from present tense to past tense when there is a good reason for doing so.

Examples: We walked through the forest, and we will see a bear. (Incorrect)
          We walked through the forest and we saw a bear. (Correct)

EXAMPLES

1. <u>Almost every time</u> Jack <u>drives</u> the family car, he <u>has left</u> it completely
          A   B   C
<u>empty of gasoline.</u> <u>No error.</u>
          D   E

   Explanation: The underlined error is choice (B); <u>drives</u> should be <u>has driven</u>.

2. If we could <u>only enjoy</u> the pleasures of our youth <u>again</u>, we <u>may find</u> that we
                    A   B   C
<u>have not forgotten</u> them after all. <u>No error.</u>
          D   E

   Explanation: The underlined error is choice (C); <u>may</u> should be <u>might</u>.

---

1. This morning, all banks in the New York <u>district announce</u> that interest
          A   B

    <u>rates</u> for all home loans would be raised to <u>8%</u>. <u>No error</u>.
     C   D   E

2. The chief strongly opposes the <u>idea of putting</u> a single police officer
                                       A

    in <u>cars</u> that <u>would be cruising</u> at night in <u>high crime districts</u>. <u>No error</u>.
        B   C   D   E

3. According to the schedule posted <u>on the skater's</u> bulletin board, <u>there are</u>
                                    A   B

    three exhibitions before the season officially began but only <u>one after the playoffs</u>
                                                                 C

    had been completed <u>by the entire league</u>. <u>No error</u>.
                                 D   E

4. If <u>John Paul Jones</u> had not been <u>victorious in his</u> naval battles, the
             A   B

    United States <u>will have</u> been a second-rate power <u>on the seas forever</u>.
                      C   D

    <u>No error</u>.
     E

Answer Explanations

1. **(B)** <u>Announce</u> should be <u>announced</u>; correct tense sequence with <u>would be raised</u>.

2. **(C)** <u>Would</u> should be <u>will</u>; correct tense sequence with <u>opposes</u>.

3. **(B)** <u>Are</u> should be <u>were</u>; correct tense sequence with <u>had been completed</u>.

4. **(C)** <u>Will</u> should be <u>would have</u>; correct tense sequence after <u>had not been</u>.

Errors in Word Choices, Diction, and Idioms

An error in diction means that the writer has selected the incorrect word. An error in word choice means that the writer has selected a word that means almost what he or she wanted to say but not quite.

An error in idiom means that the writer has selected the wrong word to complete the idiom that he or she wanted to use.

EXAMPLES

1. She looked at both pictures carefully; she could not decide which was the
                         A   B   C

   most beautiful. No error.
    D   E

   Explanation: The underlined error is choice (D); most should be more.

2. While Karen was setting out on the porch, she saw Wayne and
                 A   B

   Daryl walking slowly toward her from town. No error.
       C   D   E

   Explanation: The underlined error is choice (A); setting should be sitting.

3. When the baby woke up from his nap, he made alot of noise, jumping up and
            A   B   C   D

   down in his crib. No error.
         E

   Explanation: The underlined error is choice (C); alot should be a lot.

4. Without no warning at all, the kitten pounced on the stuffed mouse and shook
           A   B   C

   it vigorously, tearing it to shreds. No error.
           D   E

   Explanation: The underlined error is choice (A); no should be any.

5. The company is having some difficulty of promoting its new cereal; children
                           A   B   C

   must be sold the idea of switching brands. No error.
     D   E

   Explanation: The underlined error is choice (A); of should be in.

6. Every day this summer, all the children in the neighborhood have gone to the
     A   B   C

   village pool, where they have swimmed for several hours. No error.
                 D   E

   Explanation: The underlined error is choice (D); swimmed should be swam or swum.

7. After all the <u>votes have been</u> counted and <u>the winner</u> <u>declared</u>, the new
           A   B   C

   president will be <u>formerly inducted</u> into office. <u>No error.</u>
                D   E

   Explanation: The underlined error is choice (D); <u>formerly</u> should be <u>formally</u>.

8. When <u>gold was discovered</u> in California in 1849, <u>there was</u> a mad stampede
            A   B

   <u>by people</u> to both buy land in the area <u>or lease claims</u> near Sutter's Mill.
     C   D

   <u>No error.</u>
    E

   Explanation: The underlined error is choice (D); <u>or</u> should be <u>and</u>.

9. No matter how hard the teacher <u>tries to teach</u> the class, her
                              A

   efforts have <u>little affect</u> upon the students <u>who refuse</u> to study the assigned
         B   C   D

   materials. <u>No error.</u>
          E

   Explanation: The underlined error is choice (C); <u>affect</u> should be <u>effect</u>.

10. With his great strength, Samson <u>could of beaten</u> any opponent in the wrestling
            A   B

    arena, if he <u>had not</u> <u>cut his hair.</u> <u>No error.</u>
            C   D   E

    Explanation: The underlined error is choice (B); <u>of</u> should be <u>have</u>.

Now, try your hand at the following twenty-five sentences:

1. After Mother <u>had tucked</u> us into bed and kissed <u>us</u> good night, we <u>continued</u>
                A   B   C

   talking when we should <u>of closed our</u> eyes and gone to sleep. <u>No error.</u>
                      D   E

2. No matter <u>how hard</u> I try to finish an assignment, I <u>cannot do</u> it
              A   B

   <u>if there is</u> anything <u>laying around</u> that I can play with. <u>No error.</u>
     C   D   E

3. My uncle Jack, who <u>was setting</u> on the porch and enjoying <u>a cold drink</u>,
     A   B   C

    called out and told <u>me</u> to be careful about running into the street
                        D

    without looking. <u>No error.</u>
                     E

4. <u>I will</u> neither give you money to waste on that <u>junk or</u> offer any further
    A   B

    advice <u>if you</u> <u>proceed</u> against my wishes. <u>No error.</u>
            C   D   E

5. <u>Most all voters</u> <u>who support</u> conservative political candidates <u>also support</u>
       A   B   C

    many conservative <u>organizations that</u> have grown in membership within
                       D

    the past decade. <u>No error.</u>
                E

6. <u>Because it was</u> the best offer that had been made, the owner decided to
       A

    except $100,500 for his home <u>although</u> it was worth more on <u>today's</u>
      B   C   D
    market. <u>No error.</u>
              E

7. He <u>is tired</u> of picking up all the dirty clothes <u>that</u> his roommate leaves
       A   B

    <u>laying</u> on the bathroom floor <u>every morning</u>. <u>No error.</u>
     C   D   E

8. George Gershwin, composer of many of the songs <u>by which American</u>
                                                    A

    popular music has gained a reputation <u>for greatness</u>, was <u>unhappy</u> and
                                    B   C

    dissatisfied <u>by his early works</u> and studied to improve his compositions.
                  D

    <u>No error.</u>
      E

9. Jealousy <u>has been called</u> the <u>more disastrous</u> of all the human emotions
               A   B

    <u>that can wrack</u> the mind, <u>often susceptible</u> to all kinds of fears and
         C   D

    anxieties. <u>No error.</u>
               E

10. Portia Jones, <u>one of the smartest lawyers</u> in the United States, <u>has</u> often
                                  A   B

    remarked that <u>most all criminals</u> <u>really want</u> to be kept in jail. <u>No error.</u>
                     C   D   E

11. <u>Between the several</u> choices on the menu, <u>I can hardly</u> decide <u>whether</u> I will
            A   B   C

    order roast beef, fried chicken, broiled fish, <u>or baked ham.</u> <u>No error.</u>
                                           D   E

12. It is <u>really pitiful</u> to <u>see a small child</u> die <u>without never having</u> lived <u>long</u>
           A   B   C   D

    enough to accomplish anything. <u>No error.</u>
                                   E

13. Ely Culbertson, <u>a famous professional</u> bridge player, said that thirteen
                           A

    <u>spades</u> dealt in one hand is the <u>most unique unusual bridge</u> hand he ever
     B   C

    <u>saw.</u> <u>No error.</u>
     D   E

14. No team <u>ever wants</u> to <u>loose a game,</u> even though <u>it seems that</u> some teams
             A   B   C

    make many foolish mistakes and appear <u>to throw a game away.</u> <u>No error.</u>
                                        D   E

15. When the play <u>had less and less people</u> in its audience <u>as its run</u> grew
                       A   B

    longer, the producers <u>began to consider</u> the feasibility of trying to
                       C

    extend its run beyond six months. <u>No error.</u>
     D   E

16. <u>Most historians now</u> agree that the true story about John Smith and
            A

    Pocahontas <u>has never been</u> told; maybe <u>some of them</u> are <u>even real sorry</u>
                B   C   D

    that the facts are still hidden. <u>No error.</u>
                            E

17. While <u>the driver was</u> <u>very carefully moving</u> ahead on the expressway
                 A   B

    ramp, <u>she did not notice</u> that black Cadillac that was <u>speeding in back</u> of
           C   D

    her. <u>No error.</u>
     E

18. Your letter in regards to my delinquent bill has been sent to my attorneys for
                    A   B
    possible suit for slander because it contains several insinuations that are
                   C   D
    untrue. No error.
            E

19. The opera diva always enjoyed a few quit moments alone
                                    A
    in her dressing room before the performance started so that she could
            B   C
    appear on stage calm and relaxed. No error.
                     D   E

20. There is that bird again, diving at us from her nest in the elm tree,
                 A   B
    trying to peck us on the head, and then flying off somewheres else to be
             C   D
    safe from our retaliation. No error.
                               E

21. The baby-sitter says that we may have no more cookies
                        A
    without we come into the house, do our homework thoroughly, and
            B   C
    ask politely if there are any more cookies in the jar. No error.
                  D   E

22. In his statement at the press conference, the president inferred that
        A   B
    opposition to his foreign policy could be found only among those who
                                                      C
    had not voted for him in the election. No error.
                     D   E

23. Now that I have reached the age of eighty-two, I find that I can't hardly do
                              A   B
    many of the things that were very easy for me when I was sixteen and
                                  C
    still vigorous. No error.
    D   E

24. Although I enjoyed the exotic dinner we were served in San Francisco's
                                                          A
    most famous Chinese restaurant, I felt badly because I knew that I had
              B   C
    eaten more than I should have. No error.
               D   E

25. With a valid passport, an American citizen can go <u>anywheres in the world</u>,

                                                       A

   <u>to any country</u> that will give him or her permission to enter <u>except a few</u>

    B   C

   nations that the State Department has ruled <u>"out of bounds"</u> for American

                                                 D

   tourists. <u>No error.</u>

          E

Answer Explanations

1. **(D)** <u>Of</u> should be <u>have</u>.

2. **(D)** <u>Laying</u> should be <u>lying</u>.

3. **(B)** <u>Setting</u> should be <u>sitting</u>.

4. **(B)** <u>Or</u> should be <u>nor</u>.

5. **(A)** <u>Most</u> should be <u>almost</u>.

6. **(B)** <u>Except</u> should be <u>accept</u>.

7. **(C)** <u>Laying</u> should be <u>lying</u>.

8. **(D)** Should be <u>with</u> not <u>by</u> his works.

9. **(B)** <u>More</u> should be <u>most</u>.

10. **(C)** <u>Most</u> should be <u>almost</u>.

11. **(A)** <u>Between</u> should be <u>among</u>.

12. **(C)** <u>Never</u> should be <u>ever</u>.

13. **(C)** Eliminate <u>unique</u>.

14. **(B)** <u>Loose</u> should be <u>lose</u>.

15. **(A)** <u>Less and less</u> should be <u>fewer and fewer</u>.

16. **(D)** <u>Real</u> should be <u>really</u>.

17. **(D)** <u>In back of</u> should be <u>behind</u>.

18. **(A)** <u>Regards</u> should be <u>regard</u>.

19. **(A)** <u>Quit</u> should be <u>quiet</u>.

20. **(D)** <u>Somewheres</u> should be <u>somewhere</u>.

21. **(B)** <u>Without</u> should be <u>unless</u>.

22. **(B)** <u>Inferred</u> should be <u>implied</u>.

23. **(B)** Eliminate <u>hardly</u>.

24. **(C)** <u>Badly</u> should be <u>bad</u>.

25. **(A)** <u>Anywheres</u> should be <u>anywhere</u>.

Errors in Parallelism

When two or more ideas fulfill the same function in a sentence, they should be stated in the same grammatical form. This practice is called *parallelism*. Parallelism is most commonly required when two or more items are connected with the conjunctions *and, but, or, either-or, neither-nor*.

Examples: My son enjoys swimming, reading, and a walk in the park. (Incorrect)
My son enjoys swimming, reading, and walking in the park. (Correct)

EXAMPLES

1. As the locomotive left the station, it jerked them so that the passengers were
   A   B
   thrown from their seats and who fell on the floor. No error.
   C   D   E

   Explanation: The underlined error is choice (D); the sentence parallels a verb phrase (thrown from their seats) with a dependent clause, beginning who fell. The correct phrasing should be and fell.

2. Almost everyone enjoys watching a baseball game on television, having a picnic
   A   B
   in peaceful park, or to visit some strange place abroad. No error.
   C   D   E

   Explanation: The underlined error is choice (C); the sentence parallels two verbals (watching and having) with an infinitive to visit. The correct phrasing should be or visiting.

Now, try your hand with the following four sentences:

1. Dustin Hoffman, one of Hollywood's great stars, made his reputation
                    A
   playing a confused young man, a tubercular panhandler, and he also has
            B   C
   enacted other roles. No error.
          D   E

2. No one can decide between two alternatives to raise money: either the
             A   B
   club should sponsor a cookie sale or stage a festival in the town's
        C   D
   auditorium. No error.
              E

3. In the 1970s, <u>many college</u> students protested social conditions by
                        A
    sitting <u>in various</u> campus buildings, by burning campus structures,
                    B
    <u>and they have also intimidated</u> <u>members of the administration</u>. <u>No error.</u>
                    C   D   E

4. <u>Rosie O'Donnell</u>, a stand-up comedienne <u>and who has</u> written a book
            A   B
    of jokes for children, has now <u>made a name for herself</u> as the host of two
                                            C
    <u>daytime talk shows.</u> <u>No error.</u>
            D   E

Answer Explanations

1. **(C)** The sentence parallels two nouns with an independent clause. The correct word-
    ing is <u>and other roles</u>.

2. **(D)** The same construction (a complete clause) should appear after both <u>either</u> and <u>or</u>.

3. **(C)** The sentence parallels two prepositional phrases with an independent clause. The
    correct wording is <u>by intimidating</u>.

4. **(B)** The sentence parallels a noun with a dependent clause. The correct wording is
    <u>who has</u> (omit <u>and</u>).

Dangling Elements and Misplaced Modifiers

English is flexible and allows for some variety in word order when a writer is using modifiers like adjectives, adverbs, and descriptive phrases or clauses. Confusion or ambiguity can
result, however, if a modifier is placed in the wrong location.

> **Example:** Jennie's friend told us Thursday night she would visit us. (Incorrect)
> Thursday night Jennie's friend told us she would visit us. (Correct)
> OR Jennie's friend told us she would visit us Thursday night. (Correct)

Another sentence structure problem is called the *dangling modifier.* This error arises
when a modifier—a phrase or clause—does not have a specific word in the rest of the sentence to modify. For example:

> **At the age of five, my father died.**

This sentence states that my father died when he was five years old, a biological impossibility.

> **Correction:** When I was five years old, <u>my father</u> died.

Dangling modifiers do not occur only at the beginning of sentences. For example:

> **My brother fell and broke his leg in three places, which was too bad.**

<u>Which was too bad</u> does not modify a specific word in the rest of the sentence but rather
the idea that the rest of the sentence conveys.

Study a few more examples with corrections:

Looking up, four airplanes were overhead.

This sentence suggests four airplanes were looking up.

Correction: When I looked up, I saw four airplanes overhead.

The robber who was running down the street rapidly turned the corner.

(Does rapidly modify was running or turned? The modifier dangles between the two possibilities, creating an ambiguous sentence.)

Correction: The robber who was running rapidly down the street turned the corner.
or
The robber who was running down the street turned the corner rapidly.

While washing clothes, the clock struck three.

The clock wasn't washing clothes.

Correction: While I was washing clothes, the clock struck three.

My mother won a million dollars in the lottery, which was fortunate.

The lottery itself is not fortunate.

Correction: It was fortunate that my mother won a million dollars in the lottery.

EXAMPLES

1. Rising up above the top of a very high mountain, we saw the sun make
        A   B

   its way slowly to the zenith at noon. No error.
    C   D   E

   Explanation: The underlined error is choice (A); the participial phrase cannot logically modify the first word after the comma.

2. The young man who was running down the street very rapidly turned the
                A   B   C

   corner and ran into a friend who was looking for him. No error.
          D   E

   Explanation: The underlined error is choice (C); whether the adverb modifies was running or turned is not clear.

1. Waddling up to the cold pool of water, I watched the penguin do
                      A   B

   a belly flop onto the ice and dive into the water. No error.
        C   D   E

2. Looking ahead as far as the Detroit designers can predict, the automobile
           A

   will always have four wheels, a steering wheel, two headlights, and four
          B   C   D

   wheel brakes. No error.
             E

3. Chez Raddish is a superb and inexpensive restaurant where fine food
                       A   B

   is served by waiters and waitresses in appetizing forms. No error.
      C   D   E

4. The painter broke his hip when the ladder broke, climbing slowly rung
                A   B   C

   by rung until he reached the second floor of the building. No error.
                                 D   E

Answer Explanations

1. **(A)** The introductory phrase does not modify I.

2. **(A)** The introductory participial phrase does not modify automobile.

3. **(D)** The phrase in appetizing forms is misplaced. The phrase should appear after fine food.

4. **(C)** The closest word that the participial phrase could modify is ladder. And ladders don't climb!

Incorrect Verb Forms

It is important to use the proper form of each verb for each tense. Most verbs simply add *-ed* to the present tense when forming the past tense or past participle forms.

Example: talk, talked, has talked

There are, however, many verbs that have slightly different spellings for these forms. Some verbs are called *irregular* because they vary widely from the usual forms.

Examples:

I sing	I sang	I have sung
I lay	I laid	I have laid
I lie	I lay	I have lain
I choose	I chose	I have chosen
I see	I saw	I have seen

EXAMPLES

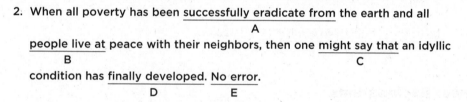

1. Alcoholics Anonymous <u>exists to rescue</u> those people who have always <u>drank</u> so
   A B

   much that they <u>cannot break</u> away from <u>their addiction alone</u>. <u>No error</u>.
   C D E

   Explanation: The underlined error is choice (B); <u>drank</u> should be <u>drunk</u>.

2. When all poverty has been <u>successfully eradicate from</u> the earth and all
   A

   <u>people live at</u> peace with their neighbors, then one <u>might say that</u> an idyllic
   B C

   condition has <u>finally developed</u>. <u>No error</u>.
   D E

   Explanation: The underlined error is choice (A); <u>eradicate</u> should be <u>eradicated</u>.

1. "The Age of Aquarius" is suppose to be an age of youth, an age of great
   A   B
   accomplishments by everyone, an age in which all of our hopes and
                     C
   aspirations will be realized. No error.
                D   E

2. Because of the high yields in the stock market, many investors
   A   B   C
   have chose to buy stocks in record numbers. No error.
   D   E

3. The driver of the car should have went right to avoid the traffic snarl,
                           A   B   C
   but he wasn't paying attention. No error.
   D   E

4. After many repetitions of the manual of arms, a raw recruit becomes use to
                           A   B
   going through the drill without thinking too hard about what
   C
   he or she is doing. No error.
   D   E

Answer Explanations

1. **(A)** Suppose should be supposed.

2. **(D)** Chose should be chosen.

3. **(A)** Went should be gone.

4. **(B)** Use should be used.

Sentence Boundaries

Writing complete sentences helps you communicate your ideas clearly. There are three types of sentence errors: *sentence fragments, comma splices,* and *run-on sentences.* To help you identify these sentence construction errors, here are three definitions and some illustrations of the errors:

1. A *complete sentence* can be defined as a group of words that has a subject and a verb and conveys a complete idea. For example:

   The child hit the ball.

That collection of words is a complete sentence; it has a subject (<u>child</u>) and a verb (<u>hit</u>). A complete sentence may be as short as this illustration or much longer, but the definition still holds: The word group conveys a complete idea.

2. A *sentence fragment* is a group of words that may look like a complete sentence but that lack a subject or a verb, or that include a word that makes the group incomplete. Look at the following examples:

Looking up at the airplanes

While the clouds turned darker and darker

A terrible experience for all of us

None of these is a complete sentence, because none of them conveys a complete idea.

3. A *run-on sentence* is defined as two complete sentences that are written as if they were one complete sentence. Here is an example:

The children worked hard they wanted to succeed.

There are two complete sentences (<u>The children worked hard</u> and <u>they wanted to succeed</u>), and English convention says that we must have some logical separation of those complete sentences. If you use a comma—<u>The children worked hard</u>, <u>they wanted to succeed</u>—you will make another error called the *comma splice*.

Here are some ways to correctly punctuate clauses.

- Use a semicolon between two sentences to show that they are related. This combination is called coordination. Here are examples:

  The baby cried; he was hungry.

  The rain clouds worried the sponsors of the fair; they were afraid rain would keep people away.

- Use a comma with a coordinating conjunction for coordination. This creates a compound sentence. The coordinating conjuctions are as follows: *but, or, yet, for, and, nor, so.* Here are examples of compound sentences:

  The job description mentioned a need for applicants to be knowledgeable of tax laws, so Humberto studied his old notes from college on the subject.

  Min needed to stay home and study for her exam, but her boss asked her to come in to work.

- Use subordinating conjunctions for subordination, thereby creating complex sentences. Some common subordinating conjunctions include *because, when, if, even though, although,* and *since.* Here are examples of complex sentences:

  Even though his favorite football team was down by four touchdowns, Rick believed there could be a fourth quarter miracle.

  Rick believed there could be a fourth quarter miracle even though his favorite football team was down by four touchdowns.

Look at some questions that might include errors in sentence construction.

1. The new Ford Focus model has captured the admiration of many automobile <u>critics, they have</u> praised its sleek lines and daring styles.
   (A) critics, they have
   (B) critics; they have
   (C) critics they have
   (D) critics, whom have
   (E) critics, she has

   Explanation: The correct answer is (B). The semicolon corrects the comma splice. (C) is incorrect because omitting punctuation creates a run-on sentence. (D) is incorrect because <u>whom</u> is the objective form of the pronoun. (E) is also incorrect because <u>she</u> (a singular) cannot refer to <u>critics</u> (plural); also, the comma splice error has not been changed.

2. Tony Blair, prime minister of Great <u>Britain, has changed</u> the course of British history within his first years in office.
   (A) Britain, has changed
   (B) Britain, who has changed
   (C) Britain; has changed
   (D) Britain has changed
   (E) Britain, whom has changed

   Explanation: The correct answer is (A). (B) and (E) are incorrect because the relative pronouns would make the sentence incomplete; <u>whom</u> is also the incorrect case. (C) is incorrect because the semicolon signals that a comma splice has been corrected, and there is no comma splice in the sentence. (D) is incorrect because there needs to be a comma to set off the appositive phrase.

Now, try several of these types of sentences, illustrating the types of items you will find on an actual CLEP test:

1. A national magazine called Jimmy Carter "the best ex-president we <u>have ever had"</u> <u>he has</u> worked on many projects to help people.

   (A) have ever had" he has
   (B) have ever had" because he has
   (C) have ever had due to the fact that
   (D) have ever had" being that he has worked
   (E) have ever had," working

2. Dustin Hoffman won an Oscar for his performance as an autistic <u>man, he lived in</u> a sheltered home for many years before being rescued by his brother.

   (A) man, he lived in
   (B) man he lived in
   (C) man who lived
   (D) man whom he had lived in
   (E) man, he will live

Answer Explanations

1. **(B)** Because makes the rest of the sentence a dependent clause. As written, it is a run-on sentence.

2. **(C)** The comma splice is eliminated. (B) is a run-on sentence. (D) uses an incorrect relative pronoun (whom). (E) is wrong because it is in the future tense, which is illogical in this sentence.

Correct Sentences

Questions on conventions of standard English include some sentences that are correct, so that the test taker must be able to distinguish errors accurately. Here are some examples.

1. Derek and José started the race this morning; we hope they will reach the
   A ⎯⎯⎯⎯   B   C
   finish line without having to quit. No error.
        D   E

2. The other night, I was reading Sylvia Plath's poetry about her experiences
   A
   when I decided that I wanted to learn more about this extraordinary
      B   C
   woman and her writing. No error.
       D   E

3. George Washington, the father of our country, had many problems with
           A   B
   the Continental Congress; many times he had to beg for funds to support
        C   D
   his starving army. No error.
           E

4. Walking up four flights of stairs is not easy for anyone who has heart
        A   B   C
   trouble or who gets tired very easily. No error.
           D   E

5. Many builders of fine furniture have used designs first created by Adams,
        A   B
   Chippendale, Duncan-Phyffe, and Morris, as well as other older furniture
                   C
   designers whose work is preserved in museums all over the world. No error.
       D   E

6. Apple pie or ice cream—which has more calories? Even the best diet
        A   B   C
   books published cannot give anyone a clear answer. No error.
           D   E

7. When the final score flashed on the scoreboard, cheers rose from the

   A B

   crowd that had been hoping for that long-awaited victory over

   C

   the traditional rival. No error.

   D E

8. According to the code of ethics that all lawyers accept, no lawyer should

   A

   take any action, within or outside the courtroom, that might damage his

   B C

   or her client's right to a fair trial. No error.

   D E

9. In any business, the workers expect to be paid promptly when pay day

   A B

   comes; none of them can finance his or her day-to-day life without such

   C D

   punctuality. No error.

   E

10. Robin Williams was famous for his expert comedy, his ability to assume a

    A B

    number of different roles, and his knack of improvising dialogue while the

    C D

    television camera is on. No error.

    E

CAUTION

On the actual CLEP examination, sentences will not be isolated by error as these practice pages and items have been organized; therefore, you will have to consider each underlined section carefully and consider the possibility that any one of the number of errors might be present. Also, do not forget that some sentences are correct and contain no error.

PRACTICE QUESTIONS FOR REVISION SKILLS

In the section on Revision Skills, you will have to answer questions that go beyond the rules of grammar and usage. You will need to understand some of the principles involved in effective writing. Here are some of the topics that may appear.

1. ORGANIZATION

Good writers make careful decisions about the order in which they present their ideas. Choosing a plan of organization that is appropriate for the audience and the topic makes the presentation much more effective.

Here are some standard types of organization commonly used in nonfiction writing:

- Chronological—arrange information in a time sequence
- Cause and effect—present information about the causes of an event
- General to specific (or specific to general)—start with the most general information and then move to a specific topic; or begin with specific ideas and move to a general conclusion
- Comparison/contrast—describe the similarities or differences between two things
- Problem/solution—explain a problem and then propose a solution

2. AUDIENCE, TONE, AND PURPOSE

Good writers pay attention to their audience, the tone of their writing, and their purpose. Knowing the intended **audience** for a piece of writing enables a writer to select the length, style, and vocabulary that best fits those readers. A writer's **tone** is the emotional attitude conveyed by the work; it might be formal or informal, playful or serious. The **purpose** of a written work is the primary reason for producing the work, the author's main goal.

3. LEVEL OF DETAIL

A writer must determine the level of detail that is appropriate for a particular paragraph or essay. If there are too many details that are unrelated to the main point, the reader will be distracted. If the writer omits details that are important in proving the main point, the reader will be unconvinced. Good writers include all the details that are necessary to establish the point, but they remove any details that have no purpose.

4. COHERENCE

Writing is coherent when it is clear and the ideas are connected properly. Many factors can improve the coherence of a passage, but there are two techniques that are especially important:

- Each paragraph should have a single focus. Every part of the paragraph should be related to the primary point that the writer is attempting to make.
- Each sentence should be connected in some way to the sentences before and after it. Writers can provide a sense of connectedness by repeating words or ideas, using parallelism, or using transition words or phrases.

5. VARIETY IN SENTENCE STRUCTURE

A skilled writer will combine various sentence structures to maintain the reader's interest. A paragraph may contain simple sentences (one independent clause), compound sentences (two independent clauses), complex sentences (an independent clause combined with one or more dependent clauses), or compound-complex sentences (two or more independent clauses combined with at least one dependent clause). Variety can also be achieved by using sentences of different lengths or different openings for the sentences.

6. MAIN IDEA, THESIS STATEMENT, AND TOPIC SENTENCES

Every written work should have a **main idea**, a central thought that serves as the main point of the essay or paragraph. In many cases, a writer will provide a **thesis statement** giving his or her opinion on the main idea of the essay.

In an essay, each paragraph should develop a focused idea that supports the thesis statement, or main idea, of the essay. Each sentence in a paragraph should be devoted to a single idea that supports the case that the writer is trying to develop. One of the sentences in each paragraph should be a summary of that paragraph; this is called the **topic sentence**. It is usually the first or last sentence of the paragraph.

7. CONSISTENCY OF VIEWPOINT

A writer may adopt one of three points of view.

- First person—written from the perspective of the writer ("I traveled to Kentucky.")
- Second person—written from the perspective of the reader ("You failed to notice the danger.")
- Third person—written from the perspective of an unseen observer, without mentioning the writer or the reader ("The actor was distracted by the applause.")

Once a writer has started a work in a particular viewpoint, he or she should not change to a different one.

Examples:
I seldom eat at a Japanese restaurant, because you might have to eat raw fish. (awkward)
I seldom eat at a Japanese restaurant, because I might have to eat raw fish. (improved)

8. TRANSITIONS

Careful writers use carefully chosen words or phrases to help readers see the logical connections between one sentence and the next.

Here are some of the more common transitions: *and, but, yet, either...or, neither...nor, as a result, for example, furthermore, however, in other words, just as, nevertheless, on the contrary, although, therefore.*

In this type of question, you are given a passage from an essay that needs revision. You will be asked questions about ways to improve specific sentences or parts of sentences or about ways to improve the passage as a whole.

DIRECTIONS: The following passages is an early drafts of an essay.

Read each passage and then answer the questions that follow. Some questions refer to particular sentences or parts of sentences and ask you to improve sentence structure or diction (word choice). Other questions refer to the entire essay or parts of the essay and ask you to consider the essay's organization, development, or effectiveness of language. In selecting your answers, follow the conventions of Standard Written English.

Questions 1–4 are based on the following passage:

(1) Revision is an important part of writing. (2) Often the writer will discover that there are problems with the arrangement of the material. (3) This may call for transpositions. (4) When this happens, you can block and copy to rearrange your sentences in better order. (5) If the problem is that the writer has taken far too many words to say whatever it is that she wanted to say in the first place, it may be that a pencil will be the only tool needed to eliminate the excess verbiage. (6) This is true even if you write with a pen. (7) Do not think that you are a failure because your first draft needs major changes. (8) Few writers have ever been so expert that they can produce exactly what they want the first time.

1. Which of the following is a valid criticism of the passage as a whole?

    (A) It is inconsistent in its use of tenses.
    (B) It is inconsistent in its use of person (pronouns).
    (C) It does not discuss a real problem.
    (D) No one writes with a pen anymore.
    (E) It is not organized logically.

2. Which of the following is the best way to combine sentences 2 and 3 (reproduced below)?

    Often the writer will discover that there are problems with the arrangement of the material. this may call for transpositions.

    (A) Often the writer will call for transpositions to cope with problems with the arrangement of the material.
    (B) Often the writer will discover that there are problems with the arrangement of the material and that transpositions are called for.
    (C) Often the writer will discover that there are problems with the arrangement of the material, calling for transpositions.
    (D) Often the writer will discover that the problems with the arrangement of the material mean that he should call for transpositions.
    (E) Often the writer will discover that there are problems with the arrangement of the material, so he should call for transpositions.

3. Which of the following is a valid criticism of sentence 5?

    (A) It is too long.

    (B) It belongs at the end of the paragraph.

    (C) It contains a mixed metaphor.

    (D) It is too wordy.

    (E) It contains a dangling modifier.

4. What should be done with sentence 6?

    (A) It should be left as it is.

    (B) It should be omitted.

    (C) It should be moved to the end of the passage.

    (D) It should follow sentence 3.

    (E) It should follow sentence 2.

Answer Explanations

1. **(B)** Sometimes the passage uses *you* (second person) and sometimes the passage uses *the writer/she* (third person). Either one would be acceptable, but not both.

2. **(C)** This combines the sentences with no grammatical problems and avoids having the writer, rather than the arrangement of the material, call for transposition.

3. **(D)** The sentence illustrates precisely the problem it describes.

4. **(B)** The sentence is irrelevant to the topic of the passage, so it should be removed.

PRACTICE QUESTIONS FOR IMPROVING SENTENCES

The College Composition Modular Exam expands the section on Revision Skills by adding questions on Improving Sentences, These items test your ability to discern what is incorrect about the structure of a sentence. You will attempt to recognize any problems in the sentence as written that would interfere with logical communication.

DIRECTIONS: The following sentences test correctness and effectiveness of expression. In choosing your answers, follow the requirements of Standard Written English: that is, pay attention to grammar, diction (choice of words), sentence construction, and punctuation.

In the following sentences, part of each sentence is underlined. Beneath each sentence you will find five versions of the underlined part. The first option repeats the original; the other four options present different versions.

Choose the option that best expresses the meaning of the original sentence. If you think the original is better than any of the alternatives, choose the first option; otherwise, choose one of the other options. Your choice should produce the most effective sentence—one that is clear and precise, without awkwardness or ambiguity.

EXAMPLES

1. The reason the company failed was because the president spent too much money.
   - (A) The reason the company failed was because
   - (B) The company failed because
   - (C) Because the company failed
   - (D) Because the reason was the company failed
   - (E) The company failed was because

   Explanation: The correct answer is (B). The other choices are wordy or create illogical sentences.

2. When four years old, my father died.
   - (A) When four years old
   - (B) When four year's old
   - (C) When he was four years old
   - (D) When I was four years old
   - (E) At the age of four

   Explanation: The correct answer is (D). The underlined section in the original sentence is a dangling modifier, and only answer (D) solves that problem.

3. Football teams pay athletes tremendous sums of money each year, the fans pay large sums for seats in the stadium.
   - (A) year, the fans pay large sums
   - (B) year, the fans paying large sums
   - (C) year, for the fans pay large sums
   - (D) year; the fans paying large sums
   - (E) year, when the fans pay large sums

   Explanation: The correct answer is (C). The original sentence contains a comma splice, and only (C) corrects the problem logically.

4. The lazy old <u>man was lying under his favorite tree, sipping</u> his favorite soft drink, and reading his favorite novel for the fifth time.
   (A) man was lying under his favorite tree, sipping
   (B) man was laying under his favorite tree, sipping
   (C) man was lying under his favorite tree sipping
   (D) man laid under his favorite tree, sipping
   (E) man lied under his favorite tree, sipping

   Explanation: The correct answer is (A). (B) is incorrect; <u>laying</u> is the wrong word choice. (C) is incorrect; the comma after <u>tree</u> is omitted, distorting the parallelism of the original. (D) is incorrect; <u>laid</u> is the wrong word choice. (E) is also incorrect; <u>lied</u> is the wrong word choice.

5. <u>People who attend baseball games often do not know enough about the fine points of offense and defense to enjoy them.</u>
   (A) People who attend baseball games often do not know enough about the fine points of offense and defense to enjoy them.
   (B) People who attend baseball games do not know a sufficient amount about the fine points of offense and defense to appreciate them.
   (C) Some people who attend baseball games do not know enough about the fine points of offense and defense to enjoy the skill of the players.
   (D) People who attend baseball games often do not know enough about them to enjoy the fine points of offense and defense.
   (E) People who attend baseball games do not understand the fine points of offense and defense.

   Explanation: The correct answer is (C). (A) and (B) has <u>them</u>, which is a vague pronoun. (D) has the same problem even though <u>them</u> is moved within the sentence. (E) changes the meaning of the original too much.

Now that you have tried some items of this type, try six more.

---

1. The wooden house had once been a showpiece of antebellum architecture, <u>but time and tide had reduced the structure to wrack and ruin.</u>

   (A) but time and tide had reduced the structure to wrack and ruin
   (B) but time had reduced the structure to wrack and ruin
   (C) but time and tide had reduced the structure to ruin
   (D) but time reduced the structure to a ruin
   (E) but time had reduced the structure to a ruin

2. <u>Bill had to be administered to by a doctor when his admittance to law school was refused.</u>

   (A) Bill had to be administered to by a doctor when his admittance to law school was refused.
   (B) Bill had to be treated by a doctor when his admission to law school was refused.
   (C) Bill had to be treated by a doctor when his admittance to law school was refused.
   (D) Bill had to be administered to by a doctor when his admission to law school was refused.
   (E) Bill was administered to by a doctor when his admittance to law school was refused.

3. Our neighborhood ice cream vendor was refused a license <u>because he sold banana splits to customers that were rotten.</u>

   (A) because he sold banana splits to customers that were rotten
   (B) because he sold banana splits to customers who were rotten
   (C) because he sold banana splits that were rotten to customers
   (D) because he sold banana splits who were rotten to customers
   (E) because he sold rotten banana splits to customers

4. We could only wonder if he were going to attend college <u>this fall, or if he was planning to seek</u> immediate employment.

   (A) this fall, or if he was planning to seek
   (B) fall, or he was planning to seek
   (C) fall, or if he were planning to seek
   (D) fall or was planning to seek
   (E) fall; or he was planning to seek

5. Running the rapids <u>of the Colorado River in a small raft are considered</u> one of the greatest sporting thrills available to anyone.

   (A) the Colorado River in a small raft are considered
   (B) the Colorado River in a small raft is considered
   (C) the Colorado River with a small raft are considered
   (D) the Colorado River in small rafts are considered
   (E) the Colorado's River in a small raft is considered

6. <u>Each of you can do the problem if you will put your</u> mind to work and not give up too easily.

   (A) Each of you can do the problem if you will put your
   (B) Each of you can do the problem if they will put their
   (C) Each and everyone of you can finish the problem if they will put their
   (D) Each and everyone one of them can finish the problems if you will put their
   (E) Everyone of you can finish the problems if they will put their

Answer Explanations

1. **(E)** Wrack and ruin and time and tide are clichés. Only choices (D) and (E) eliminate them; choice (D), however, introduces another error, an error in verb tense.

2. **(B)** Administered and admittance are errors in diction. (B) is correct.

3. **(E)** That was rotten (which modifies banana splits) is a misplaced modifier in any position except choice (E).

4. **(C)** Was must be changed to were to make the two parts of the sentence parallel in construction.

5. **(B)** Running … raft is the subject of the sentence; therefore, are must be is.

6. **(A)** The sentence is correct as it stands.

PRACTICE QUESTIONS ON ABILITY TO USE SOURCE MATERIALS

Research: The Basic Process

Writing a research paper is one of the foundational skills required of most college students. Whether you are studying astrophysics or American history, your professor is likely to assign a research paper. It is for this reason that the CLEP College Composition Exam includes a section on research skills.

A research paper is a formal presentation of information you have gathered on a particular topic. You are expected to follow sound principles of research, and to follow carefully the guidelines for a particular format in presenting the material.

What skills are required to write a research paper? You must be able to find information, evaluate the information, and use it to support the thesis of your paper. You must be able to use the information to construct a logical case for your idea. You must also be able to support each point with documented evidence, providing sources for the information you use.

What are the main features of a typical research paper?

Research papers are composed of three sections: (1) opening material, such as a title page and/or outline; (2) the body of the paper; and (3) a list of sources. You will also use a system for indicating the source of each quotation or fact in the body of the paper. This documentation system will involve a set of parenthetical references, or a set of footnotes or endnotes.

You should become familiar with the MLA, APA, and Chicago formats for research paper documentation:

1. MLA DOCUMENTATION

One of the most common systems of documenting sources is the Modern Language Association (MLA) format.

In this system, the writer places a short note in parentheses immediately after each quotation or other significant piece of information. Typically, the note simply identifies the source by giving the author's last name and the page number.

Example

(McCullough 425)

Obviously, this note does not provide enough information to lead a reader to the original source; it simply gives enough to find a complete entry in the Works Cited page at the end of the paper.

Examples of Works Cited entries:

Book by one author

McCullough, David. *Truman*. New York: Simon & Schuster, 1992. Print.

Article in a magazine

Lipman, Marvin. "The Pros and Cons of Denial." *Consumer Reports*. March 2011: 16. Print.

Article on a website

Zax, David. "The Scurlock Studio: Picture of Prosperity." Smithsonian.com. Feb. 2011. www.smithsonianmag.com/people-places/The-Scurlock-Studio-Picture-of-Prosperity.html. Web.

Article in a scholarly journal

Bagch, Alaknanda. "Conflicting Nationalisms: The Voice of the Subaltern in Mahasweta Devi's Bashai Tudu." *Tulsa Studies in Women's Literature*. 15.1 (1996):41–50. Print.

Note: 15 refers to the volume number, and 1 refers to the issue of the journal.

Complete information on the MLA format may be found in:

Gibaldi, Joseph, and Walter S. Achtert. *MLA Handbook for Writers of Research Papers*. Latest edition. New York: Modern Language Association.

2. APA DOCUMENTATION

The American Psychological Association (APA) format is often used for research papers in the social sciences.

In this system, the writer places a short note in parentheses immediately after each quotation or other significant information. The note usually identifies the source by giving the author's last name, the year of publication, and the page number.

Example

(McCullough, 1992, p. 425)

As in the MLA system, this note provides only enough information to enable the reader to identify an entry in the Reference List page at the end of the paper.

Example of Reference List entries:

Book by one author

McCullough, D. (1992) *Truman*. New York: Simon & Schuster.

Article in a magazine

> Lipman, M. (2011, March). The pros and cons of denial. *Consumer Reports*, p. 16.

Article on a website

> Zax, D. (2011, February). *The Scurlock Studio: Picture of Prosperity*. Retrieved April 4, 2011, from Smithsonian Web site: www.smithsonianmag.com/people-places/The-Scurlock-Studio-Picture-of-Prosperity.html

Article in a scholarly journal

> Physiol, J. (2011). Epithelial Acetycholine. *The Journal of Physiology*, 589(4), 771–772.

Note: 589 is the volume, and 4 is the issue of the journal.

Complete information on the APA format may be found in:

> American Psychological Association. *Publication Manual of the American Psychological Association*. Latest edition. Washington, D.C.: American Psychological Association.

3. CHICAGO MANUAL OF STYLE DOCUMENTATION

The Chicago Manual of Style system was once the most common format for college research papers. It is sometimes grouped with the Turabian system, which is very similar.

In this system, the writer places a raised (superscript) number immediately after each quotation or other significant piece of information. The number matches a numbered footnote (at the bottom of the page) or endnote (on a separate page at the end of the paper). The first footnote referring to a particular source gives full information on that source; subsequent references to the same source use abbreviations or shortened formats. A Bibliography containing complete information on all sources is placed at the end of the paper.

Example of citation in text:

> Churchill wrote: "He seems a man of exceptional character."[7]

Example of footnotes or endnotes:

Book by one author

> 7. McCullough, David. *Truman* (New York: Simon & Schuster, 1992), p. 425.

Article in a magazine

> 21. Lipman, Marvin. "The Pros and Cons of Denial." *Consumer Reports*. (March 2011): 16.

Article on a website

> 14. David Zax, "The Scurlock Studio: Picture of Prosperity," (posted February 2010), Smithsonian.com, www.smithsonianmag.com/people-places/The-Scurlock-Studio-Picture-of-Prosperity.html (accessed April 4, 2011).

Examples of Bibliography entries:

Book by one author

McCullough, David. *Truman*. New York: Simon & Schuster, 1992.

Article in a magazine

Lipman, Marvin. "The Pros and Cons of Denial." *Consumer Reports* (March 2011): 16–17.

Article on a website

Zax, David. "The Scurlock Studio: Picture of Prosperity." Posted February 2010). Smithsonian.com. www.smithsonianmag.com/people-places/The-Scurlock-Studio-Picture-of-Prosperity.html (accessed April 4, 2011).

Article in a scholarly journal

Pinaud, Raphael. "Genome of a Songbird Unveiled." *Journal of Biology* 9, no. 19 (2010):3–5.

Note: 9 is the volume number, and 19 is the issue.

Complete information on the Chicago/Turabian system may be found in:

The Chicago Manual of Style. Latest edition. Chicago: University of Chicago Press.

Turabian, Kate L. *A Manual for Writers of Term Papers, Theses, and Dissertations*. Latest edition. Chicago: University of Chicago Press.

Information on these systems of documentation is also available in most standard textbooks in college composition, or in specialized works such as Peter Markman, Alison L. Heney, Roberta Markman, and Marie L. Waddell. *10 Steps in Writing the Research Paper*. 7th ed. Hauppauge, NY: Barron's, 2011.

DIRECTIONS: The following questions test your familiarity with basic research, reference, and composition skills. Some questions refer to passages, whereas other questions are self-contained. For each question, choose the best answer.

Questions 1–2 are based on the following passage:

Aeschylus, *EHS kuh luhs* (525–356 B.C.) was the earliest writer of Greek tragedy whose plays exist in complete form. He wrote more than 80 plays, of which seven survive. These seven plays reveal a deeply patriotic and religious artist who brought Greek tragedy to maturity. Before Aeschylus, tragedies had a single actor who could only respond to the questions or suggestions of the chorus. Aeschylus increased the number of actors to two, which created dialogue that permitted interaction between characters.

Aeschylus's plots are simple. Most of them center on a conflict between an individual's will and the divine powers that rule the world. Aeschylus wrote tragedy in a grand manner, with a richness of language and complexity of thought that only the English playwright William Shakespeare has rivaled. Aeschylus's greatest work is the *Oresteia* (456 B.C.), which consists of three plays forming one drama. They are *Agamemnon, The Libation Bearers*, and *The*

Eumenides (The Furies). In these plays, Aeschylus turned the violence after the return of King Agamemnon from Troy into a drama about the reconciliation of human suffering with divine power. Aeschylus's other surviving plays are *The Persians* (472), *Seven Against Thebes* (467), *The Suppliants* (463?), and *Prometheus Bound*, which was probably written late in Aeschylus's life. Aeschylus was born into a prominent family in Eleusis, near Athens.

Luci Berkowitz

See also Drama [Greek drama]

Source: The World Book Encyclopedia.
Chicago: World Book, 2003, p. 90.

1. What information is provided by the phrase "See also Drama [Greek drama]"?

    (A) The location of a related article elsewhere in the encyclopedia
    (B) The location of a website with additional information
    (C) The section of the encyclopedia in which this article is found
    (D) A suggestion for further research in other sources
    (E) The source of the information in the article

2. Which statement is NOT supported by this article?

    (A) The *Oresteia* was probably the earliest of Aeschylus's surviving plays.
    (B) No complete plays written earlier than Aeschylus have survived.
    (C) All the surviving plays of Aeschylus are tragedies.
    (D) Aeschylus wrote only seven plays.
    (E) Aeschylus originated the use of two actors in Greek plays.

---

3. In the following Works Cited entry for a journal article, what information is given by the number *55*?

    Shields, David S. "Happiness in Society: The Development of an Eighteenth-Century American Poetic Ideal." *American Literature* 55 (December 1983): 541–545.

    (A) The page number of the entry
    (B) The volume of the journal
    (C) The date of publication
    (D) The year when the quote was first stated
    (E) The section of the journal

4. Which of the following sources would be most useful for research on the establishment of the United Nations?

    (A) The United Nations website
    (B) A textbook on international relations
    (C) A journal article on the origin of nation-states
    (D) An interview with a staff member from the U.S. State Department
    (E) The biography of the first head of the United Nations

Answer Explanations

1. **(A)** This reference tells the researcher that additional information is available in the article titled "Drama [Greek drama]," which appears elsewhere in the same encyclopedia set.

2. **(D)** Aeschylus wrote 80 plays, though only seven of them have survived. The other statements are all clearly supported by the article.

3. **(B)** Professional journals and other periodicals are often listed in *volumes*, because libraries have customarily stored back issues in the form of bound volumes. A volume might include all the issues for one year or a portion of a year. This entry refers to an article from Volume 55 of the journal *American Literature*.

4. **(A)** The United Nations website can be expected to contain authoritative information on the origin and nature of the organization. Since it is the official voice of the United Nations, this site would include primary documents. Choice C does not apply to this topic, because nation-states were a feature of society in ancient Greece, while the United Nations was founded shortly after the end of World War II. Choice B is too general, and would not focus on the United Nations. A State Department staff person (Choice D) would not necessarily be well informed about an event that happened more than 60 years ago. Choice E would be a source of interesting information, but would not be organized in a way that provides easy access to a systematic discussion of the United Nations.

PRACTICE QUESTIONS FOR RHETORICAL ANALYSIS

In the section on Rhetorical Analysis, you will be called on to answer questions that examine your understanding of a writer's purpose and the characteristics of good writing. Some of the most important areas to understand follow:

1. RHETORICAL EFFECTS AND STYLE

Rhetoric refers to the effective use of language to persuade. The Greek philosopher Aristotle outlined a classic analysis of three approaches to persuasion:

Ethos—an appeal based on the authority of the writer. When people believe that a writer is competent and trustworthy, they are likely to believe the message.
Pathos—an appeal to the emotions of the audience. A writer may present material designed to produce anger, admiration, fear, or other emotions that will motivate readers to respond.
Logos—an appeal to the reason of the audience. Such an appeal will employ logical reasoning based on various types of evidence.

Writers also use a wide range of techniques to present their ideas in an effective, readable style. Samples of skillful writing will often employ some of these features.

- Conciseness vs. wordiness—use only as many words as are necessary to make your point.
- Active vs. passive—in most cases, active verbs are more effective than passive verbs.
- Fresh vs. cliché—some expressions have been used so long and so often that they are no longer effective.

   Example: in this day and age, light as a feather

- Literal vs. figurative—figurative descriptions can be extremely effective, as long as the reader understands them.

2. USE OF LANGUAGE

Competent writers choose their words carefully, avoiding anything that will distract their readers and hinder their effectiveness. Among the most common pitfalls are the following:

- Use of excessively formal or informal language—Consider the audience and the occasion, and adopt a level of formality that is appropriate. It is particularly important to avoid sudden shifts back and forth between formal and informal expressions.
- Use of jargon—*Jargon* refers to technical terms used in a particular trade or field of study or to words that have a "private meaning" as used by a specific group of people. Using jargon can be helpful when everyone in the conversation knows the meaning of the words, but it throws up barriers to communication when the intended audience is unfamiliar with the terms used.
- Use of slang or excessive colloquialisms—In academic writing, it is better to use Standard Written English, employing words that might be found in a dictionary. Avoid words that are used only by specific age groups or cultural backgrounds; such terms are often misunderstood by the broader reading public.

3. CRITICAL THINKING AND LOGIC

A careful reader must develop the skills of critical thinking, so that he or she can recognize and evaluate the arguments used by writers. Several factors are important in learning how to recognize a good argument.

First, recognize the difference between facts and opinions. A **fact** is a statement that can be verified as true. One can simply check a reliable source to determine its accuracy. An **opinion** is a statement that may or may not be true. A writer may claim that it is true, but others may disagree. And it is important to note that it is not always easy to draw the line between the two. One writer may present something as a fact without acknowledging important reasons for questioning the idea.

Second, look for the assumptions that a writer brings to an argument. Everyone makes statements that seem so obvious to them that they see no need to provide evidence to support the ideas. For example, someone might say, "The sun rises in the East." This is such a universal occurrence that there is no need to argue for it. It is important to examine assumptions to determine whether they are justified. If someone claims, "Teenage drivers are too immature to be trusted with a license to drive with other teenagers in the car," he or she is probably assuming that most teenagers are immature, and that the presence of other young people in the car will make the problem of distraction even worse. There may be room for debate about these assumptions, and a careful reader will look for evidence to support the ideas.

Third, watch for common logical fallacies.

- Ad hominem arguments—attacking the person who makes a statement rather than the statement itself.

  Example: "You can't listen to his argument for strict enforcement of drug laws. That hypocrite thinks nothing of disregarding our traffic laws!"

- Straw man arguments—distorting the opposing position to make it easier to attack.

  > Example: A government official might announce that the city will have to look for ways to reduce funding for parks and recreation. An opponent might then argue that it is wrong to allow the park system to fall into disrepair and neglect—not at all what the first official said.

- *Post hoc ergo propter hoc* arguments—assuming that one event is the cause for a second event simply because one happened before the other. The Latin term means "after this, therefore because of this."

  > Example: "Cancer rates have increased since the Industrial Revolution, so cancer is caused by modern industry."

- Circular reasoning—making an argument by restating your premise in different words, rather than actually providing evidence for it.

  > Example: "You should major in biology when you go to the university, because biology is the best major for you."

- Hasty generalization—assuming that something is universally true based on an inadequate sample.

  > Example: "I was overcharged for a poorly done auto repair by our local Auto Pro shop. I'll never take my car to another Auto Pro shop anywhere in the country."

The questions in this section ask you to read a brief passage and answer questions that test your awareness of a writer's purpose and of characteristics that are important to good writing.

DIRECTIONS: The following questions test your ability to analyze writing. Some questions refer to passages, whereas other questions are self-contained. For each question, choose the best answer.

Questions 1–6 are based on the following passage:

(1) My basement is designed to be a family room, although we do not usually use it that way. (2) My desk is down here where it is cool, quiet, and away from the noise of the street outside the house. (3) My living room has three large windows which look out on my neighbors' driveway; thus, I can keep up with their comings and goings all hours of the day. (4) In my basement, I have my computer, all the files I need to do my writing, and a radio which I keep tuned to a good FM station. (5) I can get more work done if I have some "white noise" to block out the interference of other noises in the house. (6) When I withdraw to the basement to read papers or write, my family knows that they are not to disturb me except in case of an extreme emergency like the house catching on fire or something like that. (7) I also have my library stored down here so that I can reach for a book that I might need to refer to when I read or write. (8) There is also a bed; sometimes I get tired of typing and want to stretch out for a few minutes to rest my weary back and fingers.

1. What should be done with sentence 3?

   (A) It should begin the passage.
   (B) It should be omitted.
   (C) It should come after sentence 5.
   (D) It should come after sentence 8.
   (E) It should be combined with sentence 4.

2. Which of the following should be done with sentence 5?

   (A) It should be omitted.
   (B) It should be reduced to a clause, beginning *if,* and joined to sentence 7.
   (C) It should begin with *and* and be joined to sentence 8.
   (D) It should come at the beginning of the passage.
   (E) It should begin with *because* and be joined to sentence 4.

3. A logical concluding sentence for this passage would be which of the following?

   (A) My library is the most important thing in my life.
   (B) I spend many happy hours in my living room, watching my neighbors.
   (C) My basement is the center of my professional life; without it, I would be forced to write less than I do.
   (D) My basement is furnished with early American antiques.
   (E) My FM radio provides me with many hours of amusement.

4. The paragraph is an example of

   (A) descriptive writing
   (B) argumentative writing
   (C) comparison/contrast writing
   (D) writing that is too detailed to be interesting
   (E) fiction writing

5. The tone of the paragraph is

   (A) very formal
   (B) impressionistic
   (C) stentorian
   (D) relaxed and informal
   (E) satiric

6. From the paragraph, a reader might infer that the writer's profession is

   (A) nursing
   (B) teaching
   (C) radio announcing
   (D) preaching
   (E) automobile repairman

Answer Explanations

1. **(B)** This sentence shifts from the basement to the living room, and the whole paragraph is about the basement; thus, sentence 3 is irrelevant to the paragraph.

2. **(E)** (A) is incorrect, because sentence 5 adds important information. (B) and (C) would create illogical sentences. (D) is incorrect, because sentence 5 would not be a good topic sentence for the whole paragraph.

3. **(C)** All of the other choices focus on minor points in the paragraph; only (C) summarizes the paragraph effectively.

4. **(A)** The large number of descriptive details about the room lead to no other possible conclusion.

5. **(D)** The tone of a piece of writing is the author's attitude toward the material; the attitude here seems conversational.

6. **(B)** The number of specific references to writing and reading papers and consulting books makes this the most logical conclusion.

WRITING THE ESSAYS

Part 2 of the College Composition Exam requires you to write two essays on assigned topics, selecting a position and presenting arguments to demonstrate your point.

DIRECTIONS: You will have 30 minutes to plan and write the first essay, which is based on your own reading, experience, and observations.

You will have 40 minutes to complete the second essay, which asks you to read and synthesize two sources that are provided, using them as part of the argument of your essay.

Although the time restrictions are tight, you can improve your ability to write good essays by following certain simple strategies of organizing your thoughts and developing them into a brief example of your writing ability. It is important to express your thoughts on the topic clearly and exactly, and to make them interesting to the reader. Be specific, using supporting examples whenever appropriate. Remember that how well you write is more important than how much you write.

How can you organize your thoughts, support them with facts and examples, and demonstrate your writing skills in such a short time? The following suggestions may be helpful to you.

1. The assigned topics will often ask you to agree or disagree with a statement, often a controversial one. For example, you may be assigned a statement like this:

   Everything the government does for its citizens can be done better by private businesses. Agree or disagree.

   With time so limited, you *must* decide almost immediately whether you will support the statement or argue against it.

2. Since you have only a few minutes to think of reasons why you agree or disagree with the topic statement, you must go quickly to the core of the problem. Take a few minutes to think of several arguments to support your position. Pick three good points that will be easy to expand with good examples. Do not waste time nit-picking your brain. Quickly jot down three good reasons on the margin of your exam booklet, and then write a thesis sentence. An example of such a sentence might be: "I believe that many of the most important goals in a democracy can best be achieved by the government, not by private business; these goals include ensuring the purity of food and pharmaceutical drugs, controlling environmental pollution, and protecting the individual rights of all Americans."

3. Write your first paragraph. This should begin with a sentence or two that will catch the reader's attention and introduce your topic. Then present your thesis sentence.

4. In the second paragraph, present one of your supporting arguments. For the topic used in this sample, this might be the need to have the government monitor the purity of food and drugs. Make the point that private business, if left unregulated, might find it more profitable to cut corners and take chances with the public health. Add examples of the dangers such a policy might unleash.

5. Use your third and fourth paragraphs to present your other supporting arguments. You could discuss environmental pollution in the third paragraph and individual rights in the fourth, again pointing out the dangers of a world without environmental regulation and laws to protect the rights of all citizens. It is useful to answer the most powerful argument that can be made against your position. You can devote one of the supporting paragraphs to this task, or you can deal with it at the beginning of your closing paragraph.

6. In the fifth paragraph, sum up your argument briefly. Remember, it does not matter what your opinion is or whether the grader agrees with you. You will be judged only on the quality of your organizational and writing skills. Keep your organization simple and direct. Avoid repetition and wasted effort as much as possible, and stay precisely on the subject as outlined in your thesis sentence.

Sample First Essay

The following section contains three essays written on an assigned topic, providing models of well-written and poorly written essays.

> **DIRECTIONS:** Write an essay in which you discuss the extent to which you agree or disagree with the statement below. Support your discussion with specific reasons and examples from your reading, experience, or observations.

SAMPLE TOPIC

The government is too large and ineffective, and many of its functions would be better carried out by the private sector.

SAMPLE ESSAY 1

Anyone who listens to radio talk shows and reads letters to the editor these days knows that many people are angry with the "government." They seem to believe that private business can do anything the government does in a more efficient manner. I disagree. I believe that many of the most important goals in a democracy can best be achieved by the government, not by private business; these goals include insuring the purity of food and pharmaceutical drugs, controlling environmental pollution, and protecting the individual rights of all Americans.

Recent news stories about deaths from such bacteria as E. coli and salmonella show the importance of sanitary standards in the food business and the need for regulation by laws and inspections. Can we depend on a private business to regulate itself, without any monitoring? Most restaurants and delis try to prepare and serve products that will not harm their customers' health, but some might try to cut costs by taking chances that could prove fatal. Just as important is the federal government's examination of new prescription drugs to determine if they will be safe. Could we always trust the pharmaceutical companies, who are racing to be the first to market a new superdrug, to make such decisions? I prefer to trust the government.

Environmental pollution is a worldwide problem that must be solved if civilization as we know it is to survive for the next millennium. The purity of the air we breathe and the water we drink has a powerful adversary: industrial waste. Properly treating and disposing of such waste is expensive, and some businesses would prefer to ignore the problem. Only the government has the clout to force compliance with clean air and clean water standards. Only the government is willing to spend money on city transportation systems to reduce the number of cars and commuters that spoil the city air.

One of the most important parts of the Constitution of the United States is the Bill of Rights. Our democracy rests on the concept that every citizen has the basic right to "life, liberty, and the pursuit of happiness." Without the government, how long would it have taken for society to extend the right to vote to all its people? How long would it have taken for private business, without the laws enforced by the government, to give women equal rights in the workplace, including protection from sexual harassment?

There are some who argue that the government is too big, too wasteful of our taxes, and sometimes even repressive. Certainly there are worst-case scenarios that seem to offer evidence of these excesses. But in the matters of protecting the public health, the environment, and the basic human rights, I would prefer that the government take the major role. I think that to do otherwise would "put the foxes in charge of the henhouse," to use a wise rural axiom.

Probable score: 5 or 6. *Essays in this high range show a high degree of competence and control, are well organized and clearly focused, and contain varied and appropriate detail. They also, of course, demonstrate the effective use of language and a mastery of grammar and mechanics.*

I am angry, and many people that I know are angry. Why are we so irate? It is because the government is taking so much of our money in taxes and wasting it on big-spending programs that could be handled more efficiently by private enterprise, which is the anchor of our democratic system of government. Anyone who reads the papers and is aware of what is going on knows that nowadays private companies are building and running prisons, setting up school systems, and delivering mail and packages far cheaper than the government can do these jobs. Besides that, these companies make a profit.

Every time I see a commercial on TV that has somebody running for office, I hear them say they are tough on crime. They should be. Crime is one of our country's greatest problems. To solve it we need to put more people in prison and lock the door on them for a long time. Do we want to trust the government to build prisons and staff them with guards? I don't think so. Let's put the job on the company with the lowest bid and save a big chunk of tax money.

What is the biggest cost in any county or city? It is education. The biggest share of taxes paid to local governments goes to building schools and paying schoolteachers. Let's turn the job over to private business. They know how to downsize and save money. They can begin with a whole new staff of teachers who are not in a union and who would love to have teaching jobs with summers off.

Have you tried to send a package or an overnight letter lately? If you used the post office you were in trouble. If you sent it by any of the companies that do the job efficiently and well, you were pleased with the result. Look at the way our postage is going up. Now it costs 49 cents to send a letter. How much will it be in the future? Who knows? If it were left to good old healthy competition and private enterprise, American business would find a way to keep the cost low.

Now you know why I am angry, along with many other people. When are we going to wake up and vote to cut down on the size of our government? When are income taxes going to be cut? This will only happen when we turn over more governmental jobs to private enterprise.

Probable score: 3–4. *Essays in the middle range show adequate competence, are organized, and are without serious grammatical errors. The topic is treated somewhat superficially, however, and the use of the language does not demonstrate a very high degree of skill.*

SAMPLE ESSAY 3

Everybody is talking about goverment. What is goverment? Do we have to have it? What would we do if we don't have it? I heard something once that say that goverment is by the people and for the people, something like that. Does that mean we get bossed by the people? What do the goverment do for the people?

I guess I am a person that don't like goverment. Don't like nobody telling me what to do. When to do it. What I can't do and can do.

Maybe we need the goverment for some things. A few things. Like the arm forces. If this country was like attacked by some other country or something, the arm forces could run them off. If we didn't have no goverment, we wouldn't have no arm forces.

Maybe we ought to let some smart people try to figure out how to do without goverment. I could live with that.

Probable score: 1. *The College Board Official Study Guide describes essays in the low range (1–2) as demonstrating "clear deficiencies." "They often fail to focus on the topic; they are thinly developed; diction is immature and awkward; and errors abound in grammar, mechanics, and syntax. The paper earning a score of 1 either fails to develop the topic or contains such an accumulation of errors that meaning is seriously obscured."*

Exercises in Preplanning

The following exercises will help you become more efficient at quickly constructing a thesis sentence and planning your essay. Limiting yourself to no more than 5 minutes each, read the following essay topics and write three topic thesis sentences similar to the one used in Sample Essay 1.

a. It's better to grow up in a small town than in a city. Agree or disagree.
b. Sports are overemphasized in high school budgets. Agree or disagree.
c. There is a very old proverb that reads: "He who hesitates is lost." Agree or disagree with this idea.
d. Articles in recent psychological journals theorize that the characters and personalities of teenagers are influenced more by peer groups and other forces outside the home than by parents. Agree or disagree.
e. Should women in the military be allowed to serve in combat?

Here is one more sample essay. How would you grade it?

SAMPLE TOPIC

"The disadvantages of playing team sports in high school outweigh the advantages."
If you prefer, write on the advantages outweighing the disadvantages.

SAMPLE ESSAY 4

Many people believe that playing sports in high school will make you popular with the opposite sex, make you locally famous when you perform well and win the game for your team, and make you rich when you turn professional and sign a multimillion dollar contract. There is a possibility that all three of these results will come true, but the better chance is that team sports will take important time away from your education, lure you into an impossible dream of professional success, and even leave you with injuries that will affect your activities throughout life.

There are only 24 hours in a day, and if you spend three of these hours every weekday practicing a team sport, you have less time for the real purpose of high school: education. Much of the practice in team sports consists of running through repetitious drills. Physical tasks are repeated again and again until they become second nature. After practice and after games, most players are physically exhausted, unable to spend much quality time on their studies. Some ambitious people, who hope to one day enter a profession like law, may have to choose between high school sports or their lifelong dream.

Some players are so convinced they will become wealthy through professional sports that they focus only on athletics. They will later be unqualified to study for any high-level job because they are only proficient in one area: sports. The problem is that only a very few players go on to play in the pros. Putting all your eggs in the one basket called professional sports can lead to a life of frustration and disappointment.

I believe that a high school player has a greater chance of sustaining a nagging injury than of signing a professional contract. The knees are particularly vulnerable in contact sports like football. Also, young athletes beef up their torsos with exercise and even steroids in an effort to succeed in high school team sports. Many of these people become overweight after their athletic days are over and are vulnerable to all the health problems of carrying around too much fat.

I know that team sports can develop a sense of unselfish regard for the team instead of focusing on individual achievements. I know that one can learn discipline in this kind of athletic endeavor. But I also know that one can learn self-discipline by working hard on academic courses, which can open doors to college, graduate study, and to meaningful, life-fulfilling jobs. In my mind, the disadvantages of playing team sports in high school far outweigh the advantages.

Sample Second Essay

The second essay in the College Composition Exam asks you to write an essay with slightly different requirements. Rather than drawing exclusively from your personal experience, you will demonstrate your ability to understand and use source material. Two excerpts from source material on the topic will be provided for you, and you will be asked to use both excerpts in your essay.

The following material will allow you to preview the instructions for a sample essay of this type.

DIRECTIONS: The following assignment requires you to write a coherent essay in which you synthesize the two sources provided. Synthesis refers to combining the sources and your position to form a cohesive, supported argument. You must develop a position and incorporate both sources. **You must cite the sources whether you are paraphrasing or quoting.** Refer to each source by the author's name, the title, and any other information that adequately identifies it.

INTRODUCTION

The United States of America is a nation of immigrants, but the flow of immigration has varied widely over the course of its history. Recent decades have seen a large increase in both legal and illegal arrivals, resulting in steady growth in the percentage of the population who are not native-born Americans. This demographic has led to controversy over a web of issues: economic impact, the job market, welfare, and education. There is a wide divergence in opinion about the benefits or disadvantages of such a large influx of immigrants.

ASSIGNMENT

Read the following sources carefully. Then write an essay in which you develop a position on the question of whether immigration should be encouraged or discouraged. Should America adopt an open-door policy, or should immigration be more tightly restricted? Be sure to incorporate and cite both of the accompanying sources as you develop your position.

Giuliani, Rudolph W. Lecture. Kennedy School of Government, Cambridge, MA. 10 Oct. 1996. Cited in *Immigration and Illegal Aliens: Burden or Blessing*. Farmington Hills, MI: Gale, 2004, p. 110.

The following passage is excerpted from a speech by Rudy Giuliani, former mayor of New York.

My grandfather, Rodolfo Giuliani, arrived in New York City without much money in his pocket, but with a dream in his heart. And his dream of freedom and success became my dream. His dream of opportunity and achievement was shared by millions of immigrants from every part of the world. Their dreams transformed New York City, Boston, and Los Angeles. Their dreams became the American dream.

Each one of us owes so much to immigrants. That's why anti-immigration movements eventually die out. In the past we have always returned to the recognition that new Americans are good for our country. We realize that any effort to eliminate immigration or unfairly burden immigrants could destroy the very process that is the key to American success.

America became the most successful nation in history because of our constant process of re-evaluation, reform, and revitalization, a process that is driven by immigrants who come here to create better lives for themselves and their children. We are constantly being reinvented, not just by the free flow of ideas but by the free flow of people. This process has really defined the United States. It makes us what we are.

Kennan, George. "Immigration to the United States Should be Reduced." Reprinted from *Around the Cragged Hill: A Personal and Political Philosophy*. New York: Norton, 1993. Cited in Bender, David. *Immigration Policy*. San Diego, CA: Greenhaven Press, 1995, pp. 18–19.

The following passage is excerpted from a book by George Kennan, an American diplomat and foreign policy expert.

Just as water seeks its own level, so relative prosperity, anywhere in the world, tends to suck in poverty from adjacent regions to the lowest levels of employment. But since poverty is sometimes a habit, sometimes even an established way of life, the more prosperous society, by indulging this tendency, absorbs not only poverty into itself but other cultures in the bargain, and is sometimes quite overcome, in the long run, by what it has tried to absorb. . . .

It is obviously easier, in the short run, to draw cheap labor from adjacent pools of poverty, such as North Africa or Central America, than to find it among one's own people. And to the millions of such prospective immigrants from poverty to prosperity, there is, rightly or wrongly, no place that looks more attractive than the United States. . . .

There will be those who will say, "Oh, it is our duty to receive as many as possible of these people and to share our prosperity with them, as we have so long been doing." But suppose there are limits to our capacity to absorb. Suppose the effect of such a policy is to create, in the end, conditions within this country no better than those of the places the mass of the immigrants have left, the same poverty, the same distress. What we shall then have accomplished is not to have appreciably improved conditions in the Third World . . . but to make this country itself a part of the Third World. . . .

The following sample essay demonstrates one way in which this material could be used.

SAMPLE ESSAY 5

The Statue of Liberty stands as a symbol of America, the land of opportunity and freedom, and countless immigrants have come to this country seeking a new start. Coming to America has been a good thing for the immigrant, but has it been a good thing for America?

Rudy Giuliani, former mayor of New York, claims in a lecture at the Kennedy School of Government (cited in <u>Immigration and Illegal Aliens: Burden or Blessing</u>. Gale, 2004.) that immigration is the driving force that has moved America to greatness. One of the pivotal features of American society has been its openness to change and innovation. Thousands left the rigid class structure of European society to come to a new world where there was room for fresh ideas, where ambitious men and women could find a place to pursue their dreams. Immigrants carried the ideals that powered American growth and greatness, and they still bring that priceless energy with them today. Who comes to American shores? Those with the initiative and courage to leave their old life and start a new one. Such people are the ones who can contribute to America's future.

On the other hand, diplomat George Kennan in his book, <u>Around the Cragged Hill: A Persaonl and Political Philosophy</u>, warns that there are limits to our ability to absorb too many new arrivals. Even though we have the best of intentions, we must recognize that there are limits to our ability to help immigrants find a place and adjust to this new life. We might compare it to a family who have such open hearts that they frequently invite the neighbors over to grill a burger. Such hospitality is commendable, but if 70 hungry people showed up every night, the impact on the hosts would be disastrous.

I believe that America should keep its doors open to the world as much as possible, because such an attitude is part of our heritage. It is a good thing, and it is one of our commendable traits. But we must balance that open-hearted attitude with the common sense to recognize our limits. Striking the right balance will never be easy, and it will always be controversial; but it is necessary.

The criteria for scoring the second essay are similar to those for the first essay. In addition to the factors previously mentioned, scorers will examine your essay to see whether you:

- Cite your sources appropriately
- Synthesize both sources effectively, with a convincing link between the sources and the position you are supporting

---

ESSAY WRITING HINTS

1. Read the question very carefully. Notice the limitations of the topic (e.g., "Choose one side of this question") and any other instructions.
2. Allow a brief time (perhaps 5 minutes) to think about what you will say, and to decide how you will organize your ideas.
3. Jot down on the bottom of the instruction sheet important points that you want to include.
4. Bear in mind that there is no requirement as to length. A good essay of reasonable length will be rated higher than a poor one that is twice as long.
5. When you express a generalization, be sure to back it up with examples or other supporting evidence.
6. Allow 3–4 minutes at the end of the test period to read your essay critically. Look for misspellings, grammatical errors, ambiguities, and wordiness.

CONCLUSION

After you have worked through the sample questions in this chapter, you should be prepared for a whole CLEP Examination in College Composition. Two such examinations are given in the next chapter, models of those that you may encounter on an actual CLEP test. Again, we must caution you to ask the college to which your scores will be sent which version of the examination you are required to take—the College Composition Exam or the College Composition Modular Exam. Good luck on this examination!

COLLEGE COMPOSITION

1. Ⓐ Ⓑ Ⓒ Ⓓ Ⓔ
2. Ⓐ Ⓑ Ⓒ Ⓓ Ⓔ
3. Ⓐ Ⓑ Ⓒ Ⓓ Ⓔ
4. Ⓐ Ⓑ Ⓒ Ⓓ Ⓔ
5. Ⓐ Ⓑ Ⓒ Ⓓ Ⓔ
6. Ⓐ Ⓑ Ⓒ Ⓓ Ⓔ
7. Ⓐ Ⓑ Ⓒ Ⓓ Ⓔ
8. Ⓐ Ⓑ Ⓒ Ⓓ Ⓔ
9. Ⓐ Ⓑ Ⓒ Ⓓ Ⓔ
10. Ⓐ Ⓑ Ⓒ Ⓓ Ⓔ
11. Ⓐ Ⓑ Ⓒ Ⓓ Ⓔ
12. Ⓐ Ⓑ Ⓒ Ⓓ Ⓔ
13. Ⓐ Ⓑ Ⓒ Ⓓ Ⓔ
14. Ⓐ Ⓑ Ⓒ Ⓓ Ⓔ
15. Ⓐ Ⓑ Ⓒ Ⓓ Ⓔ
16. Ⓐ Ⓑ Ⓒ Ⓓ Ⓔ
17. Ⓐ Ⓑ Ⓒ Ⓓ Ⓔ
18. Ⓐ Ⓑ Ⓒ Ⓓ Ⓔ
19. Ⓐ Ⓑ Ⓒ Ⓓ Ⓔ
20. Ⓐ Ⓑ Ⓒ Ⓓ Ⓔ
21. Ⓐ Ⓑ Ⓒ Ⓓ Ⓔ
22. Ⓐ Ⓑ Ⓒ Ⓓ Ⓔ
23. Ⓐ Ⓑ Ⓒ Ⓓ Ⓔ

24. Ⓐ Ⓑ Ⓒ Ⓓ Ⓔ
25. Ⓐ Ⓑ Ⓒ Ⓓ Ⓔ
26. Ⓐ Ⓑ Ⓒ Ⓓ Ⓔ
27. Ⓐ Ⓑ Ⓒ Ⓓ Ⓔ
28. Ⓐ Ⓑ Ⓒ Ⓓ Ⓔ
29. Ⓐ Ⓑ Ⓒ Ⓓ Ⓔ
30. Ⓐ Ⓑ Ⓒ Ⓓ Ⓔ
31. Ⓐ Ⓑ Ⓒ Ⓓ Ⓔ
32. Ⓐ Ⓑ Ⓒ Ⓓ Ⓔ
33. Ⓐ Ⓑ Ⓒ Ⓓ Ⓔ
34. Ⓐ Ⓑ Ⓒ Ⓓ Ⓔ
35. Ⓐ Ⓑ Ⓒ Ⓓ Ⓔ
36. Ⓐ Ⓑ Ⓒ Ⓓ Ⓔ
37. Ⓐ Ⓑ Ⓒ Ⓓ Ⓔ
38. Ⓐ Ⓑ Ⓒ Ⓓ Ⓔ
39. Ⓐ Ⓑ Ⓒ Ⓓ Ⓔ
40. Ⓐ Ⓑ Ⓒ Ⓓ Ⓔ
41. Ⓐ Ⓑ Ⓒ Ⓓ Ⓔ
42. Ⓐ Ⓑ Ⓒ Ⓓ Ⓔ
43. Ⓐ Ⓑ Ⓒ Ⓓ Ⓔ
44. Ⓐ Ⓑ Ⓒ Ⓓ Ⓔ
45. Ⓐ Ⓑ Ⓒ Ⓓ Ⓔ
46. Ⓐ Ⓑ Ⓒ Ⓓ Ⓔ

47. Ⓐ Ⓑ Ⓒ Ⓓ Ⓔ
48. Ⓐ Ⓑ Ⓒ Ⓓ Ⓔ
49. Ⓐ Ⓑ Ⓒ Ⓓ Ⓔ
50. Ⓐ Ⓑ Ⓒ Ⓓ Ⓔ
51. Ⓐ Ⓑ Ⓒ Ⓓ Ⓔ
52. Ⓐ Ⓑ Ⓒ Ⓓ Ⓔ
53. Ⓐ Ⓑ Ⓒ Ⓓ Ⓔ
54. Ⓐ Ⓑ Ⓒ Ⓓ Ⓔ
55. Ⓐ Ⓑ Ⓒ Ⓓ Ⓔ
56. Ⓐ Ⓑ Ⓒ Ⓓ Ⓔ
57. Ⓐ Ⓑ Ⓒ Ⓓ Ⓔ
58. Ⓐ Ⓑ Ⓒ Ⓓ Ⓔ
59. Ⓐ Ⓑ Ⓒ Ⓓ Ⓔ
60. Ⓐ Ⓑ Ⓒ Ⓓ Ⓔ
61. Ⓐ Ⓑ Ⓒ Ⓓ Ⓔ
62. Ⓐ Ⓑ Ⓒ Ⓓ Ⓔ
63. Ⓐ Ⓑ Ⓒ Ⓓ Ⓔ
64. Ⓐ Ⓑ Ⓒ Ⓓ Ⓔ
65. Ⓐ Ⓑ Ⓒ Ⓓ Ⓔ
66. Ⓐ Ⓑ Ⓒ Ⓓ Ⓔ
67. Ⓐ Ⓑ Ⓒ Ⓓ Ⓔ
68. Ⓐ Ⓑ Ⓒ Ⓓ Ⓔ
69. Ⓐ Ⓑ Ⓒ Ⓓ Ⓔ

70. Ⓐ Ⓑ Ⓒ Ⓓ Ⓔ
71. Ⓐ Ⓑ Ⓒ Ⓓ Ⓔ
72. Ⓐ Ⓑ Ⓒ Ⓓ Ⓔ
73. Ⓐ Ⓑ Ⓒ Ⓓ Ⓔ
74. Ⓐ Ⓑ Ⓒ Ⓓ Ⓔ
75. Ⓐ Ⓑ Ⓒ Ⓓ Ⓔ
76. Ⓐ Ⓑ Ⓒ Ⓓ Ⓔ
77. Ⓐ Ⓑ Ⓒ Ⓓ Ⓔ
78. Ⓐ Ⓑ Ⓒ Ⓓ Ⓔ
79. Ⓐ Ⓑ Ⓒ Ⓓ Ⓔ
80. Ⓐ Ⓑ Ⓒ Ⓓ Ⓔ
81. Ⓐ Ⓑ Ⓒ Ⓓ Ⓔ
82. Ⓐ Ⓑ Ⓒ Ⓓ Ⓔ
83. Ⓐ Ⓑ Ⓒ Ⓓ Ⓔ
84. Ⓐ Ⓑ Ⓒ Ⓓ Ⓔ
85. Ⓐ Ⓑ Ⓒ Ⓓ Ⓔ
86. Ⓐ Ⓑ Ⓒ Ⓓ Ⓔ
87. Ⓐ Ⓑ Ⓒ Ⓓ Ⓔ
88. Ⓐ Ⓑ Ⓒ Ⓓ Ⓔ
89. Ⓐ Ⓑ Ⓒ Ⓓ Ⓔ
90. Ⓐ Ⓑ Ⓒ Ⓓ Ⓔ

Sample College Composition Examinations

5

This chapter includes two sample examinations, each with an answer key, scoring chart, and answer explanations. Take the first exam, check your answers, determine your raw score, and record it on the Progress Chart provided on page 12. Then, as you gain familiarity with the test, take the other examination and see your scores climb.

SAMPLE COLLEGE COMPOSITION EXAMINATION 1

There are two CLEP Exams in College Composition

- **COLLEGE COMPOSITION EXAM.** The College Composition Exam consists of two parts: the first part involves 50 multiple-choice questions, and the second part involves two essays.
- **COLLEGE COMPOSITION MODULAR EXAM.** The College Composition Modular Exam normally consists of two parts: the first part involves 90 multiple-choice questions, and the second part generally involves one or two essays, determined by the policies of the college granting credit.

PART ONE TIME LIMIT: 50 MINUTES

PART ONE AND PART TWO TIME LIMIT: 90 MINUTES

Sample Exam 1 is divided into two parts. Part One includes 50 questions that represent the types of questions found in the College Composition Exam. Part Two contains an additional 40 questions. The combination of Part One and Part Two represents the number and types of questions found in the College Composition Modular Exam.

If you intend to take the College Composition Exam, you may complete Part One and ignore Part Two.

If you intend to take the College Composition Modular Exam, you should complete both Part One and Part Two.

Part One

This part of Sample Exam 1 consists of 50 questions, and you have 50 minutes to complete it. If you plan to take the College Composition Exam, you should complete only Part One of this test. If you plan to take the College Composition Modular Exam, you should do Part One, then go on to complete Part Two. You may also proceed to Part Two if you simply wish to get extra practice in answering the questions.

> **DIRECTIONS:** Read each sentence carefully, paying attention to the underlined portions. Assume that elements of the sentence that are not underlined are correct and cannot be changed. In choosing answers, follow the requirements of Standard Written English.
>
> If there is an error, select the <u>one underlined part</u> that must be changed to make the sentence correct.
>
> If there is no error, select "No error," answer (E).

1. The Red Cross first aid manual <u>provides the following</u> instructions for an
                                                    A
   emergency treatment of a heart attack victim: <u>loose his or her clothing,</u>
                                                              B
   cover <u>him</u> or her with a blanket, and <u>give no medication</u> until a doctor
         C   D
   arrives. <u>No error.</u>
            E

2. <u>After the professor</u> conferred with me about my paper, <u>pointing out to me</u>
         A   B
   all the errors I made, <u>I could only</u> agree that my work <u>was not affective.</u>
                               C   D
   <u>No error.</u>
     E

3. A good umpire should <u>always be disinterested</u> in the game <u>whose rules</u> he
                           A   B
   is there to interpret for the <u>players; he must</u> maintain complete <u>partiality</u>
                                  C   D
   to avoid being charged with unfair decisions. <u>No error.</u>
                                               E

4. When Willie Mays <u>was a small boy</u>, he wanted very badly <u>to play baseball</u>
                             A   B
    in the major <u>leagues</u>, but <u>proving his competence</u> in sandlot and
                        C   D
    minor leagues was the only route he could take. <u>No error</u>.
                                                                        E

5. <u>Few art critics</u> have been able to <u>except the most recent</u> exhibitions
            A   B
    arranged by the curator of the Metropolitan Museum in New York;

    charges and countercharges of <u>lack of</u> artistic discrimination have filled the
                                              C
    columns <u>of the newspapers and magazines</u>. <u>No error</u>.
                            D   E

DIRECTIONS: The following passages are early drafts of essays.

Read each passage and then answer the questions that follow. Some questions refer to particular sentences or parts of sentences and ask you to improve sentence structure or diction (word choice). Other questions refer to the entire essay or parts of the essay and ask you to consider the essay's organization, development, or effectiveness of language. In selecting your answers, follow the conventions of Standard Written English.

Questions 6–10 are based on the following draft of an essay:

(1) Although the neighbors may complain, turning the empty lot on Maple Road into a soccer field would be a good deal for the entire community.

(2) Looking to the future, more and more children are playing soccer. (3) They need a safe place to play, a place where stray balls will not go flying into neighbors' yards or through neighbors' windows. (4) The Maple Road site is ideal for this, and all the neighbors are all on the other side of the road.

(5) The field at the high school where they are playing now is not a good place because it is needed for high school sports and the children who need the soccer field are in elementary school. (6) Besides, the field at the elementary school is too small.

(7) Turning the Maple Road lot into a soccer field would be an improvement. (8) At present, it is just a piece of wasteland, and people dump their garbage there. (9) If it is turned over to the soccer league, they will keep it cleaned up.

(10) As for the worries about noise and traffic, these can be dealt with easily. (11) The people on Maple Road who are opposing this project are just being obstructionist.

6. Which of the following is the best way to revise the underlined portion of sentence 2 (reproduced below)?

Looking to the future, more and more children are playing soccer.

(A) Looking to the future, more children, we see, are going to be

(B) A look at the future shows us how many children are

(C) If we look to the future, we see that more and more children are likely to be

(D) In the future, more and more children are

(E) If we look ahead, more children have been

7. The main problem with the introductory sentence is that

(A) nobody knows where Maple Road is.

(B) the letter never explains why the soccer field would be good for the entire community.

(C) the term "community" is too vague.

(D) it fails to make clear the writer's position.

(E) the letter was not written by a resident of Maple Road.

8. In context, the best phrase to replace "they" in sentence 9 would be

(A) the neighbors

(B) local residents

(C) the members of the league

(D) the garbage collectors

(E) elementary school students

9. The final paragraph would be improved if it

(A) restated the writer's position.

(B) said specifically how the problems of noise and traffic could be solved.

(C) showed how unpleasant the residents of Maple Road are.

(D) listed the organizations in favor of the soccer field.

(E) gave examples of soccer fields that have benefited their communities.

10. Which is the best version of the underlined portion of sentence 7 (reproduced below)?

Turning the Maple Road lot into a soccer field would be an improvement.

(A) (as it is now)

(B) would improve it

(C) would bring about an improvement

(D) would improve its appearance

(E) would improve its locale

Questions 11–15 are based on the following passage:

(1) The side yard seems full of all kinds of oak trees, red, and white among them. (2) Some people find that oak trees are not evergreen, although there is one variety whose leaves turn brown, but those leaves do not leave the tree until almost spring. (3) If you look at an oak tree, you might think about some poet who has written a poem or who has talked about the wind as it moves through the oak trees in the fall. (4) Did you ever see a group of squirrels jumping around as they move nervously from limb to limb in the trees? (5) The whole side yard seems to come alive with this sudden leaping from place to place all over, for the branches seem almost unable to remain still.

(6) Once winter arrives, the scene has changed. (7) Everything is waiting for spring to come again. (8) The oaks are bare now and the leaves are not there anymore. (9) Therefore, the squirrels are gone. (10) The lively movement of summer is ended, which is because the bare branches stand stiff, barely moving in the wind.

11. Sentence 2

    (A) should be joined to sentence 1 with "and."
    (B) should be the topic sentence of the paragraph.
    (C) should be placed after sentence 5.
    (D) should be omitted.
    (E) should be joined to sentence 1 with "however."

12. Which is the best version of the underlined portion of sentence 3?

    If you look at an oak tree, you might think about some poet who has written a poem or who has talked about the wind as it moves through the oak trees in the fall.

    (A) or who has talked about (no change)
    (B) or has talked on
    (C) or some poet who has published poems about
    (D) describing
    (E) while he describes

13. Which is the best version of sentence 8 (reproduced below)?

    The oaks are bare now and the leaves are not there anymore.

    (A) (as it is now)
    (B) The oaks are bare of leaves now.
    (C) The leaves are not there on the trees anymore.
    (D) The bare oak trees no longer have any leaves.
    (E) The leaves are not there anymore, leaving the oak trees bare.

14. Which is the best version of the underlined portion of sentence 10 (reproduced below)?

    The lively movement of summer is <u>ended, which is because the bare branches</u> stand stiff, barely moving in the wind.

    (A) (as it is now)
    (B) ended, caused by the bare branches that
    (C) stilled, which is caused by the branches that are now bare and
    (D) ended: the bare branches
    (E) ended, while the bare branches

15. What is the best thing to do with the word "Therefore" in sentence 9?

    (A) Leave it as it is (no change).
    (B) Omit it, and begin the sentence with "The."
    (C) Replace it with "As a result."
    (D) Replace it with "However."
    (E) Replace it with "Although."

Questions 16–20 are based on the following passage:

(1) Lacy's wedding reception was very inexpensive. (2) As these things go. (3) We did not have a dinner at the reception. (4) Lacy, her mother, and her aunt did all the cooking ahead of time. (5) Flowers were few and simple—most of them came from our garden. (6) The bridal gown was on sale for half price. (7) The groom and ushers wore rented tuxedos that they had not purchased. (8) There was no champagne for the toast because the church does not permit alcoholic beverages in its parlor. (9) The wedding was beautiful, and the more than one hundred guests seemed to enjoy the festivities. (10) Lacy and Jared are now living in Decatur, where Jared sells insurance for a large company, which is one of the ones that specialize in life and health insurance programs.

16. What is the best way to combine sentences 1 and 2?

    (A) with a comma at the end of sentence 1
    (B) with a colon at the end of sentence 1
    (C) with a semicolon at the end of sentence 1
    (D) with "and" between them
    (E) with "but" between them

17. Which is the best version of the underlined portion of sentence 7 (reproduced below)?

The groom and ushers wore rented tuxedos that they had not purchased.

(A) (as it is now)
(B) wore tuxedos that they rented so they did not have to buy them
(C) rented their tuxedos
(D) did not buy tuxedos so they rented them
(E) rented tuxedos, which did not have to be bought

18. Which would be the best transition word or phrase to begin sentence 9?

(A) Although,
(B) Consequently,
(C) As a result,
(D) Even so,
(E) At the same time,

19. Which is the best version of the underlined portion of sentence 10 (reproduced below)?

Lacy and Jared are now living in Decatur, where Jared sells insurance for a large company, which is one of the ones that specialize in life and health insurance programs.

(A) (as it is now)
(B) company that specializes
(C) company, which is specializing
(D) company that is one of the ones that specialize
(E) company that had specializations

20. What should be done with sentence 10?

(A) It should be moved to the beginning of the passage.
(B) It should begin a second paragraph.
(C) It should be shorter and less detailed.
(D) It should come immediately after sentence 2.
(E) It should be combined with sentence 1.

Questions 21–25 are based on the following passage:

(1) In fact, this play piled up more continuous performances in the same theater than any play in American theatrical history. (2) *The Fantasticks*, a musical, ran at a small off-Broadway theater for about forty years. (3) An actress who made her debut in this simple musical comedy moved on to starring roles on television and in Hollywood. (4) Why this play, which was ignored by sophisticated critics when it opened, established such a record is a mystery to many people. (5) The story line is a kind of fairy tale, this is not very distinctive music, and the lyrics are full of clichés. (6) And the musical continued to attract audiences. (7) People who had gone to see it as children took their own children to it. (8) Couples who had attended in their youth celebrated their silver wedding anniversaries with a return visit. (9) It became a kind of good luck charm—as long as *The Fantasticks* was still running, all was right with the world.

21. What should be done with sentence 2?

    (A) It should be at the beginning of the passage.
    (B) It should be at the end of the passage.
    (C) It should be placed immediately after sentence 4.
    (D) It should be omitted.
    (E) It should be left as it is.

22. What would be the best choice to replace "And" at the beginning of sentence 6?

    (A) Therefore
    (B) But
    (C) Thus
    (D) In this case
    (E) Finally

23. Which is the best version of the underlined portion of sentence 5 (reproduced below)?

    The story line is a kind of fairy tale, this is not very distinctive music, and the lyrics are full of clichés.

    (A) (as it is now)
    (B) this is not distinctive music
    (C) the music is not very distinctive
    (D) the music is distinguishable
    (E) this is terrible music

24. Which would be the best way to join sentences 7 and 8?

   (A) with a colon
   (B) with a comma followed by "but"
   (C) with a semicolon followed by "however,"
   (D) with a comma
   (E) with a semicolon

25. What punctuation mark could replace the dash in sentence 9 without changing the meaning of the sentence?

   (A) a period
   (B) a comma
   (C) a semicolon
   (D) a colon
   (E) a comma followed by "because"

DIRECTIONS: The following questions test your familiarity with basic research, reference, and composition skills. Some questions refer to passages, while other questions are self-contained. For each question, choose the best answer.

Questions 26–28 are based on the following passage:

587 Monk Parakeet
Myiopsitta monachus

Description: 11" (28 cm). Bright green above and pale gray below, with scalloping on throat; dark blue primaries; long and pointed tail.

Voice: Loud, harsh, screeching *eeeh-eeeh.*

Habitat: City parks, suburban yards, and semi-open country.

Nesting: 5 or 6 white eggs in a huge, bulky stick nest, placed in a tree or on top of a power pole, or attached to a building wall. Nest is domed and has entrances to egg chambers on sides and bottom.

Range: Introduced from southern South America, and now established in northeastern United States and Florida.

   This noisy but attractive parrot was first reported in the wild in the late 1960s, presumably having escaped from a shipment at New York's Kennedy Airport. Since that time, it has spread to surrounding regions. Its huge stick nests, used both for breeding and roosting, are conspicuous and may contain from one to as many as six pairs of birds.

> Source: Bull, John and John Farrand, Jr.
> *National Audubon Society Field Guide to*
> *North American Birds: Eastern Region.* Rev. ed.
> New York: Alfred A. Knopf, 1994. pp. 539–540.

26. Which of the following statements is NOT supported by the information above?

    (A) Monk parakeets are a type of parrot.
    (B) Monk parakeets are found in urban, suburban, and rural areas.
    (C) Monk parakeets are now found in large numbers in the northeastern United States.
    (D) Monk parakeets were not found wild in North America before the 1960s.
    (E) Monk parakeets sometimes share a nest with other pairs of the same species.

27. Which information about the source is NOT normally included in a bibliography entry?

    (A) The inclusion of *Jr.* as part of the author's name
    (B) The city of publication
    (C) The page number of the entry
    (D) The notice of a revised edition
    (E) The subtitle that appears after the colon

28. In the citation, what information is provided by *Myiopsitta monachus*?

    (A) The scientific name for the monk parakeet
    (B) The Latin translation of monk parakeet
    (C) The original source of information about the monk parakeet
    (D) The Library of Congress heading for information about the monk parakeet
    (E) The order and family of the monk parakeet

---

29. A book's index is most useful for

    (A) seeing the sources of quotations used in the book.
    (B) finding sources of additional information on a topic.
    (C) viewing the structure of a book's argument.
    (D) explaining specialized terms used in the book.
    (E) finding the references to a specific topic in the book.

30. Which of these is a standard guide for finding articles in journals and magazines?

    (A) *Guide to Reference Books*
    (B) *Encyclopedia Britannica*
    (C) *Reader's Guide to Periodical Literature*
    (D) *The New York Times*
    (E) *The Congressional Record*

Questions 31–34 are based on the following passage:

(1) Rwanda gained its independence from Belgium on July 1, 1962. (2) The Hutus, being the majority, soon won many of the parliament seats during the first elections. (3) Thousands of Tutsis then fled to neighboring countries, fearing persecution. (4) The Hutus soon became the favored party in Rwanda and received special treatment from the new government.

(5) During the years between 1962 and 1990, the exiled Tutsis formed an army called the Rwandan Patriotic Front (RPF). (6) In 1990 the RPF invaded Rwanda, causing three years of civil war to follow. (7) But in August 1993, peace treaties called the Arusha Accords were signed (Fisanick, 2004, p. 9). (8) The Arusha Accords may have temporarily stopped the violence, but they did nothing to heal the growing hatred between the Hutus and Tutsis.

(9) The rising tension soon manifested itself in the Rwandan Genocide of 1994. (10) On April 6, 1994, Rwandan President, Hutu, Juvenal Habyarimana's airplane was shot down over the capital city of Kigali. (11) The next day, thousands of Hutus formed militias, calling themselves the Interhamwe. (12) They then began slaughtering Tutsis with the suspicion that it was the Tutsis who shot down President Habyarimana's plane (Fisanick, 2004, p. 10-11). (13) The RPF once again invaded the country from the north and headed towards the nation's capital. (14) Over a period of 100 days, an estimated one million were slaughtered across the country. (15) Finally, between July and August of 1994 the RPF seized the capital city of Kigali. (16) This caused nearly two million Hutus to flee the country and brought the genocide to an end (Rusesabagina, 2003, p. 169).

References:
Fisanick, C. (2004). *The Rwanda Genocide*. San Diego, CA: Greenhaven.
Rusesabagina, P. and Zoellner, T. (2003). *An ordinary man: An autobiography*. New York: Penguin.

31. The parenthetical reference at the end of sentence 7 appears at the end of the material drawn from that source. In which sentence does the material from that source begin?

(A) Sentence 1
(B) Sentence 3
(C) Sentence 5
(D) Sentence 7
(E) No indication is given.

32. What is the best way to phrase the italicized portion of sentence 10? (10) On April 6, 1994, *Rwandan President, Hutu, Juvenal Habyarimana's airplane* was shot down over the capital city of Kigali.

    (A) Rwandan President, Hutu, Juvenal Habyarimana's airplane [original]

    (B) an airplane carrying Rwandan President, Hutu, Juvenal Habraimana

    (C) Hutu President Juvenal Habyarimana of Rwanda's airplane

    (D) an airplane carrying the Hutu President of Rwanda, Juvenal Habyarimana

    (E) Rwandan President Juvenal Habyarimana's Hutu airplane

33. Which of the following pieces of information, if added to the first paragraph, would most effectively advance the writer's argument?

    (A) The Hutus and Tutsis were neighboring tribes with a long history of rivalry.

    (B) The Belgians controlled one of the largest colonial empires in Africa.

    (C) The new government was structured on the model of the British Parliament.

    (D) Belgium provided substantial financial aid to the new country.

    (E) Neighboring nations such as Kenya and Sudan achieved independence during the same decade.

34. One way in which the format of the references would change if the entries were converted to the MLA format is that

    (A) the city of publication would be listed at the end

    (B) the date of publication would be listed as the end

    (C) the date of publication would be listed just before the city of publication

    (D) the author's first name would be listed before the last name

    (E) the city of publication would be omitted

---

35. Which of these is a primary source for a research paper on the writing style of Charles Dickens?

    (A) Transcript of a panel discussion by three Dickens scholars

    (B) *An Literary Analysis of Dickens* by Reginald Smith

    (C) "Charles Dickens" – article in the *World Book Encyclopedia*

    (D) *A Christmas Carol* by Charles Dickens

    (E) A biography of Dickens

36. What is a paraphrase?

    (A) A summary of a long passage

    (B) A quotation with a couple of words changed

    (C) A quotation with several words or a couple of phrases changed

    (D) A restatement of a direct quotation that uses few of the exact words and phrases of the original

    (E) A commentary on an original passage

37. In a bibliography, the name of the publisher appears

    (A) just after the date of publication
    (B) just after the title
    (C) just after the city of publication
    (D) at the beginning of the second line
    (E) at the end of the entry

DIRECTIONS: The following questions test your ability to analyze writing. Some questions refer to passages, whereas other questions are self-contained. For each question, choose the best answer.

Questions 38–44 are based on the following passage:

(1) *Sesame Street* revolutionized the whole idea of television programming for children. (2) Until this program was produced and aired by the Public Broadcasting System, parents had no real options for children's television viewing except *Captain Kangaroo*, violent and crude cartoons on Saturday morning, and a few locally originated programs. (3) But *Sesame Street* is different. (4) Not only does it provide entertainment for viewers but it also provides educational opportunities for children under about ten. (5) The Sesame Street Generation, as some teachers are calling the group of children now in high school, know their numbers and the letters of the alphabet as well as many other facts about life. (6) Perhaps the most important lessons taught by this program derive from its interracial cast, for this program demonstrates that people of all races can live and play together without racially based friction. (7) Whatever this program has cost has been money well spent.

38. Sentences 2 and 3 might be combined. Which of the following is the correct form of the combination?

    (A) originated programs, *Sesame Street*
    (B) originated programs, however, *Sesame Street*
    (C) originated programs, but *Sesame Street*
    (D) originated programs, and *Sesame Street*
    (E) originated programs with the exception of *Sesame Street*

39. What should be done with sentence 5?

    (A) It should be left as it is.
    (B) It should be omitted.
    (C) It should be placed after sentence 7.
    (D) It should be combined with sentence 2.
    (E) It should be after sentence 1.

40. Which of the following might better replace sentence 7 as a conclusion to the passage?

    (A) *Sesame Street* has revolutionized children's television.
    (B) *Sesame Street* is an excellent television program.
    (C) The *Sesame Street* Generation will take over the world when it grows up.
    (D) The Public Broadcasting System should be congratulated for providing such an excellent television program as *Sesame Street*.
    (E) The money which the Public Broadcasting System has spent on *Sesame Street* may have some questionable returns.

41. Sentence 6 provides

    (A) irrelevant information for the reader.
    (B) a second reason for public acclamation of *Sesame Street*.
    (C) a plea for funds from the public to support the program.
    (D) a justification for racial intolerance.
    (E) praise for the cast's ability to react to children.

42. The topic sentence of the paragraph is

    (A) 1
    (B) 2
    (C) 3
    (D) 4
    (E) 5

43. According to the paragraph, *Sesame Street* is a television program recommended for

    (A) adults only
    (B) for adolescent boys
    (C) for teenage girls
    (D) for mature teens
    (E) for children up to age ten

44. Which of the following is a valid criticism of the phrase "facts about life" in sentence 5?

    (A) It is ungrammatical.
    (B) It violates parallel construction.
    (C) It is vague and ambiguous.
    (D) It gives *Sesame Street* more credit than it deserves.
    (E) It is too formal to fit the tone of the passage.

Questions 45–50 are based on the following passage:

(1) For over a century, Helen Jackson's romantic story of Spanish and Indian life in California has been widely read and is now an American classic. (2) Originally published in 1884, *Ramona* has been issued in various editions, with a total of 135 printings. (3) *The Atlantic Monthly* has termed the story "one of the most artistic creations of American literature," while the late Charles Dudley Warner called it "one of the most charming creations of modern fiction." (4) Born in 1831, Mrs. Jackson was an ardent champion of the Native Americans to the end of her life, in 1885. (5) Three times, *Ramona* has been produced as a motion picture, been played on the stage, adapted for a pageant and may eventually be utilized for a grand opera.

Introduction to a 1935 reprint of *Ramona*

45. The function of sentence 1 is

    (A) to justify reprinting an 1884 novel in 1935.
    (B) to define the phrase *American classic.*
    (C) to identify Helen Jackson.
    (D) to arouse the readers' interest in buying the book.
    (E) to introduce the exotic (Spanish and Native American life in California) subject matter of the book.

46. Sentence 2

    (A) says that the book is one of the greatest novels ever written.
    (B) congratulates the author for writing such a best-seller.
    (C) reveals the plot of the book.
    (D) documents the enormous popularity of the book.
    (E) shows that the author of the introduction has not done much research.

47. The quotations in sentence 3

    (A) are so brief as to be meaningless.
    (B) provide concrete support for the figures in sentence 2.
    (C) shift the introduction from the quantity of sales to the quality of the novel.
    (D) play on the sympathy of the reader when Ms. Jackson's death in 1885 is mentioned.
    (E) shift the central idea of the passage too quickly.

48. The function of sentence 5 is to

    (A) add more figures to those of sentence 2.
    (B) add information that does not mean much to the modern reader.
    (C) say that popularity is a criterion for quality.
    (D) imply that any book that has been made into a movie has to be good.
    (E) provide more evidence of the book's popularity.

49. Sentence 4

   (A) should be eliminated.
   (B) gives a brief overview of Ms. Jackson's life.
   (C) should have been used as the topic sentence of the passage.
   (D) should be combined with sentence 1.
   (E) explains Mrs. Jackson's interest in Indians.

50. The passage concentrates

   (A) on Mrs. Jackson's life.
   (B) on *Ramona's* popularity.
   (C) on critics' opinions of *Ramona.*
   (D) on Spanish and Native American life in California.
   (E) on historical facts that are boring.

Part Two

This part of Sample Exam 1 consists of 40 questions, and you have 40 minutes to complete it. If you plan to take the College Composition Exam, you need to complete only Part One of this test. However, if you plan to take the College Composition Modular Exam, you should go on to complete Part Two. The combination of Parts One and Two is equivalent to the College Composition Modular Examination. You may also complete Part Two if you simply wish to get extra practice in answering the questions.

DIRECTIONS: Read each sentence carefully, paying attention to the underlined portions. Assume that elements of the sentence that are not underlined are correct and cannot be changed. In choosing answers, follow the requirements of Standard Written English.

If there is an error, select the <u>one underlined part</u> that must be changed to make the sentence correct.

If there is no error, select "No error," answer (E).

51. Justification for his allegations <u>came from him and I</u>, as <u>the only two</u>
                                              A   B
     witnesses to <u>the bizarre crime</u> the criminal committed against the
                            C
     defendant <u>as she walked</u> by the packing house last night. <u>No error.</u>
                        D   E

52. <u>In a convoluted style</u>, the novel tells the tragic story <u>of a father's</u>
        A   B

inhumanity to his daughter, a mother's rejection of her son, and

the <u>strong trust</u> that developed <u>between the alienated</u> boy and girl.
       C   D

<u>No error.</u>
  E

53. We could <u>only ask ourselves</u> how any sane man could <u>have choosen such</u>
          A   B

an ugly suit to wear <u>when</u>, rich as he is, he could have had the pick
                  C

<u>of any of</u> the suits in the finest men's stores in the community. <u>No error.</u>
  D   E

54. That an artist <u>like Pablo Picasso</u> priced his paintings at more <u>than</u>
         A   B

$100,000 each and actually sold as many <u>as he released</u> to the markets
                                         C

<u>seem too</u> fantastic to be believed. <u>No error.</u>
  D   E

DIRECTIONS: The following sentences test correctness and effectiveness of expression. In choosing your answers, follow the requirements of Standard Written English; that is, pay attention to grammar, diction (choice of words), sentence construction, and punctuation.

In each of the following sentences, part of the sentence or the entire sentence is underlined. Beneath each sentence you will find five versions of the underlined part. The first option repeats the original; the other four options present different versions.

Choose the option that best expresses the meaning of the original sentence. If you think the original is better than any of the alternatives, choose the first option; otherwise, choose one of the other options. Your choice should produce the most effective sentence—one that is clear and precise, without awkwardness or ambiguity.

55. <u>There were fewer people in the auditorium than</u> we had expected; there were seats for everyone.

(A) There were fewer people in the auditorium than
(B) There were no more people in the auditorium than
(C) In the auditorium, there were a lot more people than
(D) There were more people in the auditorium than
(E) A great deal fewer people showed up in the auditorium as

56. Attending college is a dream <u>which many of today's young people have had</u>.

    (A) which many of today's young people have had
    (B) which many of today's young people has had
    (C) which many of today's young people is having
    (D) which many of today's young people have been having
    (E) which many of today's young people had been having

57. A good plumber can connect one pipe <u>with another so completely that</u> there will be no leak from the joint.

    (A) with another so completely that
    (B) into another with such a high degree of skill as
    (C) with another so that there will be completely
    (D) with another with such little skill that
    (E) with another with such accuracy that

58. My old dog <u>Skippy, who is out there lying in the sun</u>, has served me well for the past twelve years.

    (A) Skippy, who is out there lying in the sun,
    (B) Skippy that foolishly is not lying in the sun
    (C) Skippy, on the alert out there in the sun,
    (D) Skippy, working hard for his daily cookie treats,
    (E) Skippy whom we found out in the bright sun of noon

59. Many <u>others who are not so fortunate</u> will lose all the money they have invested in oil well speculation.

    (A) others who are not so fortunate
    (B) others who have had more fortunes
    (C) others who are not as fortunate
    (D) others whom we find to be among the more unfortunate
    (E) others who have had too many fortunes

60. Frightened by the sound of footsteps, the puppy <u>ran upstairs and hide in the closet</u>.

    (A) ran upstairs and hide in the closet
    (B) ran upstairs, having hidden in the closet
    (C) ran upstairs; they went away
    (D) ran upstairs, which was hiding in the closet
    (E) ran upstairs and hid in the closet

61. The more money Mr. Getty accumulated, <u>the more he wanted</u>.

    (A) the more he wanted
    (B) he increased his desires
    (C) the more he accumulated
    (D) the greater quantity he desired
    (E) the larger in number became his disciples

62. No one doubts Lorraine Hansbury's skill as a <u>dramatist; but there is some critics who believe</u> her plays lack poetic dialogue and skillful exposition.

   (A) dramatist; but there is some critics who believe
   (B) dramatist; they say
   (C) dramatist, although some critics believe
   (D) dramatist, believing
   (E) dramatist, who some critics believe

63. The bus driver is always <u>pleasant to we riders even though</u> he must become impatient with some of us who never have the correct change.

   (A) pleasant to we riders even though
   (B) pleasant to us riders although
   (C) pleasant to us riders so that
   (D) pleasantly to us riders even though
   (E) impatient to those riders who

64. <u>The clever orator's presenting a specious argument caused her audience to become restless and inattentive.</u>

   (A) The clever orator's presenting a specious argument caused her audience to become restless and inattentive.
   (B) When the clever orator presented a specious argument, her audience became restless and inattentive.
   (C) The clever orator's presentation of a specious argument, causing her audience to become restless and inattentive.
   (D) The clever orator presenting a specious argument was when her audience became restless and inattentive.
   (E) The clever orator presented a specious argument because her audience became restless and inattentive.

65. <u>That type of person always</u> strongly resents any attempt by anyone to limit his actions.

   (A) That type of person always
   (B) That type of person who always
   (C) That type person that
   (D) He was that type of person who always
   (E) He is that type of persons

66. Because he was speeding, Jerry <u>was picked up</u> by the police.

   (A) was picked up
   (B) was arrested, and they were picked up
   (C) was arrested; then held
   (D) who was arrested
   (E) was arrested without charge

67. While glancing through today's newspaper, I read that the cost of living has risen another four points.

    (A) While glancing through today's newspaper, I read that the cost of living has risen another four points.
    (B) Glancing through today's newspaper, the cost of living has risen another four points.
    (C) Today's newspaper contained an item that the cost of living has risen another four points.
    (D) The cost of living having risen another four points, I read in today's newspaper.
    (E) I was glancing through today's newspaper when the cost of living rose another four points.

68. Each time Billy Joel sitting down at the piano, he plays at least one of his own songs.

    (A) Billy Joel sitting down
    (B) Billy Joel who sits down
    (C) Billy Joel while sitting down
    (D) Billy Joel, sitting down
    (E) Billy Joel sits down

69. While making a pathetic attempt to explain their behavior to the policeman, the young thief and his accomplices was caught in a web of contradictions.

    (A) thief and his accomplices was caught
    (B) thief and his accomplices who were caught
    (C) thief and his accomplices were caught
    (D) thief along with his accomplices were caught
    (E) thief who had a few accomplices were caught

70. Brianne remains convinced that she is as successful if not more successful than her friend Ariel.

    (A) Brianne remains convinced that she is as successful if not more successful than her friend Ariel.
    (B) Brianne remains convinced that she is as successful as, if not more successful than, her friend Ariel.
    (C) Brianne is convinced that Ariel is much more successful than she is.
    (D) Ariel is really much more successful than Brianne.
    (E) Brianne may be more successful than her friend Ariel.

Questions 71–72 are based on the following passage:

(1) Japan has a variety of climatic zones because of its spread over a wide latitude. (2) It tends to be rainy with high humidity levels, but is generally temperate. (3) Tokyo lies at a latitude of 36° north, and is therefore comparable with Athens or Los Angeles. (4) Regional variations in climate are extensive, ranging from very cool in Hokkaido to subtropical in Kyushu. (5) Climate also varies with altitude and with location on the Pacific or Sea of Japan coast. (6) Northern Japan has warm summers but long, cold winters with heavy snow, while southwestern Japan has long, hot, and humid summers with mild winters. (7) The climate in the summer months (June to September) is typified by hot, wet weather brought by tropical airflows from the Pacific Ocean and Southeast Asia. (8) These airflows bring substantial amounts of rain, and there is a clearly defined rainy season which begins in early June and continues for about one month. (9) This is followed by hot, sticky weather. (10) Every year, Japan is struck by typhoons (usually around five or six per year) between early August and the end of September, and these sometimes result in significant damage. (11) The annual rainfall averages between 100 and 200 cm. (12) In winter, low pressure areas over the Pacific Ocean cause cold air to flow eastwards over Japan, bringing freezing temperatures and heavy snowfalls to the central mountain ranges facing the Sea of Japan, with clear skies on the Pacific coast.

Source: Roberts, David and Elizabeth Roberts.
Live and Work in Japan. Oxford: Vacation Work, 2004.

71. Which of the following statements is supported by the information above?

(A) Japan has a climate very similar to that of Los Angeles.
(B) Hokkaido has long, cold winters.
(C) Typhoons are mostly a problem in the central mountain ranges.
(D) The rainy season runs from July to August.
(E) Tokyo is at the southern end of Japan.

72. What information would be most helpful to an American reader if added to sentence 11?

(A) the minimum and maximum rainfall
(B) the location where rainfall is measured
(C) the minimum rainfall
(D) the maximum rainfall
(E) conversion of rainfall from metric measurements to inches

---

73. What feature of this selection from a Works Cited page should be changed to put it in proper MLA format?

Morris, Edmund. The Rise of Theodore Roosevelt. New York: Random House, 1979.

Edmund Morris. Theodore Rex. NewYork: Random House, 2001.

(A) replace the author's name with three hyphens in the second entry
(B) reverse the order of the entries
(C) add the page numbers of the passages cited
(D) change to single spacing
(E) place the date of publication just after the title

74. Which source is most likely to be biased in favor of limits on malpractice suits?

(A) an interview with a lawyer specializing in malpractice suits
(B) a report from the United States Department of Health
(C) an article on a website for surgeons
(D) the transcript of a debate on the issue of limiting malpractice suits
(E) a book on the history of malpractice

Questions 75–77 are based on the following passage:

(1) Julius Caesar's political career began in the year 69 B.C. when he was elected to the position of *quaestor.* (2) Four years later he was elected to the position of *aedile,* where he was able to become popular by spending money lavishly. (3) During this time he became the *propraetor,* or governor, of Farther Spain, which enabled him to obtain the wealth that he would need later on in life. (4) Around the same time that he became the governor of Farther Spain, he also became a general in the army. (5) In the year 55 B.C. he became co-ruler of Rome with two men named Pompey and Crassus. (6) In the year 45 B.C. he was appointed dictator for life by the Roman Senate. (7) Pompey and Caesar fought for the throne in 48 B.C. (8) Crassus had already died from natural causes. (9) Caesar knew how to manipulate public opinion: in his wars in Gaul and Britain, he only sent back only positive reports to the people in Rome. (10) As dictator he rid the government of much of its corruption. (11) Also, many non-Italians were granted citizenship. (12) He also took the title *Imperator,* because the people did not like the title "king." (13) Later, in the year 44 B.C., a group of conspirators led by a man named Brutus killed him (Fisher 89–91).

Works cited: Fisher, David. *World History for High Schools.* 2nd ed. Asheville, NC: Southern University Press, 1976.

75. What changes in this passage would be necessary to change the documentation from a parenthetical citation to an endnote?

    (A) add a note at the bottom of the page with the author's last name and the page number of the citation

    (B) omit the parenthetical citation and replace it with a raised numeral

    (C) add a note at the bottom of the page with full information on the source

    (D) omit the parenthetical citation and replace it with a numeral in parentheses

    (E) omit the parenthetical citation and replace with "Note 1" in brackets

76. What was the writer's purpose in sentence 11?

    (A) to demonstrate the authority Caesar wielded as a dictator

    (B) to show how Caesar reduced corruption

    (C) to continue listing the most important changes made by Caesar

    (D) to provide an additional example of actions designed to increase Caesar's popularity

    (E) to explain Caesar's rise to power

77. According to this passage, what was the primary advantage gained by Caesar from his early appointments to office?

    (A) wealth

    (B) military rank

    (C) powerful friends

    (D) political experience

    (E) knowledge of the Empire beyond Rome

---

78. What sources should be included in the Works Cited page?

    (A) all the sources actually cited in the paper

    (B) the most important sources cited in the paper

    (C) all the sources consulted in writing the paper

    (D) the sources recommended for further study

    (E) all the sources available on the topic

79. Which of these is an effective way of showing when an indirect quotation begins?

    (A) double-spacing the information cited

    (B) placing the information cited in quotation marks

    (C) underlining the information cited

    (D) mentioning the author's name at the beginning of the information cited

    (E) beginning a new paragraph with the information cited

80. Which of these is NOT the proper format for a quotation of more than four lines?

   (A) put it in quotation marks
   (B) indent the entire quotation
   (C) indent the first line the same amount as the other lines
   (D) place any parenthetical citation at the end of the quotation
   (E) double space before and after the quotation

DIRECTIONS: The following questions test your ability to analyze writing. Some questions refer to passages, whereas other questions are self-contained. For each question, choose the best answer.

Questions 81–86 are based on the following passage:

(1) Some critics have said that the short story is dying as a literary form, that magazines no longer print them or pay as much money for those that do get printed, and that writers would rather not tie themselves down to such a restricted length. (2) But critics have said the same thing recently about poetry, about serious drama, and about novels that concern themselves with subjects other than sexual activities between men and women or two women and two men. (3) The short story has survived for about 250 years as a recognizable literary genre, and there are those who look to the Hebrew books about Esther and Ruth as among the earliest short stories. (4) But as long as *The New Yorker, The Atlantic, Harper's,* and other literary mass-market magazines publish short stories, they will be read. (5) For the past ten years, some of the best short stories could be found in *Playboy* and *Esquire,* and we recommend the printed pages (but not necessarily the *Playboy* centerfold) of these magazines as excellent sources of good short stories.

81. Sentence 1

   (A) is a good example of a periodic sentence.
   (B) violates the principles of good organization by having three negative statements in a row.
   (C) contains three clauses that function as objects of *have said.*
   (D) seems to overload the reader's mind with facts.
   (E) does not attempt to define the short story as a literary genre.

82. Sentences 2 and 4

   (A) begin with *but,* but do not violate any of the rules of sentence structure.
   (B) use *but* as a rather weak word for emphasis.
   (C) use *but* to establish a comparison with what the preceding sentences say.
   (D) are not effective, and the author should have revised them before publication.
   (E) probably seem confusing to an average reader.

83. The single purpose of sentence 3 in the paragraph is

   (A) to demonstrate the author's superior knowledge.
   (B) to prove that the short story is not dead as a literary genre
   (C) to provide the reader with information that he does not need or want.
   (D) to give a very brief history of the short story.
   (E) to make a point that any good critic can recognize.

84. What should be done with sentence 2?

   (A) But should be changed to Needless to say.
   (B) But should be changed to Let us, however, keep the following in mind.
   (C) It should be broken into two separate sentences.
   (D) It should be omitted.
   (E) It should be left as it is.

85. Sentences 4 and 5

   (A) could be logically combined with some rearrangements of the words.
   (B) lavish special praise on magazines of limited circulation.
   (C) single out two magazines for praise; yet, some people have called these magazines obscene.
   (D) seem too dry and dull for the subject.
   (E) recommend several sources of good short stories.

86. Which of the following versions of the underlined portion of sentence 5 (reproduced below) would CHANGE the meaning of the paragraph?

   For the past ten years, some of the best short stories could be found in Playboy *and* Esquire, *and we recommend the printed pages (but not necessarily the* Playboy *centerfold) of these magazines as excellent sources of good short stories.*

   (A) and we recommend the printed pages of these magazines as excellent sources of good short stories.
   (B) and we recommend these magazines as excellent sources of good short stories.
   (C) and we recommend that you read these good short stories.
   (D) and some people actually read them.
   (E) and we recommend the excellent short stories in these magazines.

Questions 87–90 are based on the following passage:

(1) I think states should change the legal driving age from 16 to 18. (2) Some will surely say I take this stand because my own daughter will soon be 16. (3) While this may be true, I believe there are benefits to an older licensing age that we can all see—with kids being the obvious exception.

(4) First of all, the difference in maturity level between a 16-year-old and an 18-year-old is monstrous. (5) In my case, it was the difference between being a sophomore in high school and being out on my own with a job and an apartment. (6) In other cases, it would be like comparing a freshman to a senior, and everyone can remember how much maturing goes on in those few years. (7) Since licensed drivers not only have their own lives but the lives of others in their hands, a few more years of maturity could really pay off.

(8) We all know the old adage "Practice makes perfect." (9) With the legal age raised to 18, young drivers could hold permits for an entire year versus the current six months. (10) This would be an extra six months of driving with a licensed and experienced driver in the car beside them.

(11) Finally, everyone can agree that saving money is a good thing. (12) Our insurance prices are based on many factors: number of accidents in your area, who is on the road in your area, how many cars are on the road in your area, and many others. (13) Raising the legal driving age will reduce the factors that raise our insurance rates.

(14) It is true that my daughter will be of legal driving age soon and I would like to keep her "Daddy's little girl" as long as possible. (15) But we can all, including young people, benefit from a higher legal driving age. (16) In the end, it is the state's responsibility to ensure the safety of our streets, and new licensees with two more years of maturity and double the amount of practice time guarantees just that.

87. What additional information would strengthen the argument in sentences 12 and 13?

(A) Statistics on the number of teenage drivers on the road
(B) Evidence that insurance companies all use the same factors in setting rates
(C) Evidence that driving age is connected to the factors involved in insurance prices.
(D) Statistics on the number of 16- and 17-year-old drivers on the road
(E) Comparative rates in various states

88. What is the purpose of sentences 2 and 14?

   (A) To explain the writer's interest in the issue
   (B) To show the writer's concern for his daughter
   (C) To demonstrate the writer's maturity
   (D) To answer the objection that the writer is biased
   (E) To present the writer's credentials

89. Which of these choices is the clearest statement of the idea in sentence 15?

   (A) But all of us, including young people, can benefit.
   (B) But we, including young people, can benefit.
   (C) Therefore, all of us can benefit, including young people.
   (D) Although all of us, including young people, can benefit.
   (E) But we can all, including young people, benefit. [original]

90. Which is the most accurate word to describe the difference in maturity levels between 16-year-olds and 18-year-olds in sentence 4?

   (A) minimal
   (B) monstrous
   (C) surprising
   (D) instructive
   (E) immense

If there is still time remaining, you may review your answers.

ANSWER KEY
Sample Examination 1

COLLEGE COMPOSITION

1.	**B**	24.	**E**	47.	**C**	70.	**B**
2.	**D**	25.	**D**	48.	**E**	71.	**B**
3.	**D**	26.	**C**	49.	**B**	72.	**E**
4.	**E**	27.	**C**	50.	**B**	73.	**A**
5.	**B**	28.	**A**	51.	**A**	74.	**C**
6.	**C**	29.	**E**	52.	**E**	75.	**B**
7.	**B**	30.	**C**	53.	**B**	76.	**D**
8.	**C**	31.	**E**	54.	**D**	77.	**A**
9.	**B**	32.	**D**	55.	**A**	78.	**A**
10.	**D**	33.	**A**	56.	**A**	79.	**D**
11.	**D**	34.	**B**	57.	**E**	80.	**A**
12.	**D**	35.	**D**	58.	**A**	81.	**C**
13.	**B**	36.	**D**	59.	**C**	82.	**A**
14.	**D**	37.	**C**	60.	**E**	83.	**D**
15.	**B**	38.	**C**	61.	**A**	84.	**E**
16.	**A**	39.	**A**	62.	**C**	85.	**E**
17.	**C**	40.	**D**	63.	**B**	86.	**D**
18.	**D**	41.	**B**	64.	**B**	87.	**C**
19.	**B**	42.	**A**	65.	**A**	88.	**D**
20.	**B**	43.	**E**	66.	**A**	89.	**A**
21.	**A**	44.	**C**	67.	**A**	90.	**E**
22.	**B**	45.	**D**	68.	**E**		
23.	**C**	46.	**D**	69.	**C**		

SCORING CHART

After you have scored your Sample Examination 1, enter the results in the chart below; then transfer your score to the Progress Chart on page 12.

Total Test	Number Right	Number Wrong	Number Omitted
90			

ANSWER EXPLANATIONS

1. **(B)** <u>Loose</u> should be <u>loosen</u>, the correct form of the verb.

2. **(D)** <u>Affective</u> is an incorrect word—use <u>effective</u>.

3. **(D)** <u>Partiality</u>—should be <u>impartiality</u>.

4. **(E)** The sentence is correct.

5. **(B)** <u>Except</u> should be <u>accept</u>.

6. **(C)** This choice avoids both the dangling modifier and an illogical sequence of tenses.

7. **(B)** An introduction should be supported by what follows.

8. **(C)** In the original, the pronoun *they* in sentence 9 has no antecedent. In context, (C) provides the most logical choice.

9. **(B)** Simply saying that a problem can be easily solved is not likely to reassure those who are troubled by the problem. Because the purpose of the letter is to convince people that the writer's position is correct or desirable, the most effective addition to this paragraph would be a solution to the major problem raised by the opposition.

10. **(D)** The problem with the original sentence is vagueness. (D) makes clear the kind of improvement the writer is suggesting.

11. **(D)** The information in this sentence has nothing to do with the rest of the passage, so the sentence should be left out.

12. **(D)** This is the most logical and least wordy choice.

13. **(B)** The problem with the original is wordiness. (B) solves this problem more gracefully than the other choices.

14. **(D)** The second part of the sentence is an illustration of the first, not a reason for it. A colon between the two makes this relationship clear.

15. **(B)** Because sentence 9 is simply another part of the description of the winter scene, no transition word is needed here.

16. **(A)** Sentence 2 is a parenthetical comment that should be added to sentence 1 with no stronger punctuation than a comma.

17. **(C)** This choice avoids the unnecessary wordiness of the other choices.

18. **(D)** This is the only choice that makes clear the logical connection between sentence 9 and the earlier parts of the passage.

19. **(B)** This choice avoids the wordiness that characterizes the others.

20. **(B)** Because this sentence introduces a new topic, it belongs in a new paragraph.

21. **(A)** Sentence 2 is clearly the topic sentence, and also provides the reference for *this play* in sentence 1. The specific reference should always come first.

22. **(B)** The relationship between sentence 5 and sentence 6 is one of contrast, so *but* would be the logical conjunction to join them.

23. **(C)** This puts the parallel thoughts in parallel construction.

24. **(E)** Two independent but comparable sentences can be joined by a semicolon.

25. **(D)** A dash and a colon are both acceptable ways to introduce an explanation.

26. **(C)** The entry says that they are found in the northeastern United States, but it says nothing about the number of birds in that area.

27. **(C)** Page numbers are included in parenthetical citations in the text of a paper, but entries for books in the bibliography do not include page numbers.

28. **(A)** This Latin name is the scientific name for the bird, giving the genus and species.

29. **(E)** An index provides a list of all the pages in a book where specific topics may be found. It does not include references to other works. A table of contents outlines the structure of the overall argument of a book (choice C), while a glossary explains specialized terms (choice D). Sources of quotations (choice A) may be found in the bibliography or works cited page.

30. **(C)** The *Reader's Guide to Periodical Literature* is the best-known standard source for articles in journals and magazines.

31. **(E)** The writer did not provide a definite indication of where the material from this source began. Good writers often use quotation marks or mention the author at the beginning of the material derived from a source, so that the reader knows how much information is covered by a parenthetical reference or footnote.

32. **(D)** Choice D makes it clear that the word Hutu is a description of the Rwandan President. The other choices are either unclear or awkward.

33. **(A)** Readers may not be familiar with the Hutus and Tutsis, so a brief explanation would help to explain the conflict between the two tribes.

34. **(B)** Works Cited entries in the MLA format place the date of publication at the end of the entry, whereas the APA format inserts the date immediately after the name of the author.

35. **(D)** A primary source is written by the author himself, as in the case of *The Christmas Carol*. Books or articles written by others who discuss the author are secondary sources.

36. **(D)** A student who paraphrases a source is presenting the material in his own words, rather than the words of the original author.

37. **(C)** Bibliographies are the lists of sources in the University of Chicago format, and in that format the publisher appears just after the city of publication.

38. **(C)** None of the other choices is grammatically correct.

39. **(A)** Sentence 5 should remain where it is. In sentence 4, the educational benefits of *Sesame Street* are mentioned, making it logical to move to a discussion of schools in sentence 5.

40. **(D)** Since cost was not mentioned elsewhere in the paragraph, it would be better to replace sentence 7 with a concluding sentence that did more to sum up the paragraph.

41. **(B)** The second reason provided in sentence 6 is the advocacy of racial harmony.

42. **(A)** Sentence 1 states the main idea that the rest of the paragraph goes on to discuss and is, therefore, the topic sentence of the paragraph.

43. **(E)** Sentence 4 says that the program "provides educational opportunities for children under about ten."

44. **(C)** The phrase is not only vague but also suggests "facts of life," implying a discussion of sex that is not offered on *Sesame Street.*

45. **(D)** The writer has chosen two impressive facts about the book to arouse the reader's interest and has added a little color, as well, by mentioning that it is a romantic story of Spanish and Indian life.

46. **(D)** Sentence 2 offers further proof that the book has continuously been well-received.

47. **(C)** The writer is covering varied ideas in his or her praise of the book. In sentence 3, the writer uses the quotes to show that the book is not only popular, but that the critics find it to be of substance.

48. **(E)** The writer uses the information in sentence 5 as yet another means of showing the book's popularity.

49. **(B)** Sentence 4 gives a brief overview of Mrs. Jackson's life.

50. **(B)** Throughout the passage, fact after fact is given to show *Ramona's* popularity.

51. **(A)** I should be me—the objective case form.

52. **(E)** The sentence is correct.

53. **(B)** Choosen should be chosen.

54. **(D)** Seem should be seems—the subject is the whole clause, therefore singular.

55. **(A)** Choices (B), (C), (D), and (E) are either wordy or change the meaning of the original.

56. **(A)** The original sentence is correct; the other choices contain errors in verb forms.

57. **(E)** Choice (A) uses the word "completely," a poor word choice to describe the plumbing ability under discussion; (B) is wordy; (C) is illogical; (D) changes the meaning too much.

58. **(A)** Choice (B) contradicts meaning of original sentence; (C) and (D) change the meaning too much; (E) introduces an irrelevant idea.

59. **(C)** Choice (A) <u>so</u> is an incorrect idiom; (B) confuses <u>fortunate</u> and <u>fortune</u>; (D) is wordy; (E) also confuses <u>fortune</u> and <u>fortunate</u>.

60. **(E)** Choice (A) <u>hide</u> should be <u>hid</u>; (B) <u>having hidden</u> is a dangling modifier; (C) and (D) have incorrect clauses.

61. **(A)** The other choices introduce grammatical errors of several kinds.

62. **(C)** Choice (A) has <u>is</u>, an error in subject-verb agreement; (B) <u>they</u> is a vague pronoun; (D) introduces a dangling modifier; (E) <u>who</u> has no verb to complete its meaning.

63. **(B)** Choice (A) <u>we</u> is incorrect case form; (C) is illogical; (D) incorrectly uses the adverb <u>pleasantly</u> instead of the adjective <u>pleasant</u>; (E) changes the meaning of the sentence.

64. **(B)** Choice (A) is illogical; (C) is a sentence fragment; (D) <u>was when</u> is an incorrect idiom; (E) <u>because</u> indicates a false cause-effect relationship.

65. **(A)** Choices (B) and (C) create sentence fragments; (D) creates a tense shift; (E) <u>persons</u> is an incorrect plural.

66. **(A)** Choice (B) presents information redundantly; (C) the semicolon is incorrect; (D) forms a sentence fragment; (E) is illogical.

67. **(A)** Choice (B) the introductory phrase is a dangling modifier; (C) is incomplete, for the sense of the original sentence is incomplete; (D) the introductory phrase is a dangling modifier; (E) implies a false sequence of events.

68. **(E)** The other choices are illogical or grammatically incorrect.

69. **(C)** Choice (A) <u>was</u> is an error in subject-verb agreement; (B) would be a sentence fragment; (D) and (E) <u>were</u> is incorrect subject-verb agreement.

70. **(B)** Choice (A) <u>as successful if</u> is an incorrect idiom; (C), (D) and (E) distort the original meaning.

71. **(B)** Sentence 4 says that Hokkaido has a very cool climate, and sentence 6 states that northern Japan has long, cold winters. It is a reasonable deduction to say that Hokkaido is in northern Japan, so the statement about cold winters would apply.

72. **(E)** Many Americans are not accustomed to the metric system, so they find it more difficult to understand rainfall measured in centimeters.

73. **(A)** When a Works Cited page lists two sources by the same author, the second entry replaces the author's name with a series of hyphens.

74. **(C)** Surgeons are at risk of being sued, so they would be likely to favor limits on such lawsuits. The other choices would be either neutral or opposed to limits on malpractice suits.

75. **(B)** When using a system that employs endnotes for documentation, a writer places a raised number (superscript) at the end of the quotation. This number corresponds to a full description of the source, which appears on a separate page at the end of the paper.

76. **(D)** The writer introduced Caesar's attempts to influence public opinion in sentence 9, and gave an example in sentence 10 of one measure he took to gain popularity. Sentence 11 continues with an additional example.

77. **(A)** Sentences 2 and 3 both specify wealth as the most notable benefit derived from his early offices. As aedile, he was able to spend lavishly; as propraetor of Farther Spain, he accumulated ample funds to spend to further his career.

78. **(A)** The Works Cited page should list all the sources actually cited in the paper. In formats where a bibliography is used, a student could add an expanded list of useful reference sources beyond those actually cited in the paper.

79. **(D)** Quotation marks are not appropriate for an indirect quotation, so the most effective way to show the beginning of the material is to introduce it by mentioning the author. Example: Senator Johnson explained in his autobiography that . . . .

80. **(A)** Long quotations should be double spaced, and the entire quotation should be indented. They should not, however, be placed in quotation marks.

81. **(C)** Critics "have said" the short story is dying; critics "have said" magazines do not print them anymore; critics "have said" writers do not want to work with a restricted length.

82. **(A)** It is perfectly correct to begin a sentence with *but* as is done here in Sentences 2 and 4.

83. **(D)** Actually, the entire passage is an attempt to prove that the short story is not dead as a literary genre. Sentence 3 helps do this by giving a factual, historical detail to support the thesis.

84. **(E)** The sentence should be left as it is.

85. **(E)** One way the author tries to prove the point that the short story is not dead is to use the fact that several renowned magazines currently publish them. By naming these magazines, the author inadvertently recommends several sources of good short stories.

86. **(D)** The surprise in the passage is that good short stories can be found in these magazines, not that people read them.

87. **(C)** The writer lists several factors that affect the cost of insurance, but does not show that any of them are linked with the driving age.

88. **(D)** Both sentences refer to the fact that teenagers might consider the writer to be biased because he is a parent, not a teen.

89. **(A)** This choice places the phrase "including young people" where it is most clearly connected to the phrase it modifies: "all of us." Choice B is grammatically correct, but changes the emphasis of the original statement.

90. **(E)** The writer is arguing that the difference in maturity between 16- and 18-year-olds is very large. *Immense* expresses this concept precisely, while *monstrous* adds an extraneous idea of something grotesque or unnatural. The other choices change the meaning of the sentence.

ANSWER SHEET
Sample Examination 2

COLLEGE COMPOSITION

1. Ⓐ Ⓑ Ⓒ Ⓓ Ⓔ
2. Ⓐ Ⓑ Ⓒ Ⓓ Ⓔ
3. Ⓐ Ⓑ Ⓒ Ⓓ Ⓔ
4. Ⓐ Ⓑ Ⓒ Ⓓ Ⓔ
5. Ⓐ Ⓑ Ⓒ Ⓓ Ⓔ
6. Ⓐ Ⓑ Ⓒ Ⓓ Ⓔ
7. Ⓐ Ⓑ Ⓒ Ⓓ Ⓔ
8. Ⓐ Ⓑ Ⓒ Ⓓ Ⓔ
9. Ⓐ Ⓑ Ⓒ Ⓓ Ⓔ
10. Ⓐ Ⓑ Ⓒ Ⓓ Ⓔ
11. Ⓐ Ⓑ Ⓒ Ⓓ Ⓔ
12. Ⓐ Ⓑ Ⓒ Ⓓ Ⓔ
13. Ⓐ Ⓑ Ⓒ Ⓓ Ⓔ
14. Ⓐ Ⓑ Ⓒ Ⓓ Ⓔ
15. Ⓐ Ⓑ Ⓒ Ⓓ Ⓔ
16. Ⓐ Ⓑ Ⓒ Ⓓ Ⓔ
17. Ⓐ Ⓑ Ⓒ Ⓓ Ⓔ
18. Ⓐ Ⓑ Ⓒ Ⓓ Ⓔ
19. Ⓐ Ⓑ Ⓒ Ⓓ Ⓔ
20. Ⓐ Ⓑ Ⓒ Ⓓ Ⓔ
21. Ⓐ Ⓑ Ⓒ Ⓓ Ⓔ
22. Ⓐ Ⓑ Ⓒ Ⓓ Ⓔ
23. Ⓐ Ⓑ Ⓒ Ⓓ Ⓔ

24. Ⓐ Ⓑ Ⓒ Ⓓ Ⓔ
25. Ⓐ Ⓑ Ⓒ Ⓓ Ⓔ
26. Ⓐ Ⓑ Ⓒ Ⓓ Ⓔ
27. Ⓐ Ⓑ Ⓒ Ⓓ Ⓔ
28. Ⓐ Ⓑ Ⓒ Ⓓ Ⓔ
29. Ⓐ Ⓑ Ⓒ Ⓓ Ⓔ
30. Ⓐ Ⓑ Ⓒ Ⓓ Ⓔ
31. Ⓐ Ⓑ Ⓒ Ⓓ Ⓔ
32. Ⓐ Ⓑ Ⓒ Ⓓ Ⓔ
33. Ⓐ Ⓑ Ⓒ Ⓓ Ⓔ
34. Ⓐ Ⓑ Ⓒ Ⓓ Ⓔ
35. Ⓐ Ⓑ Ⓒ Ⓓ Ⓔ
36. Ⓐ Ⓑ Ⓒ Ⓓ Ⓔ
37. Ⓐ Ⓑ Ⓒ Ⓓ Ⓔ
38. Ⓐ Ⓑ Ⓒ Ⓓ Ⓔ
39. Ⓐ Ⓑ Ⓒ Ⓓ Ⓔ
40. Ⓐ Ⓑ Ⓒ Ⓓ Ⓔ
41. Ⓐ Ⓑ Ⓒ Ⓓ Ⓔ
42. Ⓐ Ⓑ Ⓒ Ⓓ Ⓔ
43. Ⓐ Ⓑ Ⓒ Ⓓ Ⓔ
44. Ⓐ Ⓑ Ⓒ Ⓓ Ⓔ
45. Ⓐ Ⓑ Ⓒ Ⓓ Ⓔ
46. Ⓐ Ⓑ Ⓒ Ⓓ Ⓔ

47. Ⓐ Ⓑ Ⓒ Ⓓ Ⓔ
48. Ⓐ Ⓑ Ⓒ Ⓓ Ⓔ
49. Ⓐ Ⓑ Ⓒ Ⓓ Ⓔ
50. Ⓐ Ⓑ Ⓒ Ⓓ Ⓔ
51. Ⓐ Ⓑ Ⓒ Ⓓ Ⓔ
52. Ⓐ Ⓑ Ⓒ Ⓓ Ⓔ
53. Ⓐ Ⓑ Ⓒ Ⓓ Ⓔ
54. Ⓐ Ⓑ Ⓒ Ⓓ Ⓔ
55. Ⓐ Ⓑ Ⓒ Ⓓ Ⓔ
56. Ⓐ Ⓑ Ⓒ Ⓓ Ⓔ
57. Ⓐ Ⓑ Ⓒ Ⓓ Ⓔ
58. Ⓐ Ⓑ Ⓒ Ⓓ Ⓔ
59. Ⓐ Ⓑ Ⓒ Ⓓ Ⓔ
60. Ⓐ Ⓑ Ⓒ Ⓓ Ⓔ
61. Ⓐ Ⓑ Ⓒ Ⓓ Ⓔ
62. Ⓐ Ⓑ Ⓒ Ⓓ Ⓔ
63. Ⓐ Ⓑ Ⓒ Ⓓ Ⓔ
64. Ⓐ Ⓑ Ⓒ Ⓓ Ⓔ
65. Ⓐ Ⓑ Ⓒ Ⓓ Ⓔ
66. Ⓐ Ⓑ Ⓒ Ⓓ Ⓔ
67. Ⓐ Ⓑ Ⓒ Ⓓ Ⓔ
68. Ⓐ Ⓑ Ⓒ Ⓓ Ⓔ
69. Ⓐ Ⓑ Ⓒ Ⓓ Ⓔ

70. Ⓐ Ⓑ Ⓒ Ⓓ Ⓔ
71. Ⓐ Ⓑ Ⓒ Ⓓ Ⓔ
72. Ⓐ Ⓑ Ⓒ Ⓓ Ⓔ
73. Ⓐ Ⓑ Ⓒ Ⓓ Ⓔ
74. Ⓐ Ⓑ Ⓒ Ⓓ Ⓔ
75. Ⓐ Ⓑ Ⓒ Ⓓ Ⓔ
76. Ⓐ Ⓑ Ⓒ Ⓓ Ⓔ
77. Ⓐ Ⓑ Ⓒ Ⓓ Ⓔ
78. Ⓐ Ⓑ Ⓒ Ⓓ Ⓔ
79. Ⓐ Ⓑ Ⓒ Ⓓ Ⓔ
80. Ⓐ Ⓑ Ⓒ Ⓓ Ⓔ
81. Ⓐ Ⓑ Ⓒ Ⓓ Ⓔ
82. Ⓐ Ⓑ Ⓒ Ⓓ Ⓔ
83. Ⓐ Ⓑ Ⓒ Ⓓ Ⓔ
84. Ⓐ Ⓑ Ⓒ Ⓓ Ⓔ
85. Ⓐ Ⓑ Ⓒ Ⓓ Ⓔ
86. Ⓐ Ⓑ Ⓒ Ⓓ Ⓔ
87. Ⓐ Ⓑ Ⓒ Ⓓ Ⓔ
88. Ⓐ Ⓑ Ⓒ Ⓓ Ⓔ
89. Ⓐ Ⓑ Ⓒ Ⓓ Ⓔ
90. Ⓐ Ⓑ Ⓒ Ⓓ Ⓔ

SAMPLE COLLEGE COMPOSITION EXAM 2

SAMPLE COLLEGE COMPOSITION EXAMINATION 2

There are two CLEP Exams in College Composition

- **COLLEGE COMPOSITION EXAM.** The College Composition Exam consists of two parts: the first part involves 50 multiple-choice questions, and the second part involves two essays.
- **COLLEGE COMPOSITION MODULAR EXAM.** The College Composition Modular Exam normally consists of two parts: the first part involves 90 multiple-choice questions, and the second part generally involves one or two essays, determined by the policies of the college granting credit.

PART ONE TIME LIMIT: 50 MINUTES
PART ONE AND PART TWO TIME LIMIT: 90 MINUTES

Sample Exam 2 is divided into two parts. Part One includes 50 questions that represent the types of questions found in the College Composition Exam. Part Two contains an additional 40 questions. The combination of Part One and Part Two represents the number and types of questions found in the College Composition Modular Exam.

If you intend to take the College Composition Exam, you may complete Part One and ignore Part Two.

If you intend to take the College Composition Modular Exam, you should complete both Part One and Part Two.

Part One

This part of Sample Exam 2 consists of 50 questions, and you have 50 minutes to complete it. If you plan to take the College Composition Exam, you should complete only Part One of this test. If you plan to take the College Composition Modular Exam, you should do Part One, then go on to complete Part Two. You may also proceed to Part Two if you simply wish to get extra practice in answering the questions.

DIRECTIONS: Read each sentence carefully, paying attention to the underlined portions. Assume that elements of the sentence that are not underlined are correct and cannot be changed. In choosing answers, follow the requirements of Standard Written English.

If there is an error, select the <u>one underlined part</u> that must be changed to make the sentence correct.

If there is no error, select "No error," answer (E).

---

1. When <u>they fought</u> in the field, the <u>armies of</u> the two countries
          A   B

    <u>battled bravely</u> until <u>the war is over.</u> <u>No error.</u>
        C   D   E

2. The police officer <u>spoke harshly</u> to <u>he and I</u> about driving <u>too fast</u> on the
                   A   B   C

    residential <u>street and in</u> a school zone. <u>No error.</u>
            D   E

3. The president <u>of the board</u> of directors announced in Philadelphia today
                A

    that the company would <u>neither accede</u> to the monetary <u>demands of the</u>
                          B   C

    strikers nor accept any further delays by union leaders <u>in accepting</u> a
                                                  D

    settlement of the dispute. <u>No error.</u>
                      E

4. <u>Listening with rapt</u> attention while the orchestra was performing
        A

    <u>Beethoven's Fifth Symphony,</u> the concert hall was filled with <u>fashionably</u>
               B   C

    dressed music lovers who <u>followed the conductor's</u> every beat. <u>No error.</u>
                            D   E

5. The Pulitzer Prize Committee awarded $\underline{\$25,000}$ to Scott Adams
                                        A
   $\underline{\text{being as how}}$ the group voted his $\underline{\text{drawings in a national}}$ newspaper the
                    B   C
   best cartoons published in $\underline{\text{America that year}}$. $\underline{\text{No error}}$.
                                          D   E

DIRECTIONS: The following passages are early drafts of essays.

Read each passage and then answer the questions that follow. Some questions refer to particular sentences or parts of sentences and ask you to improve sentence structure or diction (word choice). Other questions refer to the entire essay or parts of the essay and ask you to consider the essay's organization, development, or effectiveness of language. In selecting your answers, follow the conventions of Standard Written English.

Questions 6–11 are based on the following passage:

(1) For years now, presidents and others have been saying that we must win the war against drugs. (2) Drugs are destroying whole neighborhoods. (3) They are killing our young people. (4) Drugs also cause crime, and people can get rich easily selling drugs, and because there are enormous amounts of money involved they get into fights and that causes all kinds of violence. (5) Drug dealers kill not only each other but sometimes they also kill innocent bystanders, even small children.

(6) Our national leaders have urged us to wage war on this problem to cure the plague that is haunting us. (7) But urging users to say "no" hasn't worked. (8) Building new jails and hiring more police officers hasn't worked. (9) Telling users of the dangers of drugs hasn't worked. (10) What will?

(11) No one can be sure, but there have been plenty of suggestions ranging all the way from the recommendation that all casual users suffer the same legal penalties as pushers do to the legalization of drugs often with the caveat that there should of course be strict controls on the sale of these drugs so that they aren't sold to children and used to try to get additional people addicted.

(12) Everyone agrees that there is an emergency situation, but no one—not the administration, not Congress, not the American taxpayer—seems to be willing to spend the billions of dollars that are necessary to halt the widespread use of drugs.

6. What would be the best thing to do with sentence 1?

   (A) Leave it as it is.
   (B) Move it to the end of the first paragraph.
   (C) Move it to the beginning of the second paragraph.
   (D) Move it to the end of the passage.
   (E) Delete it.

7. Which is the best version of the underlined portion of sentence 4 (reproduced below)?

   Drugs also cause crime, and people can get rich easily selling drugs, and because there are enormous amounts of money involved they get into fights and that causes all kinds of violence.

   (A) (as it is now)
   (B) people sell drugs even though the enormous amounts of money cause
   (C) competition among drug dealers for the enormous sums of money involved leads to
   (D) seeking to get rich by selling drugs, the enormous amounts of money involved cause
   (E) seeking to get rich quick by selling drugs makes people get into fights over money that cause

8. A valid criticism of sentence 6 is that

   (A) it is too informal.
   (B) it contains a mixed metaphor.
   (C) it is irrelevant to the topic.
   (D) it fails to say what should be done.
   (E) the drug problem should not concern national leaders.

9. Which of the following is a valid criticism of sentence 11?

   (A) It doesn't give any solutions.
   (B) It should make clear which side the author is on.
   (C) It tries to put too much information in a single sentence and should be broken up into two or more sentences.
   (D) Logically, it belongs after sentence 12.
   (E) It has a problem with subject-verb agreement.

10. Which of the following words or phrases could be used to replace "caveat" in sentence 11 without changing the meaning of the sentence?

    (A) warning
    (B) intention
    (C) bearing in mind
    (D) possibility
    (E) purpose

11. Which of the following would be the best way to improve the final paragraph?

    (A) Add the author's personal experiences with drugs.
    (B) Delete the references to Congress and the president.
    (C) Explain how drugs affect the central nervous system.
    (D) Explain why it is necessary to spend billions of dollars.
    (E) Add a ringing denunciation of drug pushers.

(1) Junipers are the most versatile plants we sell and are well suited to the New England climate. (2) They need to be planted in a sunny spot. (3) They tolerate relatively poor soil. (4) They tolerate salt air. (5) In addition, they will grow in windy sites. (6) All our plants are sold "B&B." (7) This means they are field-grown plants that are dug, balled, and wrapped in burlap. (8) There are three different types of junipers. (9) Ground cover types are good for steep slopes and around buildings. (10) They don't need a whole lot of maintenance. (11) Many of them will re-root wherever their stems touch the ground. (12) Spreading types work well in mass plantings where large areas need to be covered. (13) For example, you could plant them along a highway. (14) They also look attractive in mixed plantings with other evergreens. (15) They look attractive as foundation plants next to a house. (16) Upright types make attractive hedges or windbreaks when used in group plantings. (17) They are good for backgrounds or you can use them as individual specimens. (18) Ground cover types should be planted two to three feet apart. (19) Upright types should be planted four feet apart when used for hedges.

12. If this passage were to be divided into two paragraphs, which sentence should begin the second paragraph?

(A) sentence 3
(B) sentence 7
(C) sentence 8
(D) sentence 12
(E) sentence 16

13. Which of the following would be the best way to combine sentences 1 and 2?

(A) Junipers, which are the most versatile plants we sell and are well suited to the New England climate, but they need to be planted in a sunny spot.
(B) Junipers are the most versatile plants we sell and are well suited to the New England climate because they need to be planted in a sunny spot.
(C) Junipers are the most versatile plants we sell and are well suited to the New England climate if planted in a sunny spot.
(D) Junipers are the most versatile plants we sell, well suited to the New England climate, and planted in a sunny spot.
(E) Junipers, the most versatile plants we sell, are well suited to the New England climate if they need to be planted in a sunny spot.

SAMPLE COLLEGE COMPOSITION EXAM 2

14. Which of the following is the best way to combine sentences 3, 4, and 5?

    (A) They tolerate relatively poor soil; they tolerate salt air; in addition, they will grow in windy sites.

    (B) They tolerate relatively poor soil, salt air, and windy sites.

    (C) They tolerate relatively poor soil and salt air when grown in windy sites.

    (D) They tolerate relatively poor soil, and they tolerate salt air, and they will grow in windy sites.

    (E) They tolerate relatively poor soil and salt air; in addition, they will grow in windy sites.

15. Which is the best version of the underlined portion of sentence 10 (reproduced below)?

They don't need a whole lot of maintenance.

    (A) (as it is now)

    (B) to be given a whole lot of

    (C) lots of

    (D) much

    (E) many

16. Which is the best version of the underlined portion of sentence 17 (reproduced below)?

They are good for backgrounds or you can use them as individual specimens.

    (A) (as it is now)

    (B) or when used as

    (C) or are good as

    (D) or they are used as

    (E) or as

17. Which of the following pairs of sentences could most logically be combined?

    (A) sentences 7 and 8

    (B) sentences 11 and 12

    (C) sentences 12 and 13

    (D) sentences 15 and 16

    (E) sentences 17 and 18

Questions 18–21 are based on the following passage:

(1) Many students now that they are entering college for the first time are confused by the attitude of the many faculty members who teach them. (2) Many college professors lecture about their many different subjects and assume, sometimes incorrectly, that new students understand the vocabulary that the professor uses, can define the terms from unfamiliar subjects, and that they know how to take notes adequately. (3) These skills are not those that most high school teachers teach or expect. (4) Both the professors and the students are frustrated because they do not understand each other in the classroom. (5) Many students hesitate to ask questions in class or during conferences, and they continue to be confused when they listen to the lectures. (6) One thing colleges could do to fix up this problem is to offer a summer seminar in study skills for inexperienced students. (7) Those who take the class would gain valuable knowledge and develop skills that would be helpful to them throughout their college years. (8) Some colleges hesitate to offer such instruction because they say, "Here is the information you need, provided in the way we best provide it."

18. Which is the best version of the underlined portion of sentence 1 (reproduced below)?

    Many students now that they are entering college for the first time are confused by the attitude of the many faculty members who teach them.

    (A) (as it is now)
    (B) now they are entering
    (C) entering
    (D) that enter
    (E) now that they may be entering

19. Which is the best version of the underlined portion of sentence 2 (reproduced below)?

    Many college professors lecture about their many different subjects and assume, sometimes incorrectly, that new students understand the vocabulary that the professor uses, can define the terms from unfamiliar subjects, and that they know how to take notes adequately.

    (A) (as it is now)
    (B) and that know how
    (C) and that know
    (D) that know
    (E) and know how

20. A valid criticism of the first two sentences is that they

    (A) do not introduce the topic
    (B) are inconsistent in their verb tenses
    (C) repeat the word "many" too often
    (D) use pronouns with no logical antecedents
    (E) use an overly formal vocabulary

21. If this passage were to be divided into two paragraphs, which sentence should begin the second paragraph?

    (A)   sentence 3

    (B)   sentence 4

    (C)   sentence 5

    (D) sentence 6

    (E) sentence 7

Questions 22–25 are based on the following passage:

(1) If you drive from Florence to Arezzo through the Casentino, you will pass through a number of interesting places. (2) You take the main road to Pontassieve and then turn off onto the road for Vallombrosa. (3) The Casentino is the upper valley of the Arno. (4) The road to Vallombrosa goes through the villages of Pelago and Tosi. (5) After driving through a forest filled with pine, oak, and beech trees, you subsequently return to the main road just before Consuma. (6) Vallombrosa is now a popular summer resort. (7) Milton visited here when he was a young man, staying in the guest house of the famous and historic monastery of the Vallombrosan Order. (8) Just past Consuma, you will go across a mountain pass, and then one takes the road on the left to Pratovecchio and Stia. (9) The ruins of a twelfth-century castle that once belonged to the Guidi family lies near Pratovecchio. (10) Dante stayed with them when he was exiled from Florence. (11) Pratovecchio and Stia are two large villages in the Casentino. (12) Next the main road goes through Poppi and Bibbiena. (13) Poppi is a pretty little village and Bibbiena is the main town of the area. (14) You then go down across the plain and finally arrive at Arezzo.

22. One problem with sentence 8 is an inconsistency in

    (A)   tenses

    (B)   directions

    (C)   pronouns

    (D)   spelling

    (E)   sentence structure

23. In the context of the passage as a whole, the best choice to replace "a number of interesting places" in sentence 1 would be

    (A)   numerous interesting places

    (B)   a variety of interesting places

    (C)   a vast array of places of historic and literary interest

    (D)   the whole of Italian history

    (E)   a number of places of literary and historic interest

24. Which of the following would be the best way to combine sentences 9 and 10 (reproduced below)?

The ruins of a twelfth-century castle that once belonged to the Guidi family lies near Pratovecchio. Dante stayed with them when he was exiled from Florence.

(A) Near Pratovecchio lie the ruins of a twelfth-century castle that once belonged to members of the Guidi family, who sheltered Dante when he was exiled from Florence.

(B) The ruins of a twelfth-century castle that once belonged to the Guidi family lies near Pratovecchio; Dante stayed with them when he was exiled from Florence.

(C) The ruins of a twelfth-century castle that once belonged to the Guidi family lies near Pratovecchio, with whom Dante stayed when he was exiled from Florence.

(D) Dante took shelter with the Guidi family when he was exiled from Florence, and the ruins of a twelfth-century castle that once belonged to them lies near Pratovecchio.

(E) The ruins of a twelfth-century castle lies near Pratovecchio that once belonged to the Guidi family, who sheltered Dante when he was exiled from Florence.

25. Sentence 11 could most logically be combined with

(A) sentence 1
(B) sentence 3
(C) sentence 8
(D) sentence 10
(E) sentence 12

DIRECTIONS: The following questions test your familiarity with basic research, reference, and composition skills. Some questions refer to passages, while other questions are self-contained. For each question, choose the best answer.

Questions 26–27 are based on the following selection from a bibliography, using the University of Chicago documentation format:

Lamott, Anne. *Bird by Bird: Some Instructions on Writing and Life.* New York: Anchor Books, 1994.

Tolkien, J. R. R. *The Hobbit or There and Back Again.* Rev. ed. New York: Ballantine Books, 1937.

Zinsser, William. *Writing Well: An Informal Guide to Writing Nonfiction.* 3rd ed. New York: Harper & Row, 1985.

26. One feature of these entries that is NOT true of the MLA format is

    (A) page numbers are not given
    (B) no indication of source as print or electronic
    (C) author's last name comes first
    (D) listed in alphabetical order by author's last name
    (E) city of publication is followed by a colon

27. What is the meaning of the abbreviation "Rev. ed."?

    (A) Revised by editor
    (B) Revised edition
    (C) Review edition
    (D) Reverse edition
    (E) Reviewed by editor

---

28. Which of the following should be in quotation marks?

    (A) The name of a magazine
    (B) The name of a ship
    (C) The title of a painting
    (D) The title of a short poem
    (E) The name of a play

Questions 29–31 are based on the following passage:

A prominent statue sits at the center of the United Nations headquarters in New York City (United Nations, 2001). The statue depicts a man beating a sword into a plow, a reference to a statement by the Old Testament prophet Micah: "They will beat their swords into plowshares . . .Nation will not take up sword against nation, nor will they train for war anymore" (Micah 4:3). The United Nations was founded in 1945 on the premise of "Never again." Two world wars had taken millions of lives and devastated the world in the first half of the twentieth century. To prevent similar conflicts from breaking out, and to "save succeeding generations from the scourge of war" (United Nations, 1945), scores of countries banded together and ratified the Charter of the United Nations. Their criteria for achieving this goal was clear and simple: "to reaffirm faith in fundamental human rights, in the dignity and worth of the human person," and "to establish conditions under which justice and respect for the obligations arising from treaties and other sources of international law can be maintained." (United Nations, 1945)

References:
United Nations. (1945, June). *Preamble, Charter of the United Nations.* Retrieved March 3, 2011, from *http://www.un.org/aboutun/charter/*
United Nations. (2001). Swords into Plowshares. *United Nations.* Retrieved January 17, 2011, from *http://www.un.org/pubs/cyberschoolbus/untour/subswo.htm*

29. What information is given by the numeral 2001 in the second references entry?

    (A) The date when the United Nations was founded

    (B) The date when the information was accessed

    (C) The call number according to the Library of Congress catalog system

    (D) The call number according to the Dewey Decimal System

    (E) The date when the document was published

30. The statue beating a sword into a plow is a symbolic representation of

    (A) the importance of agriculture

    (B) the goal of exchanging war for peace

    (C) the military power of the United Nations

    (D) the danger of nuclear armaments

    (E) the power of change

31. What event or events most directly led to the founding of the United Nations?

    (A) The establishment of NATO

    (B) The Great Depression

    (C) The rise of Hitler

    (D) The Berlin Wall

    (E) World War I and World War II

Questions 32–34 are based on the following passage:

In the time of the Romans, the land around the present site of Brouage lay under water, submerged beneath the great gulf of Saintonge. The coast of France was nine miles away, on a ring of rising land to the east. As the gulf receded, it left a muddy mix of water and clay that was called *broue*. The lowlands that emerged from the sea were called *brouage*, which came to mean an area of mudflats and salt marsh.[3]

From an early date, villages began to rise on this new land, and one of them was also called Brouage. It was a small trading town, and its most valuable commodity was salt—a gift of the sea and the sun to the people of this region. Salt was mined from deposits in coastal marshes, and evaporated from brine in open pans. It was vital for the preservation of food, and so much in demand that it was called the "white gold" of medieval Europe. Salt also became important in another way. Monarchs were quick to discover that it could easily be taxed. The result was the hated *gabelle*, the infamous salt tax that became a major source of revenue for the old regime in France, and a leading cause of revolution in 1789.[4]

[3]Nathalie Fiquet, "Brouage in the Time of Champlain: A New Town Open to the World" in Raymonde Litalien and Denis Vaugeois, eds. *Champlain: The Birth of French America.* (Montreal, 2004), 39.
[4]Martinet, Micheline, *The Adventure of the Sea.* (Paris, 1995), 335.

Source: David Hackett Fischer, *Champlain's Dream.* NY: Simon & Schuster, 2008, p. 16.

32. What is the significance of the raised numeral *3* at the end of the first paragraph?

    (A) It refers to an earlier draft of the paper.

    (B) It refers to the endnote at the conclusion of the paper.

    (C) It refers to an entry in the Works Cited page.

    (D) It refers to an entry in the bibliography.

    (E) It refers to the footnote at the bottom of the page.

33. According to this passage, the word *brouage* is

    (A) the tax on salt.

    (B) an area of mud and marshes.

    (C) a Roman seaport.

    (D) a French term for salt.

    (E) a section of seacoast.

34. Which information is missing from both footnotes?

    (A) City of publication

    (B) Date of publication

    (C) Name of publisher

    (D) Page number

    (E) Date of access

---

35. Which of the following is NOT a characteristic of footnotes?

    (A) They are listed on a separate page at the end of the paper.

    (B) They are numbered sequentially.

    (C) They are listed at the bottom of the page containing the citation.

    (D) Each one is keyed to a superscript number in the text.

    (E) Each one includes the page number, if available.

36. The most comprehensive source to check for the names of Russian poets is

    (A) an encyclopedia article on Russian literature.

    (B) an anthology of world literature.

    (C) a magazine article on contemporary Russian poets.

    (D) a textbook on the history of Russia since the Revolution.

    (E) a transcript of an interview with a leading Russian poet.

37. An abstract from a journal article is most useful for

    (A) learning the philosophical ideas behind the article.

    (B) finding resource materials on the topic.

    (C) discovering statistical information about the topic.

    (D) deciding if the article would be helpful.

    (E) examining biographical material about the author.

Questions 38–44 are based on the following passage:

(1) Combine the sugar and flour in a large bowl, and stir well. (2) In a saucepan, combine the butter, water, cocoa, and salt; bring to a boil. (3) Stir hot mixture into sugar-flour combination, and beat well. (4) Add eggs, one at a time, beating well after each egg has been added. (5) Dissolve baking soda in buttermilk, and stir well. (6) Stir in vanilla, and beat the batter for one minute. (7) Pour batter into baking pan, and place in oven. (8) Bake for twenty minutes or until a toothpick stuck into cake comes out clean. (9) Remove from oven and cool in baking pan for at least one hour. (10) Frost cake with a favorite icing. (11) Cut into squares and serve cold.

38. The paragraph is

    (A) a recipe for preparing a cake

    (B) a guide to making a fancy dessert

    (C) directions for making a cake

    (D) a section of a comparison/contrast composition

    (E) obviously from a gourmet's cookbook

39. All of the sentences

    (A) are actually sentence fragments because each has no subject

    (B) use the imperative mood of the verbs

    (C) are too short to be helpful to a cook

    (D) use the declarative mood of the verb

    (E) use the past tense of the verbs

40. One unique feature of paragraphs of this type is that

    (A) sentences can be used in any order

    (B) sentences provide several different bits of information

    (C) there is a definite sentence of conclusion

    (D) there is no expressed topic sentence or central idea

    (E) all of the sentences have a different construction

41. Sentences 1 through 6 assume that

    (A) the paragraph has been preceded by a list of ingredients with the amount of each one specified

    (B) the reader is an experienced cook

    (C) only children will use this recipe

    (D) the reader can interpret things for himself/herself

    (E) cakes are very easy to make

42. Sentence 8 is inadequate for this type of paragraph because

    (A) it is broken into two parts with the comma
    (B) the oven temperature is not given
    (C) the reader is told to do two things
    (D) the sentence is too short
    (E) the sentence conveys little information

43. One advantage of well-written paragraphs of this type is that the reader

    (A) does not have to read every word
    (B) does not need to do anything
    (C) is not expected to understand what is written
    (D) cannot make a serious mistake
    (E) is not required to interpret what is written

44. Which type of organization is most important for a paragraph of this type?

    (A) chronological
    (B) similarities followed by differences
    (C) differences followed by similarities
    (D) most to least important
    (E) least to most important

Questions 45–50 are based on the following passage:

(1) From my study window, I can see a grassy courtyard with some blooming flowers around the sides. (2) Across the courtyard is another apartment with a balcony which is larger than the one I have. (3) Usually, children are playing under the trees, and in the afternoons the noise of their activities is often distractive to my work. (4) From my balcony, I can see seven other balconies of varying sizes as well as seven patios that are attached to the apartments on the first floor. (5) Every Monday or Tuesday, depending upon the weather, several employees of the lawn upkeep service mow the grass, trim the shrubs, rake the clippings, and rake the area under the plants. (6) Just outside my study is a large oak tree that shades the windows from the afternoon sun; farther over in the courtyard are two more oak trees that are as tall as the two-story buildings. (7) Some tenants have planted petunias, marigolds, impatiens, and other annuals in flower boxes or at the edges of patios so that we have flowering plants to enjoy until frost comes. (8) One of the trees, a red maple, has already started the annual fall leaf color change so that in a couple of weeks we can hope for reds and browns in the branches to contrast with the green in the grass. (9) Then frost comes . . .

45. Sentence 1 lets the reader assume that

    (A) the paragraph will describe the courtyard.
    (B) the writer will develop some abstract idea about the courtyard.
    (C) the courtyard has some deep significance to the writer.
    (D) the paragraph will go from a general statement to something more specific.
    (E) the courtyard is not very attractive to the viewer.

46. Sentence 5

    (A)   seems a practical statement about the courtyard.

    (B)   demonstrates the apartment manager's concern for the unemployed.

    (C)   changes the subject too abruptly and should be omitted.

    (D)   produces the reason the author should remain in the apartment.

    (E)   praises the services of the lawn upkeep company.

47. Sentence 3 implies that

    (A)   the author does not like children.

    (B)   children enjoy the grassy courtyard.

    (C)   children cannot be trusted in the courtyard.

    (D)   the author has a job that requires peace and quiet.

    (E)   children should be encouraged in their activities.

48. In sentence 7, the names of the plants that are in the courtyard illustrate what is said in

    (A)   sentence 2.

    (B)   sentence 1.

    (C)   sentence 6.

    (D)   sentence 5.

    (E)   sentence 8.

49. Sentence 8 relates most closely to what other sentence?

    (A)   sentence 3

    (B)   sentence 4

    (C)   sentence 2

    (D)   sentence 9

    (E)   sentence 6

50. The effect of sentence 9, incomplete as it is, is

    (A)   to summarize what the paragraph is all about.

    (B)   to signal the reader that the paragraph is exaggerated.

    (C)   to cast a coat of gloom on the mood of the paragraph.

    (D)   to lighten the whole mood of the paragraph.

    (E)   to show how the author can use an incomplete sentence ineffectively.

Part Two

This part of Sample Exam 2 consists of 40 questions, and you have 40 minutes to complete it. If you plan to take the College Composition Exam, you need to complete only Part One of this test. However, if you plan to take the College Composition Modular Exam, you should go on to complete Part Two. The combination of Parts One and Two is equivalent to the College Composition Modular Examination. You may also complete Part Two if you simply wish to get extra practice in answering the questions.

DIRECTIONS: Read each sentence carefully, paying attention to the underlined portions. Assume that elements of the sentence that are not underlined are correct and cannot be changed. In choosing answers, follow the requirements of Standard Written English.

If there is an error, select the <u>one underlined part</u> that must be changed to make the sentence correct.

If there is no error, select "No error," answer (E).

---

51. Senator Snodgrass <u>must have</u> a very poor speech writer; <u>his inferences are</u>
            A   B
 always so subtle that the listener has to be <u>wary of drawing</u> hasty
                                                 C
 conclusions <u>about what</u> he thinks he heard the senator say. <u>No error.</u>
              D   E

52. No <u>privately owned</u> telephone company in the United States <u>can deny</u> <u>its</u>
           A   B   C
 employees <u>the right to join whatever</u> union they choose. <u>No error.</u>
                   D   E

53. <u>True successful businesspersons</u> may belabor Congress for raising taxes on
               A
 their profits beyond <u>what they believe</u> they can afford to pay, but they can
                                   B
 <u>only admit</u> that <u>high taxes are necessary</u> during a period of increasing
           C   D
 deficits. <u>No error.</u>
           E

54. If <u>a local arrangements committee</u> can secure suitable hotel
              A
 accommodations <u>at reasonable rates</u>, the board of <u>directors plan on having</u>
                      B   C
 its annual <u>stockholders meeting</u> in Cleveland, Ohio. <u>No error.</u>
              D   E

DIRECTIONS: The following sentences test correctness and effectiveness of expression. In choosing your answers, follow the requirements of Standard Written English; that is, pay attention to grammar, diction (choice of words), sentence construction, and punctuation.

In each of the following sentences, part of the sentence or the entire sentence is underlined. Beneath each sentence you will find five versions of the underlined part. The first option repeats the original; the other four options present different versions.

Choose the option that best expresses the meaning of the original sentence. If you think the original is better than any of the alternatives, choose the first option; otherwise, choose one of the other options. Your choice should produce the most effective sentence—one that is clear and precise, without awkwardness or ambiguity.

55. To make their children realize the significance of wise decision making, sometimes parents should let them stew in the juice of their own concoction.

 (A) let them stew in the juice of their own concoction
 (B) let them suffer the consequences of their actions
 (C) let them stew in their own consequences
 (D) reduce the penalties for deviant behavior
 (E) throw a lifeline to rescue them from the sea of despond

56. The government has passed a law regulating the sale of dangerous drugs to teenagers, therefore, prescriptions from licensed physicians are now required before a druggist can dispense them.

 (A) to teenagers, therefore, prescriptions
 (B) to teenagers, therefore; prescriptions
 (C) to teenagers; therefore, prescriptions
 (D) to teenagers, so therefore, prescriptions
 (E) to teenagers; and therefore prescriptions

57. Andy Warhol was a man of many talents; he painted many strange and unusual pictures, wrote a novel based on the experiences of his coterie, and he produced several experimental films for commercial distribution.

 (A) of his coterie, and he produced
 (B) of his coterie, and produced
 (C) of his coterie; and he has produced
 (D) of his coterie and have produced
 (E) of his coterie and he has produced

58. Many others <u>who are not so fortunate</u> will lose all the money they have invested in junk bonds.

    (A) others who are not so fortunate
    (B) others who is not so fortunate
    (C) others who is not as fortunate
    (D) others whom is not so fortunate
    (E) others whom are not so fortunate

59. The bus driver was always <u>pleasant to we riders even</u> though he must become impatient with some of us who never have the correct change.

    (A) pleasant to we riders even
    (B) pleasant to us riders even
    (C) pleasant to our riders even
    (D) pleasant to no riders
    (E) pleasant to their riders

60. Since Old Mother <u>Hubbard hadn't scarcely enough</u> food for herself, her friends wondered how she expected to feed a pet from her meager supply.

    (A) Hubbard hadn't scarcely enough
    (B) Hubbard had scarcely enough
    (C) Hubbard has scarcely enough
    (D) Hubbard had scarce enough
    (E) Hubbard scarcely have enough

61. While I was looking through the morning newspaper, <u>I read where the cost of living</u> had risen another four points, mainly because food prices had gone up again.

    (A) I read where the cost of living
    (B) I read when the cost of living
    (C) I read that the cost of living
    (D) I read because the cost of living
    (E) I read after the cost of living

62. City leaders will review all existing plans and make necessary updates and revisions as needed <u>to insure that all plans will work together</u> to accomplish the long-term vision for the city.

    (A) to insure that all city workers will blend together
    (B) to make sure that all plans work together
    (C) to ensure that all city workers work together
    (D) to ensure that all plans will work together
    (E) to ensure that the combined plans will function smoothly

63. Reading a good novel can be as great a pleasure as seeing a professional football game on television or catching a four-pound trout in a clear stream in Michigan.

(A) game on television or catching a four-pound trout
(B) game on television or to catch a four-pound trout
(C) game in television or catching a four-pound trout
(D) game on television or caught a four-pound trout
(E) game on television or to caught a four-pound trout

64. In her lecture, the novelist eluded to difficulties with her publisher who insisted that all controversial material be removed from her manuscript.

(A) In her lecture, the novelist eluded to difficulties
(B) In her lecture, the novelist alluded to difficulties
(C) In her lecture, the novelist avoided her difficulties
(D) In her lecture, the novelist inferred to difficulties
(E) In her lecture, the novelist conferred to difficulties

65. The jury found the manager of the office so equally guilty as the clerk of the large establishment.

(A) so equally guilty as the clerk
(B) so much equally guilty as the clerk
(C) as equally guilty just as the clerk
(D) as guilty as the clerk
(E) as if equally guilty as the clerk

66. Luckily, the arsonist was arrested before he set any more serious fires by the policeman who took him to jail.

(A) was arrested before he set any more serious fires by the policeman who took him to jail
(B) was arrested by the policeman who took him to jail after he set more serious fires
(C) was arrested by the policeman who took him to jail before he could set any more serious fires
(D) the policeman arrested him before he could set any more serious fires
(E) was taken to jail by the policeman before he could set any more serious fires

67. I shopped in all the stores on Michigan Avenue before I found the exquisite old antique umbrella stand I wanted to give Masaki for a birthday present.

(A) the exquisite old antique umbrella stand I wanted to give
(B) the exquisite antique umbrella stand I wanted to give
(C) the elaborate old antique umbrella stand I wanted to give
(D) the exquisite antique old stand I wanted to give
(E) the exquisite old stand for antique umbrellas I wanted to give

68. A good assistant can relieve an administrator of much of the paperwork <u>that must be handled</u> within any large organization to expedite its day to day operations.

   (A) that must be handled
   (B) that should have been handled
   (C) that must have been handled
   (D) that has got to be handled
   (E) that have to be handled

69. The majority political party could not <u>except the conditions of the minority,</u> and the coalition of parties collapsed.

   (A) except the conditions of the minority
   (B) reciprocate the conditions of the minority
   (C) calibrate the conditions of the minority
   (D) restrict the conditions of the minority
   (E) accept the conditions of the minority

70. Working hard is not difficult for those <u>people whom are accustomed to</u> getting up early and coming home after dark.

   (A) people whom are accustomed to
   (B) people whom is accustomed to
   (C) people who are accustomed to
   (D) people that are accustomed to
   (E) people whose are accustomed to

DIRECTIONS: The following questions test your familiarity with basic research, reference and composition skills. Some questions refer to passages, whereas other questions are self-contained. For each question, choose the best answer.

<u>Questions 71–72</u> are based on the following passage:

(1) In 1908, the White Star Company announced that they would craft a ship that would beat all other records. (2) The *Titanic* was the result—a ten million dollar project. (3) It was said to be "the greatest ship afloat" (*Sinking* 215). (4) In fact, Mrs. Albert Caldwell asked one of the deck hands if the *Titanic* was really unsinkable, as everyone had said, and he replied, "Yes, lady, God himself could not sink this ship" (Lord 50). (5) The captain even said that he couldn't imagine anything happening to the ship because "modern shipbuilding has gone beyond that" (Lord 37). (6) There was never a ship that gave her passengers a sense of more calm and confidence than the *Titanic*.

Lord, Walter. *A Night to Remember*. New York: Henry Holt and Company, 1955.
The Sinking of the Titanic and Great Sea Disasters. San Antonio: Vision Forum, 1998.

71. What is the proper format for an entry in the Works Cited page if no author is given in the original source?

    (A) Insert "Anonymous" where the author is normally listed
    (B) List the title of the source first
    (C) List the publisher first
    (D) End the entry with the notation "Author unknown."
    (E) Insert "n.a." after the title

72. In sentence 1, what is the most effective way to end the sentence?

    (A) a ship that would beat all other records
    (B) a ship that would break all records for luxury, size, speed, and safety
    (C) a ship that would beat all other ships
    (D) a ship that would surpass all other ships
    (E) a ship that would break records in every area

---

73. Which of these parenthetical citations is the correct way in MLA format to list a source when the Works Cited list contains more than one work by this author?

    (A) (Baxter, *Saint's Rest* 72)
    (B) (Baxter 72)
    (C) (Baxter 1783, p. 72)
    (D) (Baxter, The Saint's Everlasting Rest 72)
    (E) (Baxter, *Saint's Rest*, 1783, 72)

74. In an encyclopedia, a cross-reference

    (A) provides a sample of an opposing argument
    (B) lists the location of additional information in other books or periodicals
    (C) gives alternate definitions for a technical term
    (D) identifies a related article in the same encyclopedia
    (E) records the source of the current article

75. The correct spacing for a Works Cited page is

    (A) center all entries on the page
    (B) double-space between entries, but single-space between the lines of an entry
    (C) single-space between entries, but double-space between the lines of an entry
    (D) single-space between the lines of an entry and between entries
    (E) double-space between the lines of an entry and between entries

76. Sources dating from the period of the Roman Empire would be most appropriate for a study of

    (A) the origins of Christianity
    (B) the Roman Catholic Church in the Middle Ages
    (C) trends in Italian cuisine
    (D) Romanian architecture
    (E) the unification of Italy

slip[1] /slip/ *v* (**slipped, slip·ping, slips**) **1** *vti* **MOVE SMOOTHLY** to move or make something move smoothly and easily and usually with a sliding motion ° *It slips easily in and out of its case.* **2** *vti* **PUT ON OR TAKE OFF** to put on or take off something quickly and easily **3** *vi* **LOSE YOUR FOOTING** to lose your footing or grip on a slippery surface ° *I slipped and fell.* **4** *vi* **MOVE FROM ITS PROPER POSITION** to slide or move accidentally out of the proper or desired position ° *This strap keeps slipping off my shoulder.* **5** *vti* **BE FORGOTTEN** to be forgotten or overlooked by somebody ° *It slipped my mind.* **6** *vi* **GO QUIETLY** to go somewhere in a quiet, furtive, or unnoticed way ° *He slipped out while nobody was looking.* **7** *vt* **PASS SOMETHING SECRETLY** to give somebody something furtively or secretly ° *I saw the man slip her an envelope.* **8** *vi* **ERR** to make a mistake or to do something wrong ° *You must have slipped up when you were making a note of the number.* **9** vi **GET WORSE** to decline from a previous standard, e.g., of performance or awareness ° *He's slipping—two years ago he would have spotted that mistake at once.* ° *She's in danger of slipping back into her bad old ways.* **10** *vt* **TO DISLOCATE A BONE** to dislocate or displace a bone, especially in the spine **11** *vti* **DISENGAGE THE CLUTCH** to disengage the clutch of a motor vehicle or be disengaged **12** *vi* **FAIL TO ENGAGE** to fail to engage properly, usually because of wear (*refers to mechanical parts*) **13** *vt* **LET A RESTRAINING CABLE GO** to let a line or cable that is securing a vessel to a mooring or anchor fall over the side **14** *vti* **RELEASE** to release an animal from a restraint, or be released in this way ■ *n* **1** **ACT OF SLIPPING** an act of slipping, especially a sudden slide on a slippery surface **2** **ERROR** an error or oversight **3** **LAPSE** a moral lapse or instance of misconduct **4** **UNDERGARMENT** a light sleeveless woman's undergarment worn under a dress **5** NAUT = **slipway** **6** **DEFORMATION OF A CRYSTAL** the deformation of a metallic crystal by shearing along a plane **7** **CLOTH COVERING** a cloth covering for something **8** AIR = **sideslip** *n.* **2** [13C. Probably < Middle Dutch or Middle Low German *slippen*.] ◊ **give somebody the slip** to get away from somebody who is chasing or pursuing you ◊ **let slip 1** to say something without meaning to, or reveal something that should be kept secret **2** to allow somebody or something to escape ◊ **slip one over on somebody** to trick or deceive somebody (*informal*)

Source: *Microsoft Encarta College Dictionary.*
New York: St. Martin's Press, 2001, p. 1360.

77. What is the origin of the word *slip*?

    (A) Middle Dutch or Low German in the 13th century

    (B) Variation on the word *slide*

    (C) Nautical terminology

    (D) Middle English in the 15th century

    (E) A noun meaning a moral lapse

78. What is the purpose of the phrases in all capitals?

    (A) To distinguish between the word's use as a noun or as a verb

    (B) To give a full definition of the word

    (C) To give an example of the word's use

    (D) To give a brief summary of the meaning

    (E) To provide a paraphrase of the word

79. What is the meaning of the abbreviation *vt*?

    (A) Verb: transitive

    (B) Verb: technical

    (C) Older terminology (from Latin *veteris terma*)

    (D) Variant term

    (E) Verbal term

80. In the APA system of documentation, what is the proper title for the list of sources at the end of the paper?

    (A) References

    (B) Works Cited

    (C) Bibliography

    (D) Annotated Bibliography

    (E) Glossary

DIRECTIONS: The following questions test your ability to analyze writing. Some questions refer to passages, whereas other questions are self-contained. For each question, choose the best answer.

Questions 81–86 are based on the following passage:

(1) It has become conventional that every president of the United States, once he becomes an ex-president, expects that the taxpayers will build a library or some other building in his honor. (2) These monuments usually cost well into the eight figures to construct, and the upkeep (maintenance, employees to serve the institution, etc.) is always a few more million annually. (3) For example, the Jimmy Carter library in Atlanta created some controversy, because architects planned a broad highway leading to the building. (4) The people who lived in the neighborhood protested that traffic would disturb the peace and quiet they had enjoyed before the building was completed. (5) With the protests and threatened lawsuits, we seem to have another example of NIMBY—"Not In My Backyard," which seems to afflict many people when their health, safety, or convenience is disturbed. (6) A similar protest occurred when a garbage dump for toxic wastes was proposed for a forest preserve area in Illinois. (7) Thus, often we are provided with undesirable options: either to build a building to honor an ex-president with all that follows that decision or to refuse the honor of having a tourist attraction in the neighborhood.

81. Sentence 6

   (A) produces a necessary interruption in the paragraph.
   (B) should be omitted as irrelevant to the paragraph's meaning.
   (C) provides another example of NIMBY.
   (D) confuses the tone of the paragraph with the word *garbage*.
   (E) questions the practice of building libraries to honor ex-presidents.

82. Sentence 1

   (A) is the basic generalization for the whole paragraph.
   (B) is too long to be a good topic sentence.
   (C) contains a grammatical error—*It*.
   (D) presents a rationale that opposes building presidential libraries.
   (E) protects the rights of anyone to oppose presidential libraries.

83. In sentence 2, the word *monuments* suggests that

   (A) presidential libraries are a good thing.
   (B) ex-presidents have not already been honored enough by their former office.
   (C) libraries are a legitimate means of honoring ex-presidents.
   (D) ex-presidential libraries provide examples of wasted money and unnecessary expenses.
   (E) the American people enjoy honoring ex-presidents.

84. Sentence 3

   (A) moves from the development of the generalization in sentence 1 to a specific example.
   (B) signals the reader too blatantly with *For example*.
   (C) implies that only Jimmy Carter's monument was too expensive.
   (D) begins with harsh criticism of the people of Atlanta.
   (E) attempts to inspire the reader to protest the situation.

85. Sentences 3, 4, and 5

   (A) follow logically from what is set out in sentence 2.
   (B) define the concept of NIMBY not too clearly.
   (C) provides a unified example to support sentence 1.
   (D) acts as a contradiction to sentence 1.
   (E) seem to shift the point from presidential libraries to another subject.

86. Which of the following best describes the type of prose found in this passage.

   (A) expository
   (B) descriptive
   (C) narrative
   (D) argumentative
   (E) persuasive

Questions 87–90 are based on the following passage:

(1) The key to the heart of a nation can be found in its books and pamphlets. (2) In America, where we fight our battles not with swords and guns but with words and information, there is a wide diversity of literature, reflecting the attitudes and beliefs of a multiplicity of people. (3) Solomon Short once said, "I'm all in favor of keeping dangerous weapons out of the hands of fools. Let's start with typewriters." (4) Well, typewriters may no longer be in style, but we have much wider avenues of publication today, including computers, the Internet, and CDs.

(5) It can be amazing to see the effects the ideas listed in one pamphlet or book can have on a country. (6) Take, for example, the publication of *Common Sense* by Thomas Paine in the 1770s. (7) Here just a small pamphlet excited the emotions in the hearts of thousands and millions of people. (8) Soon the whole nation had espoused its ideas, talking about them everywhere—on the streets, in the taverns, at the dinner table. (9) These ideas wakened a group of sleeping people, eventually leading them to declare themselves an independent nation, the United States of America.

(10) Today, although pamphlets may not be so much in use, we use other methods to communicate our ideas. (11) Television and the Internet are among the most effective methods. (12) It is remarkable what one popular television advertisement can effect. (13) One clever advertisement done in the last election served to propel a candidate from almost the bottom of the chart to 30% of the vote on primary day. (14) This demonstrates how powerful modern media are. (15) We must guard against letting these precious resources become dominated by fools.

87. Which of these phrases would be most effective in sentence 7?

    (A) thousands and millions
    (B) thousands
    (C) the majority of people
    (D) all the people
    (E) certain people

88. What is the writer's purpose in sentence 4?

    (A) To correct the error of mentioning typewriters
    (B) To expand the application of the quotation to more current types of communication
    (C) To add a conversational, informal tone
    (D) To demonstrate that typewriters are no longer commonly used
    (E) To explain the meaning of the quotation from Solomon Short

89. What example did the writer use to support the idea that written words can influence an entire country?

(A) A pamphlet titled *Common Sense*
(B) A political advertisement
(C) A television advertisement
(D) A book titled *Common Sense*
(E) A quotation from Solomon Short

90. What is the most serious potential problem in sentences 1 and 2?

(A) Sentence 1 is too short.
(B) Sentence 2 is too long.
(C) They contain a mixed metaphor.
(D) Books are no longer the key to a nation's heart.
(E) Swords are no longer used in combat.

STOP

If there is still time remaining, you may review your answers.

ANSWER KEY
Sample Examination 2

COLLEGE COMPOSITION

1.	**D**	24.	**A**	47.	**D**	70.	**C**
2.	**B**	25.	**C**	48.	**B**	71.	**B**
3.	**E**	26.	**B**	49.	**E**	72.	**B**
4.	**A**	27.	**B**	50.	**C**	73.	**A**
5.	**B**	28.	**D**	51.	**B**	74.	**D**
6.	**E**	29.	**E**	52.	**E**	75.	**E**
7.	**C**	30.	**B**	53.	**A**	76.	**A**
8.	**B**	31.	**E**	54.	**C**	77.	**A**
9.	**C**	32.	**E**	55.	**B**	78.	**D**
10.	**A**	33.	**B**	56.	**C**	79.	**A**
11.	**D**	34.	**C**	57.	**B**	80.	**A**
12.	**C**	35.	**A**	58.	**A**	81.	**C**
13.	**C**	36.	**A**	59.	**B**	82.	**A**
14.	**B**	37.	**D**	60.	**B**	83.	**D**
15.	**D**	38.	**C**	61.	**C**	84.	**A**
16.	**E**	39.	**B**	62.	**E**	85.	**E**
17.	**C**	40.	**D**	63.	**A**	86.	**A**
18.	**C**	41.	**A**	64.	**B**	87.	**B**
19.	**E**	42.	**B**	65.	**D**	88.	**B**
20.	**C**	43.	**E**	66.	**C**	89.	**A**
21.	**D**	44.	**A**	67.	**B**	90.	**C**
22.	**C**	45.	**A**	68.	**A**		
23.	**E**	46.	**C**	69.	**E**		

SCORING CHART

After you have scored your Sample Examination 2, enter the results in the chart below; then transfer your score to the Progress Chart on page 12.

Total Test	Number Right	Number Wrong	Number Omitted
90			

ANSWER EXPLANATIONS

1. **(D)** *Is* is present tense and does not logically follow <u>fought</u> and <u>battled</u>, past tense.

2. **(B)** <u>He</u> and <u>I</u> are wrong pronoun forms; the objective case should be <u>him</u> and <u>me</u>.

3. **(E)** Sentence is correct.

4. **(A)** A dangling modifier.

5. **(B)** Incorrect idiom.

6. **(E)** What is said in sentence 1 is repeated in sentence 6. The rest of the first paragraph has no direct connection with sentence 1.

7. **(C)** This is the clearest and most concise version.

8. **(B)** In this sentence, the drug problem is treated first as an enemy in a war, then as a plague, and finally as a ghost. It is best to stick to one metaphor at a time.

9. **(C)** Too many different points in a single sentence lead to confusion.

10. **(A)** *Warning* is a synonym for *caveat*.

11. **(D)** Because the writer has already said that no one knows what to do about the drug problem, the paragraph needs to explain why it will not be a waste of money to spend billions of dollars.

12. **(C)** This sentence begins a new topic—types of junipers.

13. **(C)** This version avoids the awkward or illogical constructions in the other choices.

14. **(B)** This version puts the similar ideas concisely in parallel form.

15. **(D)** The original is too colloquial to fit the tone of the passage as a whole. (D) is the only acceptable alternative.

16. **(E)** This choice avoids excess words and maintains the parallel construction.

17. **(C)** The example in sentence 13 can easily be combined into sentence 12.

18. **(C)** There is no need for the extra words in any of the other choices.

19. **(E)** This is the only version that keeps the parallel construction.

20. **(C)** There is nothing grammatically wrong with repeating a word, and sometimes a writer will do it for rhetorical effect. In this case, however, the repetition calls unnecessary attention to an unimportant word.

21. **(D)** The first part of the passage describes the problem. Sentence 6 begins the discussion of a possible solution that could logically be a new paragraph.

22. **(C)** Most of the passage is written in the second person (*you*), but the second part of sentence 8 switches to the third person (*one*). Either *one* or *you* would be perfectly acceptable, but the author must use the same case throughout.

23. **(E)** Specific is almost always better than vague. This makes choice (E) preferable to choices (A) or (B). Choices (C) and (D) claim more than the rest of the passage can justify.

24. **(A)** This is the only choice that is clear, grammatically correct, and free from misplaced or dangling modifiers.

25. **(C)** Identification of the villages should be provided when they are first mentioned.

26. **(B)** In the MLA format, the last item in the entry identifies the format: print, DVD, Web.

27. **(B)** *Rev. ed.* is the abbreviation for "revised edition."

28. **(D)** A short poem should be listed with quotation marks, as is the case for magazine articles or chapters of a book. Italics are normally used for all the other choices.

29. **(E)** The date that appears near the beginning of the entry in the APA format represents the date when the source was originally published or posted to the Web site. The date when the source was retrieved or accessed appears later in the entry.

30. **(B)** A sword is a customary symbol for war, whereas a plow represents the peaceful activity of agriculture. Reshaping a sword into a plow is an apt symbol for exchanging war for the benefits of peace.

31. **(E)** The United Nations was founded in the aftermath of World War I, and especially World War II, as an attempt to provide peaceful ways to deal with conflicts between nations.

32. **(E)** A raised, or superscript, number is a reference to a footnote or endnote. The sample provides footnotes directly following the quotation, rather than relegating them to a separate page; so choice E is preferred.

33. **(B)** *Brouage* is defined in the article as an area of mudflats and salt marsh. It also became the name of a village, but none of the other choices given is correct.

34. **(C)** Neither footnote contains the name of the publisher, but all the other items of information do appear.

35. **(A)** Endnotes are listed on a separate page at the end of a paper, but footnotes appear at the bottom of the page where the information is cited in the paper.

36. **(A)** An encyclopedia article on Russian literature would normally include the names of the most significant Russian poets. Choice B covers literature from all languages and eras, so its coverage of Russian poets would be minimal. Choices C and D both deal with only recent literature, so they would not cover the full range of Russian literature.

Choice E would be unlikely to be comprehensive, since it would focus on only one writer.

37. **(D)** An abstract is a brief summary of a journal article, appearing at the beginning of the article. By reviewing the abstract, a reader can get a brief look at the topics considered in the full article; this makes it easy to decide whether further study of this source would be profitable.

38. **(C)** Since the amounts for the ingredients are missing, this is not a complete recipe.

39. **(B)** All of the sentences use the imperative mood, the "you" being understood.

40. **(D)** Because this is a set of directions for baking a cake, there is no need for a topic sentence.

41. **(A)** Without a list specifying the amount of each ingredient, the directions would be meaningless.

42. **(B)** Without instructions about the proper oven temperature, the instructions in sentence 8 are not useful.

43. **(E)** The information is straightforward and, therefore, requires no interpretation on the reader's part.

44. **(A)** When you are giving instructions on how to do something, the only logical form of organization is step by step, or chronological.

45. **(A)** The narrative tone as well as the sense of the sentence makes the reader expect that a description of the courtyard will follow.

46. **(C)** The change from the mostly tranquil description of the courtyard to the activity of the gardeners disrupts the mood the author is creating.

47. **(D)** The author's statement about the children playing has neither negative nor positive implications. But the author's need for quiet is evident, since the noise of the children distracts the author from his work.

48. **(B)** In sentence 1, the author says he can see "blooming flowers." In sentence 7, he gives specific names of flowers to illustrate his point.

49. **(E)** Sentences 6 and 8 both describe the trees in the courtyard.

50. **(C)** Until this last sentence, the mood of the paragraph has been one of tranquillity and joy in the beauty of nature. The mood changes to one of gloom with the mention of frost and the visions that come with it.

51. **(B)** Inferences should be implications.

52. **(E)** Sentence is correct.

53. **(A)** True should be truly, the adverbial form.

54. **(C)** Plan on having is a poor idiom; uses plans to have.

55. **(B)** The original sentence contains a cliché; (B) corrects the problem.

56. **(C)** The comma in the original sentence is a comma splice.

57. **(B)** Error in parallelism—the section beginning <u>and he</u> is an independent clause but the preceding section contains no subject.

58. **(A)** The original sentence is correct.

59. **(B)** <u>We</u> should be <u>us</u>, the objective case.

60. **(B)** <u>Hadn't scarcely</u> is a double negative.

61. **(C)** <u>Where</u> is an incorrect word choice—<u>that</u> is correct.

62. **(E)** The proper term is <u>ensure</u>, not <u>insure</u>. The repetition of "work" and "workers" is awkward, and plans do not literally work together. (E) explains the idea most clearly.

63. **(A)** The original sentence is correct.

64. **(B)** Incorrect word choice, <u>eluded</u> should be <u>alluded</u>.

65. **(D)** The correct pair of conjunctions is <u>as . . . as</u>.

66. **(C)** A misplaced and ambiguous modifier—(C) corrects the problem.

67. **(B)** <u>Old</u> and <u>antique</u> are repetitious; (B) solves the problem.

68. **(A)** The original sentence is correct.

69. **(E)** <u>Except</u> has to be <u>accept</u>.

70. **(C)** <u>Whom</u> should be <u>who</u>, the correct case form.

71. **(B)** When no information on authorship is available, the Works Cited entry should begin with the title of the source. If the title page of a book actually says, "Anonymous," it would be appropriate to begin the entry with "Anonymous."

72. **(B)** Choice B provides a logical transition into a paragraph that deals largely with the safety of the vessel. The other choices are vague or illogical.

73. **(A)** The Works Cited list is part of the MLA system for documentation. In this system, parenthetical references in the text should list the author's last name. If two or more sources by the same author appear, a key word or two from the title should be listed.

74. **(D)** Any cross-reference in an encyclopedia article will direct the reader to other articles in the same encyclopedia on related topics.

75. **(E)** A Works Cited page in the MLA format should be completely double-spaced, both between entries and within an entry.

76. **(A)** The origins of Christianity date back to the Roman Empire period, beginning in the first century A.D. The Middle Ages are several centuries later, so choice B is incorrect. Choices C and D both refer to contemporary themes, and the unification of Italy mentioned in Choice E occurred in the late 1800s.

77. **(A)** This information is given near the end of the dictionary entry. 13C refers to the thirteenth century, and the origin is suggested as the Middle Dutch or Middle German word *slippen.*

78. **(D)** The phrases in all capitals give a brief, simple summary of the word's meaning. A more detailed, precise definition follows.

79. **(A)** This dictionary uses the abbreviations *vt, vi,* and *vti* to indicate verbs that are transitive, intransitive, or both. Transitive verbs can take a direct object; intransitive verbs occur without a direct object.

80. **(A)** The APA list of sources at the end of a paper is called "References." In the MLA format, such a list is called "Works Cited," and the University of Chicago system employs a "Bibliography."

81. **(C)** Sentence 6 provides another example of NIMBY, only this time a garbage dump rather than a library causes protest.

82. **(A)** Sentence 1 makes the basic generalization that is expanded on in the rest of the paragraph.

83. **(D)** The word *monuments* is used here in a negative sense to suggest that the real reason the libraries are being built is to memorialize ex-presidents.

84. **(A)** Sentence 3 is a good example of moving from a generalization to a specific by the use of concrete examples.

85. **(E)** Sentences 3, 4, and 5 shift the discussion from presidential libraries to NIMBY.

86. **(A)** The passage is providing information, and is therefore expository.

87. **(B)** Choice A—"thousands and millions"—is needlessly repetitious. Choice D is inaccurate, because it is virtually impossible for a whole nation to reach total agreement. Choices B and D go beyond the information available to make unsubstantiated claims about the total number who were convinced. Choice B can clearly be supported with evidence.

88. **(B)** The writer is aware that typewriters are no longer in common use, and sentence 4 attempts to deal with this problem by broadening the quotation to include more contemporary forms of communication.

89. **(A)** Although other examples were given, only *Common Sense* was directly linked to the idea that written words can influence an entire country.

90. **(C)** The sentences contain a mixed metaphor: a key unlocking a heart, blended with a battle image of swords and guns.

The Humanities Examination

ANSWER SHEET
Trial Test

HUMANITIES

1. Ⓐ Ⓑ Ⓒ Ⓓ Ⓔ
2. Ⓐ Ⓑ Ⓒ Ⓓ Ⓔ
3. Ⓐ Ⓑ Ⓒ Ⓓ Ⓔ
4. Ⓐ Ⓑ Ⓒ Ⓓ Ⓔ
5. Ⓐ Ⓑ Ⓒ Ⓓ Ⓔ
6. Ⓐ Ⓑ Ⓒ Ⓓ Ⓔ
7. Ⓐ Ⓑ Ⓒ Ⓓ Ⓔ
8. Ⓐ Ⓑ Ⓒ Ⓓ Ⓔ
9. Ⓐ Ⓑ Ⓒ Ⓓ Ⓔ
10. Ⓐ Ⓑ Ⓒ Ⓓ Ⓔ
11. Ⓐ Ⓑ Ⓒ Ⓓ Ⓔ
12. Ⓐ Ⓑ Ⓒ Ⓓ Ⓔ
13. Ⓐ Ⓑ Ⓒ Ⓓ Ⓔ
14. Ⓐ Ⓑ Ⓒ Ⓓ Ⓔ
15. Ⓐ Ⓑ Ⓒ Ⓓ Ⓔ
16. Ⓐ Ⓑ Ⓒ Ⓓ Ⓔ
17. Ⓐ Ⓑ Ⓒ Ⓓ Ⓔ
18. Ⓐ Ⓑ Ⓒ Ⓓ Ⓔ
19. Ⓐ Ⓑ Ⓒ Ⓓ Ⓔ
20. Ⓐ Ⓑ Ⓒ Ⓓ Ⓔ
21. Ⓐ Ⓑ Ⓒ Ⓓ Ⓔ
22. Ⓐ Ⓑ Ⓒ Ⓓ Ⓔ
23. Ⓐ Ⓑ Ⓒ Ⓓ Ⓔ
24. Ⓐ Ⓑ Ⓒ Ⓓ Ⓔ
25. Ⓐ Ⓑ Ⓒ Ⓓ Ⓔ
26. Ⓐ Ⓑ Ⓒ Ⓓ Ⓔ
27. Ⓐ Ⓑ Ⓒ Ⓓ Ⓔ
28. Ⓐ Ⓑ Ⓒ Ⓓ Ⓔ
29. Ⓐ Ⓑ Ⓒ Ⓓ Ⓔ
30. Ⓐ Ⓑ Ⓒ Ⓓ Ⓔ
31. Ⓐ Ⓑ Ⓒ Ⓓ Ⓔ
32. Ⓐ Ⓑ Ⓒ Ⓓ Ⓔ
33. Ⓐ Ⓑ Ⓒ Ⓓ Ⓔ
34. Ⓐ Ⓑ Ⓒ Ⓓ Ⓔ
35. Ⓐ Ⓑ Ⓒ Ⓓ Ⓔ
36. Ⓐ Ⓑ Ⓒ Ⓓ Ⓔ
37. Ⓐ Ⓑ Ⓒ Ⓓ Ⓔ
38. Ⓐ Ⓑ Ⓒ Ⓓ Ⓔ

39. Ⓐ Ⓑ Ⓒ Ⓓ Ⓔ
40. Ⓐ Ⓑ Ⓒ Ⓓ Ⓔ
41. Ⓐ Ⓑ Ⓒ Ⓓ Ⓔ
42. Ⓐ Ⓑ Ⓒ Ⓓ Ⓔ
43. Ⓐ Ⓑ Ⓒ Ⓓ Ⓔ
44. Ⓐ Ⓑ Ⓒ Ⓓ Ⓔ
45. Ⓐ Ⓑ Ⓒ Ⓓ Ⓔ
46. Ⓐ Ⓑ Ⓒ Ⓓ Ⓔ
47. Ⓐ Ⓑ Ⓒ Ⓓ Ⓔ
48. Ⓐ Ⓑ Ⓒ Ⓓ Ⓔ
49. Ⓐ Ⓑ Ⓒ Ⓓ Ⓔ
50. Ⓐ Ⓑ Ⓒ Ⓓ Ⓔ
51. Ⓐ Ⓑ Ⓒ Ⓓ Ⓔ
52. Ⓐ Ⓑ Ⓒ Ⓓ Ⓔ
53. Ⓐ Ⓑ Ⓒ Ⓓ Ⓔ
54. Ⓐ Ⓑ Ⓒ Ⓓ Ⓔ
55. Ⓐ Ⓑ Ⓒ Ⓓ Ⓔ
56. Ⓐ Ⓑ Ⓒ Ⓓ Ⓔ
57. Ⓐ Ⓑ Ⓒ Ⓓ Ⓔ
58. Ⓐ Ⓑ Ⓒ Ⓓ Ⓔ
59. Ⓐ Ⓑ Ⓒ Ⓓ Ⓔ
60. Ⓐ Ⓑ Ⓒ Ⓓ Ⓔ
61. Ⓐ Ⓑ Ⓒ Ⓓ Ⓔ
62. Ⓐ Ⓑ Ⓒ Ⓓ Ⓔ
63. Ⓐ Ⓑ Ⓒ Ⓓ Ⓔ
64. Ⓐ Ⓑ Ⓒ Ⓓ Ⓔ
65. Ⓐ Ⓑ Ⓒ Ⓓ Ⓔ
66. Ⓐ Ⓑ Ⓒ Ⓓ Ⓔ
67. Ⓐ Ⓑ Ⓒ Ⓓ Ⓔ
68. Ⓐ Ⓑ Ⓒ Ⓓ Ⓔ
69. Ⓐ Ⓑ Ⓒ Ⓓ Ⓔ
70. Ⓐ Ⓑ Ⓒ Ⓓ Ⓔ
71. Ⓐ Ⓑ Ⓒ Ⓓ Ⓔ
72. Ⓐ Ⓑ Ⓒ Ⓓ Ⓔ
73. Ⓐ Ⓑ Ⓒ Ⓓ Ⓔ
74. Ⓐ Ⓑ Ⓒ Ⓓ Ⓔ
75. Ⓐ Ⓑ Ⓒ Ⓓ Ⓔ
76. Ⓐ Ⓑ Ⓒ Ⓓ Ⓔ

77. Ⓐ Ⓑ Ⓒ Ⓓ Ⓔ
78. Ⓐ Ⓑ Ⓒ Ⓓ Ⓔ
79. Ⓐ Ⓑ Ⓒ Ⓓ Ⓔ
80. Ⓐ Ⓑ Ⓒ Ⓓ Ⓔ
81. Ⓐ Ⓑ Ⓒ Ⓓ Ⓔ
82. Ⓐ Ⓑ Ⓒ Ⓓ Ⓔ
83. Ⓐ Ⓑ Ⓒ Ⓓ Ⓔ
84. Ⓐ Ⓑ Ⓒ Ⓓ Ⓔ
85. Ⓐ Ⓑ Ⓒ Ⓓ Ⓔ
86. Ⓐ Ⓑ Ⓒ Ⓓ Ⓔ
87. Ⓐ Ⓑ Ⓒ Ⓓ Ⓔ
88. Ⓐ Ⓑ Ⓒ Ⓓ Ⓔ
89. Ⓐ Ⓑ Ⓒ Ⓓ Ⓔ
90. Ⓐ Ⓑ Ⓒ Ⓓ Ⓔ
91. Ⓐ Ⓑ Ⓒ Ⓓ Ⓔ
92. Ⓐ Ⓑ Ⓒ Ⓓ Ⓔ
93. Ⓐ Ⓑ Ⓒ Ⓓ Ⓔ
94. Ⓐ Ⓑ Ⓒ Ⓓ Ⓔ
95. Ⓐ Ⓑ Ⓒ Ⓓ Ⓔ
96. Ⓐ Ⓑ Ⓒ Ⓓ Ⓔ
97. Ⓐ Ⓑ Ⓒ Ⓓ Ⓔ
98. Ⓐ Ⓑ Ⓒ Ⓓ Ⓔ
99. Ⓐ Ⓑ Ⓒ Ⓓ Ⓔ
100. Ⓐ Ⓑ Ⓒ Ⓓ Ⓔ
101. Ⓐ Ⓑ Ⓒ Ⓓ Ⓔ
102. Ⓐ Ⓑ Ⓒ Ⓓ Ⓔ
103. Ⓐ Ⓑ Ⓒ Ⓓ Ⓔ
104. Ⓐ Ⓑ Ⓒ Ⓓ Ⓔ
105. Ⓐ Ⓑ Ⓒ Ⓓ Ⓔ
106. Ⓐ Ⓑ Ⓒ Ⓓ Ⓔ
107. Ⓐ Ⓑ Ⓒ Ⓓ Ⓔ
108. Ⓐ Ⓑ Ⓒ Ⓓ Ⓔ
109. Ⓐ Ⓑ Ⓒ Ⓓ Ⓔ
110. Ⓐ Ⓑ Ⓒ Ⓓ Ⓔ
111. Ⓐ Ⓑ Ⓒ Ⓓ Ⓔ
112. Ⓐ Ⓑ Ⓒ Ⓓ Ⓔ
113. Ⓐ Ⓑ Ⓒ Ⓓ Ⓔ
114. Ⓐ Ⓑ Ⓒ Ⓓ Ⓔ

115. Ⓐ Ⓑ Ⓒ Ⓓ Ⓔ
116. Ⓐ Ⓑ Ⓒ Ⓓ Ⓔ
117. Ⓐ Ⓑ Ⓒ Ⓓ Ⓔ
118. Ⓐ Ⓑ Ⓒ Ⓓ Ⓔ
119. Ⓐ Ⓑ Ⓒ Ⓓ Ⓔ
120. Ⓐ Ⓑ Ⓒ Ⓓ Ⓔ
121. Ⓐ Ⓑ Ⓒ Ⓓ Ⓔ
122. Ⓐ Ⓑ Ⓒ Ⓓ Ⓔ
123. Ⓐ Ⓑ Ⓒ Ⓓ Ⓔ
124. Ⓐ Ⓑ Ⓒ Ⓓ Ⓔ
125. Ⓐ Ⓑ Ⓒ Ⓓ Ⓔ
126. Ⓐ Ⓑ Ⓒ Ⓓ Ⓔ
127. Ⓐ Ⓑ Ⓒ Ⓓ Ⓔ
128. Ⓐ Ⓑ Ⓒ Ⓓ Ⓔ
129. Ⓐ Ⓑ Ⓒ Ⓓ Ⓔ
130. Ⓐ Ⓑ Ⓒ Ⓓ Ⓔ
131. Ⓐ Ⓑ Ⓒ Ⓓ Ⓔ
132. Ⓐ Ⓑ Ⓒ Ⓓ Ⓔ
133. Ⓐ Ⓑ Ⓒ Ⓓ Ⓔ
134. Ⓐ Ⓑ Ⓒ Ⓓ Ⓔ
135. Ⓐ Ⓑ Ⓒ Ⓓ Ⓔ
136. Ⓐ Ⓑ Ⓒ Ⓓ Ⓔ
137. Ⓐ Ⓑ Ⓒ Ⓓ Ⓔ
138. Ⓐ Ⓑ Ⓒ Ⓓ Ⓔ
139. Ⓐ Ⓑ Ⓒ Ⓓ Ⓔ
140. Ⓐ Ⓑ Ⓒ Ⓓ Ⓔ
141. Ⓐ Ⓑ Ⓒ Ⓓ Ⓔ
142. Ⓐ Ⓑ Ⓒ Ⓓ Ⓔ
143. Ⓐ Ⓑ Ⓒ Ⓓ Ⓔ
144. Ⓐ Ⓑ Ⓒ Ⓓ Ⓔ
145. Ⓐ Ⓑ Ⓒ Ⓓ Ⓔ
146. Ⓐ Ⓑ Ⓒ Ⓓ Ⓔ
147. Ⓐ Ⓑ Ⓒ Ⓓ Ⓔ
148. Ⓐ Ⓑ Ⓒ Ⓓ Ⓔ
149. Ⓐ Ⓑ Ⓒ Ⓓ Ⓔ
150. Ⓐ Ⓑ Ⓒ Ⓓ Ⓔ

Trial Test

This chapter contains a Trial Test in Humanities. Take this Trial Test to learn what the actual exam is like and to determine how you might score on the exam before any practice or review.

The CLEP Exam in Humanities measures your knowledge of literature and the arts—the visual arts such as painting and sculpture, music, the performing arts such as drama, dance, and architecture.

Number of Questions: 150

TIME LIMIT: 90 MINUTES

DIRECTIONS: Each of the questions or incomplete statements below is followed by five suggested answers or completions. Select the one that is best in each case.

1. Expressionism in art has most to do with

   (A) the intellect
   (B) the emotions
   (C) the dream world
   (D) geometric forms
   (E) decorative line

2. The Impressionists were least concerned with

   (A) the effects of light
   (B) informal treatment of subject matter
   (C) painting out of doors
   (D) interpenetration of forms
   (E) broken application of color

3. The length of a vibrating string or a column of air and the pitch either produces constituted the beginning of the science of

   (A) logarithms
   (B) rhythms
   (C) acoustics
   (D) theory
   (E) fuguery

4. The man who, practically single-handedly, unified the ballet and founded French opera was

   (A) Lully
   (B) Glinka
   (C) Gluck
   (D) Massenet
   (E) Offenbach

5. An important architect of the Romantic period was

   (A) Walter Gropius
   (B) Christopher Wren
   (C) James Wyatt
   (D) Joseph Paxton
   (E) Henri Labrouste

6. Ibsen did not write

   (A) plays about contemporary people
   (B) plays with realistic settings
   (C) plays employing well-made structure
   (D) comedies of manners
   (E) thesis plays

7. The release of emotions and the attaining of tranquillity therefrom in the theater is called

   (A) pyramidal plot structure
   (B) the author's use of hubris
   (C) the audience escaping dull lives by identifying with kings, aristocrats, and famous people
   (D) empathy
   (E) catharsis

8. One of the most characteristic types of 18th-century literature was the

   (A) novella
   (B) epic
   (C) nature poem
   (D) periodical essay
   (E) thesis play

9. Harriet Beecher Stowe unwittingly became a pioneer when she wrote the "propaganda novel"

   (A) *Erewhon*
   (B) *A Man's Woman*
   (C) *The Female Quixote*
   (D) *Uncle Tom's Cabin*
   (E) *The Mysterious Stranger*

10. "Brush my brow with burnished bronze" is an example of

   (A) alliteration
   (B) consonance
   (C) dissonance
   (D) onomatopoeia
   (E) free verse

11. Stravinsky's "Rite of Spring"

   (A) is a Baroque-style program piece
   (B) was called the destruction of music
   (C) is representative of the Classical styles
   (D) is in sonata-allegro form
   (E) is a symphony

12. An instrumental form usually associated with opera is

   (A) the overture
   (B) the symphony
   (C) the suite
   (D) the tone poem
   (E) the cadenza

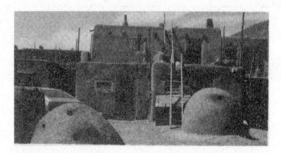

13. The type of architecture shown is found in

   (A) India
   (B) Greece
   (C) The United States
   (D) Russia
   (E) Iran

14. Paintings that reflect an interest in the fantastic, dream associations, and the impossible are most likely to have been executed by

(A) Cézanne, van Gogh, Toulouse-Lautrec
(B) Gris, Braque, Picasso
(C) Dali, Miró, de Chirico
(D) Pollack, Motherwell, Mondrian
(E) Renoir, Degas, Seurat

15. Confucius, Buddha, and Socrates, all born at the time when "the human mind seems first to have turned over in its sleep," lived in approximately

(A) 1200–1100 B.C.
(B) 2500–2400 B.C.
(C) 5000–4000 B.C.
(D) 800–700 B.C.
(E) 600–400 B.C.

Questions 16 and 17 refer to the following quotation.

"O mother, mother, make my bed,
O make it soft and narrow:
Since my love died for me today,
I'll die for him tomorrow."

16. Which of the following describes these lines?

(A) a couplet
(B) a triolet
(C) a quatrain
(D) a tercet
(E) a sestet

17. The lines are from the ballad

(A) "Sir Patrick Spens"
(B) "Barbara Allen"
(C) "Lord Randall"
(D) "The Three Ravens"
(E) "Robin Hood and the Three Squires"

18. Pop art refers to

(A) musical themes
(B) abstract Expressionism
(C) contemporary materialism and commercialism
(D) the religious revival in contemporary art
(E) a return to Classicism

19. The first to dedicate their art to the beauty of the human form were the

(A) Egyptians
(B) Renaissance artists
(C) Romans
(D) Greeks
(E) French Impressionists

20. Frank Lloyd Wright's basic role in architecture was

(A) to build a structure that was inexpensive
(B) to use a minimum of materials
(C) to build a structure in harmony with the past
(D) to build a structure that looked as if it grew out of the ground
(E) to build a structure that overpowers man and nature

21. Albert Camus said that capital punishment is

(A) necessary and desirable
(B) necessary but undesirable
(C) murder
(D) a 20th-century innovation
(E) both (A) and (C)

22. One of the greatest of the Middle High German epics is

(A) *The Nibelungenlied*
(B) *The Story of Sigurd the Volsung*
(C) *Beowulf*
(D) *The Vikings at Helgeland*
(E) *The Valkyrie*

23. A famous piece of music often associated with graduation exercises was written by

    (A) Elgar
    (B) Condon
    (C) Gluck
    (D) Palestrina
    (E) Haydn

24. A famous jazz drummer of the 1940s was

    (A) F. Waller
    (B) B. Davidson
    (C) E. Condon
    (D) J. Teagarden
    (E) M. Feld

25. Shakespeare is noted for all but one of the following:

    (A) comedies
    (B) tragedies
    (C) bourgeois dramas
    (D) histories
    (E) tragicomedies

26. An outdoor amphitheater seating 20,000 people that has been the scene of ballets and popular concerts directed by world-famous orchestral conductors is the

    (A) Rose Bowl
    (B) Snow Bowl
    (C) Hollywood Bowl
    (D) Musitoreum
    (E) Sunshine Theater

27. The "father" of Greek tragedy was

    (A) Aristotle
    (B) Sophocles
    (C) Euripides
    (D) Aeschylus
    (E) Aristophanes

28. All but one of the following are parts of the Greek theater:

    (A) eccyclema
    (B) skene
    (C) deus ex machina
    (D) orchestra
    (E) movable panels

29. All of the following are films directed by Ingmar Bergman *except*

    (A) *Persona*
    (B) *Winter Light*
    (C) *The Seventh Seal*
    (D) *The Magic Flute*
    (E) *The 400 Blows*

30. The term "Western man" or "Western civilization" refers to

    (A) the Western hemisphere
    (B) our present cultural tradition going back about 4,000 years
    (C) a force of history that always moves to the west
    (D) Europe
    (E) Canada and the United States

31. Richard Strauss is best known for his

    (A) fugues
    (B) motets
    (C) waltzes
    (D) madrigals
    (E) tone poems

32. Albert Camus, French existentialist writer, believed that the only real philosophical problem was that of suicide. What Shakespearean character expresses this same thought?

    (A) Iago
    (B) Cleopatra
    (C) Hamlet
    (D) Caliban
    (E) Julius Caesar

33. Cubism is indebted to the pioneering work of

(A) Pollack
(B) Cézanne
(C) van Gogh
(D) Munch
(E) Hals

34. Which one of the following is not a stylistic (formal) element of Cubism?

(A) compressed or "flat" space
(B) multiple perspective
(C) atmospheric perspective
(D) interpenetration of line, color, and shape
(E) an equal stress on negative and positive areas

35. The term *clerestory* would most likely be used by a(n)

(A) poet
(B) architect
(C) sculptor
(D) painter
(E) musician

36. All of the following short stories were written by Edgar Allan Poe *except*

(A) "The Fall of the House of Usher"
(B) "The Murders in the Rue Morgue"
(C) "Rappaccini's Daughter"
(D) "The Purloined Letter"
(E) "The Cask of Amontillado"

37. Sculpture is the art of

(A) making lifelike figures
(B) making statues of heroes
(C) making memorials to heroes
(D) cutting stone and marble
(E) composing in mass and space

38. The philosopher famous for the doctrine that "to be is to be perceived" is

(A) Berkeley
(B) Leibniz
(C) Hegel
(D) Plato
(E) Hume

39. The beginning of the Renaissance may be traced to the city of

(A) Rome
(B) San Miniate
(C) Venice
(D) Florence
(E) Athens

40. The "School of Lyon" was

(A) a 16th-century group of Neo-Platonist and Petrarchan poets
(B) an 18th-century artistic movement
(C) the college attended by Hugo and de Maupassant
(D) a chamber music society founded by Massenet
(E) an attempt to establish a classical spirit in French painting

41. The first important American naturalistic novel, *Maggie: A Girl of the Streets*, was written by

(A) Anderson
(B) Garland
(C) Norris
(D) Crane
(E) Robinson

42. The painters Renoir, Monet, and Pissaro were

(A) Expressionists
(B) Cubists
(C) Mannerists
(D) Impressionists
(E) Surrealists

43. The Romans made special use of

    (A) post and lintel construction
    (B) friezes carved over temple doorways
    (C) the rounded arch
    (D) the pointed arch
    (E) tempera painting

44. In music, a smooth transition from key to key is known as

    (A) modulation
    (B) constructioning
    (C) harmony
    (D) invention
    (E) translation

45. All of the following deal with the Trojan War or the men who fought in that war *except*

    (A) *The Odyssey*
    (B) *Agamemnon*
    (C) *The Iliad*
    (D) *Oedipus the King*
    (E) *The Aeneid*

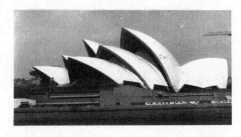

46. This well-known landmark is found in

    (A) New York Harbor
    (B) Ceylon
    (C) India
    (D) Australia
    (E) Japan

47. The first major American author to be born west of the Mississippi was

    (A) William Dean Howells
    (B) Walt Whitman
    (C) Carl Sandburg
    (D) Mark Twain
    (E) Ellen Glasgow

48. "Twas brillig, and the slithy toves, Did gyre and gimble in the wabe," is an example of

    (A) *vers de société*
    (B) nonsense verse
    (C) a limerick
    (D) shaped verse
    (E) Goliardic verse

49. Farcical interludes in dramas

    (A) developed during the Middle Ages
    (B) dealt with sin
    (C) were essentially romantic comedies
    (D) developed during the Renaissance
    (E) adhered to the unities of time, place, and action

50. *The Decameron*, like *The Canterbury Tales*, has a specific dramatic framework. However, instead of pilgrims journeying to Canterbury, *The Decameron* has seven women and three men withdrawing from their native city for what purpose?

    (A) To seek the Holy Grail
    (B) To visit the Pope
    (C) To see Charles the Great
    (D) To make pilgrimage to the tomb of Abelard
    (E) To escape the Black Death

51. "All pigs are equal, but some pigs are more equal than others" is a line from what novel?

    (A) *Lassie, Come Home*
    (B) *The Red Pony*
    (C) *Federico and his Falcon*
    (D) *Animal Farm*
    (E) *A Day at the Zoo*

52. An American tap dancer who appeared in musical comedies, revues, and motion pictures is

    (A) Mikhail Baryshnikov
    (B) Ray Jones
    (C) Adolph Bolm
    (D) David Klein
    (E) Ray Bolger

53. "The Grand Canyon Suite" was composed by

(A) Anton Dvorák
(B) George M. Cohan
(C) Edward McDowell
(D) Aaron Copland
(E) Ferde Grofé

54. The medieval architect symbolized God's presence in the cathedral by

(A) creating great areas of interior space
(B) embellishing the surface with great columns and lacy decorations
(C) creating the choir and high altar areas
(D) combining the arts of painting and free-standing sculpture
(E) placing gargoyles atop the roof to ward off evil spirits

55. "The lost generation" refers to those who lived during the period

(A) 1900–1915
(B) 1920–1940
(C) 1940–1950
(D) 1950–1960
(E) 1960–1970

56. A leader of the "beat generation" was

(A) Ernest Hemingway
(B) John Steinbeck
(C) Jack Kerouac
(D) Ring Lardner
(E) Flannery O'Connor

57. A short narrative from which a moral can be drawn is

(A) a parable
(B) an anecdote
(C) an abstraction
(D) an aphorism
(E) a frame story

58. Lascaux and Altamira are

(A) two French Gothic cathedrals
(B) two painters working in a surrealistic style
(C) caves in which prehistoric paintings have been found
(D) mythological subjects used by Pierre Cot in "The Tempest"
(E) leaders in the Fauve movement

59. A feeling of unrest and tension in a painting can be achieved by a powerful emphasis upon

(A) horizontal line
(B) vertical line
(C) parallel line
(D) diagonal line
(E) linear grid pattern

60. The way in which we perceive abstractly is largely determined by

(A) cultural conditioning
(B) memory learning
(C) individual genes
(D) intellectual association
(E) abstract behavior patterns

61. One of the first American "troubadors" and minstrels was

(A) Vachel Lindsay
(B) Edward McDowell
(C) John Knowles Pain
(D) Aaron Copland
(E) Stephen Foster

62. An early American statesman, writer, inventor, and foreign correspondent, also known as the first American music critic, was

(A) Paul Revere
(B) Cotton Mather
(C) Benjamin Franklin
(D) Thomas Jefferson
(E) Patrick Henry

63. "I have measured out my life with coffee spoons," said

   (A) Benjamin Compson
   (B) Lady Brett Ashley
   (C) Scarlet O'Hara
   (D) Phillip Jordan
   (E) J. Alfred Prufrock

64. A "mystery circle" may best be described as

   (A) based upon scriptures
   (B) basically religious
   (C) short biblical plays produced outside the church
   (D) performed by the guilds
   (E) all of the above

65. Which of the following has been hailed as a great novel of the women's movement?

   (A) *The Golden Notebook* by Doris Lessing
   (B) *Emma* by Jane Austen
   (C) *Wise Blood* by Flannery O'Connor
   (D) *Fluff* by Virginia Woolf
   (E) *Swain* by Carolyn Kimball

66. A satire on the medieval chivalric code is

   (A) *Don Quixote*
   (B) *Gulliver's Travels*
   (C) *Candide*
   (D) *Idylls of the King*
   (E) *Erewhon*

67. One of the most popular English painters of the 18th century, noted for his society portraits, was

   (A) John Singleton Copley
   (B) Sir Edward Burne-Jones
   (C) Thomas Gainsborough
   (D) John Constable
   (E) William Blake

68. Included among Johann Sebastian Bach's great works is

   (A) "The Well-Tempered Clavier"
   (B) "The Pathétique Sonata"
   (C) *The Student Prince*
   (D) "The Unfinished Symphony"
   (E) *Der Rosenkavalier*

69. Included among Beethoven's great works is

   (A) "The Symphonie Espagnole"
   (B) "The Moonlight Sonata"
   (C) "The Mass in B Minor"
   (D) *Messiah*
   (E) "The Minute Waltz"

70. Nicknamed "Red," the man who became famous for his novels about "main street" America was

   (A) Ernest Hemingway
   (B) John Steinbeck
   (C) Sinclair Lewis
   (D) Upton Sinclair
   (E) Booth Tarkington

71. The creative process is

   (A) limited to art
   (B) limited to art and music
   (C) limited to the humanities
   (D) limited to the arts and sciences
   (E) not limited to any one area

72. Of the Greek playwrights, Euripides is considered the most "modern" because he

   (A) usually disregards the unities
   (B) concentrates on message rather than moments
   (C) does not use women as protagonists
   (D) stresses his belief in reform
   (E) is most psychological in his treatment of conflict

73. Of which playwright is the following true: Nearly every character in his plays is at one time or another the hero of a tiny "microcosmic" drama that has a beginning, middle, and an end in itself, but does not become the basis for the total plot?

(A) George Bernard Shaw
(B) Henrik Ibsen
(C) Arthur Miller
(D) Anton Chekov
(E) Oscar Wilde

74. The opera *I Pagliacci* was written by

(A) Puccini
(B) Leoncavallo
(C) Mascagni
(D) Verdi
(E) Mozart

75. In music, this sign ♭ is called a

(A) flat
(B) sharp
(C) bass clef
(D) treble clef
(E) time signature

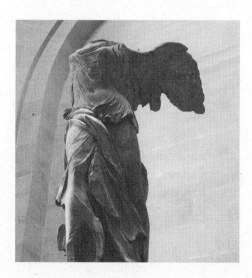

76. The photograph above is

(A) Nike of Samothrace
(B) Venus de Milo
(C) Mercury
(D) Apollo Belvedere
(E) Dionysius

77. The audiences who attended Shakespeare's plays were

(A) aristocrats who enjoyed occasionally letting their hair down
(B) commoners who had aristocratic taste in poetry
(C) primarily drawn from the middle classes
(D) a mixture of all classes
(E) the most tightly knit "in group" in the history of the theater

78. All of the following represent serious barriers to critical perception of plays and films *except*

(A) failing to remember that a drama is not reality
(B) viewing the drama in terms of a particular occupation with which the viewer is familiar
(C) reacting to the characterization of an ethnic type
(D) accepting the drama on its own terms without any bias
(E) entering the theater with the expectation of seeing one's moral values upheld

79. All of the following painters were called by critics "Fauve" or "wild beasts" *except*

(A) Matisse
(B) Dufy
(C) Vlaminck
(D) Rouault
(E) Gauguin

80. The chief exponent of pointillism was

(A) Cézanne
(B) Monet
(C) de Chirico
(D) Courbet
(E) Seurat

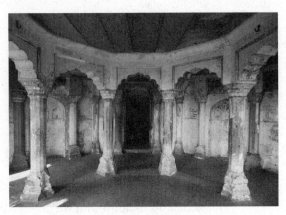

© Charlene Winfred

81. The photograph shows an interior of Amber Fort. What styles of ornamentation can be seen here?

(A) Buddhist and Hindu
(B) Ottoman and Persian
(C) Hindu and Mughal
(D) Moslem and Romanesque
(E) Byzantine and Moorish

82. A chromatic scale is

(A) all half steps played in order
(B) every other half step played in order
(C) no half steps played
(D) only half steps played
(E) all full steps played in order

Questions 83–85 refer to the following lines:

Come live with me, and be my love,
And we will all the pleasures prove,
That valleys, groves, hills, and fields,
Woods or steepy mountains yields.

83. These lines are from

(A) "The Passionate Shepherd to His Love"
(B) "The Shepherd's Wife's Song"
(C) "A Strange Passion of a Lover"
(D) one of Shakespeare's sonnets
(E) "Troilus and Cressida"

84. The lines were written by

(A) William Shakespeare
(B) Christopher Marlowe
(C) John Lyly
(D) T.S. Eliot
(E) Alexander Pope

85. The verse form is a

(A) couplet
(B) sestina
(C) sonnet
(D) quatrain
(E) cinquaine

86. Most basic to a fundamental appreciation of art are

(A) seeing and feeling
(B) words and descriptions
(C) knowing the life of the artist and understanding his or her ethnic background
(D) understanding the theories of art and their corollaries
(E) courses in art history

87. "Comfort ye, comfort ye, my people," saith your God. "Speak ye comfortably to Jerusalem, and cry unto her, that her warfare is accomplished, that her iniquity is pardoned."

The source of this quotation, which is a portion of the libretto of Handel's *Messiah* and was taken directly from the Bible, was

(A) Amos
(B) Misab
(C) Isaiah
(D) Ezekiel
(E) Hosea

Questions 88–90 refer to the following groups of people:

(A) John Williams, Burt Bacharach, Henry Mancini
(B) Sir George Solti, André Previn, Leonard Bernstein
(C) John Steinbeck, William Faulkner, Sinclair Lewis
(D) Andy Warhol, Joan Miró, Claes Oldenburg
(E) Twyla Tharp, Michael Bennett, Gower Champion

88. Which is a group of contemporary symphony conductors?

89. Which is a group of novelists who won the Nobel Prize for Literature?

90. Which is a group of choreographers for Broadway musicals of the 1970s and 1980s?

91. *The Great Gatsby* was written by

(A) Emerson
(B) Lewis
(C) Dreiser
(D) Dos Passos
(E) Fitzgerald

92. Nietzsche said that the noble man

(A) never notices the unfortunate
(B) always helps the unfortunate out of pity
(C) always seeks to eradicate the unfortunate
(D) helps the unfortunate, not from pity, but rather from an impulse generated out of a superabundance of power
(E) always tries to trick the unfortunate into helping him

93. *Kiss Me Kate* is based upon William Shakespeare's play

(A) *Romeo and Juliet*
(B) *The Winter's Tale*
(C) *A Midsummer Night's Dream*
(D) *The Tempest*
(E) *The Taming of the Shrew*

94. The artist van Gogh wrote that he

(A) did his best not to put in detail
(B) avoided using black altogether
(C) could paint only when he was nervous
(D) became an artist in order to travel and see the world
(E) became an artist in order to prove he was sane

95. The musical notation  indicates

(A) the bass clef
(B) crescendo
(C) pianissimo
(D) the treble clef
(E) 1/2 time

96. A term used to describe choral music without instrumental accompaniment is

(A) cantilena
(B) a cappella
(C) enharmonic
(D) appoggiatura
(E) oratorio

97. "The greatest happiness for the greatest number" is the ethical objective of

   (A) Pragmatism
   (B) Scholasticism
   (C) Hegelianism
   (D) utilitarianism
   (E) hedonism

98. A Southern writer well known for her short stories, as well as her novels *Wise Blood* and *The Violent Bear It Away*, is

   (A) Gwendolyn Brooks
   (B) Jean Auel
   (C) Frances Cassidy
   (D) Flannery O'Connor
   (E) Elizabeth James

99. Baroque architecture is characterized by

   (A) severe simplicity
   (B) ornamentation and curved lines
   (C) post and lintel construction
   (D) steel and reinforced concrete
   (E) low, heavy domes

100. A good definition of art is

   (A) significant form
   (B) a production or procession of images expressing the personality of the artist
   (C) a reflection in visual form of the philosophy and culture of the period
   (D) nature seen through the emotion and intellect of man
   (E) all of the above

101. The first spoken line by Hamlet in the play is an aside: "A little more than kin, and less than kind." By this line, he indicates that

   (A) he already suspects Claudius of some sort of duplicity
   (B) he already knows that Claudius has killed his father
   (C) he already has designs on the throne
   (D) he is already plotting revenge
   (E) he intends to feign madness

102. The Connecticut Wits

   (A) were devoted to the modernization of the Yale curriculum and the declaration of independence of American letters from British influences
   (B) favored Unitarianism and Transcendentalism
   (C) included Timothy Dwight, john Trumbull, and Joel Barlow
   (D) all of the above
   (E) (A) and (C) above

103. A Latin-American writer, author of *One Hundred Years of Solitude*, is

   (A) Isabel Allende
   (B) Carlos Noriega
   (C) Gabriel García Márquez
   (D) Pablo Neruda
   (E) Guillermo González

104. The creator of Charlie Brown is

   (A) Bud Blake
   (B) Al Capp
   (C) Charles Schulz
   (D) Alex Kotsby
   (E) Fred Lasswell

105. "Each narrow cell in which we dwell" provides an example of

   (A) alliteration
   (B) internal rhyme
   (C) sprung rhythm
   (D) end rhyme
   (E) spondaic trimeter

106. A playwright who wrote a modern comic-psychological version of *Antigone* is

   (A) Arther Miller
   (B) Jean Anouilh
   (C) Edward Albee
   (D) Jean-Paul Sartre
   (E) Georges Clemenceau

107. This is an example of

(A) Mesopotamian sculpture
(B) Egyptian sculpture
(C) Indian sculpture
(D) prehistoric sculpture
(E) modern sculpture

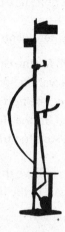

Estate of David Smith,
courtesy of Marlborough Gallery, New York

108. Molière's audiences were predominantly

(A) peasants
(B) a great cross-section of the population
(C) people pretending to a higher station in life
(D) aristocrats
(E) middle class only

109. Edgar Allan Poe believed a short story should

(A) be sufficiently short to permit the reader to finish the work in a single sitting
(B) have a surprise ending
(C) delight and instruct the reader
(D) have complicated characters
(E) be realistic

110. The French word *genre* means

(A) plot
(B) category
(C) climax
(D) story
(E) introduction

111. What Renaissance writer do you associate with the Abbey of Theleme?

(A) Castiglione
(B) Shakespeare
(C) Ariosto
(D) Rabelais
(E) Cervantes

112. Ursula K. LeGuin is regarded primarily as a writer of

(A) poetry
(B) romantic fiction
(C) mysteries
(D) spy stories
(E) science fiction

113. A 19th-century novelist who anticipated many 20th-century discoveries and inventions was

(A) T.H. Huxley
(B) Mary Shelley
(C) Thomas Hardy
(D) Jules Verne
(E) Bram Stoker

114. According to tradition, who wrote *The Odyssey* and *The Iliad*?

(A) Achilles
(B) Tacitus
(C) Homer
(D) Vergil
(E) Thucydides

115. A form of music drama without stage action, of which Handel became a master, is the

(A) oratorio
(B) opera
(C) cantata
(D) castrati
(E) duet

116. The conductor's copy of the notes contains all the notes for each player in the orchestra. It is called the

    (A) score
    (B) libretto
    (C) manuscript
    (D) theme
    (E) thesis

117. The theme of John Steinbeck's *In Dubious Battle* is

    (A) the exodus of the Okies from Oklahoma
    (B) the growth of labor unions in America
    (C) the frustration of the war in Vietnam
    (D) the blacks' fight for freedom
    (E) World War II

118. An Aeschylean dramatic pattern made possible the first true plays because it introduced

    (A) villainy
    (B) humanism
    (C) plausibility
    (D) conflict between two characters
    (E) the family theme

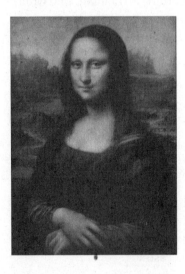

119. The portrait above was painted by

    (A) da Vinci
    (B) Delacroix
    (C) van Gogh
    (D) Michelangelo
    (E) Dali

120. A pieta portrays

    (A) the dead Christ held by Mary
    (B) the canonization ceremony of a saint in the Roman Catholic Church
    (C) the Archangel Gabriel telling Mary that she will give birth to the Son of God
    (D) Christ's death on the cross
    (E) the birth of Jesus Christ in a stable

121. Why did Jason set sail on his fateful voyage?

    (A) To search for the Golden Fleece
    (B) To make war on Sparta
    (C) To destroy the port of Colchis
    (D) To search for the Holy Grail
    (E) To put a stop to pirateering

122. Most scholars believe that the Dead Sea scrolls were part of the library of some

    (A) Buddhists
    (B) Platonists
    (C) Essenes
    (D) Pharisees
    (E) Sadducees

123. The architect associated with St. Paul's Cathedral is

    (A) Inigo Jones
    (B) Christopher Wren
    (C) Le Corbusier
    (D) Frank Lloyd Wright
    (E) Walter Gropius

124. The opening scene of Shakespeare's *Henry IV, Part I* establishes for the audience that

    (A) all is well in England
    (B) a pilgrimage to the Holy Land is in progress
    (C) it is raining
    (D) the king has two major problems confronting him
    (E) the king is dead

125. Byzantine art was a major contribution to the world because of its

(A) sculpture
(B) portraits
(C) armor
(D) mosaics
(E) glassware

126. The variety of styles in modern art is a reflection of

(A) the complexity of modern life
(B) a lack of purpose
(C) a loss of values
(D) foreign influence
(E) our susceptibility to sensationalism and fads

127. In formal science, *all* statements are

(A) intuitively true
(B) given meaning by induction
(C) hypothetically true
(D) empirically true
(E) given meaning by experiment

128. The poem "Trees" was written by

(A) E.E. Cummings
(B) Edna St. Vincent Millay
(C) Joyce Kilmer
(D) Lawrence Ferlinghetti
(E) John Frederick Nims

129. Voltaire's Candide journeyed from continent to continent to find his elusive Cunegonde, whose chief virtue was

(A) beauty
(B) physical indestructibility
(C) piety
(D) faithfulness
(E) mental alertness

130. *The Tales of Hoffmann* was written by

(A) De Maistre
(B) Bierce
(C) Poe
(D) Hoffmann
(E) Irving

131. The operatic score for *The Tales of Hoffmann* was written by

(A) Offenbach
(B) Adam
(C) Rimsky-Korsakov
(D) Schubert
(E) Schumann

132. When the Christian Church came into power after the fall of the Roman Empire, it

(A) used professional actors to perform plays
(B) urged the wealthy to sponsor acting groups
(C) emphasized the "here" rather than the "hereafter"
(D) abolished all theatrical activities
(E) began putting on plays in the church itself

133. The death of Seneca in A.D. 65 marks the

(A) end of the Roman Empire
(B) beginning of creative playwrighting
(C) end of creative playwrighting until the Middle Ages
(D) beginning of the Middle Ages
(E) birth of comedy

134. Which of the following, written during the Revolutionary period, is often considered the first American novel?

(A) *McTeague*
(B) *Moby Dick*
(C) *Huckleberry Finn*
(D) *Golden Wedding*
(E) *The Power of Sympathy*

135. The Artful Dodger is a character in the novel

(A) *Oliver Twist*
(B) *The Little Prince*
(C) *Hard Times*
(D) *David Copperfield*
(E) *Vanity Fair*

136. One of the greatest jazz musicians of all time is

    (A) "Dizzy" Gillespie
    (B) Ray Charles
    (C) Pete Seeger
    (D) Arthel Watson
    (E) David Byrne

137. John Milton in *Paradise Lost* attempted to

    (A) justify the ways of men to God
    (B) justify the ways of God to men
    (C) explain evil
    (D) show that Satan and God have equal powers
    (E) explain why good and evil are necessary

138. The two great Italian writers of the 14th century were

    (A) Petrarch and Pirandello
    (B) Petrarch and Boccaccio
    (C) Dante and Fellini
    (D) Boccaccio and Silone
    (E) Machiavelli and Borgia

139. The ghost advises Hamlet, concerning his mother, to

    (A) make certain that she does not escape death
    (B) bring her to public trial and let the people of Denmark decide her fate
    (C) wash her incestuous sheets
    (D) allow heaven to decide her fate
    (E) deny her Christian burial so that her soul will wander forever, as his is doomed to do

140. A sonata is a musical composition for instruments. A cantata is

    (A) a slow symphony
    (B) an aria
    (C) a slow madrigal
    (D) a choral work
    (E) a round

141. "But I will start afresh and make dark things plain. In doing right by Laius, I protect myself . . . ," said

    (A) Phoebus
    (B) Oedipus
    (C) Ismene
    (D) Creon
    (E) Jocasta

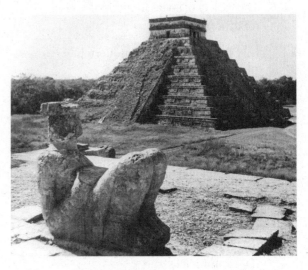

Ruth S. Ward

142. The photograph above pictures

    (A) an Egyptian temple
    (B) an Etruscan temple
    (C) a Mayan temple
    (D) a Greek temple
    (E) a Roman temple

143. A chilling modern novel by Margaret Atwood is

    (A) *A Handmaid's Tale*
    (B) *Fear of Flying*
    (C) *The House of Sorrows*
    (D) *The Eiger Sanction*
    (E) *As I Lay Dying*

144. The rhyme scheme of Dante's *Divine Comedy* in its original Italian is

    (A) sestina
    (B) terza rima
    (C) sonnet
    (D) ballade
    (E) rondeau

145. The magnificent achievements of Gothic art are found especially in

(A) the structures of the great cathedrals
(B) the carving of statues on the porches of these cathedrals
(C) the beauty of stained glass
(D) the invention of the flying buttress
(E) all of the above

146. All of the following Americans were awarded the Nobel Prize for Literature *except*

(A) Pearl S. Buck
(B) William Faulkner
(C) Robert Frost
(D) Ernest Hemingway
(E) Eugene O'Neill

147. A soliloquy is

(A) A short speech delivered to the audience while other characters are on stage
(B) a few moments of pantomime by the main character in a play
(C) a speech of some length spoken directly to the audience while the character speaking is alone on stage
(D) a verbal exchange between two characters on stage
(E) a short, comic speech by the protagonist

148. Which of the following painters produced a number of canvasses of jungle plants and animals?

(A) Henri Rousseau
(B) Paul Cézanne
(C) Jackson Pollock
(D) Mary Cassatt
(E) Andy Warhol

149. Which of the following conductors began with opera and for many years headed the New York Philharmonic?

(A) George Szell
(B) Sir John Barbarolli
(C) Herbert von Karajan
(D) Arturo Toscanini
(E) André Previn

150. A handkerchief plays a key role in which of the following tragedies?

(A) *All for Love*
(B) *Othello*
(C) *King Lear*
(D) *Antony and Cleopatra*
(E) *Macbeth*

STOP

If there is still time remaining, you may review your answers.

ANSWER KEY
Trial Test

HUMANITIES

1.	**B**	39.	**D**	77.	**D**	115.	**A**
2.	**D**	40.	**A**	78.	**D**	116.	**A**
3.	**C**	41.	**D**	79.	**E**	117.	**B**
4.	**A**	42.	**D**	80.	**E**	118.	**D**
5.	**C**	43.	**C**	81.	**C**	119.	**A**
6.	**D**	44.	**A**	82.	**A**	120.	**A**
7.	**E**	45.	**D**	83.	**A**	121.	**A**
8.	**D**	46.	**D**	84.	**B**	122.	**C**
9.	**D**	47.	**D**	85.	**D**	123.	**B**
10.	**A**	48.	**B**	86.	**A**	124.	**D**
11.	**B**	49.	**A**	87.	**C**	125.	**D**
12.	**A**	50.	**E**	88.	**B**	126.	**A**
13.	**C**	51.	**D**	89.	**C**	127.	**E**
14.	**C**	52.	**E**	90.	**E**	128.	**C**
15.	**E**	53.	**E**	91.	**E**	129.	**B**
16.	**C**	54.	**A**	92.	**D**	130.	**D**
17.	**B**	55.	**B**	93.	**E**	131.	**A**
18.	**C**	56.	**C**	94.	**E**	132.	**D**
19.	**D**	57.	**A**	95.	**D**	133.	**C**
20.	**D**	58.	**C**	96.	**B**	134.	**E**
21.	**C**	59.	**D**	97.	**D**	135.	**A**
22.	**A**	60.	**A**	98.	**D**	136.	**A**
23.	**A**	61.	**E**	99.	**B**	137.	**B**
24.	**E**	62.	**C**	100.	**E**	138.	**B**
25.	**C**	63.	**E**	101.	**A**	139.	**D**
26.	**C**	64.	**E**	102.	**E**	140.	**D**
27.	**D**	65.	**A**	103.	**C**	141.	**B**
28.	**E**	66.	**A**	104.	**C**	142.	**C**
29.	**E**	67.	**C**	105.	**C**	143.	**A**
30.	**B**	68.	**A**	106.	**B**	144.	**B**
31.	**E**	69.	**B**	107.	**E**	145.	**E**
32.	**C**	70.	**C**	108.	**D**	146.	**C**
33.	**B**	71.	**E**	109.	**A**	147.	**C**
34.	**C**	72.	**E**	110.	**B**	148.	**A**
35.	**B**	73.	**D**	111.	**D**	149.	**D**
36.	**C**	74.	**B**	112.	**E**	150.	**B**
37.	**E**	75.	**A**	113.	**D**		
38.	**A**	76.	**A**	114.	**C**		

SCORING CHART

After you have scored your Trial Test, enter the results in the chart below, then transfer your score to the Progress Chart on page 12. As you complete the Sample Examinations later in this part of the book, you should be able to achieve increasingly higher scores.

Total Test	Number Right	Number Wrong	Number Omitted
150			

ANSWER EXPLANATIONS

1. **(B)** Expressionism in the arts was a movement during the latter part of the 19th and early part of the 20th centuries that emphasized the objective expression of inner experience through color, brushstrokes, symbols, and abstract shapes.

2. **(D)** The Impressionists were a group of late-19th-century painters who created a general impression of a scene or object by the use of color juxtapositions and small strokes to simulate actual reflected light.

3. **(C)** Acoustics is the study of sound.

4. **(A)** Jean Baptiste Lully (c. 1633–1687) was an Italian operatic composer who has been called "the father of French opera." In 1653 he was made court composer by Louis XIV, for whom he composed many ballets.

5. **(C)** James Wyatt (1746–1813) restored English Gothic cathedrals at Lincoln and Salisbury and built several buildings at Magdelen College, Oxford.

6. **(D)** A "comedy of manners" is a type of social farce. Ibsen wrote plays of a more serious nature.

7. **(E)** Aristotle said that the primary purpose of tragedy is to create a catharsis, or purgation, of the emotions.

8. **(D)** The best-known essayists of this period were Joseph Addison and Richard Steele, who contributed to both the *The Tattler* and *The Spectator*.

9. **(D)** *Uncle Tom's Cabin* ran as a serial in the *National Era*, an abolitionist paper, from June 1851 to April 1852, and was later published as a book.

10. **(A)** Alliteration is the occurrence in a phrase or line of speech or writing of two or more words having the same initial sound, as the "b" sound in "brush," "brow," "burnished," and "bronze."

11. **(B)** The ballet "The Rite of Spring" was first produced by Diaghileff's Ballets Russes in Paris in 1913. It raised a storm of protest and was performed only six times.

12. **(A)** An overture is an instrumental introduction to an opera.

13. **(C)** The photograph shows a pueblo in Taos, New Mexico.

14. **(C)** Dali, Miró, and de Chirico are three artists noted for their Surrealist paintings.

15. **(E)** This is a historical fact.

16. **(C)** A quatrain is a stanza or poem of four lines.

17. **(B)** "Barbara Allen" is an ancient British folk ballad.

18. **(C)** Pop art frequently depicts such things as Campbell's soup cans, flashy cars, and movie stars.

19. **(D)** The Greeks are noted for their graceful statues depicting the human body.

20. **(D)** Wright believed that a building should be built of the materials native to the area and should blend in with its particular surroundings.

21. **(C)** Camus says this in many essays, but no more strongly than in his "Reflections on the Guillotine."

22. **(A)** *The Nibelungenlied*, of unknown origin, was probably composed between the 12th and 14th centuries.

23. **(A)** This is the famous "Pomp and Circumstance" overture.

24. **(E)** None of the others were jazz drummers.

25. **(C)** Shakespeare never wrote dramas about the middle class.

26. **(C)** The Hollywood Bowl opened in California in 1922.

27. **(D)** Aeschylus, the Athenian tragic poet, was the first of the three great tragedians, the others being Sophocles and Euripides.

28. **(E)** No scenery or props were employed by the Greeks in the open, outdoor theater.

29. **(E)** The Swedish director Ingmar Bergman directed all of these films with the exception of *The 400 Blows*, which was directed by François Truffaut, a French filmmaker. Bergman's films deal with themes such as faith, betrayal, and death.

30. **(B)** This is a standard definition of "Western man" or "Western civilization."

31. **(E)** A tone poem is an elaborate orchestral composition, usually in one movement, having no fixed form and based upon some nonmusical, poetic or descriptive theme. Strauss' best-known tone poem is "Thus Spake Zarathustra."

32. **(C)** Hamlet's famous "to be or not to be" soliloquy addresses this problem.

33. **(B)** Paul Cézanne (1839–1906) was a French post-Impressionist painter. He was noted for the use of very vivid colors, and for a striving for depth in place of flatness, which he achieved by very dark shadows and outlines.

34. **(C)** Cubism is a school of modern art characterized by the use of cubes and other abstract geometric forms rather than by a realistic representation of nature.

35. **(B)** A clerestory is an outside wall of a room or building that is carried above an adjoining roof and pierced with windows.

36. **(C)** "Rappaccini's Daughter" is a short story written by the American author Nathaniel Hawthorne (1804–1864).

37. **(E)** Not all sculpture is a realistic portrayal of the human being; stone and marble can be cut for flooring and may be functional, but not necessarily artistic.

38. **(A)** George Berkeley (1685–1753) denied the independent existence of matter. His was the philosophy of subjective idealism, or immaterialism.

39. **(D)** Florence is a city in Tuscany, Italy. Among those who added luster to its name were the artist Michelangelo and the writers Dante and Boccaccio.

40. **(A)** The principal members of the School of Lyon, headed by Maurice Scève, were Antoine Heroet, Pernette de Guillet, and Louise Labè, all poets.

41. **(D)** Stephen Crane (1871–1900) was an American novelist, poet, and journalist. His *Red Badge of Courage* is a well-known tale of the American Civil War.

42. **(D)** Renoir, Monet, and Pissaro were 19th-century painters who attempted to create a general impression of a scene or object by the use of unmixed primary colors and small strokes to simulate actual reflected light.

43. **(C)** This is noticeable in Roman roads and aqueducts as well as in buildings.

44. **(A)** Modulation, in music, is defined as a shifting from one key to another by the transitional use of a chord common to both.

45. **(D)** *Oedipus the King*, a play written by Sophocles, concerns Oedipus, who killed his father and married his mother.

46. **(D)** The photograph is of the Opera House in Sydney, Australia.

47. **(D)** Mark Twain was the pseudonym of Samuel L. Clemens, who was born in Florida, Missouri, in 1835 and spent his childhood in Hannibal, Missouri.

48. **(B)** This example of nonsense verse is from the poem "Jabberwocky," by Lewis Carroll, and is to be found in *Through the Looking Glass*.

49. **(A)** With the fall of the Roman Empire, Christian forces had succeeded in driving the actors out of Rome. Modern drama, including farcical interludes, had its origins in the Middle Ages.

50. **(E)** The Black Death was an epidemic of plague in the 14th century.

51. **(D)** *Animal Farm* is a political satire by George Orwell.

52. **(E)** Bolger, the only tap dancer of the group, appeared in the musical *On Your Toes* and the motion picture *The Wizard of Oz*.

53. **(E)** Ferde Grofé was an American composer and arranger who became famous when he orchestrated Gershwin's *Rhapsody in Blue* in 1924. He also wrote other music describing the American scene, including "The Grand Canyon Suite."

54. **(A)** The great areas of interior space created the feeling of human insignificance and God's infinite and all-powerful presence.

55. **(B)** Some authors pictured the effects of the Great Depression and laborers brutalized by machines.

56. **(C)** Kerouac's novel *On the Road* ushered in a new movement in American literature.

57. **(A)** A parable is sometimes a religious lesson as well.

58. **(C)** Altamira is in northern Spain, and Lascaux is in south-central France.

59. **(D)** This is a basic principle of art.

60. **(A)** Modern psychologists and sociologists have demonstrated that cultural conditioning determines the way we perceive.

61. **(E)** Stephen Foster (1826–1864) was the composer of "Old Folks at Home," "Oh Susannah," "My Old Kentucky Home," and many other songs.

62. **(C)** Benjamin Franklin (1706–1790) was one of the most versatile of the early American founding fathers.

63. **(E)** The line comes from T.S. Eliot's poem "The Love Song of J. Alfred Prufrock."

64. **(E)** The mystery plays were the forerunner of modern drama.

65. **(A)** Lessing's *The Golden Notebook* appeared at the beginning of the Women's Liberation Movement in 1962.

66. **(A)** *Don Quixote*, the best-known work of Miguel de Cervantes, is a satire.

67. **(C)** Among Gainsborough's best-known works are "Mrs. Siddons" and "The Blue Boy."

68. **(A)** "The Well-Tempered Clavier," sometimes called "the Well-Tempered Clavichord," consists of forty-eight preludes and fugues.

69. **(B)** None of the other works was written by Beethoven.

70. **(C)** Among Lewis' best known novels are *Main Street* and *Babbitt*.

71. **(E)** The creative process can occur in any field.

72. **(E)** Aeschylus and Sophocles were more conservative and traditional in their approach.

73. **(D)** The Russian author Anton Chekhov (1860–1904) is noted for presenting small "slices of life" in his plays.

74. **(B)** Leoncavallo wrote several operas, but only *I Pagliacci* was successful.

75. **(A)** A flat is a musical note one-half step lower than a specified note or tone.

76. **(A)** This famous Greek statue is presently to be seen in the Louvre in Paris.

77. **(D)** Shakespeare's plays contain elements such as song, dance, and ghostly apparitions because it was necessary for him to appeal to a diverse audience.

78. **(D)** In other words, the viewer must enter the theater with an open mind.

79. **(E)** Paul Gauguin was a French landscape and figure painter best known for his paintings of Tahitian subjects.

80. **(E)** Pointillism is characterized by the application of paint in small dots and brushstrokes so as to create an effect of blending and luminosity.

81. **(C)** Amber Fort, Rajasthan state, India, is known for its unique artistic style, blending Hindu and Mughal elements.

82. **(A)** This answer is true by definition.

83. **(A)** The poem was first published in *The Passionate Pilgrim* in 1599.

84. **(B)** The poem was published after Marlowe's death.

85. **(D)** A quatrain is a stanza of four lines.

86. **(A)** The appreciation of art is basically an emotional, sensory experience.

87. **(C)** Isaiah was one of the greatest of the Hebrew prophets.

88. **(B)** The other groups consist of those who are not symphony conductors.

89. **(C)** The others are not writers.

90. **(E)** The others are not choreographers.

91. **(E)** F. Scott Fitzgerald is probably the best-known writer of the "roaring 20s."

92. **(D)** Nietzsche wrote about the will to power, and the superman who, he believed, is to come.

93. **(E)** Kate is the name of the female lead in Shakespeare's play.

94. **(E)** Van Gogh became an artist, but he did not prove his point.

95. **(D)** This is a traditional musical notation.

96. **(B)** This is a definition of a cappella.

97. **(D)** Utilitarians hold that human behavior should be directed toward maximizing human happiness. Jeremy Bentham and John Stuart Mill were two leading proponents of utilitarianism.

98. **(D)** Mary Flannery O'Connor (1925–1964) lived most of her life in Milledgeville, Georgia.

99. **(B)** This ornate style in art and architecture developed in Europe about 1550 to 1700.

100. **(E)** "Art" is an abstract concept, and therefore may have many definitions.

101. **(A)** Hamlet's mother, Gertrude, is married to Claudius, but Hamlet mistrusts him.

102. **(E)** This group, also called the Hartford Wits, flourished in the late 18th and early 19th centuries.

103. **(C)** Márquez, author of *One Hundred Years of Solitude*, was awarded the Nobel Prize for literature in 1982.

104. **(C)** Schulz is the creator of the comic strip *Peanuts*.

105. **(C)** Sprung rhythm is a forcefully accentual verse rhythm in which a stressed syllable is followed by an irregular number of unstressed or slack syllables to form a foot having a metrical value equal to that of the other feet in the line.

106. **(B)** Anouilh's play is also entitled *Antigone*.

107. **(E)** Metal is a popular medium for modern sculptors.

108. **(D)** Molière's attacks on bourgeois morality greatly appealed to his aristocratic audience.

109. **(A)** Poe, one of the first great American short story writers, coined this criterion.

110. **(B)** This is a translation from the French. A genre of literature, for example, is the novel.

111. **(D)** François Rabelais (1494–1553) entered a monastery but later abandoned monasticism. His best-known work is *Gargantua and Pantagruel.*

112. **(E)** LeGuin's *The Left Hand of Darkness* is considered a classic in its field.

113. **(D)** Perhaps Verne's best-known work is *20,000 Leagues Under the Sea,* in which he anticipated the invention of the submarine.

114. **(C)** There is no proof, but tradition does hold that Homer was the author.

115. **(A)** Handel's most famous oratorios are on biblical subjects, such as *Esther, Deborah,* and *Samson.*

116. **(A)** The score is the written form of a musical composition. The conductor's copy is complete.

117. **(B)** This book shows how labor was oppressed by management in the early days of unionization.

118. **(D)** These characters are termed the protagonist and the antagonist. Without conflict, there can be no drama.

119. **(A)** The painting is of La Gioconda, popularly known as the Mona Lisa.

120. **(A)** The Pietà is a subject in Christian art depicting the Virgin Mary cradling the dead body of Jesus.

121. **(A)** Jason stole the Golden Fleece from Aeetes, with the help of Aeetes' daughter, Medea.

122. **(C)** Most scholars identify the Dead Sea scrolls with an ancient Jewish sect called the Essenes.

123. **(B)** Sir Christopher Wren (1632–1723) was one of the foremost architects of his day. All of his buildings exhibit elegance, vigor, and dignity.

124. **(D)** The king had learned of uprisings in both Scotland and Wales.

125. **(D)** A mosaic is a decorative design or picture made by setting small colored pieces, such as tile, in mortar.

126. **(A)** All the answers to the above are true, but only partial, explanations. "A," "the complexity of modern life," encompasses all of them and more.

127. **(E)** Formal science relies heavily upon experimentation for proof of a hypothesis.

128. **(C)** Kilmer's "Trees" is often recited on Arbor Day.

129. **(B)** Cunegonde's many experiences would have killed a weaker individual.

130. **(D)** Ernst Hoffmann (1776–1822) was a German musician, artist, and Romantic writer, who is one of the masters in the field of fantastic prose.

131. **(A)** Jacques Offenbach (1819–1880), a French composer of light operas, is best known for his adaptation of Hoffmann's stories.

132. **(D)** The Roman Church abolished all "immoral activities," theater among them.

133. **(C)** There was no theater under the Roman Church during the Dark Ages in Europe.

134. **(E)** This is the only work mentioned that was written during the Revolutionary period.

135. **(A)** *Oliver Twist* was written by Charles Dickens in 1838.

136. **(A)** John Brinks "Dizzy" Gillespie, along with Charlie Parker, created the style of jazz known as "bebop."

137. **(B)** Milton said this in *Paradise Lost*.

138. **(B)** The others are Italian, but not all are 14th-century writers.

139. **(D)** Hamlet had been contemplating murder, but he listened to the ghost.

140. **(D)** A cantata is a vocal and instrumental composition comprising choruses, solos, and recitatives.

141. **(B)** Laius, king of Thebes, was the father of Oedipus, who killed him.

142. **(C)** Mayan architecture is to be found in sections of Mexico and Central America.

143. **(A)** Only *A Handmaid's Tale* was written by Margaret Atwood, a contemporary Canadian author.

144. **(B)** Terza rima is composed of tercets that are not separate stanzas, because each is joined to the one preceding and the one following by a common rhyme: aba, bcb, cdc, ded, etc.

145. **(E)** All of the above are to be found in Gothic cathedrals.

146. **(C)** Robert Frost, one of America's most admired poets, never received the Nobel Prize.

147. **(C)** This is the answer by definition of "soliloquy."

148. **(A)** Henri Rousseau was a French primitive painter best known for his "Sleeping Gypsy" and "The Jungle."

149. **(D)** The others either did not begin with opera, did not head the New York Philharmonic, or did neither.

150. **(B)** It is Desdemona's handkerchief that spurs Othello to such jealousy that he kills her.

Background and Practice Questions

7

DESCRIPTION OF THE HUMANITIES EXAMINATION

The CLEP General Examination in Humanities measures your general knowledge of literature and the arts. It covers material that is generally taught in lower-division college courses designed to survey the humanities. The exam is given in two parts, each consisting of approximately 70 questions and each requiring 45 minutes to complete. See the following chart for approximate percentages of examination items:

Humanities Exam

	Content and Item Types	Time/Number of Questions

50%	Literature
	    10% Drama
	    10–15% Poetry
	    15–20% Fiction
	    10% Nonfiction (including Philosophy)
		150 questions
		90 minutes

50%	The Arts
	    20% Visual arts (painting, sculpture)
	    15% Performing arts (music)
	    10% Performing arts (film, dance)
	    5% Visual arts (architecture)	

The questions on this exam include aspects of the humanities that may not have been covered in courses you have taken in school. Your ability to answer these questions will depend on the extent to which you have maintained a general interest in the arts and kept current by reading widely; attending movies, theater, and concerts; visiting museums; and watching television.

A knowledge of foreign languages is not required to prepare for this exam. All literary works included are readily available in English translations.

The ability to read music is not necessary to answer the questions about music.

Although a few questions may appear rather technical, remember that no one is expected to have complete mastery of all fields of the humanities.

THE KINDS OF QUESTIONS THAT APPEAR ON THE EXAMINATION

There are two important aspects of the examination questions: (1) the knowledge and abilities they test for and (2) the formats in which they are presented.

Knowledge and Abilities Required

The questions require factual answers, not answers which depend upon your emotional responses or aesthetic tastes. Some questions cover material with which you should be familiar from course work. For other questions, the correct answer can be derived from your ability to analyze artistic creations, to recognize certain basic artistic techniques, and to make analogies between two works of art. You will be expected to identify literary passages and authors. In some cases, you will be presented with pictures of works of art that you will be expected to identify by artist, period, or in some other way.

The following questions illustrate the various types of questions you will encounter on the exam.

KNOWLEDGE OF FACTUAL INFORMATION

Questions 1–3 refer to the following groups of people.

(A) John Williams, Burt Bacharach, Henry Mancini
(B) Sir George Solti, Andre Previn, Leonard Bernstein
(C) John Steinbeck, William Faulkner, Sinclair Lewis
(D) Andy Warhol, Joan Miro, Claes Oldenburg
(E) Twyla Tharp, Michael Bennett, Gower Champion

1. Which is a group of contemporary symphony conductors?

2. Which is a group of novelists who won the Nobel Prize for Literature?

3. Which is a group of choreographers for Broadway musicals of the 1970s and 1980s?

RECOGNITION OF TECHNIQUES AND IDENTIFICATION WITH ARTISTS AND PERIODS

Questions 4–6 refer to the following lines.

> Come live with me, and be my love,
> And we will all the pleasures prove,
> That valleys, groves, hills, and fields,
> Woods or steepy mountains yields.

4. These lines are from

(A) "The Passionate Shepherd to His Love"
(B) "The Shepherd's Wife's Song"
(C) "A Strange Passion of a Lover"
(D) one of Shakespeare's sonnets
(E) "Troilus and Cressida"

5. The lines were written by

   (A) William Shakespeare
   (B) Christopher Marlowe
   (C) John Lyly
   (D) T.S. Eliot
   (E) Alexander Pope

6. The verse form is a

   (A) couplet
   (B) sestina
   (C) sonnet
   (D) quatrain
   (E) cinquaine

ANALYSIS OF ARTISTIC CREATIONS

7.   LADY BRACKNELL: "Do you smoke?"
                JACK: "Well, yes, I must admit I smoke."
      LADY BRACKNELL: "I am glad to hear it. A man should always have an
                       occupation of some sort."

This dialogue from Oscar Wilde's *The Importance of Being Earnest* illustrates

   (A) sympathy
   (B) empathy
   (C) scorn
   (D) comic pathos
   (E) linguistic wit

Answers

1. **B**   2. **C**   3. **E**   4. **A**
5. **B**   6. **D**   7. **E**

STUDY SOURCES

If you would like to review some of the information that you may already have studied or fill in some gaps in your formal education, we recommend the following as excellent sources:

Literature

Abrams, M.H. *The Norton Anthology of English Literature.* 4th ed. New York: W.W. Norton and Co., Inc., 1979.

Baker, Nancy L. *A Research Guide for Undergraduate Students: English and American Literature.* 2nd ed. New York: Modern Language Association of America, 1985.

Brooks, Cleanth, et al., eds. *American Literature: The Makers and the Making.* 4 volumes. New York: St. Martin's Press, Inc., 1974.

Grant, Michael. *Myths of the Greeks and Romans.* New York: New American Library, 1975.

Heiney, D.W. and L.H. Downs. *Contemporary Literature of the Western World.* 4 volumes. Hauppauge, NY: Barron's Educational Series, Inc., 1974.

Perrine, Laurence. *Sound and Sense: An Introduction to Poetry.* 5th ed. New York: Harcourt Brace Jovanovich, Inc., 1977.

The Arts

Apel, Willi. *Harvard Dictionary of Music.* 2nd ed. Cambridge, MA: Harvard University Press, 1969.

Grout, Donald. *A History of Western Music.* 3rd ed. New York: W.W. Norton and Co., Inc., 1980.

Janson, H.W. *History of Art: A Survey of the Major Visual Arts from the Dawn of History to the Present Day.* 2nd ed. New York: Harry N. Abrams, Inc., 1977.

Whiting, Fran M. *An Introduction to the Theatre.* 4th ed. New York: Harper and Row Pubs., Inc., 1978.

In addition to these specific works, you might consult the excellent series of dictionaries for the various art forms published by Oxford University Press in New York. For very recent information, you might consult the music, art and book reviews and film criticisms that appear regularly in such publications as *Playboy, Esquire, Saturday Review, The National Review, The New Republic, The New York Times, The New York Review of Books, The New Yorker, The Film Quarterly,* and other periodicals.

For practice, we will now give you some sample questions in each of the areas that the CLEP Humanities Examination will cover; these questions should be considered typical.

PRACTICE QUESTIONS ON THE HUMANITIES

Literature

DIRECTIONS: Each of the questions or incomplete statements below is
answers or completions. Select the one that is best in each case.

1. What 17th-century poet attempted to
   "justify the ways of God to man"?

   (A) John Bunyan
   (B) Samuel Johnson
   (C) John Dryden
   (D) John Milton
   (E) John Donne

2. In poetry, the invention or use of a word
   whose sound echoes or suggests its meaning
   is called

   (A) amphibrach
   (B) sprung rhythm
   (C) onomatopoeia
   (D) zeugma
   (E) sententia

3. A Japanese poem of seventeen syllables is
   the

   (A) kyogen
   (B) haiku
   (C) sentyu
   (D) tanka
   (E) renka

4. The Greek theater contained all but one of
   the following:

   (A) masks
   (B) boots
   (C) proscenium
   (D) movable props
   (E) song and dance

5. A well-known 19th-century symbol
   is "Afternoon of a Faun." This poem was
   written by

   (A) Baudelaire
   (B) Rimbaud
   (C) Valéry
   (D) Mallarmé
   (E) Claudel

6. A pastoral elegy, bewailing the death of
   Edward King, is

   (A) "In Memoriam"
   (B) "Lycidas"
   (C) "Thyrsis"
   (D) "Il Penseroso"
   (E) "Adonais"

7. An example of an Old English folk epic is

   (A) *The Canterbury Tales*
   (B) *The Iliad*
   (C) *Beowulf*
   (D) *A Midsummer Night's Dream*
   (E) *Paradise Lost*

8. The essence of comedy is

   (A) satire
   (B) surprise
   (C) mistaken identity
   (D) disguise
   (E) incongruity

9. The Greek word for "overweening pride" is

   (A) hamartia
   (B) catharsis
   (C) anagnorisis
   (D) peripety
   (E) hubris

ord *utopia* comes from a 16th-century
k by

(A) Sir Thomas More
(B) Thomas à Becket
(C) Samuel Beckett
(D) William Shakespeare
(E) Ben Jonson

11. A famous contemporary of John Dryden was

(A) Alexander Pope
(B) Ben Jonson
(C) Thomas Macaulay
(D) Leigh Hunt
(E) John Milton

12. According to Aristotle, tragedy evokes pity
and fear and produces a

(A) catharsis
(B) dénouement
(C) climax
(D) recognition
(E) kothurnos

13. A Japanese play that exists as a harmony
of all theatrical elements—poetry, music,
dance, costume, mask, setting, and the
interaction of performance—is the

(A) kabuki
(B) shinto
(C) hari kiri
(D) no
(E) joruri

14. In the 16th century, people believed the
main purpose of poetry was to

(A) relieve the emotions
(B) make science bearable
(C) enliven life
(D) delight and instruct
(E) philosophize

15. Shakespeare's best-known comic character
is

(A) Titania
(B) Falstaff
(C) Henry VIII
(D) Ariel
(E) Friar Lawrence

16. A collection of medieval stories concerning a
group of people on a pilgrimage is

(A) *The Decameron*
(B) *The Canterbury Tales*
(C) *Sir Gawain and the Green Knight*
(D) *Morte d'Arthur*
(E) *Idylls of the King*

17. An American poet and novelist, awarded
the Pulitzer Prize for her novel *The Color
Purple*, is

(A) Zora Neale Hurston
(B) Ursula K. LeGuin
(C) Barbara Bellows
(D) Cynthia Blake
(E) Alice Walker

18. "All are but parts of one stupendous whole,
Whose body Nature is, and God the soul"
was written by

(A) Matthew Arnold
(B) Alexander Pope
(C) Percy B. Shelley
(D) John Milton
(E) Robert Browning

19. A well-known British writer, born in Trinidad
of Hindu parents, is

(A) Derek Walcott
(B) Malachi Smith
(C) V.S. Naipaul
(D) Abdur-Rahman Slade Hophinson
(E) Erna Brodber

20. John Donne and his followers are known to literary historians as the

    (A) metaphysical poets
    (B) Molly Maguires
    (C) cavalier poets
    (D) graveyard school
    (E) Sons of Ben

21. The "hero" of Milton's *Paradise Lost* is

    (A) Satan
    (B) man
    (C) God
    (D) Adam
    (E) Jesus

22. A convention in drama wherein a character speaks his innermost thoughts aloud while alone on stage is the

    (A) aside
    (B) prologue
    (C) soliloquy
    (D) epilogue
    (E) proscenium

23. A fire-breathing monster, part lion, part goat, and part serpent, slain by Bellerophon, was the

    (A) medusa
    (B) chimera
    (C) phoenix
    (D) minotaur
    (E) hydra

24. The writer primarily responsible for the creation of the western as a literary genre is

    (A) Louis L'Amour
    (B) Jack London
    (C) Ernest Hemingway
    (D) Ambrose Bierce
    (E) Zane Grey

25. One of the great Sanskrit epics of Western India is

    (A) *The Mahabharata*
    (B) *Siddhartha*
    (C) *The Triptaka*
    (D) *The Analects*
    (E) *The Rubáiyát*

26. A well-known contemporary of William Shakespeare was

    (A) John Milton
    (B) Dante Alighieri
    (C) Geoffrey Chaucer
    (D) Christopher Marlowe
    (E) John Dryden

27. A 20th-century novel that made the public aware of the plight of migrant laborers is

    (A) *East of Eden*
    (B) *To a God Unknown*
    (C) *Cannery Row*
    (D) *The Grapes of Wrath*
    (E) *Tortilla Flat*

28. A poet who writes of ordinary people and of nature is considered a

    (A) naturalist
    (B) realist
    (C) romanticist
    (D) medievalist
    (E) Victorian

29. The "comedy of manners" was most popular during the

    (A) 16th century
    (B) 17th century
    (C) 18th century
    (D) 19th century
    (E) 20th century

30. The first book by a black author to be selected as a Book of the Month Club selection was

    (A) *The Invisible Man*
    (B) *Black Like Me*
    (C) *Giovanni's Room*
    (D) *Black Boy*
    (E) *Native Son*

31. A Greek divinity who punished crimes, particularly those of impiety and hubris, was

    (A) Artemis
    (B) Mercury
    (C) Clio
    (D) Clytaemnestra
    (E) Nemesis

32. Which Lawrence authored *Women in Love* and *Lady Chatterley's Lover*?

    (A) T.E. Lawrence
    (B) D.H. Lawrence
    (C) Ernest Lawrence
    (D) Gertrude Lawrence
    (E) Christian Lawrence

33. In Greek mythology, Demeter is the goddess of

    (A) the moon
    (B) the earth
    (C) rivers and lakes
    (D) agriculture
    (E) the hunt

34. The only two Americans to write poems for presidential inaugurations were

    (A) Sandberg and Ginsberg
    (B) Whitman and Lowell
    (C) Millay and Dickinson
    (D) Longfellow and Poe
    (E) Frost and Angelou

35. A 20th-century writer who refused the Nobel prize for literature was

    (A) Faulkner
    (B) Sartre
    (C) Camus
    (D) Lewis
    (E) Hemingway

Questions 36–38 refer to the following poem, "The Eagle" by Alfred, Lord Tennyson.

> He clasps the crag with crooked hands;
> Close to the sun in the lonely lands,
> Ringed with the azure world, he stands.
>
> The wrinkled sea beneath him crawls;
> He watches from his mountain walls,
> And like a thunderbolt he falls.

36. Which line contains a metaphor?

    (A) line 2
    (B) line 4
    (C) line 5
    (D) line 6
    (E) all of these lines

37. Which line contains a simile?

    (A) line 1
    (B) line 2
    (C) line 3
    (D) line 5
    (E) line 6

38. Which line contains an example of alliteration?

    (A) line 1
    (B) line 3
    (C) line 4
    (D) line 5
    (E) line 6

Answers

1. **D**	6. **B**	11. **E**	16. **B**	21. **B**	26. **D**	31. **E**	36. **B**
2. **C**	7. **C**	12. **A**	17. **E**	22. **C**	27. **D**	32. **B**	37. **E**
3. **B**	8. **E**	13. **D**	18. **B**	23. **B**	28. **C**	33. **D**	38. **A**
4. **D**	9. **E**	14. **D**	19. **C**	24. **E**	29. **C**	34. **E**	
5. **D**	10. **A**	15. **B**	20. **A**	25. **A**	30. **E**	35. **B**	

Music

> **DIRECTIONS:** Each of the questions or incomplete statements below is followed by five suggested answers or completions. Select the one that is best in each case.

1. The assistant conductor or concertmaster of the orchestra is

   (A) the first chair violinist
   (B) the second chair violinist
   (C) a pianist
   (D) a harpist
   (E) standing in the wings ready to take over

2. The instrument with the stablest pitch and therefore the one asked to "sound your A" for all other players is the

   (A) piano
   (B) first violin
   (C) first oboe
   (D) clarinet
   (E) trumpet

3. The tone poem "Afternoon of a Faun" was composed by

   (A) Debussy
   (B) Liszt
   (C) Bizet
   (D) Rimsky-Korsakov
   (E) Poulenc

4. The first American music comes from the American Indian and, with its emphasis on single rhythms, American Indian music is primarily

   (A) emotional
   (B) formal
   (C) heterophonic
   (D) polyphonic
   (E) choral

5. Sir Andrew Lloyd Webber wrote the music for all of the following shows except

   (A) *Aspects of Love*
   (B) *Phantom of the Opera*
   (C) *Evita*
   (D) *Cats*
   (E) *Blood Brothers*

6. Composer of "4 minutes and 33 Seconds," in which the pianist sits at a piano for that length of time but does not play, is

   (A) Schoenberg
   (B) Bernstein
   (C) Ellington
   (D) Gershwin
   (E) Cage

7. The term "impressionism" was first applied to the music of

(A) Ravel
(B) Stravinsky
(C) Debussy
(D) Weill
(E) Schoenberg

8. The music for the ballets "Rodeo," "Billy the Kid," and "Appalachian Spring" was written by

(A) Howard Hanson
(B) George Gershwin
(C) Aaron Copland
(D) Ferde Grofé
(E) Elmer Bernstein

9. What American choreographer is best known for her "Fall River Legend" and "Rodeo"?

(A) Agnes deMille
(B) Isadora Duncan
(C) Martha Graham
(D) Loie Fuller
(E) Doris Humphrey

10. The composer of the opera *Four Saints in Three Acts*, and the recipient of the Pulitzer Prize for his score to the documentary motion picture *Louisiana Story*, is

(A) Aaron Copland
(B) Kurt Weill
(C) Erik Satie
(D) Albert Roussel
(E) Virgil Thomson

11. Running through music literature is a persistent thread that has affected, positively or negatively, the work of every composer from Bach to our 20th-century modernists. This thread is

(A) melody
(B) sonata
(C) tone-poem
(D) counterpart
(E) atonality

12. The "Unfinished Symphony" was written by

(A) Mendelssohn
(B) Schubert
(C) Brahms
(D) Tchaikovsky
(E) Chopin

13. The opera *The Barber of Seville* has music by

(A) Puccini
(B) Verdi
(C) Mendelssohn
(D) Rossini
(E) Poulenc

14. The opera *The Marriage of Figaro* has music by

(A) Mozart
(B) Haydn
(C) Verdi
(D) Rossini
(E) Puccini

15. A celebrated violinist who made his debut at Carnegie Hall at age eleven and toured the world before his twentieth birthday is

(A) Georges Enesco
(B) Aaron Copland
(C) Elmer Bernstein
(D) Yehudi Menuhin
(E) André Previn

16. We get the word *octave* from a Latin word meaning

(A) two
(B) four
(C) six
(D) eight
(E) nine

17. The direct ancestor of the symphony is the

    (A) concerto
    (B) sonata
    (C) motet
    (D) aria
    (E) overture

18. The method of four voices singing different tunes at the same time, yet linked by strict rules, is called a

    (A) motet
    (B) combo
    (C) chorus
    (D) fugue
    (E) baroque

19. Beethoven is best known for his

    (A) tone poems
    (B) operas
    (C) symphonies
    (D) waltzes
    (E) fugues

20. Many muscians agree that the greatest choral work ever written is

    (A) Beethoven's "Moonlight Sonata"
    (B) Bach's "Mass in B Minor"
    (C) Schubert's "Second Symphony"
    (D) Chopin's "Polonaise Militaire"
    (E) Bizet's *Carmen*

Answers

1. **A**	6. **E**	11. **E**	16. **D**
2. **C**	7. **C**	12. **B**	17. **E**
3. **A**	8. **C**	13. **D**	18. **A**
4. **D**	9. **A**	14. **A**	19. **C**
5. **E**	10. **E**	15. **D**	20. **B**

The Arts—Painting, Architecture, Sculpture, Dance

> **DIRECTIONS:** Each of the questions or incomplete statements below is followed by five suggested answers or completions. Select the one that is best in each case.

1. In painting, *chiaroscuro* refers to

   (A) a light-and-dark technique
   (B) brilliant colors
   (C) monochromes
   (D) perspective
   (E) a single-stroke technique

2. From 1692 to 1702 Giordano painted the ceiling of Charles II's palace, the Escorial, in

   (A) Versailles
   (B) Verona
   (C) Madrid
   (D) Rome
   (E) Milan

3. What is the main part of the interior of a church called?

   (A) The nave
   (B) The transept
   (C) The altar
   (D) The cruciform
   (E) The sacristy

4. One of the most famous modern ballet choreographers was

   (A) George Balanchine
   (B) Nicholas Sergeyev
   (C) Marius Petipa
   (D) Phillippe Taglioni
   (E) Rudolf von Laban

5. The artist famous for his painting on the ceiling of the Sistine Chapel is

   (A) Raphael
   (B) da Vinci
   (C) Michelangelo
   (D) Rembrandt
   (E) Delacroix

6. A painter noted for his madonnas is

   (A) Botticelli
   (B) van Gogh
   (C) Raphael
   (D) Picasso
   (E) Goya

7. The art of painting on freshly spread moist lime plaster with pigments suspended in a water vehicle is called

   (A) collage
   (B) pointillism
   (C) surrealism
   (D) primitivism
   (E) fresco

8. Perhaps the best known painting of Gustav Klimt is

   (A) *Ruth*
   (B) *The Last Temptation of Christ*
   (C) *Moses*
   (D) *The Kiss*
   (E) *The Thinker*

9. An artistic composition of fragments of printed matter and other materials pasted on a picture surface is called

(A) dadaism
(B) a fresco
(C) art nouveau
(D) a collage
(E) pop art

10. Perhaps the outstanding master of the engraving and the woodcut was

(A) Pieter Brueghel
(B) Albrecht Dürer
(C) William Blake
(D) Leonardo da Vinci
(E) Honoré Daumier

11. An Italian designer of the mid-20th-century known for his tiles painted to look like shelves of a bookcase was

(A) Picasso
(B) Miró
(C) Ferrari
(D) Fornasetti
(E) Pucci

12. A "Spanish" painter noted for his thin-faced, elongated individuals was

(A) Goya
(B) Velásquez
(C) El Greco
(D) Picasso
(E) Orozco

13. The first black choreographer to work at the Metropolitan Opera House was

(A) Isadora Duncan
(B) Alvin Ailey
(C) Maya Angelou
(D) Katherine Dunham
(E) Katharine Graham

14. One of the 20th century's great British sculptors is

(A) Ernst Barlach
(B) Alberto Giacometti
(C) Ossip Zadkine
(D) Jacob Epstein
(E) Alexander Calder

15. Inigo Jones was a

(A) 17th-century architect and set designer
(B) clarinetist with Bunk Johnson's orchestra
(C) Restoration playwright
(D) leading tenor with the La Scala Opera
(E) 19th-century Impressionist painter

16. The American sculptor who designed two bridges for the Peace Park in Hiroshima and the Billy Rose Sculpture Garden for the National Museum in Jerusalem is

(A) Cornell
(B) Noguchi
(C) Lipton
(D) Calder
(E) Duchamp

17. Perspective, as a unified system for representing space, was brought to perfection during the

(A) Golden Age of Greece
(B) Roman Republic
(C) Byzantine period
(D) Renaissance
(E) nineteenth century

18. One of the many artists who designed sets and costumes for Sergei Diaghilev's Ballets Russes was

(A) Claude Monet
(B) Juan Gris
(C) Jacques Lipchitz
(D) Paul Gauguin
(E) Paul Cezanne

19. An artist noted for her decorative sculpture and designs for metalwork is

(A) Esther Moore
(B) Edna St. Vincent Millay
(C) Grandma Moses
(D) Edith Sitwell
(E) Francine Smythe

20. Edvard Munch's most famous painting is

(A) *The Scream*
(B) *Venus*
(C) *The Persistence of Memory*
(D) *Guernica*
(E) *The Dream*

Answers

1. **A**	6. **C**	11. **D**	16. **B**
2. **C**	7. **E**	12. **C**	17. **D**
3. **A**	8. **D**	13. **D**	18. **B**
4. **A**	9. **D**	14. **D**	19. **A**
5. **C**	10. **B**	15. **A**	20. **A**

ANSWER SHEET
Sample Examination 1

HUMANITIES

1. Ⓐ Ⓑ Ⓒ Ⓓ Ⓔ	39. Ⓐ Ⓑ Ⓒ Ⓓ Ⓔ	77. Ⓐ Ⓑ Ⓒ Ⓓ Ⓔ	115. Ⓐ Ⓑ Ⓒ Ⓓ Ⓔ
2. Ⓐ Ⓑ Ⓒ Ⓓ Ⓔ	40. Ⓐ Ⓑ Ⓒ Ⓓ Ⓔ	78. Ⓐ Ⓑ Ⓒ Ⓓ Ⓔ	116. Ⓐ Ⓑ Ⓒ Ⓓ Ⓔ
3. Ⓐ Ⓑ Ⓒ Ⓓ Ⓔ	41. Ⓐ Ⓑ Ⓒ Ⓓ Ⓔ	79. Ⓐ Ⓑ Ⓒ Ⓓ Ⓔ	117. Ⓐ Ⓑ Ⓒ Ⓓ Ⓔ
4. Ⓐ Ⓑ Ⓒ Ⓓ Ⓔ	42. Ⓐ Ⓑ Ⓒ Ⓓ Ⓔ	80. Ⓐ Ⓑ Ⓒ Ⓓ Ⓔ	118. Ⓐ Ⓑ Ⓒ Ⓓ Ⓔ
5. Ⓐ Ⓑ Ⓒ Ⓓ Ⓔ	43. Ⓐ Ⓑ Ⓒ Ⓓ Ⓔ	81. Ⓐ Ⓑ Ⓒ Ⓓ Ⓔ	119. Ⓐ Ⓑ Ⓒ Ⓓ Ⓔ
6. Ⓐ Ⓑ Ⓒ Ⓓ Ⓔ	44. Ⓐ Ⓑ Ⓒ Ⓓ Ⓔ	82. Ⓐ Ⓑ Ⓒ Ⓓ Ⓔ	120. Ⓐ Ⓑ Ⓒ Ⓓ Ⓔ
7. Ⓐ Ⓑ Ⓒ Ⓓ Ⓔ	45. Ⓐ Ⓑ Ⓒ Ⓓ Ⓔ	83. Ⓐ Ⓑ Ⓒ Ⓓ Ⓔ	121. Ⓐ Ⓑ Ⓒ Ⓓ Ⓔ
8. Ⓐ Ⓑ Ⓒ Ⓓ Ⓔ	46. Ⓐ Ⓑ Ⓒ Ⓓ Ⓔ	84. Ⓐ Ⓑ Ⓒ Ⓓ Ⓔ	122. Ⓐ Ⓑ Ⓒ Ⓓ Ⓔ
9. Ⓐ Ⓑ Ⓒ Ⓓ Ⓔ	47. Ⓐ Ⓑ Ⓒ Ⓓ Ⓔ	85. Ⓐ Ⓑ Ⓒ Ⓓ Ⓔ	123. Ⓐ Ⓑ Ⓒ Ⓓ Ⓔ
10. Ⓐ Ⓑ Ⓒ Ⓓ Ⓔ	48. Ⓐ Ⓑ Ⓒ Ⓓ Ⓔ	86. Ⓐ Ⓑ Ⓒ Ⓓ Ⓔ	124. Ⓐ Ⓑ Ⓒ Ⓓ Ⓔ
11. Ⓐ Ⓑ Ⓒ Ⓓ Ⓔ	49. Ⓐ Ⓑ Ⓒ Ⓓ Ⓔ	87. Ⓐ Ⓑ Ⓒ Ⓓ Ⓔ	125. Ⓐ Ⓑ Ⓒ Ⓓ Ⓔ
12. Ⓐ Ⓑ Ⓒ Ⓓ Ⓔ	50. Ⓐ Ⓑ Ⓒ Ⓓ Ⓔ	88. Ⓐ Ⓑ Ⓒ Ⓓ Ⓔ	126. Ⓐ Ⓑ Ⓒ Ⓓ Ⓔ
13. Ⓐ Ⓑ Ⓒ Ⓓ Ⓔ	51. Ⓐ Ⓑ Ⓒ Ⓓ Ⓔ	89. Ⓐ Ⓑ Ⓒ Ⓓ Ⓔ	127. Ⓐ Ⓑ Ⓒ Ⓓ Ⓔ
14. Ⓐ Ⓑ Ⓒ Ⓓ Ⓔ	52. Ⓐ Ⓑ Ⓒ Ⓓ Ⓔ	90. Ⓐ Ⓑ Ⓒ Ⓓ Ⓔ	128. Ⓐ Ⓑ Ⓒ Ⓓ Ⓔ
15. Ⓐ Ⓑ Ⓒ Ⓓ Ⓔ	53. Ⓐ Ⓑ Ⓒ Ⓓ Ⓔ	91. Ⓐ Ⓑ Ⓒ Ⓓ Ⓔ	129. Ⓐ Ⓑ Ⓒ Ⓓ Ⓔ
16. Ⓐ Ⓑ Ⓒ Ⓓ Ⓔ	54. Ⓐ Ⓑ Ⓒ Ⓓ Ⓔ	92. Ⓐ Ⓑ Ⓒ Ⓓ Ⓔ	130. Ⓐ Ⓑ Ⓒ Ⓓ Ⓔ
17. Ⓐ Ⓑ Ⓒ Ⓓ Ⓔ	55. Ⓐ Ⓑ Ⓒ Ⓓ Ⓔ	93. Ⓐ Ⓑ Ⓒ Ⓓ Ⓔ	131. Ⓐ Ⓑ Ⓒ Ⓓ Ⓔ
18. Ⓐ Ⓑ Ⓒ Ⓓ Ⓔ	56. Ⓐ Ⓑ Ⓒ Ⓓ Ⓔ	94. Ⓐ Ⓑ Ⓒ Ⓓ Ⓔ	132. Ⓐ Ⓑ Ⓒ Ⓓ Ⓔ
19. Ⓐ Ⓑ Ⓒ Ⓓ Ⓔ	57. Ⓐ Ⓑ Ⓒ Ⓓ Ⓔ	95. Ⓐ Ⓑ Ⓒ Ⓓ Ⓔ	133. Ⓐ Ⓑ Ⓒ Ⓓ Ⓔ
20. Ⓐ Ⓑ Ⓒ Ⓓ Ⓔ	58. Ⓐ Ⓑ Ⓒ Ⓓ Ⓔ	96. Ⓐ Ⓑ Ⓒ Ⓓ Ⓔ	134. Ⓐ Ⓑ Ⓒ Ⓓ Ⓔ
21. Ⓐ Ⓑ Ⓒ Ⓓ Ⓔ	59. Ⓐ Ⓑ Ⓒ Ⓓ Ⓔ	97. Ⓐ Ⓑ Ⓒ Ⓓ Ⓔ	135. Ⓐ Ⓑ Ⓒ Ⓓ Ⓔ
22. Ⓐ Ⓑ Ⓒ Ⓓ Ⓔ	60. Ⓐ Ⓑ Ⓒ Ⓓ Ⓔ	98. Ⓐ Ⓑ Ⓒ Ⓓ Ⓔ	136. Ⓐ Ⓑ Ⓒ Ⓓ Ⓔ
23. Ⓐ Ⓑ Ⓒ Ⓓ Ⓔ	61. Ⓐ Ⓑ Ⓒ Ⓓ Ⓔ	99. Ⓐ Ⓑ Ⓒ Ⓓ Ⓔ	137. Ⓐ Ⓑ Ⓒ Ⓓ Ⓔ
24. Ⓐ Ⓑ Ⓒ Ⓓ Ⓔ	62. Ⓐ Ⓑ Ⓒ Ⓓ Ⓔ	100. Ⓐ Ⓑ Ⓒ Ⓓ Ⓔ	138. Ⓐ Ⓑ Ⓒ Ⓓ Ⓔ
25. Ⓐ Ⓑ Ⓒ Ⓓ Ⓔ	63. Ⓐ Ⓑ Ⓒ Ⓓ Ⓔ	101. Ⓐ Ⓑ Ⓒ Ⓓ Ⓔ	139. Ⓐ Ⓑ Ⓒ Ⓓ Ⓔ
26. Ⓐ Ⓑ Ⓒ Ⓓ Ⓔ	64. Ⓐ Ⓑ Ⓒ Ⓓ Ⓔ	102. Ⓐ Ⓑ Ⓒ Ⓓ Ⓔ	140. Ⓐ Ⓑ Ⓒ Ⓓ Ⓔ
27. Ⓐ Ⓑ Ⓒ Ⓓ Ⓔ	65. Ⓐ Ⓑ Ⓒ Ⓓ Ⓔ	103. Ⓐ Ⓑ Ⓒ Ⓓ Ⓔ	141. Ⓐ Ⓑ Ⓒ Ⓓ Ⓔ
28. Ⓐ Ⓑ Ⓒ Ⓓ Ⓔ	66. Ⓐ Ⓑ Ⓒ Ⓓ Ⓔ	104. Ⓐ Ⓑ Ⓒ Ⓓ Ⓔ	142. Ⓐ Ⓑ Ⓒ Ⓓ Ⓔ
29. Ⓐ Ⓑ Ⓒ Ⓓ Ⓔ	67. Ⓐ Ⓑ Ⓒ Ⓓ Ⓔ	105. Ⓐ Ⓑ Ⓒ Ⓓ Ⓔ	143. Ⓐ Ⓑ Ⓒ Ⓓ Ⓔ
30. Ⓐ Ⓑ Ⓒ Ⓓ Ⓔ	68. Ⓐ Ⓑ Ⓒ Ⓓ Ⓔ	106. Ⓐ Ⓑ Ⓒ Ⓓ Ⓔ	144. Ⓐ Ⓑ Ⓒ Ⓓ Ⓔ
31. Ⓐ Ⓑ Ⓒ Ⓓ Ⓔ	69. Ⓐ Ⓑ Ⓒ Ⓓ Ⓔ	107. Ⓐ Ⓑ Ⓒ Ⓓ Ⓔ	145. Ⓐ Ⓑ Ⓒ Ⓓ Ⓔ
32. Ⓐ Ⓑ Ⓒ Ⓓ Ⓔ	70. Ⓐ Ⓑ Ⓒ Ⓓ Ⓔ	108. Ⓐ Ⓑ Ⓒ Ⓓ Ⓔ	146. Ⓐ Ⓑ Ⓒ Ⓓ Ⓔ
33. Ⓐ Ⓑ Ⓒ Ⓓ Ⓔ	71. Ⓐ Ⓑ Ⓒ Ⓓ Ⓔ	109. Ⓐ Ⓑ Ⓒ Ⓓ Ⓔ	147. Ⓐ Ⓑ Ⓒ Ⓓ Ⓔ
34. Ⓐ Ⓑ Ⓒ Ⓓ Ⓔ	72. Ⓐ Ⓑ Ⓒ Ⓓ Ⓔ	110. Ⓐ Ⓑ Ⓒ Ⓓ Ⓔ	148. Ⓐ Ⓑ Ⓒ Ⓓ Ⓔ
35. Ⓐ Ⓑ Ⓒ Ⓓ Ⓔ	73. Ⓐ Ⓑ Ⓒ Ⓓ Ⓔ	111. Ⓐ Ⓑ Ⓒ Ⓓ Ⓔ	149. Ⓐ Ⓑ Ⓒ Ⓓ Ⓔ
36. Ⓐ Ⓑ Ⓒ Ⓓ Ⓔ	74. Ⓐ Ⓑ Ⓒ Ⓓ Ⓔ	112. Ⓐ Ⓑ Ⓒ Ⓓ Ⓔ	150. Ⓐ Ⓑ Ⓒ Ⓓ Ⓔ
37. Ⓐ Ⓑ Ⓒ Ⓓ Ⓔ	75. Ⓐ Ⓑ Ⓒ Ⓓ Ⓔ	113. Ⓐ Ⓑ Ⓒ Ⓓ Ⓔ	
38. Ⓐ Ⓑ Ⓒ Ⓓ Ⓔ	76. Ⓐ Ⓑ Ⓒ Ⓓ Ⓔ	114. Ⓐ Ⓑ Ⓒ Ⓓ Ⓔ	

Sample Humanities Examinations

8

This chapter contains two sample Humanities examinations, each with an answer key, scoring chart, and answer explanations. Calculate and record your scores and see your improvement on the Progress Chart on page 12.

SAMPLE HUMANITIES EXAMINATION 1

Number of Questions: 150

TIME LIMIT: 90 MINUTES

DIRECTIONS: Each of the questions or incomplete statements below is followed by five suggested answers or completions. Select the one that is best in each case.

1. The composer of *Carmina Burana* and *Die Kluge* is

 (A) Olivier Messiaen
 (B) Carl Orff
 (C) Leos Janácek
 (D) Peter Mennin
 (E) Nicolas Medtner

2. George Gershwin wrote all of the following except

 (A) *An American in Paris*
 (B) *Porgy and Bess*
 (C) *Cuban Overture*
 (D) *Rhapsody in Blue*
 (E) *The White Peacock*

3. Fernand Leger was a contemporary of

 (A) Michelangelo
 (B) da Vinci
 (C) Rubens
 (D) Braque
 (E) van Gogh

4. A major recurrent theme in the compositions of Willem de Kooning is

 (A) flowers
 (B) children
 (C) nightmares
 (D) birds
 (E) women

5. The first American writer to popularize the American Indian in literature was

 (A) Cooper
 (B) Hillerman
 (C) Twain
 (D) Irving
 (E) Longfellow

6. In a popular short story by F. Scott Fitzgerald, Bernice

   (A) runs away from school
   (B) steals a purse
   (C) elopes
   (D) bobs her hair
   (E) steals her sister's beau

7. Structural elements of architecture such as the pointed arch and the flying buttress were extensively used in the period known as

   (A) Byzantine
   (B) Gothic
   (C) Renaissance
   (D) Baroque
   (E) Victorian

8. The most intrinsically American and most durable of all motion picture genres is

   (A) romantic comedy
   (B) black comedy
   (C) musical comedy
   (D) the western
   (E) tragedy

9. "I have found that all the bronze my furnace contained had been exhausted in the head of this figure [of the statue of Perseus]. . . . It was a miracle. . . . I seemed to see in this head the head of god." This statement was made by

   (A) Grangousier
   (B) Cellini
   (C) Machiavelli
   (D) Michelangelo
   (E) Praxiteles

10. Which of the following plays was not written by Shakespeare?

    (A) *Titus Andronicus*
    (B) *Dr. Faustus*
    (C) *Love's Labour's Lost*
    (D) *The Tempest*
    (E) *Coriolanus*

11. The monarch known as the "Sun King" was

    (A) Charles II of England
    (B) Edward I of England
    (C) George VI of England
    (D) Henry IV of France
    (E) Louis XIV of France

12. The difference between sonata and sonata-allegro is

    (A) the sonata is more contrapuntal
    (B) the sonata is more homophonic
    (C) one is faster than the other
    (D) the sonata is a multi-movement work which might contain one or more movements in sonata-allegro form
    (E) the sonata-allegro form preceded the sonata

13. Impressionism in music originated in France under the leadership of

    (A) Debussy and Ravel
    (B) Poulenc and Hindemith
    (C) Stravinsky and Bartók
    (D) Debussy and Chopin
    (E) Sessions and Varese

14. Leonardo da Vinci was one of the greatest artists of the period known as

    (A) Baroque
    (B) the early Renaissance
    (C) the high Renaissance
    (D) Gothic
    (E) Byzantine

15. The word *philosophy* means literally

    (A) love of knowledge
    (B) knowledge of God
    (C) love of God
    (D) love of wisdom
    (E) science and progress

16. The play that shows the downfall of a man as a result of biological urges or his social environment is called

(A) epic theater
(B) neorealism
(C) romantic tragedy
(D) deterministic tragedy
(E) Ibsenian irony

17. The unresolved or "open" ending is one of the trademarks of

(A) Greek tragedy
(B) Restoration comedy
(C) Shakespearean comedy
(D) Roman tragedy
(E) modern plays and cinema

18. Dante's *Divine Comedy* contains how many cantos?

(A) 3
(B) 4
(C) 33
(D) 99
(E) 100

19. The origins of Baroque architecture can be traced to Sansovino, Palladio, and

(A) Bellini
(B) Michelangelo
(C) Giotto
(D) da Vinci
(E) Lorenzo

20. In the theater, a conventional character, a type that recurs in numerous works, is called

(A) a tragic hero
(B) a deus ex machina
(C) a stock character
(D) a redundant character
(E) a supernumerary character

21. The greatest ballet dancer of the beginning of the 20th century and prima ballerina of the Maryinsky Theater was

(A) Tamara Karsavina
(B) Galina Ulanova
(C) Anna Pavlova
(D) Tamara Toumanova
(E) Alexandra Danilova

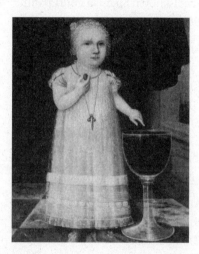

22. The photo above is an example of

(A) 17th-century art
(B) 18th-century Spanish art
(C) modern Mexican art
(D) medieval art
(E) American primitive art

23. Polyphonic texture is

(A) chordal texture
(B) unaccompanied melody
(C) accompanied melody
(D) a combination of melodies
(E) common to all forms

24. The work of the filmmaker Sanjit Ray was greatly influenced by

(A) E.M. Forster
(B) Mahatma Gandhi
(C) Rabindranath Tagore
(D) Anita Desai
(E) V.S. Naipaul

25. A Danish writer, best known for the *Seven Gothic Tales* and *Winter's Tales*, was

    (A) Isak Dinesen
    (B) Karen Petersen
    (C) Inge Johanssen
    (D) Ingeborg Carlsen
    (E) Gerte Grimm

26. A well-known Spanish court painter of the 18th century was

    (A) Velásquez
    (B) Ribera
    (C) Pisarro
    (D) Goya
    (E) Pisano

27. The Greek playwright who introduced the third actor into tragedy was

    (A) Agamemnon
    (B) Euripides
    (C) Socrates
    (D) Thespis
    (E) Clytaemnestra

28. The Romantic period of literature gave birth to a special kind of horror story, the

    (A) pastoral romance
    (B) epic
    (C) vignette
    (D) Gothic novel
    (E) dramatic monologue

29. The story of the founding of Rome by the mythical Aeneas was written by

    (A) Augustus
    (B) Vergil
    (C) Homer
    (D) Sibyl
    (E) Romulus

30. Wagner's last opera concerning the search for the Holy Grail is

    (A) *Festspielhaus*
    (B) *Cosima*
    (C) *Siegfried*
    (D) *Parsifal*
    (E) *Wahnfried*

31. Rome contributed all of the following to architecture except

    (A) an emphasis on verticality
    (B) design of significant interiors
    (C) buildings for use
    (D) the arch and vault as a building principle
    (E) the flying buttress

32. A post-Impressionist painter best known for his South Seas subjects was

    (A) Paul Gauguin
    (B) Vincent van Gogh
    (C) Toulouse-Lautrec
    (D) Paul Cezanne
    (E) Georges Seurat

33. A modern playwright who believes in "aesthetic distancing" is

    (A) Arthur Miller
    (B) Eugene O'Neill
    (C) Jean Paul Sartre
    (D) Stanley Kubrick
    (E) Bertolt Brecht

34. The central figure in the Bayeux tapestry is

    (A) Alexander the Great
    (B) William the Conqueror
    (C) Edward the Confessor
    (D) Gregory the Great
    (E) Charlemagne

35. During the Hellenic period, the great center of Greek culture was located at

(A) Alexandria
(B) Antioch
(C) Athens
(D) Rhodes
(E) Pergamon

Questions 36–38 refer to the following groups of people:

(A) Paul Klee, Marc Chagall, Pablo Picasso
(B) Samuel Barber, Alban Berg, George Gershwin
(C) Paul Johnson, Mies van der Rohe, Louis Sullivan
(D) Anne Jackson, Anne Tyler, Anne Bradstreet
(E) Amy Lowell, May Senson, Nikki Giovanni

36. Which is a group of 20th-century painters?

37. Which is a group of 20th-century American poets?

38. Which is a group of 20th-century composers of opera?

_____

39. All of the following are of the House of Atreus except

(A) Agamemnon
(B) Menelaus
(C) Orestes
(D) Iphigenia
(E) Aphrodite

40. Willy Loman is one of the most famous characters in the modern American theater. He appears in

(A) *Cat on a Hot Tin Roof*
(B) *Murder in the Cathedral*
(C) *The Sand Box*
(D) *Oklahoma!*
(E) *Death of a Salesman*

41. Which item does not belong in the following group?

(A) a priori knowledge
(B) deductive thinking
(C) intuition
(D) formal science
(E) empirical knowledge

42. Which of the following Greek divinities is not properly identified?

(A) Zeus, supreme god of the Greeks
(B) Hephaestus, messenger of the gods
(C) Aphrodite, goddess of love
(D) Artemis, goddess of the moon
(E) Apollo, god of the sun

43. A painter noted for his scenes of the American West was

(A) Thomas Hart Benton
(B) Frederick Remington
(C) Grant Wood
(D) Edward Hopper
(E) John Marin

44. "Capriccio Espagnol" and "Scheherazade" were written by

(A) Glinka
(B) Moussorgsky
(C) Tchaikovsky
(D) Borodin
(E) Rimsky-Korsakov

45. Which of the following composers served as a bridge between the Classical and Romantic periods?

    (A) Bruckner
    (B) Wagner
    (C) Tchaikovsky
    (D) Beethoven
    (E) Berlioz

46. John Steinbeck traveled America and reported on the people he met, the things he saw. His constant companion on one trip was his dog

    (A) Mitzi
    (B) Rocinante
    (C) Charlie
    (D) Joseph
    (E) Willie

47. "The Hand of God" and "The Kiss" are sculptures by

    (A) Rodin
    (B) Bertinelli
    (C) Michelangelo
    (D) Brancusi
    (E) Epstein

48. All of the following operas were written by Mozart except

    (A) *Don Giovanni*
    (B) *The Marriage of Figaro*
    (C) *Orpheus and Eurydice*
    (D) *The Magic Flute*
    (E) *Cosi fan tutte*

49. The American poet who wrote such works as "Abraham Lincoln Walks at Midnight" and "The Santa Fe Trail" was

    (A) Vachel Lindsay
    (B) William Carlos Williams
    (C) Walt Whitman
    (D) Carl Sandburg
    (E) Van Wyck Brooks

50. The medieval liturgical drama

    (A) was an outgrowth of the Roman theater
    (B) was an outgrowth of the Greek theater
    (C) sprang up independently of Roman and Greek theaters
    (D) was based upon pagan rites and rituals
    (E) owed much to such writers as Ben Jonson and William Shakespeare

51. The best known of the medieval morality plays is

    (A) *Quem Quaeritis Trope*
    (B) *The Castell of Perseverance*
    (C) *The Life of Christ*
    (D) *Hamlet*
    (E) *Everyman*

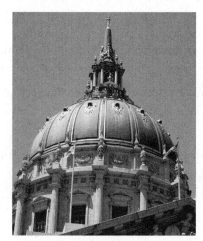

© Charlene Winfred

52. The photograph above shows the Dome of City Hall, San Francisco. What style of architecture can be seen here?

    (A) Greek Revival
    (B) Art Deco
    (C) Federal
    (D) Beaux-Arts
    (E) Georgian

53. An American author who vigorously attacked the "genteel tradition" and who took an active interest in American social problems was

   (A) Stephen Crane
   (B) Edward Arlington Robinson
   (C) Edgar Lee Masters
   (D) Theodore Dreiser
   (E) Thomas Wolfe

54. Two composers from the Baroque period are

   (A) Brahms and Berlioz
   (B) Stravinsky and Piston
   (C) Bach and Handel
   (D) Mozart and Haydn
   (E) Verdi and Puccini

55. Most jazz has a standard form of

   (A) sonata-allegro
   (B) rondo
   (C) theme and variation
   (D) fugue
   (E) canon

56. Surrealist art is associated with

   (A) frottage, the subconscious, paradox
   (B) anxiety, silence, the metaphysical
   (C) timelessness, literary origins, loneliness
   (D) fantasy, Freud, free association
   (E) all of these

57. Unlike most of the later troubadours, the *jongleurs* of the 11th century were

   (A) not of noble birth
   (B) accompanied by a small orchestra
   (C) able to sing the *chanson de geste*
   (D) more sophisticated
   (E) accompanied by two men

58. According to Plato, the principles of goodness and truth are

   (A) purely human conceptions
   (B) a result of class training
   (C) descriptions of the ways our minds work
   (D) objective realities that transcend human experience
   (E) rationalizations to conceal expediency and laziness

59. Two composers of the Italian Renaissance were

   (A) Ockeghem and Paderewski
   (B) Monteverdi and Bellini
   (C) Palestrina and Josquin
   (D) Josquin and Cellini
   (E) Parmagianino and Cavalli

60. *Metaphysics* is primarily the study of

   (A) morals
   (B) art
   (C) the composition of reality
   (D) beauty and goodness
   (E) knowledge

61. The convention by which an actor, "unnoticed" by others on the stage, makes a brief comment to the audience, is the

   (A) soliloquy
   (B) perspective
   (C) aside
   (D) periphery
   (E) denouement

62. The Globe Theater

   (A) was closed on all sides but open on top
   (B) had a stage that extended into the audience area
   (C) depended upon natural lighting
   (D) was built in 1599
   (E) all of these

63. "One that lov'd not wisely but too well," describes

    (A) Hamlet
    (B) Romeo
    (C) Cleopatra
    (D) Othello
    (E) Desdemona

64. All except one of the following 20th-century authors have used materials from their Jewish backgrounds. The one exception is

    (A) Philip Roth
    (B) Saul Bellow
    (C) Bernard Malamud
    (D) Paul Goodman
    (E) John Updike

65. The art of painting on freshly spread moist lime plaster with pigments suspended in a water vehicle is called

    (A) collage
    (B) fresco
    (C) surrealism
    (D) primitivism
    (E) pointillism

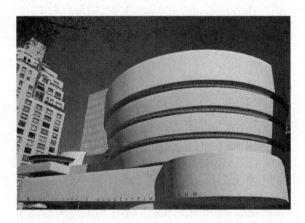

66. The building pictured above is an example of the architecture of

    (A) Christopher Wren
    (B) Inigo Jones
    (C) Frank Lloyd Wright
    (D) Joseph Paxton
    (E) Gustave Eiffel

67. Artists rediscovered man, glorified him as part of the world, and scientists discovered the world around man in the time of

    (A) the Roman Empire
    (B) the Middle Ages
    (C) the late 19th century
    (D) the Greek period
    (E) the Renaissance

68. All of the following were written by Ernest Hemingway except

    (A) *For Whom the Bell Tolls*
    (B) *The Old Lions*
    (C) *The Old Man and the Sea*
    (D) *Death in the Afternoon*
    (E) *The Sun Also Rises*

69. The Renaissance Italian author who, writing in the vernacular, opposed the extension of the pope's secular power was

    (A) Cellini
    (B) Machiavelli
    (C) Dante
    (D) Scotti
    (E) Manzoni

70. John Steinbeck once undertook a study of tide pools with Dr. Ed Ricketts, a noted marine biologist. The trip is recorded in Steinbeck's

    (A) *Two Years Before the Mast*
    (B) *Tide Pools and Sea Urchins*
    (C) *Log of the Sea of Cortez*
    (D) *The Dory*
    (E) *Innocents Abroad*

71. In Shakespeare's plays,

    (A) all the female roles were played by boys when the plays were first produced
    (B) highly stylized language was a convention of the theater
    (C) the "tragic hero" was always of noble birth
    (D) the dialogue was written in poetic forms
    (E) all of the above

72. A Roman writer of comedy was

    (A) Menander
    (B) Hrosvitha
    (C) Plautus
    (D) Seneca
    (E) Sodomaeus

73. The American author who gave the English language the word *babbitry* was

    (A) Sinclair Lewis
    (B) Robinson Jeffers
    (C) Willa Cather
    (D) Edward Arlington Robinson
    (E) John Steinbeck

Questions 74 and 75 refer to the following line of poetry:

"How do I love thee? Let me count the ways."

74. This is the opening line of

    (A) *A Midsummer's Night Dream*
    (B) "Sonnets from the Portuguese"
    (C) "Burnt Norton"
    (D) "Sestina Altaforte"
    (E) "The Ballade of Dead Ladies"

75. The poem from which the line is taken was written by

    (A) William Shakespeare
    (B) T.S. Eliot
    (C) Ezra Pound
    (D) Robert Browning
    (E) Elizabeth Barrett Browning

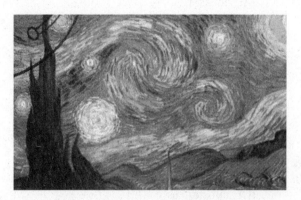

76. The photograph above is an example of a style of painting popular during which century?

    (A) 15th
    (B) 17th
    (C) 18th
    (D) 19th
    (E) 20th

77. When the ghost in *Hamlet* appeared, most people in Shakespeare's audience would have

    (A) laughed, because the supernatural was considered ridiculous
    (B) recognized the figure as a dramatic symbol
    (C) been unimpressed, since the device had been over-used
    (D) reacted in a manner that we are unable to guess
    (E) believed in the actuality of ghosts appearing on stage

78. The architect who designed the Crystal Palace was

   (A) Charles Percier
   (B) P.F.L. Fontaine
   (C) Joseph Paxton
   (D) James Wyatt
   (E) Georges-Eugene Haussmann

79. Agamemnon's wife was

   (A) Jocasta
   (B) Clytaemnestra
   (C) Cassandra
   (D) Iphigenia
   (E) Antigone

80. When we speak of the study of *axiology*, we are talking about the interpretation of

   (A) existences
   (B) essences
   (C) substances
   (D) forms
   (E) values

81. The "green ey'd monster which doth mock the meat it feeds on" is

   (A) revenge
   (B) jealousy
   (C) pride
   (D) hatred
   (E) lust

82. The Upanishads are a group of writings sacred in

   (A) Judaism
   (B) Islam
   (C) Buddhism
   (D) Hinduism
   (E) Zoroastrianism

83. The Greek chorus did not

   (A) foretell the future
   (B) explain past actions
   (C) serve as the additional character in the play
   (D) philosophize
   (E) help to move scenery

84. Creon repents and goes to free Antigone, but she has already hanged herself. This is an example of

   (A) denouement
   (B) proscenium
   (C) deus ex machina
   (D) irony
   (E) *in medias res*

85. The modern meaning of deux ex machina in relation to drama is

   (A) a wheeled platform used as part of the scenery
   (B) a god from a machine
   (C) a mechanical device for staging elaborate effects
   (D) the catastrophic event at the climax of a play
   (E) an unsatisfactory resolution to problems of plot by means of an event for which the audience has not been prepared

86. Vincent van Gogh

   (A) faithfully followed the Impressionist techniques
   (B) felt that Impressionism did not allow the artist enough freedom to express his inner feelings
   (C) believed the artist must paint only what he could see, not what appeared in the mind
   (D) founded the movement in art called "abstract art"
   (E) led 17th-century art back to natural forms of realism

87. A single melody with subordinate harmony demonstrates

   (A) polyphonic texture
   (B) homophonic texture
   (C) monophonic texture
   (D) bitonality
   (E) rondo form

88. The musical terms *consonance* and *dissonance* are most properly used in a discussion of

   (A) texture
   (B) tone color
   (C) melody
   (D) rhythm
   (E) harmony

89. Gregorian chants are examples of which textures?

   (A) monophonic
   (B) contrapuntal
   (C) polyphonic
   (D) homophonic
   (E) modern

90. Which of the following is not characteristic of the Gregorian chant?

   (A) meter
   (B) use of Latin
   (C) use of eight church modes
   (D) male choir
   (E) a capella

91. A school of art known as *Surrealism* developed in the 1920s. A forerunner of the Surrealist school and the painter of *I and My Village* was

   (A) Picasso
   (B) Chagall
   (C) Klee
   (D) Kandinsky
   (E) Beckman

92. What author, sometimes called a western realist, wrote many tales of the American West and its mining towns?

   (A) A.P. Oakhurst
   (B) Ambrose Bierce
   (C) Stephen Crane
   (D) Bret Harte
   (E) M. Shipton

93. A singer, actress, poet, and playwright, perhaps best known for her autobiographical series, which includes *I Know Why the Caged Bird Sings and Gather Together in My Name,* is

   (A) Alice Walker
   (B) Linda Reed
   (C) Maya Angelou
   (D) Patricia Goldberg
   (E) Meryl Brooks

94. "The Rhapsody in Blue" was composed by

   (A) Paul Whiteman
   (B) Oscar Levant
   (C) Leonard Bernstein
   (D) Antheil Carpenter
   (E) George Gershwin

95. The first "King of Jazz" was a New Orleans barber named

   (A) Al Hirt
   (B) Bix Beiderbecke
   (C) Sidney Bechet
   (D) Charles Bolden
   (E) Papa Celestine

96. Almost every country in Europe has a national hero who has been enshrined in epic poems and myths. The national hero of Italy is

   (A) El Cid
   (B) Orlando Furioso
   (C) Beowulf
   (D) Roland
   (E) Giovanni Magnifioso

97. "The Canticle of the Sun" was written by

(A) Dante
(B) Chaucer
(C) St. Francis of Assisi
(D) Caedmon
(E) The Venerable Bede

98. The 20th-century composer who first used the twelve-tone method was

(A) Arnold Schoenberg
(B) Leonard Bernstein
(C) John Cage
(D) George Gershwin
(E) Richard Rodgers

99. Which of the following statements is *false*?

(A) Satire is a means of showing dissatisfaction with an established institution or principle.
(B) Satire is most easily accepted by an audience holding various beliefs or beliefs different from those of the playwright.
(C) Satire was an early form of comedy.
(D) *Lysistrata* is a classic example of satire.
(E) Modern satire does not run the risk of being offensive.

100. LADY BRACKNELL: "Do you smoke?"

JACK: "Well, yes, I must admit I smoke."

LADY BRACKNELL: "I am glad to hear it. A man should always have an occupation of some sort."

The dialogue from Oscar Wilde's *The Importance of Being Earnest* illustrates

(A) sympathy
(B) empathy
(C) scorn
(D) comic pathos
(E) linguistic wit

101. Today's foremost American composer of musicals, noted for *Company, Sweeney Todd,* and *Sunday in the Park with George,* is

(A) Elmer Bernstein
(B) Stephen Sondheim
(C) Richard Rodgers
(D) Frederick Loewe
(E) Ernest Fleischman

102. Which American author, grandchild of a president, wrote a famous book about his own education?

(A) Henry Adams
(B) Robert Jackson
(C) Jonathan Tyler
(D) Elliot Roosevelt
(E) Howard Taft

103. In 1988 Toni Morrison won the Pulitzer Prize for her novel

(A) *Sula*
(B) *Song of Solomon*
(C) *I Know Why the Caged Bird Sings*
(D) *Beloved*
(E) *Tar Baby*

104. Best known for his book *I and Thou* is the philosopher

(A) Nietzsche
(B) Buber
(C) Russell
(D) Chardin
(E) Sartre

105. The Mexican painter whose murals can be seen in the Government Palace at Guadalajara is

(A) Rivera
(B) Orozco
(C) Siqueiros
(D) Hernández
(E) Cinfuentes

106. "I saw the sky descending black and white" is an example of

(A) iambic pentameter
(B) anapestic dimeter
(C) spondaic hexameter
(D) dactylic pentameter
(E) iambic tetrameter

107. Which of the following statements concerning courtly love is false?

(A) The idea was born in Provence in the 11th century.
(B) It was limited to the nobility.
(C) True love was considered impossible between husband and wife.
(D) Christian behavior was shunned.
(E) It glorified adultery.

108. The site of Apollo's great oracle was

(A) Parnassus
(B) Olympus
(C) Athens
(D) Crete
(E) Delphi

109. The "Age of Faith" is a term that best applies to the

(A) classical Greek period
(B) Baroque period
(C) Gothic period
(D) Renaissance
(E) 18th century

110. According to the Hedonist philosophers,

(A) actions are right if they tend to promote pleasure
(B) good acts depend primarily upon good intentions
(C) good cannot be separated from work
(D) duty makes an absolute demand upon us
(E) right conduct involves obedience to some established authority

111. Giotto is noted for

(A) writing a poem on a Grecian urn
(B) discovering the principle of the flying buttress
(C) the beginning of realistic painting in Western art, about 1300
(D) impressionistic painting since 1900
(E) inventing a secret process, now lost, for turning jewels into stained glass

Questions 112–114 refer to illustrations (A) through (E).

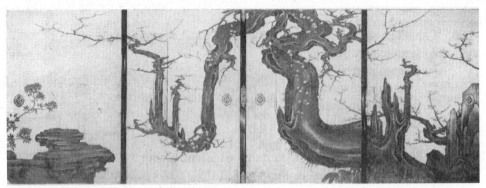

The Metropolitan Museum of Art, The Harry G.C. Packard Collection of Asian Art, Gift of
Harry G.C. Packard and Purchase, Fletcher, Rogers, Harris Brisbane Dick and Louis V. Bell Funds,
Joseph Pulitzer Bequest and The Annenberg Fund, Inc. Gift, 1975 (1975.268.48a-d)
Image © The Metropolitan Museum of Art.

(A)

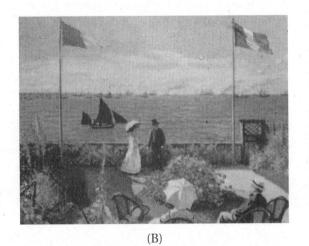

(B)

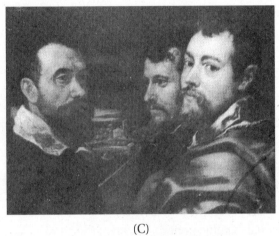

(C)

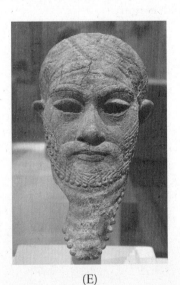

(D)

(E)

112. Which is the Rembrandt?

113. Which is Japanese?

114. Which is an example of Impressionism?

———————————

115. The image below is a photograph of

(A) the Parthenon
(B) the Coliseum
(C) Stonehenge
(D) the Temple at Karnak
(E) the Lighthouse at Knossos

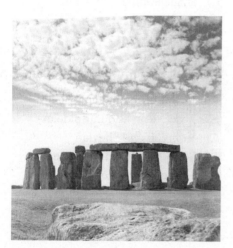

Ruth S. Ward

116. In ancient and medieval mythology, the griffin is usually represented as a

(A) winged horse
(B) cross between a lion and an eagle
(C) creature that is half man, half horse
(D) winged lion with the head of a woman
(E) devil with horns and cloven hooves

117. Deucalion is

(A) the Greek Noah
(B) the 10th book of the Bible
(C) one of the daughters of Danaus
(D) a whirlpool Odysseus encountered on his voyage
(E) the hero of the Trojan War

118. "Ding, dong, bell;
Pussy's in the well.
Who put her in?
Little Johnny Thin."

The lines above are an example of

(A) slant rhyme
(B) a run-on line
(C) sprung rhythm
(D) hidden alliteration
(E) ottava rima

119. A painter noted for his moving portraits, with bright light emerging from a dark canvas, is

(A) Pollock
(B) Picasso
(C) Rembrandt
(D) Vermeer
(E) van Gogh

120. The musical sign ♭

(A) indicates false notes: falsetto
(B) lowers the pitch of a note by a full step
(C) precedes a note to be raised a full step
(D) precedes a note to be raised by a half step
(E) lowers the pitch of a note by a half step

121. Songs that are not as unreal as operatic arias but are much more sophisticated than folk songs are called

(A) natural
(B) erotic
(C) lieder
(D) appassionata
(E) nova

122. As Candide journeyed from continent to continent, he searched for

(A) Dr. Pangloss
(B) the Oreillons
(C) Providence
(D) Cacambo
(E) Cunegonde

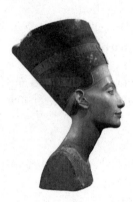

123. The photograph above is a bust of

(A) Queen Elizabeth I
(B) Queen Nefertiti
(C) the goddess Athena
(D) Buddha
(E) an unknown African warrior

124. The photograph above is an example of

(A) neolithic art
(B) Corinthian art
(C) Greek art
(D) Egyptian art
(E) Renaissance art

125. Peter Weir directed all of the following films *except*

(A) *The Truman Show*
(B) *Witness*
(C) *On the Beach*
(D) *Dead Poets Society*
(E) *Picnic at Hanging Rock*

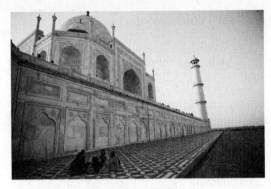

© Charlene Winfred

126. What structure is shown in the photograph above?

(A) L'Institut du Monde Arabe
(B) Mosque of Cristo de la Luz
(C) Hagia Sophia
(D) the Taj Mahal
(E) Fatehpur Sikri

127. Two principal forms of irony in tragedy are

(A) Euripidean and Sophoclean
(B) Aeschylean and Euripidean
(C) Ibsenian and Shavian
(D) Sophoclean and Aeschylean
(E) comic and tragic

128. Leitmotif means

(A) a note that is sung only once
(B) a note or theme that is repeated
(C) the leading motive
(D) an aria
(E) the first violinist is to take over leading the orchestra

129. Which of the following is not a convention of the Elizabethan theater?

(A) women's roles acted by young boys
(B) setting established by dialogue
(C) a chorus of elders
(D) poetic language
(E) the soliloquy

130. The basing of knowledge on scientific observation is best illustrated by

   (A) empiricists
   (B) rationalists
   (C) theologians
   (D) both rationalists and theologians
   (E) existentialists

131. In Greek mythology, the greatest of all musicians was

   (A) Dionysius
   (B) Musicus
   (C) Pan
   (D) Apollo
   (E) Orpheus

132. Odysseus' old nurse, who recognizes him from a scar on his leg, was named

   (A) Argus
   (B) Euryclea
   (C) Menelaus
   (D) Calliope
   (E) Nausicaa

133. What Florentine autobiographer, goldsmith, and sculptor was a child of will rather than of reason and the quintessential Renaissance man?

   (A) Cellini
   (B) Lucagnolo
   (C) Urbrino
   (D) Francesco
   (E) Machiavelli

134. *Libretto* means the

   (A) rhythm of a musical composition
   (B) words of a musical composition, especially an opera
   (C) tempo of a musical composition
   (D) directions to the conductor
   (E) full orchestra is to play

135. A 20th-century poet who left America, went to England, and became one of England's most famous citizens was

   (A) Ezra Pound
   (B) Robinson Jeffers
   (C) Archibald MacLeish
   (D) Thomas Wolfe
   (E) T.S. Eliot

136. At the end of Saint-Exupéry's fairy tale, *The Little Prince*, the little prince

   (A) dies
   (B) goes home to his planet
   (C) falls into a deep sleep
   (D) decides to remain on earth
   (E) changes into a star

137. The work of the American artist Mary Cassatt was greatly influenced by the art of

   (A) the Bauhaus school
   (B) the French Impressionists
   (C) early German Expressionists
   (D) American Abstract Expressionists
   (E) Native American art

138. A famous opera based on *Madame Butterfly* was written by

   (A) Puccini
   (B) Verdi
   (C) Strauss
   (D) Monteverdi
   (E) Offenbach

139. Which of these dances is performed by two preadolescent girls?

   (A) Legong
   (B) Bhangra
   (C) Kecak
   (D) Bharata Natyam
   (E) Noh Mai

140. Which of the following did *not* write an autobiography that became well-known?

 (A) Henry Adams
 (B) Benjamin Franklin
 (C) John Stuart Mill
 (D) Bertrand Russell
 (E) George Washington

141. The first black American writer to win the Nobel Prize for Literature was

 (A) Maya Angelou
 (B) Richard Wright
 (C) Toni Morrison
 (D) Langston Hughes
 (E) James Baldwin

142. A park dedicated to the sculptor Gustav Vigeland is to be found in

 (A) Oslo
 (B) Copenhagen
 (C) Paris
 (D) Helsinki
 (E) Stockholm

143. In music, a performer of unusual interpretive and technical skill is referred to as a(n)

 (A) savant
 (B) virtuoso
 (C) prima donna
 (D) maestro
 (E) maestoso

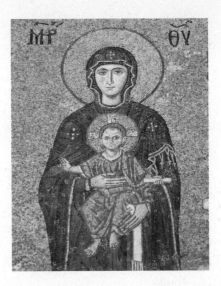

144. This art is an example of

 (A) Expressionism
 (B) Impressionism
 (C) Greek art
 (D) Byzantine art
 (E) primitive art

145. The author of the one-act plays *The Toilet* and *Dutchman* is

 (A) Thomas Wolfe
 (B) James Baldwin
 (C) Lorraine Hansbury
 (D) LeRoi Jones (Imamu Amiri Baraka)
 (E) Countee Cullen

146. The modern musical *My Fair Lady* is based upon G.B. Shaw's play

 (A) *Man and Superman*
 (B) *Back to Methusaleh*
 (C) *Pygmalion*
 (D) *Candida*
 (E) *Arms and the Man*

Questions 147–149 refer to the following lines:

(A) "I have measured out my life in coffee spoons."

(B) "Do not go gentle into that good night,
Old age should burn and rave at close day;
Rage, rage, against the dying of the light."

(C) "How did they fume, and stamp, and roar, and chafe!
And swear, not Addison himself was safe."

(D) "O Captain! my Captain! our fearful trip is done,
The ship has weather'd every rack, the prize we sought is won,
The port is near, the bells I hear, the people all exulting,
While follow eyes the steady keel, the vessel grim and daring;
But O heart! heart! heart!
O the bleeding drops of red,
Where on the deck my captain lies,
Fallen cold and dead."

(E) "Shall I compare thee to a summer's day?
Thou art more lovely and more temperate."

147. Which alludes to the death of Abraham Lincoln?

148. Which is an example of a rhymed couplet?

149. Which is from a Shakespearean sonnet?

---

150. A cathedral noted for its famous rose windows is located at

(A) Canterbury
(B) Rome
(C) London
(D) Chartres
(E) Istanbul

STOP

If there is still time remaining, you may review your answers.

ANSWER KEY
Sample Examination 1

HUMANITIES

1.	B	39.	E	77.	B	115.	C
2.	E	40.	E	78.	C	116.	B
3.	D	41.	C	79.	B	117.	A
4.	E	42.	B	80.	E	118.	C
5.	A	43.	B	81.	B	119.	C
6.	D	44.	E	82.	D	120.	E
7.	B	45.	D	83.	E	121.	C
8.	D	46.	C	84.	D	122.	E
9.	B	47.	A	85.	E	123.	B
10.	B	48.	C	86.	B	124.	D
11.	E	49.	A	87.	B	125.	C
12.	D	50.	C	88.	E	126.	D
13.	A	51.	E	89.	A	127.	A
14.	C	52.	D	90.	A	128.	B
15.	D	53.	D	91.	B	129.	C
16.	D	54.	C	92.	C	130.	A
17.	E	55.	C	93.	C	131.	E
18.	E	56.	E	94.	E	132.	B
19.	B	57.	A	95.	D	133.	A
20.	C	58.	D	96.	B	134.	B
21.	C	59.	C	97.	C	135.	E
22.	E	60.	C	98.	A	136.	B
23.	D	61.	C	99.	E	137.	B
24.	C	62.	E	100.	E	138.	A
25.	A	63.	D	101.	B	139.	A
26.	D	64.	E	102.	A	140.	E
27.	B	65.	B	103.	D	141.	C
28.	D	66.	C	104.	B	142.	A
29.	B	67.	E	105.	B	143.	B
30.	D	68.	B	106.	A	144.	D
31.	E	69.	C	107.	D	145.	D
32.	A	70.	C	108.	E	146.	C
33.	E	71.	E	109.	C	147.	D
34.	B	72.	C	110.	A	148.	C
35.	C	73.	A	111.	C	149.	E
36.	A	74.	B	112.	D	150.	D
37.	E	75.	E	113.	A		
38.	B	76.	D	114.	B		

SCORING CHART

After you have scored your Sample Examination 1, enter the results in the chart below; then transfer your score to the Progress Chart on page 12.

Total Test	Number Right	Number Wrong	Number Omitted
150			

ANSWER EXPLANATIONS

1. **(B)** Carl Orff believes that music in the long-accepted classical or romantic tradition has come to an end, and since 1935 has dedicated himself to the stage.

2. **(E)** *The White Peacock* was written by Charles T. Griffes.

3. **(D)** Fernand Leger (1881–1955), a Cubist, exhibited with both Braque and Picasso.

4. **(E)** De Kooning started his first series of women in 1938.

5. **(A)** James Fenimore Cooper (1789–1851) is best remembered for his *Leatherstocking Tales.*

6. **(D)** Fitzgerald, perhaps best known for his novel *The Great Gatsby,* also wrote short stories, one of the most popular being "Bernice Bobs Her Hair."

7. **(B)** "Gothic" pertains to an architectural style prevalent in western Europe from the 12th through the 15th centuries.

8. **(D)** Other countries have attempted to make westerns, but have had, in the view of many critics, only limited success.

9. **(B)** Benvenuto Cellini (1500–1571) was an Italian sculptor, metal-worker, and author.

10. **(B)** *Dr. Faustus* was written by Christopher Marlowe.

11. **(E)** Louis XIV (1638–1715) was king of France from 1643 to 1715.

12. **(D)** This is true by definition.

13. **(A)** Impressionism was the late-19th-century movement. The other composers listed are either not French, not Impressionist composers, or not both.

14. **(C)** The Renaissance originated in Italy in the 14th century, and later spread through Europe. Leonardo da Vinci (1452–1519) lived during the peak of the Italian Renaissance.

15. **(D)** This is true by definition.

16. **(D)** The point is that man is "determined" by heredity and/or environment.

17. **(E)** During other periods in time, all plays had a beginning, a middle, and an end.

18. **(E)** The poem is divided into three canticles, each made up of thirty-three cantos, plus the first canto in "Inferno," which serves as an introduction to the entire poem.

19. **(B)** Michelangelo was the famous painter of the Sistine Chapel.

20. **(C)** Stock characters, such as the braggart soldier, the jealous husband, and the stubborn father, appear as far back as the Greek and Roman comedies.

21. **(C)** Pavlova was promoted to prima ballerina in 1906, after a performance of *Swan Lake.*

22. **(E)** This American Primitive work was painted by an unknown artist, circa 1795.

23. **(D)** This is true by definition.

24. **(C)** Sanjit Ray was an Indian filmmaker. He studied at a university founded by his eminent compatriot, the writer Rabindranath Tagore. Throughout his life, Ray was influenced by Tagore and his writing.

25. **(A)** Isak Dinesen was the pen name of Karen Dinesen von Blixen. She signed her stories "Isak," meaning "he who laughs."

26. **(D)** Goya was the leading painter, etcher, and designer of his day.

27. **(B)** None of the others were Greek playwrights.

28. **(D)** One of the most enduring popular examples of this genre is Mary Shelley's *Frankenstein.*

29. **(B)** The work is *The Aeneid.*

30. **(D)** *Parsifal* was the first presented in 1882 in Bayreuth.

31. **(E)** The flying buttress was a development in Gothic architecture.

32. **(A)** Gauguin spent many years in Tahiti, painting native subjects.

33. **(E)** Brecht has even written plays within plays within plays so that the audience is always aware it is attending a play, and not experiencing reality.

34. **(B)** The Bayeux Tapestry depicts the Norman Conquest of England and the events leading up to it.

35. **(C)** Athens was the home of the arts, mathematics, philosophy, etc.

36. **(A)** The others are not 20th-century painters.

37. **(E)** The others are not 20th-century poets.

38. **(B)** The others are not 20th-century composers of opera.

39. **(E)** Aphrodite was the Greek goddess of love.

40. **(E)** The play was written by Arthur Miller, and it ushered in a new concept of tragedy.

41. **(C)** Intuition may be defined as the power or faculty of attaining to direct knowledge or cognition without rational thought. All the other terms imply rational thought.

42. **(B)** Hephaestus was the Greek god of fire and metalcraft.

43. **(B)** Remington is especially noted for his cowboys, Indians, and soldiers.

44. **(E)** Rimsky-Korsakov (1844–1908) was a Russian composer.

45. **(D)** Ludwig van Beethoven (1770–1827) studied with Mozart and Haydn and influenced the later Romantic composers.

46. **(C)** The book Steinbeck wrote was entitled *Travels with Charlie.*

47. **(A)** Auguste Rodin (1840–1917), the great French artist, was perhaps the greatest sculptor of his time.

48. **(C)** *Orpheus and Eurydice* was written by Gluck.

49. **(A)** Vachel Lindsay (1897–1931) was an American poet noted for his individualistic style, characterized by jazz-like rhythm.

50. **(C)** The medieval liturgical drama developed during the celebration of the mass.

51. **(E)** *Everyman* is a 15th-century allegorical play. Everyman, the hero, is summoned by Death to appear before God. Of all his friends and virtues, only Good Deeds may accompany him.

52. **(D)** San Francisco City Hall was destroyed in the 1906 earthquake and was rebuilt in the Beaux-Arts style.

53. **(D)** Two of Dreiser's best known novels are *An American Tragedy* and *Sister Carrie.*

54. **(C)** The other composers are not both from the Baroque period.

55. **(C)** Each time a musician plays a jazz work, he or she interprets the piece. Jazz is notoriously individualistic and variable.

56. **(E)** To select but one of the other answers would be to only partially explain Surrealism.

57. **(A)** These early medieval minstrels came from the lower classes. They usually accompanied themselves on a simple musical instrument, such as a lute.

58. **(D)** This is one of the basic tenets of Platonism.

59. **(C)** This is the only example of two composers, both Italian and of the Renaissance period.

60. **(C)** Metaphysics is the branch of philosophy concerned with the ultimate nature of reality.

61. **(C)** This is true by definition. The aside differs from the soliloquy in that, in the latter, the character reveals his thoughts in the form of a monologue, without addressing a listener.

62. **(E)** To ignore any of the above would be to give an incomplete answer.

63. **(D)** This line is spoken after the death of Othello, and refers to his intense passion for Desdemona, which led to his murdering her in a fit of jealousy.

64. **(E)** Updike's best known works are *Rabbit, Run* and *Rabbit Redux.*

65. **(B)** This is true by definition.

66. **(C)** Wright was a modern architect who believed in functional buildings, made of materials native to the region.

67. **(E)** The clue is in the word *rediscovered.* Renaissance means rebirth or revival of interest in learning.

68. **(B)** Hemingway was a famous 20th-century American writer who won the Nobel Prize for literature.

69. **(C)** Dante's best-known work is *The Divine Comedy.*

70. **(C)** The Sea of Cortez, in Mexico, sometimes called the Gulf of California, separates Baja California from Sonora.

71. **(E)** The others are true, but only partial answers.

72. **(C)** Plautus and Terence were the great Roman writers of comedy.

73. **(A)** The word was coined from the title of Lewis' novel *Babbitt.* Babbitry can be defined as "narrow-minded materialism."

74. **(B)** The sonnet sequence that opens with the line quoted is one of the most famous in English literature.

75. **(E)** Elizabeth Barrett wrote the sonnet sequence for her future husband, Robert Browning.

76. **(D)** The painting is *The Starry Night,* by Vincent van Gogh (1853–1890).

77. **(B)** Ghosts often appeared in Elizabethan plays as dramatic symbols. The audience was accustomed to the dramatic use of the ghost.

78. **(C)** Paxton first designed a similar but larger structure for the London Exhibition of 1851. In 1853 and 1854 he supervised the building of the Crystal Palace at Sydenham, England.

79. **(B)** Agamemnon was the leader of the Greeks in the Trojan War. Upon his return from the war Clytaemnestra and Aegisthus, her lover, murdered Agamemnon in his bath.

80. **(E)** This is true by definition.

81. **(B)** This line is from Shakespeare's *Othello.*

82. **(D)** The Upanishads are philosophical texts considered to be an early source of Hindu religion.

83. **(E)** The Greeks did not use scenery in their plays.

84. **(D)** Dramatic irony occurs when the audience understands the incongruity between a situation and the accompanying speeches while the characters in the play remain unaware of the incongruity.

85. **(E)** The modern meaning is that of a contrived or improbable conclusion.

86. **(B)** Van Gogh is generally considered a post-Impressionist.

87. **(B)** This is true by definition.

88. **(E)** Harmony, in music, refers to the structure of a musical composition from the point of view of its chordal characteristics and relationships.

89. **(A)** Gregorian chants contain a single melodic line.

90. **(A)** Gregorian chant is the monodic liturgical plainsong of the Roman Catholic Church.

91. **(B)** Chagall is also well known for his stained glass windows that adorn churches and synagogues throughout Europe and Israel.

92. **(D)** Two of Harte's best-known short stories are "The Outcasts of Poker Flat" and "The Luck of Roaring Camp."

93. **(C)** Angelou, born in Arkansas in 1928, also wrote *Singin' and Swingin' and Gettin' Merry Like Christmas* and *The Heart of a Woman.*

94. **(E)** Gershwin was also the composer of the folk opera *Porgy and Bess,* as well as many popular songs.

95. **(D)** The others are jazz figures, but none were barbers.

96. **(B)** Ariosto's "Orlando Furioso" is the best-known poem on the subject.

97. **(C)** Francis of Assisi was the founder of the Franciscan Order and one of the greatest of Christian saints.

98. **(A)** Schoenberg's twelve-tone system has become perhaps the most controversial musical development of the 20th century.

99. **(E)** Modern satire is often intentionally offensive.

100. **(E)** Wilde was noted for his linguistic wit.

101. **(B)** Sondheim's most recent works are *Into the Woods* and *Passion.* He also wrote the lyrics for *West Side Story.*

102. **(A)** The book is entitled *The Education of Henry Adams.*

103. **(D)** A novel in the "magical realism" mode, *Beloved* is based upon a true story of infanticide in Kentucky.

104. **(B)** Martin Buber's *I and Thou* posits a direct dialogue between the individual and God.

105. **(B)** Jose Clemente Orozco (1883–1949) was a painter of revolutionary murals. The imagination and emotional force of the murals in the Government Palace are impressively powerful.

106. **(A)** The iamb is a metrical foot consisting of a short syllable followed by a long or an unstressed syllable followed by a stressed. *Pentameter* means "five meters," or feet, and so iambic pentameter equals five iambs to the line.

107. **(D)** Under the rules of courtly love, the true knight was expected to be the epitome of the Christian man.

108. **(E)** Delphi is located near Mount Parnassus in ancient Greece. The legendary founder of the oracle was the goddess Gaea.

109. **(C)** The Gothic period approximates the Middle Ages. It was during this period that the Roman Catholic Church had its greatest hold on the populace.

110. **(A)** The Greek doctrine of hedonism states that pleasure is the highest good. In ancient times, hedonism was characteristic of the school of Aristippus.

111. **(C)** Giotto (c.1266–c.1337), Florentine painter and architect, was a perfector of form and movement. His faces and gestures are graceful and lifelike.

112. **(D)** The photograph is of a self-portrait by the 54-year-old Rembrandt, whose long series of self-portraits records every stage of his career.

113. **(A)** An ancient plum tree decorates these Japanese sliding screens from the study room of a Zen temple.

114. **(B)** Monet's *Terrace at Sainte-Adresse*, shown in this photograph, is an Impressionist painting.

115. **(C)** Stonehenge, a prehistoric structure, is on Salisbury Plain, in England.

116. **(B)** The origin of the griffin has been traced to the Hittites. It is also conspicuous in Assyrian and Persian sculpture.

117. **(A)** Deucalion and his wife, Pyrrha, are the principal figures in the Greek flood story.

118. **(C)** Sprung rhythm is a term for a mixed meter in which the foot consists of a stressed syllable which may stand alone, or be combined with from one to three more unstressed syllables.

119. **(C)** Rembrandt van Rijn (1606–1669), Dutch painter and etcher, was the greatest master of the Dutch school.

120. **(E)** This is a standard musical notation, a flat.

121. **(C)** The other words have nothing to do with songs.

122. **(E)** Cunegonde was the woman with whom Candide was in love.

123. **(B)** Nefertiti was an ancient Egyptian queen, wife of Akhenaton, a pharoah who ruled from 1367 to 1350 B.C.

124. **(D)** See above.

125. **(C)** The Australian Peter Weir directed all of the films except *On the Beach*, which was directed by Stanley Kramer.

126. **(D)** The Taj Mahal is an example of Mughal architecture, which combines elements from Indian, Persian, and Moslem styles.

127. **(A)** In Sophoclean irony the characters are symbols of tragic human fate. In Euripidean tragedy, the irony lies in the inner psyche of humans, who no longer struggle with fate, but fight with the demons of their own souls; each person is responsible for his or her actions.

128. **(B)** This is true by definition.

129. **(C)** The Elizabethan theater, unlike the Greek, did not make use of a chorus.

130. **(A)** Empiricism may be defined as the practice of relying upon observation and experiment, especially in the natural sciences.

131. **(E)** Orpheus was so skilled in singing and in playing the lyre that he could enchant not only men and animals, but even trees and stones.

132. **(B)** Euryclea appears in the *The Odyssey*.

133. **(A)** None of the others mentioned was as knowledgeable and talented in so many areas as Cellini.

134. **(B)** This is true by definition.

135. **(E)** T.S. Eliot is known as the author of "The Wasteland," "The Love Song of J. Alfred Prufrock," the play *Murder in the Cathedral,* and a large number of other works.

136. **(B)** Saint-Exupéry tells his reader to look up to the stars and listen for the laughter of the little prince.

137. **(B)** Mary Cassatt was for a time a part of an Impressionist group of painters in France, and much of her work was influenced by the school.

138. **(A)** Puccini's opera was first performed in 1904, and is still one of the most popular of all operas.

139. **(A)** Legong is a Balinese dance performed by two girls who have not reached puberty.

140. **(E)** George Washington did not write an autobiography. The autobiographies by the other men are regarded as important works.

141. **(C)** Nobel Laureate Toni Morrison is the author of *Song of Solomon, The Bluest Eye, Beloved,* and *Jazz.*

142. **(A)** Vigeland studied in Oslo and Copenhagen, and in Paris with Rodin. Many of his sculpted figures represent the cycle of mankind from birth to death.

143. **(B)** This is true by definition.

144. **(D)** Byzantine refers to the style developed in Byzantium from the 5th century A.D. It is characterized by formality of design, frontal, stylized presentation of figures, rich use of color, especially gold, and generally religious subject matter.

145. **(D)** The contemporary American author LeRoi Jones changed his name to Imamu Amiri Baraka when he adopted the Muslim faith.

146. **(C)** Shaw's early-20th-century *Pygmalion* is one of his most frequently performed plays. *My Fair Lady* is the musical by Lerner and Loewe.

147. **(D)** The quote is from Walt Whitman's *O Captain! My Captain!*—a poem on Lincoln's death.

148. **(C)** These two lines are an example of a heroic couplet—two rhymed lines of verse of ten syllables each, having the same meter. The example here was written by Alexander Pope, a master of the heroic couplet. It is from Pope's "An Epistle to Dr. Arbuthnot."

149. **(E)** These are the first two lines of Shakespeare's Sonnet 18.

150. **(D)** The Gothic cathedral of Chartres is in northern France.

ANSWER SHEET
Sample Examination 2

HUMANITIES

1. Ⓐ Ⓑ Ⓒ Ⓓ Ⓔ	39. Ⓐ Ⓑ Ⓒ Ⓓ Ⓔ	77. Ⓐ Ⓑ Ⓒ Ⓓ Ⓔ	115. Ⓐ Ⓑ Ⓒ Ⓓ Ⓔ
2. Ⓐ Ⓑ Ⓒ Ⓓ Ⓔ	40. Ⓐ Ⓑ Ⓒ Ⓓ Ⓔ	78. Ⓐ Ⓑ Ⓒ Ⓓ Ⓔ	116. Ⓐ Ⓑ Ⓒ Ⓓ Ⓔ
3. Ⓐ Ⓑ Ⓒ Ⓓ Ⓔ	41. Ⓐ Ⓑ Ⓒ Ⓓ Ⓔ	79. Ⓐ Ⓑ Ⓒ Ⓓ Ⓔ	117. Ⓐ Ⓑ Ⓒ Ⓓ Ⓔ
4. Ⓐ Ⓑ Ⓒ Ⓓ Ⓔ	42. Ⓐ Ⓑ Ⓒ Ⓓ Ⓔ	80. Ⓐ Ⓑ Ⓒ Ⓓ Ⓔ	118. Ⓐ Ⓑ Ⓒ Ⓓ Ⓔ
5. Ⓐ Ⓑ Ⓒ Ⓓ Ⓔ	43. Ⓐ Ⓑ Ⓒ Ⓓ Ⓔ	81. Ⓐ Ⓑ Ⓒ Ⓓ Ⓔ	119. Ⓐ Ⓑ Ⓒ Ⓓ Ⓔ
6. Ⓐ Ⓑ Ⓒ Ⓓ Ⓔ	44. Ⓐ Ⓑ Ⓒ Ⓓ Ⓔ	82. Ⓐ Ⓑ Ⓒ Ⓓ Ⓔ	120. Ⓐ Ⓑ Ⓒ Ⓓ Ⓔ
7. Ⓐ Ⓑ Ⓒ Ⓓ Ⓔ	45. Ⓐ Ⓑ Ⓒ Ⓓ Ⓔ	83. Ⓐ Ⓑ Ⓒ Ⓓ Ⓔ	121. Ⓐ Ⓑ Ⓒ Ⓓ Ⓔ
8. Ⓐ Ⓑ Ⓒ Ⓓ Ⓔ	46. Ⓐ Ⓑ Ⓒ Ⓓ Ⓔ	84. Ⓐ Ⓑ Ⓒ Ⓓ Ⓔ	122. Ⓐ Ⓑ Ⓒ Ⓓ Ⓔ
9. Ⓐ Ⓑ Ⓒ Ⓓ Ⓔ	47. Ⓐ Ⓑ Ⓒ Ⓓ Ⓔ	85. Ⓐ Ⓑ Ⓒ Ⓓ Ⓔ	123. Ⓐ Ⓑ Ⓒ Ⓓ Ⓔ
10. Ⓐ Ⓑ Ⓒ Ⓓ Ⓔ	48. Ⓐ Ⓑ Ⓒ Ⓓ Ⓔ	86. Ⓐ Ⓑ Ⓒ Ⓓ Ⓔ	124. Ⓐ Ⓑ Ⓒ Ⓓ Ⓔ
11. Ⓐ Ⓑ Ⓒ Ⓓ Ⓔ	49. Ⓐ Ⓑ Ⓒ Ⓓ Ⓔ	87. Ⓐ Ⓑ Ⓒ Ⓓ Ⓔ	125. Ⓐ Ⓑ Ⓒ Ⓓ Ⓔ
12. Ⓐ Ⓑ Ⓒ Ⓓ Ⓔ	50. Ⓐ Ⓑ Ⓒ Ⓓ Ⓔ	88. Ⓐ Ⓑ Ⓒ Ⓓ Ⓔ	126. Ⓐ Ⓑ Ⓒ Ⓓ Ⓔ
13. Ⓐ Ⓑ Ⓒ Ⓓ Ⓔ	51. Ⓐ Ⓑ Ⓒ Ⓓ Ⓔ	89. Ⓐ Ⓑ Ⓒ Ⓓ Ⓔ	127. Ⓐ Ⓑ Ⓒ Ⓓ Ⓔ
14. Ⓐ Ⓑ Ⓒ Ⓓ Ⓔ	52. Ⓐ Ⓑ Ⓒ Ⓓ Ⓔ	90. Ⓐ Ⓑ Ⓒ Ⓓ Ⓔ	128. Ⓐ Ⓑ Ⓒ Ⓓ Ⓔ
15. Ⓐ Ⓑ Ⓒ Ⓓ Ⓔ	53. Ⓐ Ⓑ Ⓒ Ⓓ Ⓔ	91. Ⓐ Ⓑ Ⓒ Ⓓ Ⓔ	129. Ⓐ Ⓑ Ⓒ Ⓓ Ⓔ
16. Ⓐ Ⓑ Ⓒ Ⓓ Ⓔ	54. Ⓐ Ⓑ Ⓒ Ⓓ Ⓔ	92. Ⓐ Ⓑ Ⓒ Ⓓ Ⓔ	130. Ⓐ Ⓑ Ⓒ Ⓓ Ⓔ
17. Ⓐ Ⓑ Ⓒ Ⓓ Ⓔ	55. Ⓐ Ⓑ Ⓒ Ⓓ Ⓔ	93. Ⓐ Ⓑ Ⓒ Ⓓ Ⓔ	131. Ⓐ Ⓑ Ⓒ Ⓓ Ⓔ
18. Ⓐ Ⓑ Ⓒ Ⓓ Ⓔ	56. Ⓐ Ⓑ Ⓒ Ⓓ Ⓔ	94. Ⓐ Ⓑ Ⓒ Ⓓ Ⓔ	132. Ⓐ Ⓑ Ⓒ Ⓓ Ⓔ
19. Ⓐ Ⓑ Ⓒ Ⓓ Ⓔ	57. Ⓐ Ⓑ Ⓒ Ⓓ Ⓔ	95. Ⓐ Ⓑ Ⓒ Ⓓ Ⓔ	133. Ⓐ Ⓑ Ⓒ Ⓓ Ⓔ
20. Ⓐ Ⓑ Ⓒ Ⓓ Ⓔ	58. Ⓐ Ⓑ Ⓒ Ⓓ Ⓔ	96. Ⓐ Ⓑ Ⓒ Ⓓ Ⓔ	134. Ⓐ Ⓑ Ⓒ Ⓓ Ⓔ
21. Ⓐ Ⓑ Ⓒ Ⓓ Ⓔ	59. Ⓐ Ⓑ Ⓒ Ⓓ Ⓔ	97. Ⓐ Ⓑ Ⓒ Ⓓ Ⓔ	135. Ⓐ Ⓑ Ⓒ Ⓓ Ⓔ
22. Ⓐ Ⓑ Ⓒ Ⓓ Ⓔ	60. Ⓐ Ⓑ Ⓒ Ⓓ Ⓔ	98. Ⓐ Ⓑ Ⓒ Ⓓ Ⓔ	136. Ⓐ Ⓑ Ⓒ Ⓓ Ⓔ
23. Ⓐ Ⓑ Ⓒ Ⓓ Ⓔ	61. Ⓐ Ⓑ Ⓒ Ⓓ Ⓔ	99. Ⓐ Ⓑ Ⓒ Ⓓ Ⓔ	137. Ⓐ Ⓑ Ⓒ Ⓓ Ⓔ
24. Ⓐ Ⓑ Ⓒ Ⓓ Ⓔ	62. Ⓐ Ⓑ Ⓒ Ⓓ Ⓔ	100. Ⓐ Ⓑ Ⓒ Ⓓ Ⓔ	138. Ⓐ Ⓑ Ⓒ Ⓓ Ⓔ
25. Ⓐ Ⓑ Ⓒ Ⓓ Ⓔ	63. Ⓐ Ⓑ Ⓒ Ⓓ Ⓔ	101. Ⓐ Ⓑ Ⓒ Ⓓ Ⓔ	139. Ⓐ Ⓑ Ⓒ Ⓓ Ⓔ
26. Ⓐ Ⓑ Ⓒ Ⓓ Ⓔ	64. Ⓐ Ⓑ Ⓒ Ⓓ Ⓔ	102. Ⓐ Ⓑ Ⓒ Ⓓ Ⓔ	140. Ⓐ Ⓑ Ⓒ Ⓓ Ⓔ
27. Ⓐ Ⓑ Ⓒ Ⓓ Ⓔ	65. Ⓐ Ⓑ Ⓒ Ⓓ Ⓔ	103. Ⓐ Ⓑ Ⓒ Ⓓ Ⓔ	141. Ⓐ Ⓑ Ⓒ Ⓓ Ⓔ
28. Ⓐ Ⓑ Ⓒ Ⓓ Ⓔ	66. Ⓐ Ⓑ Ⓒ Ⓓ Ⓔ	104. Ⓐ Ⓑ Ⓒ Ⓓ Ⓔ	142. Ⓐ Ⓑ Ⓒ Ⓓ Ⓔ
29. Ⓐ Ⓑ Ⓒ Ⓓ Ⓔ	67. Ⓐ Ⓑ Ⓒ Ⓓ Ⓔ	105. Ⓐ Ⓑ Ⓒ Ⓓ Ⓔ	143. Ⓐ Ⓑ Ⓒ Ⓓ Ⓔ
30. Ⓐ Ⓑ Ⓒ Ⓓ Ⓔ	68. Ⓐ Ⓑ Ⓒ Ⓓ Ⓔ	106. Ⓐ Ⓑ Ⓒ Ⓓ Ⓔ	144. Ⓐ Ⓑ Ⓒ Ⓓ Ⓔ
31. Ⓐ Ⓑ Ⓒ Ⓓ Ⓔ	69. Ⓐ Ⓑ Ⓒ Ⓓ Ⓔ	107. Ⓐ Ⓑ Ⓒ Ⓓ Ⓔ	145. Ⓐ Ⓑ Ⓒ Ⓓ Ⓔ
32. Ⓐ Ⓑ Ⓒ Ⓓ Ⓔ	70. Ⓐ Ⓑ Ⓒ Ⓓ Ⓔ	108. Ⓐ Ⓑ Ⓒ Ⓓ Ⓔ	146. Ⓐ Ⓑ Ⓒ Ⓓ Ⓔ
33. Ⓐ Ⓑ Ⓒ Ⓓ Ⓔ	71. Ⓐ Ⓑ Ⓒ Ⓓ Ⓔ	109. Ⓐ Ⓑ Ⓒ Ⓓ Ⓔ	147. Ⓐ Ⓑ Ⓒ Ⓓ Ⓔ
34. Ⓐ Ⓑ Ⓒ Ⓓ Ⓔ	72. Ⓐ Ⓑ Ⓒ Ⓓ Ⓔ	110. Ⓐ Ⓑ Ⓒ Ⓓ Ⓔ	148. Ⓐ Ⓑ Ⓒ Ⓓ Ⓔ
35. Ⓐ Ⓑ Ⓒ Ⓓ Ⓔ	73. Ⓐ Ⓑ Ⓒ Ⓓ Ⓔ	111. Ⓐ Ⓑ Ⓒ Ⓓ Ⓔ	149. Ⓐ Ⓑ Ⓒ Ⓓ Ⓔ
36. Ⓐ Ⓑ Ⓒ Ⓓ Ⓔ	74. Ⓐ Ⓑ Ⓒ Ⓓ Ⓔ	112. Ⓐ Ⓑ Ⓒ Ⓓ Ⓔ	150. Ⓐ Ⓑ Ⓒ Ⓓ Ⓔ
37. Ⓐ Ⓑ Ⓒ Ⓓ Ⓔ	75. Ⓐ Ⓑ Ⓒ Ⓓ Ⓔ	113. Ⓐ Ⓑ Ⓒ Ⓓ Ⓔ	
38. Ⓐ Ⓑ Ⓒ Ⓓ Ⓔ	76. Ⓐ Ⓑ Ⓒ Ⓓ Ⓔ	114. Ⓐ Ⓑ Ⓒ Ⓓ Ⓔ	

> **DIRECTIONS:** Each of the questions or incomplete statements below is followed by five suggested answers or completions. Select the one that is best in each case.

1. The first Caribbean writer to win the Nobel Prize for Literature was

    (A) Jamaica Kincaid
    (B) Derek Walcott
    (C) V.S. Naipaul
    (D) Geoffrey Philp
    (E) Ian McDonald

2. Lao Tzu, the Chinese philosopher, is regarded as the founder of

    (A) Zen
    (B) Mahayana Buddhism
    (C) Theravada Buddhism
    (D) Taoism
    (E) Shintoism

3. The seven daughters of Atlas who were changed into a cluster of stars to escape the hunter Orion were

    (A) Gorgons
    (B) Muses
    (C) Pleiades
    (D) Furies
    (E) Chimeras

4. The first black author to have a long-running Broadway hit was

    (A) Wright
    (B) Baldwin
    (C) Hughes
    (D) Hansbury
    (E) Morrison

5. Classicism is a style that embodies all of the following qualities except

    (A) balance
    (B) restraint
    (C) objectivity
    (D) form
    (E) abstraction

6. One of America's most renowned architects, designer of the JFK Library in Massachusetts, is

    (A) I.M. Pei
    (B) Jonathan Barnett
    (C) Charles Gwathmey
    (D) Frank Lloyd Wright
    (E) Richard Meier

7. One of the most popular operettas of all time, *La Grande-Duchess de Gerolstein*, was written by

    (A) Bizet
    (B) Gilbert and Sullivan
    (C) Offenbach
    (D) Lecocq
    (E) Halevy

8. The author of *Myra Breckinridge, Burr,* and *Empire* is

    (A) Gore Vidal
    (B) Kurt Vonnegut
    (C) Erich Segal
    (D) Philip Roth
    (E) Rod Steiger

9. Menotti wrote all of the following *except*

(A) *The Medium*
(B) *The Telephone*
(C) *The Rake's Progress*
(D) *The Consul*
(E) *Amahl and the Night Visitor*

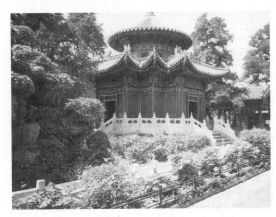

© Ruth S. Ward

10. The architecture depicted in this photograph is typical of that found in

(A) India
(B) New Zealand
(C) Russia
(D) Hungary
(E) China

11. *A priori* knowledge is

(A) knowledge obtained from sensory experience
(B) knowledge existing in the mind before sensory experience
(C) a concept stressed particularly by the empiricist
(D) a concept denied by the objective realist
(E) knowledge verified by inductive evidence

12. The conclusion of *Candide* is that

(A) "whatever is, is right"
(B) "love conquers all"
(C) "do unto others as you would have others do unto you"
(D) "we must cultivate our garden"
(E) "the end justifies the means"

13. The prefix "ur-" (as in *Ur-Faust, Ur-Hamlet*) means

(A) early or primitive
(B) alternate
(C) pirated
(D) last known
(E) composite

14. All of the following are 19th-century Russian writers except

(A) Chekhov
(B) Nabokov
(C) Tolstoy
(D) Turgenev
(E) Dostoevsky

15. The term *chamber music* can be applied to all of the following *except*

(A) quartets
(B) quintets
(C) trios
(D) symphonies
(E) duo sonatas

16. An outside wall of a room or building carried above an adjoining roof and pierced with windows is called a

(A) transept
(B) clerestory
(C) pilaster
(D) transverse arch
(E) atrium

17. A contemporary of E.A. Robinson, Edgar Lee Masters, Stephen Crane, and Theodore Dreiser, this poet holds a permanent place in American literature because his poetry is not only highly original, but also stresses the problems of his age. He is

(A) Robert Morse Lovett
(B) Walt Whitman
(C) Vachel Lindsay
(D) Robinson Jeffers
(E) William Vaughn Moody

18. This female satirist, known especially for her novels *Ethan Frome* and *The Age of Innocence*, was influenced by Henry James, and her interests were centered mainly in the changing society of New York City. She is

(A) Edith Wharton
(B) Lily Bart
(C) Zelda Fitzgerald
(D) Dorothy Parker
(E) Willa Cather

19. The blind seer who appears in several Greek tragedies is

(A) Tiresias
(B) Homer
(C) Clytaemnestra
(D) Oedipus
(E) Agamemnon

20. A large composition for voices and orchestra, usually based on a religious text, is

(A) an aria
(B) an oratorio
(C) a capella
(D) a madrigal
(E) a mass

21. France's two greatest writers of classical tragedy were

(A) Molière and Rostand
(B) Corneille and Racine
(C) Jarry and Racine
(D) Molière and Corneille
(E) Balzac and Hugo

22. The author of *The Flies and The Clouds* was

(A) Beckett
(B) Sartre
(C) Menander
(D) Aristophanes
(E) Molière

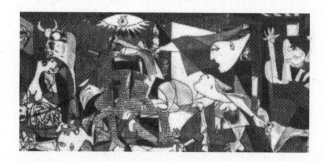

23. The painting above is

(A) Whistler's *Arrangement in Gray and Black*
(B) Klee's *Around the Fish*
(C) Picasso's *Guernica*
(D) Durer's *Four Horsemen of the Apocalypse*
(E) Poussin's *Triumph of Neptune and Amphitrite*

24. Of the following statements concerning a literary work read in translation, which is true?

   (A) It cannot escape the linguistic characteristics of the language into which it is turned.
   (B) Often one loses the *shade* of meaning when translating from an ancient language.
   (C) The translated work reflects the individuality of the age in which it is done.
   (D) Both A and B
   (E) All of the above

25. The author of "Waltzing Matilda" and "The Man from Snowy River" was the Australian poet

   (A) Hart Crane
   (B) "Banjo" Paterson
   (C) Lincoln Steffens
   (D) T.S. Eliott
   (E) Allen Ginsberg

26. The musical notation ♭: represents

   (A) the bass clef
   (B) the treble clef
   (C) sharp
   (D) flat
   (E) diminuendo

27. "Interpretation is the revenge of the intellectual upon art."

   "So successful has been the camera's role in beautifying the world that photographs, rather than the world, have become the standard of the beautiful."

   The quotations above are both from the writings of

   (A) Pauline Kael
   (B) Susan Sontag
   (C) Norman Mailer
   (D) Woody Allen
   (E) Thomas Pynchon

28. In the theater, the exploitation of "tender" emotions for their own sake—that is, whether motivated by the action or not—is called

   (A) virtue
   (B) temperamentality
   (C) melodrama
   (D) drama
   (E) sentimentality

29. If you raise a musical note from G to G sharp, or lower a note from E to E flat, you are practicing

   (A) staffing
   (B) writing musical shorthand
   (C) lengthening the composition
   (D) harmonizing
   (E) alteration

30. When the fingers of the hand that holds the bow are used to pluck the strings of an instrument, we call this

   (A) fortissimo
   (B) dissonance
   (C) pizzicato
   (D) diminuendo
   (E) espressivo

31. Perhaps the "perfect courtier" of the Renaissance was

   (A) Castiglione
   (B) Shakespeare
   (C) Maddox of Leicester
   (D) Henry VIII
   (E) Andrew the Chaplain

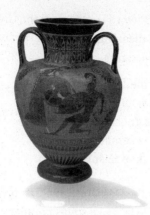

32. The beaker in the photograph above is

    (A) Egyptian
    (B) Peruvian
    (C) Byzantine
    (D) Roman
    (E) Greek

Questions 33–35 refer to the following quotation:

"All nature is but Art, unknown to thee;
All Chance, Direction, which thou canst not
    see;
All Discord, Harmony not understood;
All partial Evil, universal Good:
And, spite of Pride, in erring Reason's spite,
One truth is clear, *Whatever is, is Right.*"

33. The preceding lines are from

    (A) Yeats' "Sailing to Byzantium"
    (B) Tennyson's "In Memoriam"
    (C) Whitman's "Song of Myself "
    (D) Wordsworth's "Ode on Intimations of
        Immortality"
    (E) Pope's "Essay on Man"

34. The verse form is the

    (A) sestina
    (B) ballad
    (C) heroic couplet
    (D) sonnet
    (E) haiku

35. The meter is

    (A) iambic pentameter
    (B) trochaic dimeter
    (C) anapestic tetrameter
    (D) iambic tetrameter
    (E) trochaic pentameter

36. The philosopher Nietzsche, from whom the
    Nazis derived some of their doctrines, taught
    that the basic human motivation is

    (A) intellectual curiosity
    (B) sensual pleasure
    (C) the desire for wealth
    (D) sex
    (E) the will to power

37. Two 20th-century composers of atonal
    music are

    (A) Bartók and Schoenberg
    (B) Stravinsky and Debussy
    (C) Ives and Wagner
    (D) Prokofiev and Poulenc
    (E) Rimsky-Korsakov and Rachmaninoff

38. The novels of Honoré de Balzac are known
    collectively as

    (A) *"Père Goriot" and Other Stories*
    (B) *The Collected Works of Honoré
        de Balzac*
    (C) *The Human Tragedy*
    (D) *The Human Comedy*
    (E) *Tales of the Tatras*

39. Which one of the following was a
    Renaissance painter?

    (A) Degas
    (B) Picasso
    (C) Michelangelo
    (D) Goya
    (E) Gainsborough

40. "To be, or not to be," is the beginning of a famous soliloquy from

   (A) *Dr. Faustus*
   (B) *Romeo and Juliet*
   (C) *Tamburlaine*
   (D) *Othello*
   (E) *Hamlet*

41. Just as Aristophanes used satire and humor to attack the existing society in early Athens, so did an American author use these media to express the discrepancy between American expectations and the very disturbing reality of his times. He is

   (A) Charles Brockden Brown
   (B) Augustus Longstreet
   (C) Robert Frost
   (D) Edwin Arlington Robinson
   (E) Mark Twain

42. A period of enthusiasm for the classics in art, architecture, literature, drama, etc., is known as

   (A) the Age of Enlightenment
   (B) the Neo-Classic Age
   (C) Romantic Age
   (D) the Classical Age
   (E) the Renaissance

43. The painter who became interested in politics and who, under Napoleon, became First Painter of the Empire was

   (A) Goya
   (B) Gros
   (C) Géricault
   (D) Ingres
   (E) David

44. Which word comes from the Greek term meaning "unknown" or "without knowledge"?

   (A) metaphysics
   (B) axiology
   (C) agnosticism
   (D) pragmatism
   (E) skepticism

45. After the Dark Ages, the first professional people to make songs popular were called

   (A) troubadours
   (B) barbershop quartets
   (C) castrati
   (D) church choirs
   (E) motets

46. In Greek drama, the protagonist's tragic flaw is frequently pride; in a Greek comedy, it is often

   (A) anguish
   (B) single-mindedness
   (C) open-mindedness
   (D) lust
   (E) super-intellectualism

47. Stimulated by the Cubist style, the Italian artists who introduced the additional concept of movement in "space-time" were the

   (A) Expressionists
   (B) Impressionists
   (C) Non-objectivists
   (D) Futurists
   (E) Romanticists

48. Henri Matisse is to Fauvism what Edvard Munch is to

   (A) Impressionism
   (B) Surrealism
   (C) Cubism
   (D) German Expressionism
   (E) *Die Brücke*

49. Franz Liszt

    (A) used classical forms in his music
    (B) experimented with atonal music
    (C) used romantic forms such as the tone poem
    (D) was a virtuoso performer on the violin
    (E) rejected the ideals of romanticism

50. In Greek legend, who killed his father, married his mother, and became King of Thebes?

    (A) Polynices
    (B) Agamemnon
    (C) Laius
    (D) Oedipus
    (E) Jason

51. Johann Strauss is best known for his

    (A) waltzes
    (B) tone poems
    (C) fugues
    (D) sonatas
    (E) symphonies

52. Often considered the "showpiece of French realism" is

    (A) Flaubert's *Madame Bovary*
    (B) Balzac's *Eugénie Grandet*
    (C) Hugo's *Les Misérables*
    (D) Zola's *Nana*
    (E) Voltaire's *The Huron*

53. In an orthodox sense, Arabic literature begins with

    (A) *The Rubáiyát*
    (B) *The Koran*
    (C) *The Book of the Dead*
    (D) *The Ramayana*
    (E) *The Mahabharata*

Questions 54 and 55 refer to the photograph below.

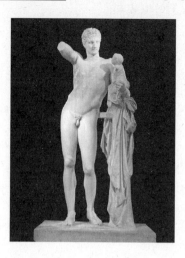

54. The work pictured is

    (A) Michelangelo's "David"
    (B) Michelangelo's "Pietá"
    (C) "The Nike of Samothrace"
    (D) Brancusi's "Father and Son"
    (E) Praxiteles' "Hermes"

55. If you wanted to see sculpture of this type in the city where it was created, you would visit

    (A) Paris
    (B) Washington, D.C.
    (C) Rome
    (D) Athens
    (E) Munich

56. The view that the mind is passive, or a *tabula rasa* upon which experience writes, and that the senses are more reliable than reason, was held by

    (A) Hegel
    (B) Socrates
    (C) Locke
    (D) Kant
    (E) Plato

57. According to legend, what was the cause of the Trojan War?

   (A) Argos's need for more land
   (B) the sacrifice of Iphigenia
   (C) the adultery of Clytaemnestra
   (D) the murder of Aegisthus
   (E) the kidnapping of Helen by Paris

58. *The Executions of May Third, 1808* was painted by

   (A) Goya
   (B) Canova
   (C) Vignon
   (D) Ingres
   (E) David

59. A writer who exerted a profound influence on the development of the American short story was William Sidney Porter, better known as

   (A) Artemus Ward
   (B) Josh Billings
   (C) Edgar Allan Poe
   (D) Mark Twain
   (E) O. Henry

60. An American author best known for his depictions of the old French Quarter of New Orleans, ante-bellum plantations, and the survival of the chivalric code in the South is

   (A) Rhett Butler
   (B) George Washington Cable
   (C) Joel Chandler Harris
   (D) William Faulkner
   (E) Joseph Lee

61. The most sensitively expressive of all musical instruments made by the family of Stradivari is the

   (A) drum
   (B) violin
   (C) cymbal
   (D) oboe
   (E) piano

62. A contemporary of Johann Sebastian Bach, though not as great an innovator, nevertheless one of the most successful of the world's serious composers, was

   (A) Beethoven
   (B) Mendelssohn
   (C) Handel
   (D) Silbermann
   (E) Schmidt

63. The one-eyed giant whom Odysseus met on his voyage was named

   (A) Dryope
   (B) Polyphemus
   (C) Aeolus
   (D) Circe
   (E) Medea

64. The proximity of the audience to the players influenced some of the theatrical devices used by Shakespeare and made feasible

   (A) the soliloquy
   (B) the appearance of boys in feminine roles
   (C) the use of special effects
   (D) music with dance sequences
   (E) the use of pantomime

65. The three hideous sisters of Greek mythology, one of whom (Medusa) was killed by Perseus, were called

   (A) Gorgons
   (B) Sphinxes
   (C) Furies
   (D) Sirens
   (E) Charities

66. The music Beethoven wrote for the theater was all of the following except

   (A) based on a theme of the quest for individual liberty
   (B) based on the cause of popular freedom
   (C) reflective of high moral purpose
   (D) religious in nature
   (E) based on an ideal of human creativity

67. In poetry, the omission of one or more final unstressed syllables is called

    (A) anacrusis
    (B) catalexis
    (C) feminine rhyme
    (D) masculine rhyme
    (E) caesura

68. Penelope's chief suitor was named

    (A) Telemachus
    (B) Oedipus
    (C) Creon
    (D) Telegonus
    (E) Antinous

69. Because of his innovations of style, his free hand with form, and his use of extra-musical devices, the man often called the first Romantic composer is

    (A) Liszt
    (B) Beethoven
    (C) Haydn
    (D) Mozart
    (E) von Weber

70. The great French tragic dramatist of the Neo-Classic period was

    (A) Racine
    (B) Pascal
    (C) Molière
    (D) La Fontaine
    (E) Sainte-Beuve

71. A stale phrase used where a fresh one is needed is

    (A) parallelism
    (B) a cliché
    (C) denouement
    (D) poetic license
    (E) a pun

72. Poetry that is not so much read as looked at is called

    (A) structured poetry
    (B) nonsense verse
    (C) gnomic poetry
    (D) euphuistic verse
    (E) concrete verse

73. Shelley's elegy on the death of John Keats is

    (A) "In Memoriam"
    (B) "Adonais"
    (C) "Thyrsis"
    (D) "Lycidas"
    (E) "Stanzas Written in Dejection near Naples"

74. Thomas Henry Huxley was

    (A) primarily a man of letters
    (B) author of *Brave New World*
    (C) devoted to the popularization of science
    (D) noted for his florid, romantic style
    (E) the founder of *The Spectator*

75. A florid, ornate portion of prose or poetry, which stands out by its rhythm, diction, or figurative language, is called

    (A) pure poetry
    (B) a purple passage
    (C) quantitative verse
    (D) prosody
    (E) hyperbole

76. Which of the following philosophers is *not* generally considered to be an idealist?

    (A) Immanuel Kant
    (B) Friedrich Hegel
    (C) Plato
    (D) Bishop Berkeley
    (E) Bertrand Russell

77. A well-known sonneteer of the 14th century was

(A) Petrarch
(B) Dante
(C) Shakespeare
(D) Shelley
(E) Boccaccio

78. Today's audiences would find strange the theater for which Shakespeare wrote because they

(A) prefer to attend matinees
(B) are not accustomed to intermissions
(C) prefer simple sets and costumes
(D) are not used to listening to such complex language
(E) are less well educated

79. The literal meaning of the word "Renaissance" is

(A) rebirth
(B) clarification
(C) analysis
(D) enlightenment
(E) question

80. Canio is the famous clown from the opera

(A) *I Pagliacci*
(B) *Rigoletto*
(C) *Cavalleria Rusticana*
(D) *Gianni Schicchi*
(E) *Così fan tutte*

81. The English language is most closely related to which of the following in the structure of its sentences?

(A) Latin
(B) German
(C) French
(D) Bulgarian
(E) Italian

82. The period in English literature called the "Restoration" is commonly regarded as running from

(A) 1300 to 1450
(B) 1500 to 1550
(C) 1660 to 1700
(D) 1798 to 1848
(E) 1848 to 1900

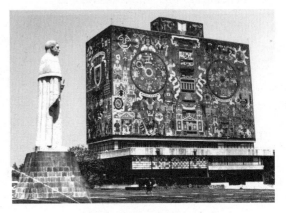

© Ruth S. Ward

83. Above is a photograph of

(A) a Greek temple
(B) a Roman temple
(C) an Egyptian temple
(D) the University of South Florida
(E) the University of Mexico

84. Walter Pater believed that one should

(A) "cultivate one's own garden"
(B) "justify the ways of God to man"
(C) "follow the sun"
(D) "burn with a hard, gem-like flame"
(E) "contemplate the Absolute"

85. The expressive combination of reinforced concrete material, cantilevered construction, and a dramatic site are characteristic of the modern architect

(A) J.J.P. Oud
(B) Walter Gropius
(C) Louis Sullivan
(D) Frank Lloyd Wright
(E) Le Corbusier

86. The "Theater of the Absurd" is basically

    (A) ridiculous
    (B) emotional
    (C) comic
    (D) tragic
    (E) intellectual

87. What daughter of an American president successfully established herself as a mystery writer?

    (A) Amy Carter
    (B) Margaret Truman
    (C) Tricia Nixon Cox
    (D) Julie Nixon Eisenhower
    (E) Lynda Johnson Robb

88. Don Quixote's horse was named

    (A) Escudero
    (B) Rocinante
    (C) Sancho Panza
    (D) Dulcinea
    (E) Gringolet

89. A modern folklorist, author of *The Hero with a Thousand Faces*, is

    (A) Jacob Grimm
    (B) Margaret Hunt
    (C) Padriac Colum
    (D) Joseph Stern
    (E) Joseph Campbell

90. Sir Arthur Conan Doyle's famous character Sherlock Holmes, the Victorian sleuth, was

    (A) based on a character from Edgar Allan Poe
    (B) known to be addicted to cocaine
    (C) believed to be Jack the Ripper
    (D) based on a well-known detective of the time, James Edmunds
    (E) killed in an airplane accident

91. The institution of the villain in drama goes back to

    (A) the Greek epics
    (B) the medieval romance
    (C) Christianity and the writings of Machiavelli
    (D) the Protestant attack on corrupt clergy
    (E) an ancient source, probably a ritual

92. The slogan of the 19th-century Aesthetic Movement was

    (A) "Art is the opiate of the masses"
    (B) "Art is life"
    (C) "Art for art's sake"
    (D) "What is art, that it should have a sake?"
    (E) "Burn with a hard, gem-like flame"

93. The most famous medieval tapestry is the

    (A) Bayeux
    (B) Byzantine
    (C) Canterbury
    (D) Hastings
    (E) Norman

94. The main difference between the Pantheon (in Italy) and the Parthenon (in Greece) is that

    (A) the Parthenon was constructed of raw concrete
    (B) the Pantheon used red bricks and mortar
    (C) the Pantheon is topped with a dome, while the roof of the Parthenon is triangular
    (D) the Parthenon used plain pillars without any ornamentation, while those in the Pantheon are elaborately decorated
    (E) the floor space in the Parthenon is about four times larger

95. The Greek tragedy *Antigone* was written by

(A) Socrates
(B) Plato
(C) Aristotle
(D) Sophocles
(E) Agamemnon

96. The poignant line "But where are the snows of yesteryear?" is from "The Ballade of Dead Ladies" by

(A) François Villon
(B) Percy Bysshe Shelley
(C) John Keats
(D) William Shakespeare
(E) Lord Byron

97. Which of the following Hindu holy books especially influenced the so-called "beat generation" of poets and novelists?

(A) *The Bhagavad-Gita*
(B) *Upanishads*
(C) *Carmina Burana*
(D) *Jaina Sutras*
(E) *Mahabharata*

98. When people started to sing different tunes together, which of the following had its beginnings?

(A) monophony
(B) jazz
(C) polyphony
(D) a capella
(E) homophony

99. A thought that does not follow logically from what has been said is

(A) non sequitor
(B) a malapropism
(C) a pun
(D) an acronym
(E) an oxymoron

100. The life of decadent Europe is contrasted unfavorably with life on an unspoiled, Eden-like island. This is indicative of an Age called

(A) Elizabethan
(B) Neo-Classic
(C) Classic
(D) Romantic
(E) Victorian

101. *Waverly, Ivanhoe,* and *Quentin Durward* were written by

(A) Sir Thomas Hardy
(B) Sir Walter Scott
(C) Henry Makepeace Thackeray
(D) Charlotte Brontë
(E) Emily Brontë

102. The medieval poem "Piers Plowman" belongs to the literature of

(A) chivalry
(B) social protest
(C) mythology
(D) social satire
(E) pastoral philosophy

103. The greatest Spanish painter of the 17th century, who worked almost exclusively on portraits of the nobility and court figures, was

(A) Velázquez
(B) Murillo
(C) Goya
(D) Utrillo
(E) El Greco

104. The French novelist George Sand was the mistress of which famous composer?

(A) Verdi
(B) Rachmaninoff
(C) Prokofiev
(D) Chopin
(E) Mahler

SAMPLE HUMANITIES EXAM 2

105. In music, gradual decrease of tempo is called

 (A) retardando
 (B) accelerando
 (C) moderato
 (D) presto
 (E) allegro

106. The philosophy best represented by the statement "true ideas are those that work" is

 (A) rationalism
 (B) positivism
 (C) empiricism
 (D) pragmatism
 (E) Thomism

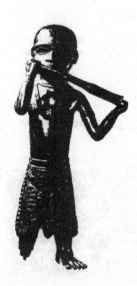

107. This is an example of

 (A) Hindu art
 (B) Chinese art
 (C) Egyptian art
 (D) primitive art
 (E) Etruscan art

108. The Russian writer thought to have coined the word "nihilist" was

 (A) Chekhov
 (B) Dostoevsky
 (C) Pushkin
 (D) Tolstoy
 (E) Turgenev

109. Which one of the following do most critics consider the greatest novel ever written?

 (A) *War and Peace*
 (B) *The Brothers Karamazov*
 (C) *The Forsyte Saga*
 (D) *The Sound and the Fury*
 (E) *Pride and Prejudice*

110. How many muses were there in Greek mythology?

 (A) 3
 (B) 4
 (C) 7
 (D) 9
 (E) 11

111. In three novels, called collectively U.S.A., this author employed interludes he dubbed "The Camera Eye" and "Newsreels." The author is

 (A) John Dos Passos
 (B) James Jones
 (C) John Steinbeck
 (D) Truman Capote
 (E) John P. Marquand

112. The "Father of the Irish Renaissance" was

 (A) George Moore
 (B) George Russell
 (C) J.M. Synge
 (D) W.B. Yeats
 (E) G.B. Shaw

113. Josiah Wedgwood began making pottery in England during which period?

 (A) Medieval
 (B) Renaissance
 (C) Neo-Classic
 (D) Romantic
 (E) Victorian

114. A contemporary choreographer whose ballets included "Fancy Free" and the dances in *West Side Story* is

    (A) Michael Kidd
    (B) Agnes de Mille
    (C) Jerome Robbins
    (D) John Cranko
    (E) Gene Kelly

115. All of the following are Italian film directors who have achieved worldwide fame since 1945 *except*

    (A) Roberto Rossellini
    (B) Michaelangelo Antonioni
    (C) Michelangelo Buonarroti
    (D) Federico Fellini
    (E) Vittorio de Sica

116. Which one of the following was *not* considered a medieval knightly virtue?

    (A) chastity
    (B) honesty
    (C) fortitude
    (D) faithfulness
    (E) duplicity

117. Chaucer wrote in the dialect of

    (A) Mercia
    (B) Wessex
    (C) Kent
    (D) Northumbria
    (E) London

Questions 118–120 refer to the following quotation:

"Ring out the old, ring in the new;
Ring, happy bells, across the snow:
The year is going, let him go;
Ring out the false, ring in the true."

118. The lines are quoted from

    (A) Tennyson's "In Memoriam"
    (B) Milton's "Lycidas"
    (C) Browning's "Pippa Passes"
    (D) Anonymous: "Christmas Bells"
    (E) Poe's "The Bells"

119. The verse form is a

    (A) sonnet
    (B) quatrain
    (C) couplet
    (D) tercet
    (E) cinquaine

120. The rhyme scheme is

    (A) a b a b
    (B) a b c d
    (C) a b b c
    (D) a b b a
    (E) a b c b

121. Impressionism found its most frequent expression in painting and music, but there was at least one sculptor who utilized the principles of Impressionism in his work:

    (A) Gustave Moreau
    (B) Odilon Redon
    (C) Giovanni Segantini
    (D) P.W. Steer
    (E) Auguste Rodin

122. A contemporary Russian novelist who experienced political difficulties with Soviet authorities because of his criticisms of Stalin and communism is

    (A) Ivan Denisovich
    (B) Konstantin Fedin
    (C) Pavel Antokolsky
    (D) Aleksandr Solzhenitsyn
    (E) Alexander Bek

123. The meter of a musical composition

    (A) has to do with regularly recurring accents

    (B) determines tempo

    (C) indicates texture

    (D) determines dynamics

    (E) is the same as rhythm

124. The most famous saint of Tibet is

    (A) Milarepa

    (B) Siddhartha

    (C) Tukela

    (D) the Dalai Lama

    (E) Naropa

125. When an author selects a title for a novel, he may quote another author. When Ernest Hemingway chose *For Whom the Bell Tolls* as the title for his novel about the Spanish Civil War, he was referring to

    (A) a poem by Andrew Marvell

    (B) a satire by Juvenal

    (C) a meditation by John Donne

    (D) a tragedy by John Ford

    (E) an essay by William Hazlitt

126. A Gilbert and Sullivan operetta that had a successful revival in London and on Broadway, and even made its way to the movie screen, is

    (A) *Iolanthe*

    (B) *The Mikado*

    (C) *The Pirates of Penzance*

    (D) *H.M.S. Pinafore*

    (E) *Ruddigore*

127. Samuel Johnson attached the label "Metaphysical Poets" to which of the following groups?

    (A) Donne, Marvell, Crashaw, and Herbert

    (B) Dryden, Pope, and Young

    (C) Greene, Jonson, and Herrick

    (D) Shakespeare, Milton, and Pope

    (E) Wordsworth, Keats, Shelley, and Byron

128. One of America's best-loved humorists, known for his satiric essays and hilarious cartoons, is

    (A) Berke Breathed

    (B) Walt Kelly

    (C) Mark Twain

    (D) William Zinsser

    (E) James Thurber

129. Which of the following lists of musical periods is arranged in the correct chronological sequence?

    (A) Renaissance, Classical, Baroque

    (B) Classical, Medieval, Romantic

    (C) Renaissance, Baroque, Romantic

    (D) Romantic, Renaissance, Baroque

    (E) Medieval, Baroque, Renaissance

130. The artist usually considered the father of modern abstract sculpture is

    (A) Brancusi

    (B) Maillol

    (C) Rodin

    (D) Lehmbruck

    (E) Archipenko

131. Most readers consider *Frankenstein* only a horror story about a fabricated monster. Few realize it has a social theme of

    (A) racial prejudice

    (B) class bigotry

    (C) the rejection by society of an individual who differs from the norm

    (D) sexual immorality

    (E) an individual's dependence upon drugs

132. *Frankenstein* was written in 1817 by

    (A) Sir Walter Scott

    (B) Horace Walpole

    (C) William Godwin

    (D) Mary Godwin

    (E) Mary Wollstonecraft Shelley

"It is an ancient Mariner
And he stoppeth one of three.
'By thy long gray beard and glittering eye,
Now wherefore stopp'st thou me?' "

133. The lines were written by

(A) Keats
(B) Eliot
(C) Coleridge
(D) Tennyson
(E) Shelley

134. The form is a

(A) tercet
(B) quatrain
(C) rondelay
(D) haiku
(E) sestina

135. The form of the whole poem is

(A) a ballade
(B) a dramatic monologue
(C) a traditional ballad
(D) a literary ballad
(E) an unconventional form which the author invented for this poem and never used again

136. The contemporary American author of *The Fire Next Time* and *Tell Me How Long the Train's Been Gone* is

(A) James Baldwin
(B) Margaret Walker
(C) LeRoi Jones (Imamu Amiri Baraka)
(D) Frederick Douglass
(E) John Williams

137. The immediate intention of the comic theater is to

(A) show the absurdity of life
(B) make us feel better
(C) drive a group of people into hysterical laughter
(D) act as an emotional tranquilizer
(E) convert the audience into giggling optimists

138. In the beginning, conductors performed their task from

(A) a podium
(B) the right side of the stage
(C) the left side of the stage
(D) an instrument, usually a clavier
(E) a pit hidden from the audience

139. "What animal goes in the morning on four feet, at noon on two, and in the evening on three?" is the riddle posed by the

(A) Griffin
(B) Jabberwock
(C) Sphinx
(D) Muses
(E) Furies

140. While David extolled the virtues and nobility of the conqueror Napoleon in his paintings, another artist depicted the sufferings of a subjugated people. He was

(A) Rodin
(B) Gros
(C) Géricault
(D) Goya
(E) Ingres

141. All of the following were essayists of the English Romantic Movement *except*

(A) De Quincey
(B) Lamb
(C) Addison
(D) Hazlitt
(E) Hunt

142. The "vast chain of being" is an important concept of the

(A) 16th century
(B) 17th century
(C) 18th century
(D) 19th century
(E) 20th century

143. The first composer to use hammering repetition as a dramatic device was

(A) Schmoll
(B) Beethoven
(C) Oberon
(D) Offenbach
(E) Stravinsky

144. A 19th-century writer noted for his short stories about life in India and his novels, poems, and children's stories was

(A) George Orwell
(B) Thomas Hardy
(C) John Masefield
(D) Joseph Conrad
(E) Rudyard Kipling

145. In the lines, "Hail to thee, blithe spirit!/Bird thou never wert," the bird referred to is a

(A) sparrow
(B) nightingale
(C) robin
(D) skylark
(E) mockingbird

146. A defector from the Soviet Union and a British dame formed one of the greatest ballet teams of all time. They were

(A) Mikhail Baryshnikov and Cyd Charisse
(B) Vaslav Nijinsky and Isadora Duncan
(C) Boris Chaliapin and Martha Graham
(D) Rudolf Nureyev and Margot Fonteyn
(E) Jacques d'Amboise and Maria Tallchief

147. Jane Austen's novels *Pride and Prejudice* and *Emma* deal with

(A) the English lower middle-class
(B) the English working class
(C) the problem of getting married
(D) child labor laws
(E) the plight of coal miners in Wales

148. Robert Browning is especially noted for his

(A) short stories
(B) dramatic monologues
(C) sonnets
(D) ballads
(E) dirges

149. The painting of Leda and the swan is associated with which Renaissance artist?

(A) Michelangelo
(B) Botticelli
(C) da Vinci
(D) Correggio
(E) Masaccio

150. In scansion of poetry, the symbol / indicates

(A) a slight pause within a line
(B) a foot
(C) read more slowly
(D) read faster
(E) stress the syllable

If there is still time remaining, you may review your answers.

ANSWER KEY
Sample Examination 2

HUMANITIES

1.	B	39.	C	77.	A	115.	C
2.	D	40.	E	78.	D	116.	E
3.	C	41.	E	79.	A	117.	E
4.	C	42.	B	80.	A	118.	A
5.	E	43.	E	81.	B	119.	B
6.	A	44.	C	82.	C	120.	D
7.	C	45.	A	83.	E	121.	E
8.	A	46.	B	84.	D	122.	D
9.	C	47.	D	85.	D	123.	A
10.	E	48.	D	86.	E	124.	A
11.	B	49.	C	87.	B	125.	C
12.	D	50.	D	88.	B	126.	C
13.	A	51.	A	89.	E	127.	A
14.	B	52.	A	90.	B	128.	E
15.	D	53.	B	91.	C	129.	B
16.	B	54.	E	92.	C	130.	A
17.	E	55.	D	93.	A	131.	C
18.	A	56.	C	94.	C	132.	E
19.	A	57.	E	95.	D	133.	C
20.	B	58.	A	96.	A	134.	B
21.	B	59.	E	97.	A	135.	D
22.	D	60.	B	98.	C	136.	A
23.	C	61.	B	99.	A	137.	B
24.	E	62.	C	100.	D	138.	D
25.	B	63.	B	101.	B	139.	C
26.	A	64.	A	102.	B	140.	D
27.	B	65.	A	103.	A	141.	C
28.	E	66.	D	104.	D	142.	C
29.	E	67.	B	105.	A	143.	B
30.	C	68.	E	106.	D	144.	E
31.	A	69.	E	107.	D	145.	D
32.	E	70.	A	108.	E	146.	D
33.	E	71.	B	109.	A	147.	C
34.	C	72.	E	110.	D	148.	B
35.	A	73.	B	111.	A	149.	C
36.	E	74.	C	112.	D	150.	E
37.	A	75.	B	113.	C		
38.	D	76.	E	114.	C		

SCORING CHART

After you have scored your Sample Examination 2, enter the results in the chart below; then transfer your score to the Progress Chart on page 12.

Total Test	Number Right	Number Wrong	Number Omitted
150			

ANSWER EXPLANATIONS

1. **(B)** Walcott's works include the long poem *Omeros,* his stage adaptation of Homer's *The Odyssey,* and his *Collected Poems,* published in 1986. He won the Nobel Prize in 1992.

2. **(D)** Lao Tzu emphasized the tao, the harmonious and inevitable way of the universe.

3. **(C)** In astronomy, the Pleiades is a star cluster in the constellation Taurus, which represents the seven sisters of Greek mythology.

4. **(C)** Langston Hughes' play *Mulatto* opened on Broadway in 1935, and played continuously for more than two years.

5. **(E)** This is true by definition.

6. **(A)** Pei also designed the East Building of the National Gallery of Art in Washington, D.C.

7. **(C)** Offenbach is also well known for his *La Vie Parisienne* and *Tales of Hoffman.*

8. **(A)** Writer and critic, much of Vidal's fiction deals satirically with history and politics.

9. **(C)** *Tile Rake's Progress* is a ballet by Gavin-Gordon.

10. **(E)** The photograph is of a pagoda. The architecture is typical of that found in the Orient.

11. **(B)** This is true by definition.

12. **(D)** These lines appear in the final chapter of Voltaire's novel.

13. **(A)** This is true by definition.

14. **(B)** Nabokov is a 20th-century writer.

15. **(D)** A large symphony orchestra is composed of string, wind, and percussion sections. The other answers refer to two to four instruments.

16. **(B)** This is true by definition.

17. **(E)** None of the other poets has all of the qualifications listed.

18. **(A)** Edith Wharton (1862–1937) was an American poet, short story writer, and novelist.

19. **(A)** Tiresias is important in many of the stories of Thebes. He is consulted also, in the underworld, by Odysseus.

20. **(B)** This is true by definition.

21. **(B)** Pierre Corneille (1606–1684) was the first of the great tragic writers of the era. Jean Racine (1639–1699) is generally described as France's greatest writer of tragedy.

22. **(D)** Aristophanes was the great Greek writer of comedy.

23. **(C)** *Guernica* depicts the ravaging of a small town by that name in Spain during the Revolution.

24. **(E)** To limit the answer to only one of the other statements would be to make an inadequate statement.

25. **(B)** Paterson, whose full name is Andrew Barton "Banjo" Paterson, is the only Australian in the group.

26. **(A)** This is a standard musical notation.

27. **(B)** Two of Susan Sontag's well-known books are *Against Interpretation* and *On Photography*. The quotations are from these books.

28. **(E)** This is true by definition.

29. **(E)** This is true by definition.

30. **(C)** This is true by definition.

31. **(A)** Baldassare Castiglione (1478–1529) wrote a handbook of manners, *The Courtier*, which was a guidebook for elegant deportment.

32. **(E)** The artistic style and decorations of the Greeks are far different from any of the others mentioned.

33. **(E)** The philosophy expressed is typical of the Neo-Classic period.

34. **(C)** Couplets are lines of poetry rhyming in pairs. The most widely used couplet form is the iambic pentameter, known as the heroic couplet.

35. **(A)** Iambic pentameter is five feet of unstressed/stressed syllables to the line.

36. **(E)** Nietzsche's *The Will to Power* was published in Germany in 1888. The first English translation appeared in 1909–10.

37. **(A)** The others are either not 20th-century composers, not composers of atonal music, or both.

38. **(D)** Honoré de Balzac (1799–1850) wrote *The Human Comedy*. The chief novels in this group are *Père Goriot* and *Eugénie Grandet*.

39. **(C)** Michelangelo (1475–1564) was the most famous artist of the Renaissance period.

40. **(E)** In his famous soliloquy, Hamlet is pondering whether or not to commit suicide.

41. **(E)** Perhaps Twain's most famous satire on contemporary society is *Huckleberry Finn*.

42. **(B)** The late 18th century and early 19th century are known as the Neo-Classic Age.

43. **(E)** Jacques Louis David (1748–1825) was one of the most famous painters of his day.

44. **(C)** This is true by definition.

45. **(A)** The troubadours were lyric poets of the 12th and 13th centuries attached to the courts of Provence and northern Italy.

46. **(B)** A character with one overriding purpose or opinion is often hilarious.

47. **(D)** Futurism, an artistic movement that originated in Italy about 1910, attempted to depict the dynamic quality of contemporary life influenced by the force and motion of modern machinery.

48. **(D)** Edvard Munch (1863–1944) was a Norwegian painter and printmaker who used intense colors and body attitudes to show love, sickness, anxiety, and death. He greatly influenced the German Expressionist movement of the early 1900s.

49. **(C)** Liszt wrote twelve tone poems, the form of which he invented.

50. **(D)** According to legend, Oedipus killed his father, married his mother, Jocasta, and had four children by her: Polynices, Eteocles, Antigone, and Ismene.

51. **(A)** Johann Strauss was a composer of comic operas, but his reputation rests on some 400 waltzes.

52. **(A)** Flaubert's *Madame Bovary*, published in 1859, was the first of the works that made him a model for later writers of the realistic school.

53. **(B)** *The Koran* is the sacred book of Islam, purportedly revealed by God to the Prophet Mohammed.

54. **(E)** Praxiteles was the most famous of the Attic sculptors.

55. **(D)** Praxiteles was from Athens, Greece.

56. **(C)** John Locke (1632–1704), an English philosopher, is best known for his *Essay Concerning the Human Understanding*, which poses the view of the tabula rasa.

57. **(E)** Paris kidnapped Helen, wife of Menelaus, king of Sparta, and brought her back to Troy. The Greek leaders rallied to aid Menelaus, and thus began the Trojan War.

58. **(A)** Goya (1746–1828) was a Spanish painter, etcher, and designer.

59. **(E)** O. Henry is noted for his surprise endings. One of his best known short stories is "The Gift of the Magi." The other writers did not use the pseudonym "O. Henry."

60. **(B)** The others were not writers of ante-bellum New Orleans chivalric literature.

61. **(B)** The Stradivarius is also perhaps the most famous and most expensive violin in the world.

62. **(C)** George Friedrich Handel (1685–1759) is perhaps best known as the composer of *The Messiah.*

63. **(B)** Polyphemus is the only cyclops Odysseus met.

64. **(A)** In the soliloquy, the actor could speak his innermost thoughts aloud.

65. **(A)** The others are mythological creatures, but no other fits the description.

66. **(D)** Beethoven was a prolific composer of symphonies, sonatas, and opera, but he did not write religious music.

67. **(B)** This is true by definition.

68. **(E)** The other characters were not suitors of Penelope.

69. **(E)** Von Weber (1786–1826) was a German who composed his first opera at age thirteen.

70. **(A)** The others were not tragic dramatists of the Neo-Classic period.

71. **(B)** This is true by definition.

72. **(E)** This is true by definition.

73. **(B)** John Keats, English Romantic poet, was a friend of Shelley.

74. **(C)** Huxley was a 19th-century evolutionist and social reformer who was instrumental in popularizing science. He was the grandfather of Aldous Huxley, author of *Brave New World*.

75. **(B)** This is true by literary definition.

76. **(E)** Although Russell was trained in the British Idealist tradition, he rebelled against it, becoming a leader of the analytic movement in philosophy.

77. **(A)** Petrarch's sonnets, mostly inspired by Laura, form one of the most splendid bodies of verse in literature. Petrarch's sonnets were first imitated in England by Sir Thomas Wyatt; the form was later used by Milton, Wordsworth, and other sonneteers.

78. **(D)** The Elizabethan audience insisted upon inflated, poetic language.

79. **(A)** This answer is true by definition.

80. **(A)** *I Pagliacci* is an opera in two acts by Leoncavallo.

81. **(B)** English is considered a Germanic language. Old English and German are similar in many respects.

82. **(C)** In English literature, the Restoration generally refers to the period from the accession of Charles II to the throne in 1660 to the death of Dryden in 1770. This period is sometimes called "The Age of Dryden."

83. **(E)** Brilliantly colored mosaics are typical of the art and architecture of the University of Mexico.

84. **(D)** Pater was an important Victorian essayist and literary critic.

85. **(D)** Wright's immensely functional, yet artistic, buildings always blend in with the environment.

86. **(E)** One must be able to intellectualize the absurdity of life in order to enjoy this type of theater.

87. **(B)** Among Ms. Truman's novels are *Murder on Embassy Row*, *Murder in Georgetown*, and *Murder in the Smithsonian*.

88. **(B)** Rocinante was a run-down nag Don Quixote rode into his famous, or infamous, battles.

89. **(E)** Campbell also authored *The Masks of God* and *Myths to Live By*.

90. **(B)** The novel and movie *The Seven-Per-Cent Solution,* concerns Holmes' addiction, and his treatment by Dr. Sigmund Freud.

91. **(C)** In Christianity, the Devil is evil incarnate. In Machiavelli's *The Prince,* his greatest work, evil is permissible, if necessary.

92. **(C)** The "art for art's sake" movement was an attempt to break away from all theories and traditions of the past.

93. **(A)** This tapestry depicts scenes of the Norman Conquest of England and the events leading up to it.

94. **(C)** Other than this distinction, the two buildings are architecturally similar in many respects.

95. **(D)** Sophocles is the only playwright in this group.

96. **(A)** François Villon (1431–1463?) was a vagabond, a rogue, and the greatest lyric poet of his time.

97. **(A)** Allen Ginsberg, one of the most popular "beat" poets, was greatly influenced by Hindu philosophy and incorporated Hindu chants into some of his poetry.

98. **(C)** *Polyphony* means the simultaneous combination of two or more independent melodic parts, especially when in close harmonic relationship.

99. **(A)** This is true by definition.

100. **(D)** The Romantic Age originated in Europe toward the end of the 18th century. It asserted the validity of subjective experience.

101. **(B)** Sir Walter Scott (1771–1832) was a British novelist and poet.

102. **(B)** "Piers Plowman" is a 14th-century English allegorical poem satirizing and attacking the clergy and exalting the simple and truthful life.

103. **(A)** Diego Velázquez (1599–1660) was perhaps the most naturalistic and objective of all the court painters.

104. **(D)** George Sand's liaison with Chopin lasted from 1837 until 1847.

105. **(A)** This is true by definition.

106. **(D)** Another word for pragmatism is *practicality.*

107. **(D)** One should notice the lack of sophistication in the sculpture.

108. **(E)** *Fathers and Sons* is the most famous nihilist novel by Turgenev.

109. **(A)** This monumental work was written by the Russian writer Tolstoy.

110. **(D)** The Muses, the nine daughters of Zeus and Mnemosyne, were originally the patronesses of literature.

111. **(A)** This trilogy is Dos Passos' most famous work.

112. **(D)** W.B. Yeats (1865–1939) was influenced by Irish folklore and mythology and the French Symbolists. He brought to the Irish literary movement a sophistication of technique it had previously lacked.

113. **(C)** "Neo-Classic" refers to the 17th and 18th centuries in Europe.

114. **(C)** The others are well known figures in the field, but Robbins' dances in *West Side Story* have become classics.

115. **(C)** Michelangelo Buonarroti is another name for Michelangelo, the famous Italian Renaissance artist.

116. **(E)** Duplicity is not a virtue.

117. **(E)** Most of the educated people in England lived in London, and Chaucer spent most of his life there.

118. **(A)** Tennyson wrote this poem to commemorate the death of his very dear friend, Arthur Hallam.

119. **(B)** Quatrain means four lines of verse.

120. **(D)** The rhyme scheme is determined by listening to the vowel sounds of the last word of each line, and lettering alphabetically; therefore, new = a; snow = b; go (which has the same vowel sound as "snow") = b, and true (which has the same vowel sound as "new") = a.

121. **(E)** Auguste Rodin (1840–1917) was a French sculptor and perhaps the strongest influence on 20th-century art.

122. **(D)** Nobel Prize–winner Solzhenitsyn has written *Gulag Archipelago, Cancer Ward,* and *One Day in the Life of Ivan Denisovich.*

123. **(A)** The meter means a division of music into measures of bars.

124. **(A)** The name Milarepa, which means "Mila who wears the cotton cloth of an ascetic," lived from 1025 to 1135. His biography, written in the 15th century, containing many spiritual songs, is one of the greatest sources of inspiration in Tibetan Buddhism.

125. **(C)** John Donne was an English poet and preacher. The meditation referred to is his 17th.

126. **(C)** W.S. Gilbert and Sir Arthur Sullivan collaborated on fourteen operettas.

127. **(A)** The most conspicuous characteristics of this group of 17th-century poets are the use of conceits, harshness of versification, and a combination of different types of emotions.

128. **(E)** James Thurber (1894–1961) was well known for his stories and cartoons depicting the battles of the sexes.

129. **(B)** Classical: pertaining to the ancient Greek or Roman period; Medieval: pertaining to the Middle Ages; Romantic: pertaining to the late 18th and early 19th century.

130. **(A)** Constantin Brancusi (1876–1957) was a Rumanian abstract sculptor.

131. **(C)** Mary Shelley intended the monster to arouse the sympathy of her readers.

132. **(E)** Mary Shelley published her novel *Frankenstein* in 1818.

133. **(C)** The poem is "The Ancient Mariner."

134. **(B)** Quatrain means four lines of verse.

135. **(D)** A literary ballad is written in deliberate imitation of the form and spirit of a folk ballad. The ballad stanza is usually a quatrain in alternate 4- and 3-stress lines, rhyming abcb.

136. **(A)** Baldwin is one of America's best known contemporary black writers.

137. **(B)** A good laugh is the best cure for many ills.

138. **(D)** A clavier is a stringed keyboard instrument, such as a harpsichord.

139. **(C)** Oedipus solved the riddle by replying, "It is man."

140. **(D)** Goya (1746–1828) was a Spanish painter, etcher, and designer, and a leading representative of the Spanish school of his day.

141. **(C)** Addison was the leading prose stylist of the early 18th century.

142. **(C)** This is a concept first stated by Aristotle.

143. **(B)** Beethoven's Fifth Symphony is the most obvious example of the use of this technique.

144. **(E)** Kipling is well known for such works as *Gunga Din*, *Kim*, and *The Jungle Book*.

145. **(D)** The lines are from the poem "To a Skylark," by Shelley.

146. **(D)** Nureyev was the only one of the group to defect from the Soviet Union; Fonteyn is the only British dame listed.

147. **(C)** Getting married was of prime consideration to a woman in Victorian England.

148. **(B)** Browning's "My Last Duchess" is perhaps his best known dramatic monologue.

149. **(C)** This painting, to date, has not been found.

150. **(E)** This is a standard accent mark used when scanning poetry.

The College Mathematics Examination

ANSWER SHEET
Trial Test

COLLEGE MATHEMATICS

1. Ⓐ Ⓑ Ⓒ Ⓓ

2.

3. Ⓐ Ⓑ Ⓒ Ⓓ

4. Ⓐ Ⓑ Ⓒ Ⓓ

5.

6. Ⓐ Ⓑ Ⓒ Ⓓ

7. Ⓐ Ⓑ Ⓒ Ⓓ

8. Ⓐ Ⓑ Ⓒ Ⓓ

9. Ⓐ Ⓑ Ⓒ Ⓓ

10.

11. Ⓐ Ⓑ Ⓒ Ⓓ

12.

13. Ⓐ Ⓑ Ⓒ Ⓓ

14. Ⓐ Ⓑ Ⓒ Ⓓ

15. Ⓐ Ⓑ Ⓒ Ⓓ

16.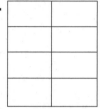

17. Ⓐ Ⓑ Ⓒ Ⓓ

18. Ⓐ Ⓑ Ⓒ Ⓓ

19. Ⓐ Ⓑ Ⓒ Ⓓ

20. Ⓐ Ⓑ Ⓒ Ⓓ

21. Ⓐ Ⓑ Ⓒ Ⓓ

22.

23. Ⓐ Ⓑ Ⓒ Ⓓ

24. Ⓐ Ⓑ Ⓒ Ⓓ

25. Ⓐ Ⓑ Ⓒ Ⓓ

26.

27. Ⓐ Ⓑ Ⓒ Ⓓ

28. Ⓐ Ⓑ Ⓒ Ⓓ

29. Ⓐ Ⓑ Ⓒ Ⓓ

30. Ⓐ Ⓑ Ⓒ Ⓓ

31. Ⓐ Ⓑ Ⓒ Ⓓ

32. Ⓐ Ⓑ Ⓒ Ⓓ

33. Ⓐ Ⓑ Ⓒ Ⓓ

34. Ⓐ Ⓑ Ⓒ Ⓓ

35. Ⓐ Ⓑ Ⓒ Ⓓ

36. Ⓐ Ⓑ Ⓒ Ⓓ

37. Ⓐ Ⓑ Ⓒ Ⓓ

38. Ⓐ Ⓑ Ⓒ Ⓓ

39. Ⓐ Ⓑ Ⓒ Ⓓ

40. Ⓐ Ⓑ Ⓒ Ⓓ

41. Ⓐ Ⓑ Ⓒ Ⓓ

42. Ⓐ Ⓑ Ⓒ Ⓓ

43. Ⓐ Ⓑ Ⓒ Ⓓ

44. Ⓐ Ⓑ Ⓒ Ⓓ

45. Ⓐ Ⓑ Ⓒ Ⓓ

46. Ⓐ Ⓑ Ⓒ Ⓓ

47. Ⓐ Ⓑ Ⓒ Ⓓ

48. Ⓐ Ⓑ Ⓒ Ⓓ

49. Ⓐ Ⓑ Ⓒ Ⓓ

50. Ⓐ Ⓑ Ⓒ Ⓓ

51. Ⓐ Ⓑ Ⓒ Ⓓ

52. Ⓐ Ⓑ Ⓒ Ⓓ

53. Ⓐ Ⓑ Ⓒ Ⓓ

54. Ⓐ Ⓑ Ⓒ Ⓓ

55. Ⓐ Ⓑ Ⓒ Ⓓ

56.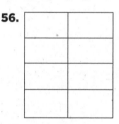

57. Ⓐ Ⓑ Ⓒ Ⓓ

58. Ⓐ Ⓑ Ⓒ Ⓓ

59. Ⓐ Ⓑ Ⓒ Ⓓ

60. Ⓐ Ⓑ Ⓒ Ⓓ

Trial Test

This chapter contains a Trial Test in College Mathematics. Take this Trial Test to learn what the actual exam is like, and to determine how you might score on the exam before any practice or review.

The CLEP General Exam in College Mathematics measures your knowledge of the mathematical skills generally covered in college-level courses for nonmath majors, including algebra and functions, counting and probability, data analysis and statistics, financial mathematics, geometry, logic and sets, and other topics and properties about the real number system.

Note that when you take the actual test, an online scientific calculator will be available. That means you'll be able to use this calculator for arithmetic (add, subtract, multiply, divide, square roots, and so on) and some special functions (such as permutations and combinations), but the calculator will not be able to draw graphs or be programmable. Although no questions actually *require* a calculator, we recommend that you use a scientific calculator when you take this Trial Test and throughout your preparation for the CLEP College Mathematics Exam.

Number of Questions: 60

TIME LIMIT: 90 MINUTES

DIRECTIONS: You will have access to an online scientific calculator during this test.

For multiple-choice questions, select the *best* of the four choices, then fill in the corresponding oval on the answer sheet. For the other questions, write your answer in the box.

Notes:

1. If the domain of a function *f* is not specified in a question, assume that it is the set of all real numbers for which *f(x)* is defined.
2. Figures are drawn to scale and lie in a plane, *unless* otherwise specified.

1. For which of these lists of numbers would the standard deviation be the largest?

   (A) {1, 3, 3, 3, 3, 3, 5}
   (B) {21, 23, 23, 23, 23, 23, 25}
   (C) {1, 1, 1, 3, 5, 5, 5}
   (D) {3, 3, 3, 3, 3, 3, 3}

2. If $f(x) = 4 - x^3$, then $f(-2)$ equals

3. If Jose must pay 8% sales tax for his $25.00 restaurant bill, how much will he pay in total?

   (A) $2.00
   (B) $27.00
   (C) $23.00
   (D) $45.00

4. In an isosceles triangle, one angle measures 38°. Which of the following could be the measures of the other two angles?

   I. 38°, 104°
   II. 71°, 71°
   III. 56°, 86°

   (A) I only
   (B) II only
   (C) III only
   (D) I or II

5. If an average grade of 60 on four tests is required to pass a course and Chris has grades of 52, 57, and 61 on the first three tests, what is the least grade she can get on the fourth test and pass the course?

   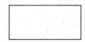

6. If $R = \{x : x < 3\}$ and $S = \{x : x \geq 0\}$, then the number of integers in $R \cup S$ is

   (A) none
   (B) two
   (C) three
   (D) infinite

7. The statement "If she has passed this test, then she'll get college credit" is true. Which of the following is also true?

   (A) If she fails this test, then she'll not get college credit.
   (B) If she does not get college credit, then she has not passed this test.
   (C) She passes this test but does not get college credit.
   (D) If she gets college credit then she has passed this test.

8. Which of the following graphs is for the line $2x + y = 2$?

(A)

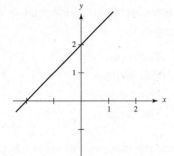

(B)

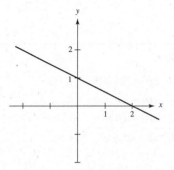

(C)

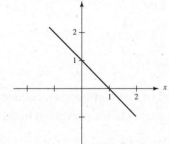

(D)

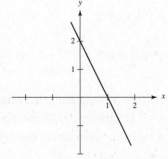

9. The pie chart below depicts a class of 40 students' favorite ice cream flavors.

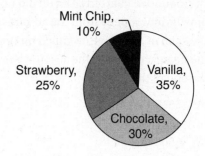

Based on this chart, how many students prefer chocolate or vanilla ice cream?

(A) 12
(B) 14
(C) 26
(D) 65

10. If $g(x)$ is a linear function such that $g(-2) = -7$ and $g(3) = 8$, then $g(1)$ equals

11. What is the area of a circle that has a diameter of 12 cm?

(A) 144π cm^2
(B) 36π cm^2
(C) 24π cm^2
(D) 6π cm^2

12. Two members of a group of 12 people are teachers. How many committees of 3 can be chosen so as to include at least one teacher?

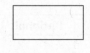

13. For her birthday Doyun got a $500 certificate of deposit which earns 4% annual interest compounded quarterly. Doyun did not add or withdraw money from the account over the span of 3 years. How much money (to the nearest cent) was the account worth at the end of the 3 years?

(A) $515.15
(B) $562.43
(C) $563.41
(D) $800.52

14. If $x^2 - x > 0$, then which of the following statements is false?

(A) $x < 0$
(B) $x > 1$
(C) $0 < x < 1$
(D) $x < 0$ or $x > 1$

15. Due to inconsistencies in the manufacturing process, a cereal box labeled as containing 40 oz of cereal actually contains anywhere from 39.6 oz to 42.2 oz. Which of the following inequalities describes the interval of all weights x, in ounces, for a box of cereal?

(A) $|39.9 - x| \leq 0.3$
(B) $|39.9 - x| \geq 0.3$
(C) $39.9 - x \leq 0.3$
(D) $39.9 - x \geq 0.3$

16. Check (✔) the appropriate boxes to indicate whether these numbers are rational or irrational.

Number(s)	Rational	Irrational
0		
x such that $x^2 = 8$		
$\frac{1}{6}$		
$\sqrt{121}$		

17. After looking over the scores on a quiz she gave in class, the teacher decides to raise everyone's score by 5 points. Which of these summaries of class performance will not change?

(A) The mean
(B) The median
(C) The mode
(D) The range

18. Given the number line shown below, which of the statements is false?

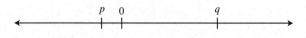

(A) $|p| - |q| < 0$
(B) $|p| + |q| > q$
(C) $|p| - |q| > p$
(D) $|p - q| > q$

19. What is 1.5% of 20?

(A) 0.03
(B) 0.3
(C) 3
(D) 30

20. Which of the following is an equation of a line parallel to the one given by $6x + 3y = 4$?

(A) $y = -2x + 7$
(B) $y = 2x + 7$
(C) $y = \frac{1}{2}x + 7$
(D) $y = -\frac{1}{2}x + 7$

21. A regulation rectangular soccer field measures 105 meters by 68 meters. How long is the diagonal of the field to the nearest whole meter?

(A) 80 meters
(B) 125 meters
(C) 173 meters
(D) 7140 meters

22. The median age for the data given is

AGE	15	18	20	22	30	31
FREQUENCY	6	2	9	2	8	1

$$\boxed{}$$

23. Which of these scatterplots demonstrates close to no relationship between the variables graphed?

(A)

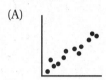

(B)

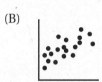

(C)

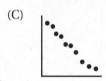

(D)

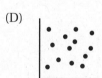

24. If function $f = \{(0,2), (1,5), (2,4), (3,6)\}$ and function $g = \{(2,3), (4,1), (6,0), (8,2)\}$, then $f \circ g(2) =$

(A) 1
(B) 4
(C) 6
(D) 12

25. For which real numbers is the function

$$f(x) = \frac{x}{x^2 - 9} \; not \text{ defined?}$$

(A) only $x = 0$
(B) only $x = 3$
(C) $x = 0$ or 3
(D) $x = 3$ or -3

26. If n is divisible both by 6 and by 10, then it must also be divisible by

$$\boxed{}$$

27. If $f(x) = ax + b$, $f(0) = 2$, and $f(1) = -1$, then

(A) $a = 3$, $b = 2$
(B) $a = 3$, $b = -2$
(C) $a = -3$, $b = 2$
(D) $a = -3$, $b = -2$

28. If m and n are real numbers, which of the following statements is false?

(A) $2^m \cdot 2^n = 2^{mn}$
(B) $(2^m)^n = 2^{mn}$
(C) $2^m \div 2^n = 2^{m-n}$
(D) $2^m \cdot 2^n = 2^{m+n}$

29. If $4,000 is placed into an account with 3.5% interest compounded continuously and no additional withdrawals or deposits are made, how long will it take for the amount in the account to reach $7,000?

(A) less than 1 year
(B) between 1 and 2 years
(C) between 15 and 16 years
(D) between 16 and 17 years

30. Which of the following has the same standard deviation as the set $\{3, 5, 6, 9\}$?

(A) $\{10, 14, 15, 16\}$
(B) $\{6, 10, 12, 18\}$
(C) $\{10, 12, 13, 16\}$
(D) $\{3, 4, 7, 9\}$

31. Which graph below represents the inequality $|x| < 2$?

(A) ← | | | (|) | | | →
-2 0 2

(B) ← | | [|] | | →
-2 0 2

(C) ← | |) | (| | →
-2 0 2

(D) ← | |] | [| | →
-2 0 2

32. If the lines given by the equations $3x + 2y = 7$ and $ax + by = 12$ are perpendicular, what are the values of a and b?

(A) $a = 2, b = -3$
(B) $a = -2, b = 3$
(C) $a = 3, b = 2$
(D) $a = -2, b = -3$

33. Which function has a graph symmetric to the origin?

(A) $y = x^2$

(B) $y = \dfrac{1}{x^2}$

(C) $y = x + 3$

(D) $y = \dfrac{1}{x}$

34. If a pizza of a certain size is cut into 8 slices, each slice has an area of 8π in^2. What is the diameter of the pizza?

(A) 4 in
(B) 8 in
(C) 16 in
(D) 64 in

35. Note: $R \cap \overline{S} = \{x | x \in R, x \notin S\}$. If $R = \{x | x$ is a real number$\}$ and S is the set of all nonnegative real numbers, then $R \cap \overline{S} =$

(A) Ø, the empty set
(B) the set of negative real numbers
(C) $\{x | x \leq 0\}$
(D) $\{0\}$

36. Suppose $f(x) = \begin{cases} x & \text{if } x \leq 1 \\ 2 - x^2 & \text{if } x > 1 \end{cases}$.

Then the graph of f is

(A)

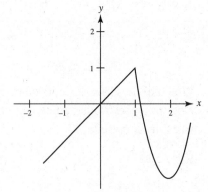

(B)

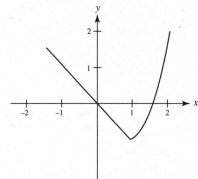

(C)

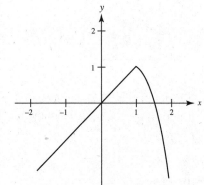

(D)

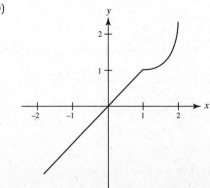

37. Which of the following is *not* the graph of a function?

(A)

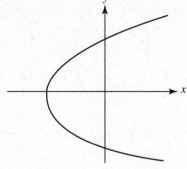

(B)

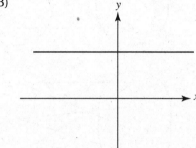

(C)

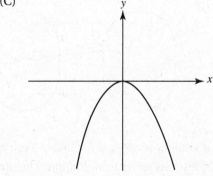

(D)

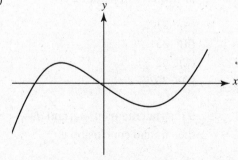

38. If the statement "Some Martians are green" is false, which of these must be true?

(A) Some Martians are not green.
(B) Some non-Martians are green.
(C) No Martians are green.
(D) All Martians are green.

39. Suppose $a < b$ (a, b real). Then it always follows that

(A) $-a > -b$
(B) $-a < -b$
(C) $-a < b$
(D) none of the preceding

Questions 40 and 41 refer to the graph below, which shows the size of the graduating senior class of a certain high school over the span of 25 years.

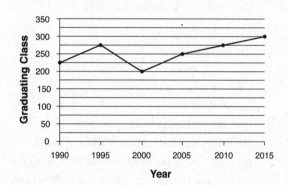

40. How many more students graduated in 2015 than graduated in 2000?

(A) 75
(B) 100
(C) 200
(D) 300

41. Which of the following is the overall percent change in the graduating class from 2005 to 2015?

(A) 10%
(B) 20%
(C) 33%
(D) 50%

42. Which pair of integers (m,n) does *not* satisfy the inequality $3m - 2n \leq 4$?

    (A) $(-4,-9)$
    (B) $(-1,2)$
    (C) $(2,1)$
    (D) $(0,-2)$

43. The negation of "if p, then q" is

    (A) If not p, then not q.
    (B) If not q, then not p.
    (C) p is true, but q is false.
    (D) If q, then p.

44. The population of a small town has been growing at a rate of 2% per year. If the population of the town in 2010 was 13,500 people, which of the following would give the town's population in 2016?

    (A) $13,500(2)^6$
    (B) $13,500(0.02)^6$
    (C) $13,500(0.98)^6$
    (D) $13,500(1.02)^6$

45. Five different algebra books, four different geometry books, and two different books on probability are to be placed on a shelf so that all the books on a particular subject are lined up together. How many ways can this be done?

    (A) 40
    (B) $40 \cdot 3!$
    (C) $5! \, 4! \, 2!$
    (D) $(5! \, 4! \, 2!)3!$

46. The notation $A \subset B$ says that "A is a subset of B." Which of the following statements is false?

    (A) Every nonempty set has at least 2 subsets.
    (B) If $P \subset Q$ then $P = Q$.
    (C) If $P = Q$ then $P \subset Q$.
    (D) The empty set is a subset of every set.

47. Which diagram does *not* define a function from $X(x_1, x_2, x_3, x_4)$ into $Y(y_1, y_2, y_3)$?

    (A)

    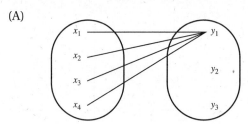

    (B)

    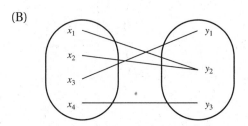

    (C)

    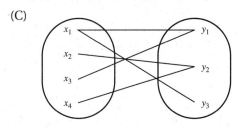

    (D)

    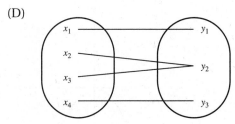

48. A student is allowed to choose 5 out of 7 questions on an examination. The number of ways it can be done is

    (A) 21
    (B) 35
    (C) 42
    (D) 2520

49. If the statements $p \to q$ and $q \to \sim r$ are true, then a valid conclusion is

    (A) $p \to r$
    (B) $\sim p \to r$
    (C) $r \to p$
    (D) $p \to \sim r$

50. Box I contains 2 red and 5 black marbles; box II contains 4 green and 2 black marbles. If 1 marble is drawn from each box the probability that they will be of different colors is

(A) $\dfrac{20}{147}$

(B) $\dfrac{5}{21}$

(C) $\dfrac{4}{7}$

(D) $\dfrac{16}{21}$

51. Which of the following is equivalent to
$\dfrac{(2\times10^2)(3\times10^3)}{4\times10^7}$?

(A) 1.5×10^{-2}
(B) 1.5×10^{-1}
(C) 1.5×10^2
(D) 1.5×10^{12}

52. If the annual interest rate of an investment is 12% compounded monthly, the effective annual percentage rate is closest to which of the following?

(A) 1.0%
(B) 12.0%
(C) 12.6%
(D) 12.7%

53. The set $\{x : x$ is an integer and $|x - 1| < 2\}$ equals

(A) $\{1, 2\}$
(B) $\{-2, -1, 1, 2\}$
(C) $\{-2, -1, 0, 1, 2\}$
(D) $\{0, 1, 2\}$

54. Joel has a coupon to his local electronics store for a certain percent off on one item. He buys a television that has a listed price of $600 but only pays $510 for it before taxes. For what percent off was the coupon valued?

(A) 15%
(B) 17.6%
(C) 85%
(D) 90%

55. The probability of Jane's winning a game of darts against Val is $\dfrac{1}{4}$. If they play three games, what is the probability that Jane will win at least one game?

(A) $\dfrac{1}{2}$

(B) $\dfrac{9}{16}$

(C) $\dfrac{37}{64}$

(D) $\dfrac{3}{4}$

56. It is known that m and n are positive integers, m is even, and n is odd. Check (✔) the appropriate boxes to indicate whether each of these numbers is even or odd.

Number	Even	Odd
$mn + 2$		
m^n		
$5n + 1$		
n^m		

57. How much—to the nearest dollar—would you need to invest in an account that pays 4% interest compounded annually in order to have $5,000 in the account after 3 years, assuming no further deposits or withdrawals?

(A) $4,435
(B) $4,440
(C) $4,445
(D) $4,805

58. If $m @ n = m^2 - 2n$, then $3 @ (2 @ 1) =$

(A) 23
(B) 9
(C) 7
(D) 5

59. At a certain high school 20% of the students are athletes, 25% are honors students, and 10% are both. The probability that a student selected at random is an athlete if he is an honors student is

(A) $\dfrac{2}{7}$

(B) $\dfrac{2}{5}$

(C) $\dfrac{1}{2}$

(D) $\dfrac{4}{5}$

60. What is the value of x in the equation
$$\dfrac{x+4}{2} = \dfrac{x+9}{3} ?$$

(A) 1
(B) 5
(C) 6
(D) 14

STOP

If there is still time remaining, you may review your answers.

ANSWER KEY
Trial Test

COLLEGE MATHEMATICS

1. **C**	17. **D**	35. **B**	53. **D**
2. **12**	18. **C**	36. **C**	54. **A**
3. **B**	19. **B**	37. **A**	55. **C**
4. **D**	20. **A**	38. **C**	56.
5. **70**	21. **B**	39. **A**	
6. **D**	22. **20**	40. **B**	
7. **B**	23. **D**	41. **B**	
8. **D**	24. **C**	42. **A**	
9. **C**	25. **D**	43. **C**	
10. **2**	26. **30**	44. **D**	
11. **B**	27. **C**	45. **D**	57. **C**
12. **100**	28. **A**	46. **B**	58. **D**
13. **C**	29. **C**	47. **C**	59. **B**
14. **C**	30. **C**	48. **A**	60. **C**
15. **A**	31. **A**	49. **D**	
16.	32. **A**	50. **D**	
	33. **D**	51. **A**	
	34. **C**	52. **D**	

56.

✔	
✔	
✔	
	✔

16.

✔	
	✔
✔	
✔	

SCORING CHART

After you have scored your Trial Test, enter the results in the chart below, then transfer your score to the Progress Chart on page 12. As you complete the Sample Examinations later in this part of the book, you should be able to achieve increasingly higher scores.

Total Test	Number Right	Number Wrong	Number Omitted
60			

NOTE

Did you omit any questions? If so, check to see which questions they were and think about how you could have answered them. Because there's no penalty for wrong answers on the CLEP, you should answer *all* the multiple-choice questions, even if you have to guess. Although guessing on the answer-in-the-box questions is more difficult, you should try to enter answers whenever possible, even if you are not sure they are correct.

ANSWER EXPLANATIONS*

1. **(C)** The mean of sets (A), (C), and (D) are all 3, but (C) has the greatest quantity of numbers farther away from the mean. Increasing all values by a constant as with (B) does not affect the standard deviation.

2. **(12)** $f(-2) = 4 - (-2)^3 = 4 - (-8) = 4 + 8 = 12.$

3. **(B)** The total bill will be $25 + 0.08 \times 25 = 25 + 2 = 27.$

4. **(D)** An isosceles triangle must have two equal angle measures.

5. **(70)** If x is the grade required on the fourth test to pass the course, then x must satisfy $\frac{52+57+61+x}{4} \geq 60$. So $170 + x \geq 240$, or $x \geq 70$.

6. **(D)** The integers in R are $\ldots, -2, -1, 0, 1, 2$. The integers in S are $0, 1, 2, 3, \ldots$. Those in $R \cup S$ are $\ldots, -2, -1, 0, 1, 2, \ldots$, namely, the entire set of integers.

7. **(B)** The contrapositive of statement $p \to q$ is $\sim q \to \sim p$.

8. **(D)** The line $2x + y = 2$ has x-intercept $+1$ and y-intercept $+2$.

*In some explanations of the Practice Sets we verify that incorrect answers are indeed incorrect—even though we have recommended that you not do this when taking the examination. Our intention here is to review and reinforce the mathematics, when time restrictions are not a factor. When working on one of the practice examinations, or on the CLEP Examination itself, time is a factor, and you should follow the instructions given on page 285 to the best of your ability. See also pages 310–311.

9. **(C)** A total of 65% of students preferred chocolate or vanilla ice cream.
$40 \times 0.65 = 26$.

10. **(2)** $g(x) = ax + b$. Then $g(-2) = -2a + b = -7$, and $g(3) = 3a + b = 8$. Subtracting, we get $-5a = -15$ and $a = 3$. Then $b = -1$ and $g(x) = 3x - 1$. So $g(1) = 2$.

11. **(B)** The area of a circle is πr^2 and the radius is half the diameter.

12. **(100)** A committee must have one or two teachers. There are $_2C_1 \cdot {}_{10}C_2$ one-teacher committees and $_2C_2 \cdot {}_{10}C_1$ two-teacher committees. The sum is $2 \cdot \dfrac{10 \cdot 9}{1 \cdot 2} + 1 \cdot 10$, or $90 + 10$. Why is $_{12}C_3 - {}_{10}C_3$ also correct?

13. **(C)** Use the formula $A = P\left(1 + \dfrac{r}{n}\right)^{nt}$ with $P = 500$, $r = 0.04$, $n = 4$, and $t = 3$.

14. **(C)** $x^2 - x = x(x - 1)$; the product is positive if $x > 1$ or if $x < 0$.

15. **(A)** Solving the inequalities yields the solution $39.6 \le x \le 42.2$, which matches the scenario described.

16.

Number(s)	Rational	Irrational
0	✔	
x such that $x^2 = 8$		✔
$\dfrac{1}{6}$	✔	
$\sqrt{121}$	✔	

Note that $\sqrt{121} = 11$, a rational number.

17. **(D)** If the lowest score and the highest score each increase by five points, the difference between them will remain the same, and therefore the range will not change. The mean, median, and mode will each increase by five points.

18. **(C)** Choose suitable values for p and q, for example, $p = -1$ and $q = 3$. You may then verify that (A), (B), and (D) are true. But (C) is false since $|-1| - |3| = -2$, which is *not* greater than -1.

19. **(B)** $20 \times 0.015 = 0.3$

20. **(A)** Parallel lines have the same slope, and the slope of the line given in the question is -2.

21. **(B)** Draw a diagram and note that the Pythagorean theorem ($a^2 + b^2 = c^2$) can be used to find the diagonal.

22. **(20)** The total number reported on (that is, the sum of the frequencies) is 28; the middle one (14th or 15th) is age 20.

23. **(D)** Plots (A) and (B) both indicate a positive relationship (the y-variable increasing along with the x-variable). Plot (C) indicates a negative relationship (the y-variable decreasing with an increasing x-variable).

24. **(C)** $g(2) = 3$, so $f \circ g(2) = f(g(2)) = f(3) = 6$.

25. **(D)** Division by zero is excluded.

26. **(30)** Since $6 = 2 \cdot 3$ and $10 = 2 \cdot 5$, n must be divisible by 2, 3, and 5.

27. **(C)** $f(0) = b = 2$; $f(1) = a + b = -1$; so $a + 2 = -1$ and $a = -3$.

28. **(A)** $2^m \cdot 2^n = 2^{m+n}$ as in (D).

29. **(C)** Use the formula $A = Pe^{rt}$ with $P = 4{,}000$ and $r = 0.035$, then try the various answer choices as values for t.

30. **(C)** Measures of spread—like the standard deviation—are unchanged by a constant increase to all data. The values in (C) have all been uniformly increased by 7.

31. **(A)** $|x| < a$ is equivalent to $-a < x < a$.

32. **(A)** Two lines are perpendicular if their slopes multiply to -1. The slope of the first line given is $-\dfrac{3}{2}$, so the perpendicular slope must be $\dfrac{2}{3}$. Investigate the given values.

33. **(D)** A graph of $y = f(x)$ is symmetric to the origin if $(-x, -y)$ lies on the graph, that is, if it satisfies the equation. Note that $(-y) = \dfrac{1}{(-x)}$ is equivalent to $y = \dfrac{1}{x}$.

34. **(C)** The area of the whole pizza is $8\pi \times 8 = 64\pi$ in^2. This gives a radius of 8 in, which doubles to 16 in for the diameter.

35. **(B)** The set $R \cap \bar{S}$ contains all the elements of R that are not in S. Here S is the set of positive real numbers and 0.

36. **(C)** The graph consists of the line through the origin with slope 1 for $x \leq 1$ and that part of the parabola (whose vertex is $(0,2)$ and which opens down) for $x > 1$.

37. **(A)** The graph of a function must pass the vertical-line test (a vertical line can intersect the graph at most at one point). Analytically, for each x in the domain, there is a *unique y*.

38. **(C)** "Some Martians are green" says that among Martians, some individuals are green. If that's false, then none of the Martians can be green.

39. **(A)** $a < b$ implies that $(b - a) > 0$, so $-a > -b$.

40. **(B)** According to the graph, 200 students graduated in 2000 and 300 students graduated in 2015.

41. **(B)** 50 more students graduated in 2015 than graduated in 2005. $50 \div 250 = 0.2 \rightarrow 20\%$. Note that the question asks about the *overall* percent change, meaning the graduating class in 2010 is not considered.

42. **(A)** Substitute the first number in the ordered pair for m, the second for n. Only for (A) is $3m - 2n$ *greater* than 4.

43. **(C)** Here is the truth table.

p	q	$p \rightarrow q$	$\sim(p \rightarrow q)$
T	T	T	F
T	F	F	T
F	T	T	F
F	F	T	F

$\sim(p \rightarrow q)$ is true only when p is true and q is false.

44. **(D)** Note that (B) and (C) give a population that is *less* than the original population and (A) gives a population that is unreasonably large.

45. **(D)** There are 5! ways to arrange the algebra books, 4! ways to arrange the geometry books, and 2! ways to arrange the probability books. The three subjects can be arranged in 3! ways.

46. **(B)** As a counterexample to statement (B), let $P = \{1,2\}$ and $Q = \{1,2,3\}$. Then $P \subset Q$ but $P \neq Q$.

47. **(C)** Note, in (C), that x_1 maps into both y_1 and y_3. Since X is a function, $X(x_1)$ must be unique.

48. **(A)** The answer is the number of combinations of 7 elements taken 5 at a time, or $_7C_5$. Since $_7C_5 = {}_7C_2$, we get $\dfrac{(7 \cdot 6)}{(1 \cdot 2)}$ or 21.

49. **(D)** If p implies q and q implies $\sim r$ then p implies $\sim r$.

50. **(D)** Compute the probability of obtaining two marbles of the same color and subtract from 1. The probability of getting 2 blacks is $\left(\dfrac{5}{7}\right)\left(\dfrac{2}{6}\right)$ or $\dfrac{5}{21}$.

The required probability is $1 - \dfrac{5}{21} = \dfrac{16}{21}$.

51. **(A)** Note that only the exponents of the 10 differ. Exponents add when their bases are multiplied and subtract when the bases are divided. $3 + 2 - 7 = -2$.

52. **(D)** Use the formula $APR = \left(1 + \dfrac{r}{n}\right)^n - 1$ with $r = 0.12$ and $n = 12$.

53. **(D)** If $|x - 1| < 2$, then x is within two units of 1; that is, $-2 < x - 1 < 2$.

54. **(A)** Take the amount of the discount, $90, and divide it by the original cost, $600.

55. **(C)** The probability that Jane will lose a game against Val is $\frac{3}{4}$, and that she will lose all three games is $\left(\frac{3}{4}\right) \cdot \left(\frac{3}{4}\right) \cdot \left(\frac{3}{4}\right)$. The probability that she will win at least one game is $1 - \left(\frac{3}{4}\right)^3$, or $\frac{37}{64}$.

56. Let $m = 2$, $n = 3$. Note that (A), (B), (C) are all even, but $3^2 = 9$.

Number	Even	Odd
$mn + 2$	✔	
m^n	✔	
$5n + 1$	✔	
n^m		✔

57. **(C)** The formula would be $5{,}000 = P(1 + 0.04)^3$. Solve for P.

58. **(D)** $3 @ (2 @ 1) = 3 @ (2^2 - 2 \cdot 1) = 3 @ 2 = 3^2 - 2 \cdot 2 = 5$.

59. **(B)** The probability that a student is an athlete if he is an honors student is the percentage of students who are both athletes and honors students out of the percentage of students who are honors students:

$$\frac{\text{probability the student is both athlete and honors student}}{\text{probability the student is an honors student}} = \frac{0.10}{0.25} = \frac{2}{5}$$

60. **(C)** Cross multiply to get $3x + 12 = 2x + 18$ and solve for x.

Background and Practice Questions

10

DESCRIPTION OF THE COLLEGE MATHEMATICS EXAMINATION

The CLEP General Examination in College Mathematics measures your knowledge of fundamental principles and concepts of mathematics. It covers material that is generally taught in a college course for nonmathematics majors. See the following chart for approximate percentages of examination items:

College Mathematics Exam

Content and Item Types	Time/Number of Questions
20% Algebra and Functions—Solving equations, linear inequalities, and systems of linear equations by analytic and graphical methods; interpretation, representation, and evaluation of functions using numerical, symbolic, and graphical methods; translations and horizontal and vertical reflections of graphs of functions, and symmetry about the x-axis, y-axis, and origin; and linear and exponential growth	60 questions 90 minutes
10% Counting and Probability—counting problems using the multiplication rule, combinations, and permutations; probability of unions, intersections, independent events, mutually exclusive events, conditional probabilities, and expected value	
15% Data Analysis and Statistics—data interpretation and representation using tables, bar graphs, line graphs, circle graphs, pie charts, scatterplots, and histograms; numerical summaries of data including mean (average), median, mode, and range; and conceptual questions about the standard deviation and normal distribution	
20% Financial Mathematics—percent change, markups, discounts, taxes, profit and loss, simple and compound interest calculations, continuous interest, effective interest rate, effective annual yield or annual percentage rate (APR), and present and future value	
10% Geometry—properties of triangles and quadrilaterals, including perimeter, area, similarity, and the Pythagorean theorem; properties of circles, including circumference, area, central angles, inscribed angles, and sectors; and parallel and perpendicular lines	

Content and Item Types	Time/Number of Questions
15% Logic and Sets—logical operations and statements, including conditional statements, conjunctions, disjunctions, negations, hypotheses, logical conclusions, converses, inverses, counterexamples, contrapositives, logical equivalences; set relationships, including subsets, disjoint sets, equality of sets, and Venn diagrams; and operations on sets, including union, intersection, complement, and Cartesian product	
10% Numbers—properties of numbers and their operations, including integers and rational, irrational, and real numbers (including recognizing rational and irrational numbers); elemental number theory (including factors and divisibility), primes and composites, odd and even integers, and the fundamental theorem of arithmetic; measurements, including unit conversion, scientific notation, and numerical precision; and absolute value	

About half of the exam asks you to solve routine, straightforward problems, while the other half requires you to do nonroutine problems that involve understanding and application of basic concepts of mathematics.

The College Mathematics Exam does not emphasize arithmetical calculations, so a calculator is not required for the examination. However, the testing software includes a scientific (nongraphing, nonprogrammable) calculator for your use during the exam. We recommend that you have a scientific calculator available as you prepare.

COMMON MATHEMATICAL SYMBOLS AND FORMULAS

Symbols Used in Arithmetic, Algebra, Geometry, and So Forth

$a = b$	a equals b
$a \neq b$	a does not equal b
$a \approx b$	a is approximately equal to b
$a > b$	a is greater than b
$a \geq b$	a is greater than or equal to b
$a < b$	a is less than b
$a \leq b$	a is less than or equal to b
$a < x < b$	x is greater than a and less than b
$|x|$	the absolute value, or magnitude, of x
$\sqrt{q}$	the square root of q
$\sqrt[3]{q}, \sqrt[4]{q}, \sqrt[n]{q},$	the cube root of q, the fourth root of q, the nth root of q
$a : b$	the ratio of a to b, "a is to b"
π	the constant pi (the ratio of the circumference of a circle to its diameter; approximately 22/7 or 3.14)
$0.\overline{18}$	the repeated decimal 0.1818...

Symbols Used in Set Theory†

$a \in S$	a is an element of set S
$a \notin S$	a is not an element of set S
$\{a, b, c\}$	the set containing the elements a, b, and c
$\emptyset$	the null or empty set
U	the universal set
$\overline{R}$ (or R' or $\tilde{R}$)	the complement of set R: the set of all elements that are not in set R
$A \cup B$	the union of sets A and B; the set of all items that appear in at least A or B
$A \cap B$	the intersection of sets A and B; the set of all items that appear in *both* A and B
$A \times B$	the Cartesian product of A and B: the set of all ordered pairs whose first element is in A and whose second element is in B
$A \cap \overline{B}$	the set of all elements that are in A but not in B

†*Most of these symbols are defined or illustrated when they first occur in the chapter.*

$A \subset B$	A is a subset of B.
	(Some authors use "$A \subset B$" to mean A is a proper subset of B and "$A \subseteq B$" to mean A is a subset, proper or improper, of B.)
$A \not\subset B$	set A is not a subset of set B

Symbols Used in Logic†

$\sim p$	not p (the negation of p)
$p \wedge q$	p and q (conjunction)
$p \vee q$	p or q (disjunction: p or q or both)
$p \rightarrow q$	if p then q; or p implies q
$p \leftrightarrow q$	p if and only if q, or p is equivalent to q

Symbols Used for Functions†

$f(x)$	A function f of a variable x (see definition of function on page 306).
$f(a)$	The value of the function $f(x)$ when x is equal to a; $f(a)$ is obtained by replacing x wherever it appears in $f(x)$ by a. For example, if
	$f(x) = x^2 - x + 1$, then
	$f(-2) = (-2)^2 - (-2) + 1 = 7.$
$f(g(x))$ or $(f \circ g)(x)$	The composite of functions f and g; $f(g(x))$ is obtained by replacing x wherever it appears in $f(x)$ by $g(x)$. For example, if $f(x) = 2x^2 - x + 3$
	and $g(x) = 4 - x$, then
	$f(g(x)) = 2(4 - x)^2 - (4 - x) + 3$
	$\qquad\quad = 2x^2 - 15x + 31$
	Note that
	$g(f(x)) = 4 - (2x^2 - x + 3)$
	$\qquad\quad = -2x^2 + x + 1.$

Symbols Used in Probability and Statistics†

$n!$	n factorial, the product of the first n positive integers:
	$n! = n(n-1)\,(n-2)\cdots 3 \cdot 2 \cdot 1$
	For example, $6! = 6 \cdot 5 \cdot 4 \cdot 3 \cdot 2 \cdot 1 = 720$.
$_nP_r$ or $P(n,r)$	The number of *permutations* (ordered arrangements) of a set of n objects taken r at a time:
	$$_nP_r = \frac{n!}{(n-r)!}$$

†*Most of these symbols are defined or illustrated when they first occur in the chapter.*

$_nC_r$ or $C(n,r)$ or $\begin{pmatrix} n \\ r \end{pmatrix}$

The number of *combinations* (selections in which order does not matter) of a set of n objects taken r at a time:

$$_nC_r = \frac{_nP_r}{r!} = \frac{n!}{r!(n-r)!}$$

$\sum\limits_{k=1}^{n} f(k)$

The sum obtained by letting k vary from 1 through n and adding up the resulting terms:

$$\sum_{k=1}^{n} f(k) = f(1) + f(2) + \cdots + f(n)$$

For example,

$$\sum_{k=1}^{4} 3(k) - 1 = 3(1) - 1 + 3(2) - 1 + 3(3) - 1 + 3(4) - 1$$
$$= 2 + 5 + 8 + 11$$
$$= 26$$

$\bar{x}$

The arithmetic mean (average) of a set of numbers (see definition of mean on page 306). If the set of numbers is $\{x_1, x_2, ..., x_n\}$, then

$$\bar{x} = \frac{\sum\limits_{k=1}^{n} x_k}{n}$$

Formulas Used in Financial Mathematics

$A = P(1 + r)^t$

The future value A of an initial principal P investment made in an account with a simple annual interest rate r, with no further withdrawals or deposits made for t years.

$A = P\left(1 + \dfrac{r}{n}\right)^{nt}$

The future value A of an initial principal P investment made in an account with annual interest rate r, compounded n times per year with no further withdrawals or deposits made for t years.

$A = Pe^{rt}$

The future value A of an initial principal P investment made in an account with annual interest rate r, compounded continuously throughout the year with no further withdrawals or deposits made for t years.

$APR = \left(1 + \dfrac{r}{n}\right)^{n} - 1$

The effective annual yield or annual percentage rate of an account with annual interest rate r, compounded n times per year.

Other Symbols†

(a,b) — The point in the plane whose x-coordinate (abscissa) is a and whose y-coordinate (ordinate) is b. Also, the ordered pair of elements a and b, where the set containing a and b is specified.

$a \, @ \, b$ — Here "@" stands for some algebraic operation; thus $a \, @ \, b$ is the element obtained by applying this operation to the ordered pair of elements (a,b). For example, if @ is ordinary subtraction on the set of integers, then

$$3 \, @ \, 7 = 3 - 7 = -4.$$

DEFINITIONS OF SOME COMMON MATHEMATICAL TERMS

prime number   A positive integer other than 1 whose only factors are 1 and itself; for example, 2, 3, 5, . . ., 23, 29, . . ., 41, 43, ... There are infinitely many primes.

composite number   A positive integer that has a factor other than 1 and itself; for example, 4, 6, 8, 9, 10, 12, ...

function   A correspondence between two sets such that each element of one set, called the *domain*, is associated with one and only one element of the other set, called the *range*.

mean   The arithmetic average of a set of values; the mean of a set is equal to the sum of all the values in the set divided by the number of values in the set.

median   The middle value of a set (or the value halfway between the two middle values) when the values are arranged in order of size. The median of the set [1, 1, 4, 6, 7, 7, 10] is 6; the median of [1, 2, 4, 6, 6, 8] is 5.

mode   The most frequent value in a set. The mode of {2, 3, 4, 4, 5, 6, 6, 6, 7, 8} is 6, because there are three 6's in the set.

range   The difference between the largest and smallest values in a set, a measure of the amount of spread in the set. The range of the set {60, 66, 67, 71, 75, 78, 80) is $80 - 60 = 20$.

standard deviation   A measure of spread in a set of values, based on the typical difference between the values and the mean. The standard deviation of the set {2, 4, 6, 8, 10} is greater than the standard deviation of the set {4, 5, 6, 7, 8}, because the values in the first set are farther from the mean of 6 than are the values in the second set.

†*Most of these symbols are defined or illustrated when they first occur in the chapter.*

COMMON GEOMETRIC FORMULAS

Sum of the angles of a triangle.

The sum is 180°.

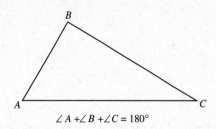

$$\angle A + \angle B + \angle C = 180°$$

Pythagorean theorem.

In a right triangle, the square of the length of the hypotenuse equals the sum of the squares of the lengths of the other two sides:

$$c^2 = a^2 + b^2$$

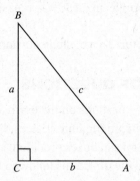

		Areas	**Perimeters**
RECTANGLE		$A = lw$	$P = 2l + 2w$
SQUARE		$A = s^2$	$P = 4s$
PARALLELOGRAM		$A = bh$	
TRIANGLE		$A = \frac{1}{2}bh$	$P = a + b + c$
TRAPEZOID		$A = \frac{1}{2}(b + b')h$	
CIRCLE		$A = \pi r^2$	$C = 2\pi r$

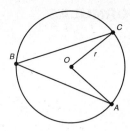

Central Angle: m$\angle AOC$ = measure of arc AC

Inscribed Angle: m$\angle ABC$ = $\frac{1}{2}$ measure of arc AC

Area of Sector: Area of circle portion defined by $\angle AOC$ is equal to $\pi r^2 \cdot \dfrac{\text{m}\angle AOC}{360°}$

TYPES OF QUESTIONS

Most of the questions on the exam are of the multiple-choice type, where you select the best answer from among four choices. For other questions, you may be asked to enter numbers or check marks in boxes provided.

Here are the directions followed by six examples, with correct answers and explanations.

DIRECTIONS: For each of the following questions select the best answer or write the correct answer in the box provided.

---

1. If $2x - y = 7$ and $3x + y = 8$, then $x + y$ equals

$$\boxed{2}$$

Answer

Solve the pair of equations simultaneously:

$$
\begin{aligned}
(1) \quad & 2x - y = 7 \\
(2) \quad & 3x + y = 8 \\
& 5x \quad\;\; = 15 \text{ (by adding (1) and (2))} \\
& x \quad\quad = 3
\end{aligned}
$$

Then, substituting for x in equation (1), we have

$$
\begin{aligned}
2(3) - y &= 7 \\
6 - y &= 7 \\
y &= -1
\end{aligned}
$$

So $x = 3$ and $y = -1$. Then $x + y = 3 + (-1) = 2$.

Note that we have inserted the answer "2" in the box provided.

2. Suppose $f(x) = \dfrac{x+1}{x-1}$. Then $f(1)$ equals

    (A) −1

    (B) 0

    (C) 2

    (D) none of these

Answer

Replacing x by 1, we get

$$f(1) = \frac{1+1}{1-1} = \frac{2}{0}.$$

Since division by zero is excluded, the function is not defined at $x = 1$.

The correct answer is D.

3. If a is negative, indicate whether each of the following numbers is positive or negative by checking ($\checkmark$) the appropriate box.

Number	Positive	Negative
a^3		
a^4		
$10 - 2a$		
$\lvert a - 100 \rvert$		

Answer

Note that the product of three negative numbers is negative, so a^3 is negative. Check the appropriate box by clicking in it. Similarly, the product of four negative numbers is positive, so a^4 is positive.

The product of two negative numbers is positive, so $-2a$ is positive, and thus $10 - 2a$ is positive.

The absolute value is defined as follows:

$$|x| = \begin{cases} x, & \text{if } x \geq 0 \\ -x, & \text{if } x < 0 \end{cases}$$

Since a is given as negative, the quantity $a - 100$ is negative. The absolute value $\lvert a - 100 \rvert$ is therefore the opposite (or negative) of the negative quantity $a - 100$, a positive number.

The correct answer is

Number	Positive	Negative
a^3		✔
a^4	✔	
$10 - 2a$	✔	
$|a - 100|$	✔	

TIPS ON ANSWERING QUESTIONS

1. As soon as you recognize the correct answer to a multiple-choice question, indicate that choice in the answer column immediately and move on to the next question. Do not try to verify that the other choices are incorrect. You may notice that this point differs from the strategy explained in Chapter 2. In that chapter, we advised you to read *all* the answers carefully before selecting your answer. This advice works well on the other exams because more than one answer might be correct. On those exams, you are asked to pick the *best* answer, even if another answer might be possible. On the math exam, however, only one answer is correct. The others are definitely wrong. Therefore, you only need to find the one correct answer; there is no need to look further. For example:

Which of the following Venn diagrams is for the set $R \cap S$?

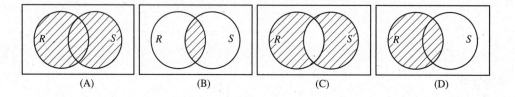

(A) (B) (C) (D)

Choice (A) is incorrect. Since choice (B) is correct, blacken space (B) on the answer sheet immediately without considering the remaining choices. Many multiple-choice questions can be answered using this strategy; for example: Which of the following statements is true (*or* false *or* impossible)? Which set is *not* empty? Which number is irrational? Which of the following graphs represents a function?

2. Be careful when solving an equation like $x^2 = 3x$. If you divide through by x, you will throw away a root. Instead, rewrite and factor as follows:

$$x^2 - 3x = 0$$
$$x(x - 3) = 0$$
$$x = 0 \text{ or } x = 3$$

3. Draw a sketch, if appropriate, and label the parts with given data or variables. To find a function or express a relation among variables, it may help to replace the variables by simple numbers.

4. Avoid excessive computation. Don't use pencil and paper unless you must. You will be allowed to use an online, scientific nongraphing, nonprogrammable calculator during the examination if you need to.

5. Do not spend too much time on any one question. If you're not sure of the answer, or if your equations or your computations seem unduly complicated, mark the question and return to it later if time permits.

6. Keep track of the time. Try to answer about 20 questions during the first 30 minutes. If you answer fewer, try to work a bit faster on the remaining questions.

7. You should not be concerned if you do not answer all the questions on the mathematics examination, because no one is expected to do all of them within the time limit. If you answer about half the questions correctly, your score will be approximately equal to the average score obtained by a test group of college sophomores with liberal arts backgrounds.

8. You are encouraged to guess whenever you do not know or are not sure of the answer since your score will be based only on the number of questions you answer correctly; you are not penalized for a wrong answer.

Try to keep in mind the tips given above and to use them when appropriate in answering the practice questions that follow.

STUDY SOURCES

Throughout this chapter, we will encourage you to develop a systematic approach to problem-solving, suggesting specific techniques and offering further hints on taking the test. You may find it helpful for your review to refer to one or more of the books listed below. These books, or others covering similar material, are available in public and school libraries.

The College Board Official Study Guide (2015) and its website at
www.collegeboard.com/clep.

Leff, Lawrence S. *Let's Review: Geometry* (2015). Hauppauge, NY: Barron's Educational Series, Inc.

Leff, Lawrence S. *EZ-101: College Algebra* (2005). Hauppauge, NY: Barron's Educational Series, Inc.

Rubinstein, Gary M. *Let's Review: Algebra I* (2015). Hauppauge, NY: Barron's Educational Series, Inc.

Waldner, Bruce. *Let's Review: Algebra 2 and Trigonometry* (2012). Hauppauge, NY: Barron's Educational Series, Inc.

PRACTICE QUESTIONS ON MATHEMATICS

In this section we will use practice questions to review the skills and content tested on the CLEP College Mathematics Examination. The topics covered are those frequently taught in college courses designed for non-mathematics majors: survey courses, courses offered to meet general education requirements, or courses designed for majors in elementary education. You will be expected to understand conventional symbols and notation, especially as used for the topics of sets, logic, and functions. Contemporary mathematical terminology and symbolism will generally be used here to provide review.

In the material that follows, practice questions are given separately for each topic covered: algebra and functions, counting and probability, data analysis and statistics, financial mathematics, geometry, logic and sets, and other topics and properties about the real-number system.

As noted earlier, most of the questions on the CLEP Examination are multiple-choice. The others require that you enter type a numerical answer or checkmark in the boxes provided.

DIRECTIONS: Answer each of the following questions. Keep track of your answers so you can compare them with the correct ones beginning on page 321.

Algebra and Functions

The subtopics are solving equations, linear inequalities, and systems of linear equations by analytic and graphical methods; interpretation, representation, and evaluation of functions using numerical, symbolic, and graphical methods; translations and horizontal and vertical reflections of graphs of functions, and symmetry about the x-axis, y-axis, and origin; and linear and exponential growth.

EXAMPLES

1. Which of these values of x is a solution to the inequality $-4x + 2 > 10$?

   (A) 3
   (B) 2
   (C) -2
   (D) -4

   Explanation: Note the inequality specifies the expression must evaluate to a number *greater than* 10. Substitute each value of x into the expression, and you'll find that options (A) and (B) evaluate to a number less than 10 and option (C) evaluates to exactly 10. Only option (D) evaluates to a number greater than 10. The correct answer is D.

2. Which ordered pair is a solution to the system of equations $y = 2x$ and $y = 3x - 2$?

   (A) (-2,4)
   (B) (2,4)
   (C) (-2,-4)
   (D) (2,-4)

Explanation: Since the equations are both solved for y, you can set them equal to each other and solve for x: $2x = 3x - 2$ yields $x = 2$, eliminating options (A) and (C). Substitute $x = 2$ back into either equation to find that $y = 4$. You can also substitute the values of x and y of each option choice into the two equations given to check their validity. The correct answer is B.

3. What is the value of y in the solution to the system of equations $x + 2y = 9$ and $x - y = 3$?

   (A) 2
   (B) 3
   (C) 5
   (D) 6

   Explanation: Multiply the second equation by two and add the two equations together to get $3x = 15 \rightarrow x = 5$. Substitute 5 for x into either equation to find that $y = 2$. The correct answer is A.

4. If $f(x) = x^3 - x - 1$, then $f(-1) =$

   Explanation: $f(-1) = (-1)^3 - (-1) - 1 = -1 + 1 - 1 = -1$.

5. If $R = \{1,2,3\}$, which of the following is a function from R into R?

   (A) $\{(1,3), (2,1)\}$
   (B) $\{(3,1), (2,3), (1,5)\}$
   (C) $\{(1,2), (2,2), (3,2)\}$
   (D) $\{(1,2), (2,3), (3,1), (3,3)\}$

   Explanation: A function from R into R may be defined as a set of ordered pairs in which each element of R must be a first element of exactly one pair, and the second element of that pair, its image, must belong to R. (A) is not a function because although $3 \in R$, it has no image; in (B), the image of 1 is 5, which is not in R; and in (D) the element 3 has two images. The correct answer is C.

6. Which of the following could be the graph of a function $y = f(x)$?

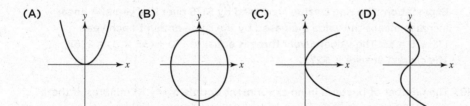

   (A)   (B)   (C)   (D)

   Explanation: If $y = f(x)$ is a function, then for each x in the domain there is a *unique* y. A vertical line can cut the graph of a function at most once. The correct answer is A.

7. Which of the following is the graph of $y = \begin{cases} x+3, & x > 0 \\ 3 & x \le 0 \end{cases}$?

(A)

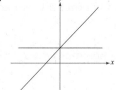

(B)

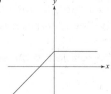

(C)

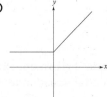

(D)

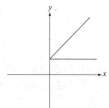

Explanation: The given function includes the horizontal line, which is the graph of $y = 3$ for $x \le 0$ (to the left of the y-axis), and the diagonal line, which is the graph of $y = x + 3$ for $x > 0$ (to the right of the y-axis). The correct answer is C.

8. If $f(x) = x^2$ and $g(x) = x - 4$, then $f \circ g(10) =$

   (A) 600
   (B) 106
   (C) 96
   (D) 36

   Explanation: $f \circ g(x)$ represents the composition of functions f and g, and may also be written $f(g(x))$. Since $g(10) = 10 - 4 = 6$, $f(g(10)) = f(6) = 6^2 = 36$. The correct answer is D.
       Alternatively, $f(g(x)) = f(x - 4) = (x - 4)^2$ and thus $f(g(10)) = (10 - 4)^2 = 36$.

9. A ring is appraised at a value of \$170. If the ring's value increases linearly and is worth \$345 five years later, how much was the ring worth in year three?

   Explanation: The ring's value increased by \$175 over five years. A linear increase means the value increased by the same amount each year: $175 \div 5 = 35$. The value in year three is equal to $170 + (35 \times 3) = 275$. The correct answer is \$275.

10. The number of bacteria in an experiment double every 10 minutes. If there were 150 bacteria in the sample at the start of the experiment, how many would there be in 1 hour?

   (A) 900
   (B) 1,500
   (C) 1,800
   (D) 9,600

   Explanation: There are 60 minutes in an hour, so the amount of bacteria will have doubled six times. $150 \times 2^6 = 9,600$. The correct answer is D.

1. If $g(x) = x^2 - 2x + 1$, then $g(-x) =$

   (A) $x^2 - 2x + 1$

   (B) $-x^2 + 2x + 1$

   (C) $x^2 + 2x + 1$

   (D) $x^2 + 2x - 1$

2. Which of the following is the graph of $x + 2y = 2$?

   (A)
   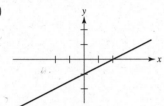

   (B)
   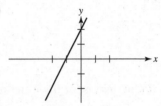

   (C)
   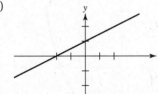

   (D)
   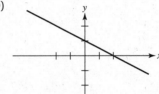

3. If $f(x) = x^2 - x + 3$, then $f(2) =$

4. If $f(x) = \dfrac{x+1}{(x-1)^3}$, then $f(0)$ equals

   (A) -1

   (B) 0

   (C) 1

   (D) none of these

5. If $f(x) = x^2 + 1$ then the domain of f is

   (A) $\{x : x > 0\}$

   (B) $\{x : -\infty < x < \infty\}$

   (C) $\{x : x \geq 0\}$

   (D) $\{x : x \geq 1\}$

6. The range of the function of question 5 is

   (A) all real numbers
   (B) all positive numbers
   (C) all numbers greater than one
   (D) all numbers y such that $y \geq 1$

7. Let $g(x) = \dfrac{x+1}{x^2 - x}$. Then the set of real numbers excluded from the domain of g is

   (A) $\{-1, 0, 1\}$
   (B) $\{0, 1\}$
   (C) $\{1\}$
   (D) $\{-1, 1\}$

8. A function $y = f(x)$ is even if $f(-x) = f(x)$. Which of the following functions is even?

   (A) $f(x) = 2x + 4$
   (B) $f(x) = x^2 + 2x$
   (C) $f(x) = 3x^2 + 5$
   (D) $f(x) = 4x$

9. The graph to the right is for the function

   (A) $2y = x^2 - 4$
   (B) $y = x^2 - 2$
   (C) $2y = x^2$
   (D) $y = x^2 - 4$

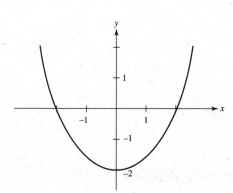

10. Which of the following points lies on the line $2x - 3y = 6$?

    (A) $(3, 2)$
    (B) $(0, 2)$
    (C) $(-3, 0)$
    (D) $(-3, -4)$

11. $f(x) = x(x - 2)$ and $g(x) = x + 1$. Then $f(g(0)) =$

12. Find $g(f(3))$ if function $f(x) = \dfrac{12}{x}$ and function g is defined by this table:

x	1	2	3	4
$g(x)$	3	4	6	9

13. If $f(x) = x^2 - 2x + c$ and $f(0) = 1$, then $c =$

14. The graph of $y = x^2 - 3$ is obtained from that of $y = x^2$ by translating the latter

   (A)   to the right 3 units
   (B)   to the left 3 units
   (C)   up three units
   (D)   down 3 units

15. If 3 markers and 2 pencils cost \$1.80 at a school store, and 4 markers and 6 pencils cost \$2.90, what is the cost of 1 marker and 1 pencil?

16. Which of the following diagrams does *not* define a function from $\{a,b,c\}$ into $\{d,e,f\}$?

   (A)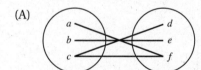

   (B)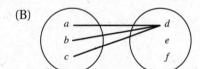

   (C)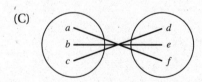

   (D)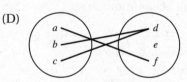

17. Let $f(x) = \begin{cases} x-1 & \text{if } x < 2 \\ x^2 - 3 & \text{if } x \geq 2 \end{cases}$. The graph of f is

(A)

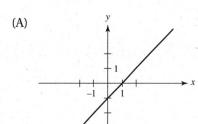

(B)

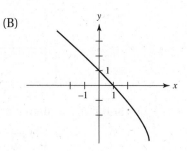

(C)

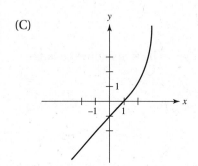

(D)

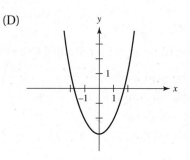

18. If $f(x) = 3x + 2$ and $g(x) = x^2 - 3$, then $f(g(x))$ equals

(A) $9x^2 + 12x + 1$

(B) $3x^2 - 7$

(C) $3x^2 - 1$

(D) $9x^2 + 6x + 1$

19. If $g(x) = 3x + k$ and $g(1) = -2$, then $g(2) =$

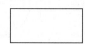

20. The graph below is for the set

(A) $\{x : -2 < x < 1\}$

(B) $\{x : x < -2, \ x = 1\}$

(C) $\{x : x > 1, \ x \neq -2\}$

(D) $\{x : x < -2 \text{ or } x > 1\}$

21. If none of the denominators below is zero, which of the following is true?

(A) $\dfrac{2p+4q}{p+2q}=2$

(B) $\dfrac{2m+p}{p+2q}=\dfrac{m+p}{q}$

(C) $\dfrac{q}{q+p}=\dfrac{1}{p}$

(D) $\dfrac{3m}{3q+p}=\dfrac{m}{q+p}$

22. The points in the interior, but not on the boundary, of the triangle in the figure satisfy

(A) $y<2-x,\ y>0,\ x>0$
(B) $y>2-x,\ y>0,\ x>0$
(C) $y\le2-x,\ y\ge0,\ x\ge0$
(D) $y<x-2,\ y>0,\ x>0$

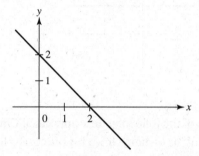

23. If $[x]$ denotes the greatest integer less than or equal to x, then $[-1.2]$ equals

24. Which of the equations below defines exactly one function $y=f(x)$ from the reals into the reals?

(A) $y^2=x^2+1$
(B) $x^3-y=4$
(C) $x-4y^2=2$
(D) $4x^2+9y^2=36$

25. Which of the following could be the graph of a function $y = f(x)$?

(A)

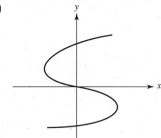

(B)

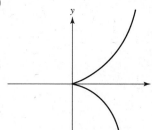

(C)

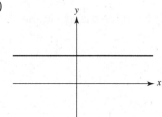

(D)

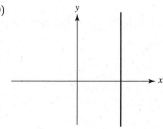

26. Which of the following descriptions of Chuck's activities may be illustrated by this graph of his distance from his office as a function of time, if he leaves his office at noon?

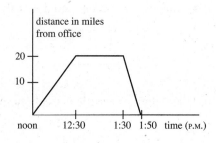

(A) Chuck drives 20 miles at 40 mph to visit his dentist, spends an hour there, then returns to his office in twenty minutes.

(B) Chuck drives at 60 mph to visit his dentist 20 miles away, spends an hour and 20 minutes there, then returns to his office in half an hour.

(C) Chuck drives 20 miles to his dentist in half an hour, spends an hour and 20 minutes there, then returns to his office in twenty minutes.

(D) At 40 mph, it takes Chuck a half hour to reach his dentist, with whom he spends an hour. Then he returns to his office in half an hour.

27. If $f(x) = x^2 - 4$ and $g(x) = \sqrt{x}$, then the composite function $(f \circ g)(x)$ is

(A) $x - 4$ (x is any real number)

(B) $x - 4$ ($x \geq 0$)

(C) $\sqrt{x^2} - 4$ ($|x| \geq 2$)

(D) $\sqrt{x^2} - 4$ ($x \geq 2$)

Answers and Explanations*

1. **(C)** $g(-x) = (-x)^2 - 2(-x) + 1 = x^2 + 2x + 1.$

2. **(D)** Checking the intercepts of the line is fastest. Here, they are $x = 2$ and $y = 1$. Only (D) qualifies.

3. **(5)** $f(2) = 2^2 - 2 + 3 = 4 - 2 + 3 = 5.$

4. **(A)** $f(0) = \dfrac{0+1}{(0-1)^3} = \dfrac{1}{-1} = -1.$

5. **(B)** A sketch of the graph may help for questions 5 and 6.

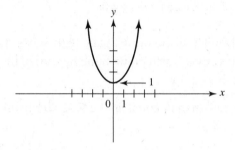

6. **(D)** See graph for question 5.

7. **(B)** Set the denominator of g equal to zero. Note that $x^2 - x = x(x-1) = 0$ when $x = 0$ or $x = 1$.

8. **(C)** Note that (A), (B), and (D) are not even. For example: $(-x)^2 + 2(-x) = x^2 - 2x \neq x^2 + 2x.$

9. **(A)** Check intercepts first. From the graph we see that $x = \pm 2$ and $y = -2$. Only $2y = x^2 - 4$ has these intercepts.

10. **(D)** The left side of the given equation must equal 6 when x and y are replaced by their coordinates.

11. **(-1)** $g(0) = 0 + 1 = 1, f(g(0)) = f(1) = 1(1-2) = 1 \cdot -1 = -1.$

12. **(9)** $f(4) = \dfrac{12}{4} = 3$, so $g(f(3)) = g(4) = 9.$

13. **(1)** $f(0) = 0^2 - 2(0) + c = 1 \rightarrow c = 1.$

14. **(D)** For a given x, each y-value of $y = x^2 - 3$ is 3 *less* than that of $y = x^2.$

15. **(0.65)** The scenario given produces the system of equations $3m + 2p = 1.80$ and $4m + 6p = 2.90$. Multiplying the entire first equation by 3 and subtracting the second equation yields the new equation $5m = 2.5$, which gives $m = 0.5$. Substitute that value back into either equation to find $p = 0.15.$

In some explanations of the Practice Sets we verify that incorrect answers are indeed incorrect—even though we have recommended that you not do this when taking the examination. Our intention here is to review and reinforce the mathematics, when time restrictions are not a factor.

16. **(A)** Note in (A) that the element c has two images, d and f. Why do diagrams (B), (C), and (D) define functions?

17. **(C)** The graph consists of part of a straight line ($y = x - 1$ if $x < 2$) and part of a parabola ($y = x^2 - 3$ if $x \geq 2$). Checking intercepts helps.

18. **(B)** $f(g(x)) = 3(x^2 - 3) + 2 = 3x^2 - 9 + 2 = 3x^2 - 7$.

19. **(1)** Since $g(1) = 3(1) + k = -2$, $k = -5$. So $g(2) = 3(2) + (-5) = 1$.

20. **(D)** The x-axis has been darkened to the left of $x = -2$ and to the right of $x = 1$. The hollow circles tell us to exclude these two points.

21. **(A)** $\dfrac{2p+4q}{p+2q} = \dfrac{2(p+2q)}{p+2q} = 2$ as long as $p + 2q \neq 0$.

22. **(A)** Since the line goes through the points (0,2) and (2,0), it has slope -1. Its equation is $y = 2 - x$. The coordinates (x,y) of each point in the interior of the triangle satisfy the inequalities $x > 0$, $y > 0$, and $y < 2 - x$.

23. **(−2)** The greatest integer less than or equal to -1.2 is -2. Verify this with a number line if necessary.

24. **(B)** When the exponent of y is 2, there may be 2 values of y for an x in the domain.

25. **(C)** The graphs in (A), (B), and (D) do not pass the vertical-line test (see example on page 313).

26. **(A)** At 40 mph it takes Chuck half an hour to drive the 20 miles to the dentist; he arrives at 12:30. His distance from his office remains constant until 1:30, hence he is at the dentist's for one hour. At 60 mph he drives the 20 miles back to his office in 20 minutes, arriving at 1:50.

27. **(B)** $(f \circ g)(x) = f(g(x)) = f(\sqrt{x}) = (\sqrt{x})^2 - 4 = x - 4$. The domain of $(f \circ g)(x)$ is the set of all x in the domain of g for which $g(x)$ is in the domain of f. Here the domain of g is $\{x \mid x \geq 0\}$, eliminating choice (A).

Counting and Probability

The subtopics include counting problems using the multiplication rule, combinations, and permutations; probability of unions, intersections, independent events, mutually exclusive events, conditional probabilities, and expected value.

EXAMPLES

1. How many ways can an 8-member council elect a chairman, a vice chairman, and a secretary if no member may hold more than one office?

   (A) $\dfrac{8!}{3!}$

   (B) $\dfrac{8!}{5!}$

   (C) $\dfrac{8!}{3!\,5!}$

   (D) 8^3

   Explanation: The chairman can be elected in 8 ways, after which the vice chairman can be elected in 7 different ways; following this, the secretary can be chosen from among 6 different people. There are then $8 \cdot 7 \cdot 6$ different ways the officers can be elected. For this question the *order* matters. An ordered arrangement of *n* objects taken *r* at a time is called a *permutation,* and is denoted by $_nP_r$ or by $P(n,r)$. Note that

   $$_nP_r = \frac{n!}{(n-r)!}$$

   This command can also be found on most scientific calculators and the online one available during the exam. If common factors are eliminated from numerator and denominator, a product of exactly *r* factors remains. Thus

   $$\frac{8!}{5!} = \frac{8 \cdot 7 \cdot 6 \cdot 5 \cdot 4 \cdot 3 \cdot 2 \cdot 1}{5 \cdot 4 \cdot 3 \cdot 2 \cdot 1} = 8 \cdot 7 \cdot 6$$

2. How many different 3-member committees can be selected from a group of 5 people?

   (A) 60
   (B) 20
   (C) 10
   (D) 5

   Explanation: This question calls for a *combination* of 5 objects taken 3 at a time; i.e., a selection where order does *not* matter. A combination of *n* objects taken *r* at a time is just the number of different *r*-element subsets that an *n*-element set has. We'll use the notation $_nC_r$; others used are $C(n,r)$, $C_{n,r}$, and $\left(\dfrac{n}{r}\right)$. Since there are *r*! permutations of each *r*-element set, we find $_nC_r$ by dividing $_nP_r$ by *r*!. Here the answer is $_5C_3$ or

   $$\frac{5!}{2!\,3!} = \frac{5 \cdot 4 \cdot 3 \cdot 2 \cdot 1}{2 \cdot 1 \cdot 3 \cdot 2 \cdot 1} = 10$$

For computation, it's easiest to remember $_5C_3$ as

$$\frac{5 \cdot 4 \cdot 3}{1 \cdot 2 \cdot 3}$$

where you have the same number of factors in the numerator as in the denominator. Or use the combination command on the calculator.

3. A box contains 4 black and 3 white chips. Two chips are selected at random. The probability that one is black and one is white is

(A) $\frac{2}{7}$

(B) $\frac{3}{7}$

(C) $\frac{4}{7}$

(D) $\frac{7}{12}$

Explanation: The probability of an event is the ratio

$$\frac{\text{number of ways the event can occur}}{\text{total number of possible outcomes}}$$

There are $4 \cdot 3$ or 12 ways of selecting 1 black chip and 1 white chip. There are $_7C_2$ or $\frac{(7 \cdot 6)}{(1 \cdot 2)}$ ways of choosing 2 chips from 7. The answer is $\frac{12}{21}$ or $\frac{4}{7}$. The correct answer is C.

4. Kids at a summer camp can sign up to play baseball or basketball or both. Of the 150 kids at the camp, 50 play baseball only, 35 play basketball only, and 30 kids do not participate in either sport. What is the probability that a randomly chosen baseball player also plays basketball?

$$\frac{\boxed{}}{\boxed{}}$$

Explanation: Make a Venn diagram to show that 35 kids play both sports. The requested conditional probability is defined as:

$$\frac{\text{number of kids who play both sports}}{\text{number of all kids who play baseball}}$$

We are told that 35 kids play basketball only, but 35 more kids play both basketball and baseball, so the total number of kids who play baseball is 70. The probability is therefore equal to $\frac{35}{70}$ or $\frac{1}{2}$.

1. The number of different license plates that start with one letter followed by three different digits selected from the set {0, 1, 2, 3, 4, 6, 6, 7, 8, 9} is

   (A) $26 \cdot 10 \cdot 10 \cdot 10$
   (B) $26 \cdot 9 \cdot 9 \cdot 9$
   (C) $26 \cdot 10 \cdot 9 \cdot 8$
   (D) $16 \cdot 9 \cdot 8 \cdot 7$

2. The number of different license plates beginning with two different letters followed by two digits either of which may be any digit other than zero is

   (A) $26^2 \cdot 8^2$
   (B) $26 \cdot 25 \cdot 9 \cdot 9$
   (C) $26^2 \cdot 9 \cdot 8$
   (D) $26^2 \cdot 9^2$

3. A box contains 6 green pens and 5 red pens. The number of ways of drawing 4 pens if they must all be green is

4. How many committees consisting of 3 girls and 2 boys may be selected from a club of 5 girls and 4 boys?

   (A) 6
   (B) 20
   (C) 60
   (D) 72

5. In how many ways can 2 or more bonus books be selected from a set of 5 offered by a book club?

6. The number of different ways a student can answer a 10-question true-false test is

   (A) 2
   (B) 20
   (C) 10^2
   (D) 2^{10}

7. A fair, six-sided cube with faces labeled with the numbers 1 through 6 is rolled. What is the probability of rolling a 5?

$$\frac{\boxed{}}{\boxed{}}$$

8. If a fair coin is tossed 3 times, then the number of different possible outcomes is

$$\boxed{}$$

9. If a fair coin and a fair cube with sides numbered 1 through 6 are tossed, then the probability that the coin shows heads and the die an even number is the fraction

$$\frac{\boxed{}}{\boxed{}}$$

10. A college that administered two tests to 100 freshmen got the following results: 14 failed both exams; 28 failed the mathematics exam; 33 failed the English exam. The number of students who passed both exams is

(A) 53
(B) 67
(C) 72
(D) 86

11. Given the data in question 10, what is the probability that a freshman failed both exams if he failed the math exam?

(A) $\frac{19}{47}$

(B) $\frac{14}{33}$

(C) $\frac{1}{2}$

(D) $\frac{28}{33}$

12. You pay $10 to buy one of 1,000 tickets for a lottery. If your ticket is chosen, you win $5,000. In dollars, what is the expected value of this lottery?

```
┌─────────┐
│         │
└─────────┘
```

13. Slips numbered 1 to 6 are placed in a bag. If two slips are drawn from the bag without replacement, then the probability that the sum will equal 7 is

    (A) $\frac{2}{5}$

    (B) $\frac{1}{3}$

    (C) $\frac{1}{5}$

    (D) $\frac{1}{15}$

14. A bag contains 2 red, 3 white, and 4 green balls. If 2 balls are drawn at random, what is the probability that at least 1 is green?

    (A) $\frac{5}{18}$

    (B) $\frac{13}{18}$

    (C) $\frac{4}{9}$

    (D) $\frac{59}{72}$

15. Based on a sample of 500,000 people, the American Cancer Society estimated that 750 people would die of cancer in 1973. The probability of death from cancer in 1973 for this sample was

    (A) 0.17
    (B) 0.015
    (C) 0.0017
    (D) 0.0015

16. The number of distinguishable permutations of letters in the word CANAL is

    (A) 31
    (B) 4!
    (C) 60
    (D) 5!

17. The eye color of students in a class is given by the chart. The probability that a person selected at random is a male or has blue eyes is

	MALES	FEMALES
BROWN EYES	6	4
BLUE EYES	3	7

(A) $\dfrac{3}{20}$

(B) $\dfrac{3}{10}$

(C) $\dfrac{1}{3}$

(D) $\dfrac{4}{5}$

18. One bag contains 5 black and 3 green marbles. A second bag has 4 black and 2 green marbles. If one marble is chosen from each bag at random, the probability that they are both green is

(A) $\dfrac{1}{8}$

(B) $\dfrac{1}{4}$

(C) $\dfrac{1}{3}$

(D) $\dfrac{5}{14}$

19. If a pair of fair cubes labeled with the numbers 1 through 6 are rolled, then the probability that the sum is greater than 9 is

(A) $\dfrac{1}{18}$

(B) $\dfrac{1}{12}$

(C) $\dfrac{1}{9}$

(D) $\dfrac{1}{6}$

20. Assume that the probability that it will rain on a day to be selected at random for a picnic is 10%. The probability that a Tuesday will be chosen and that that Tuesday will be dry is

(A) $\dfrac{10}{9}$

(B) $\dfrac{9}{10}$

(C) $\dfrac{9}{70}$

(D) $\dfrac{1}{70}$

Questions 21 and 22 are based on the following information:

> A college registrar reports the following statistics on 360 students:
>
> 200 take politics   70 take politics and biology
> 150 take biology   50 take biology and mathematics
> 75 take mathematics   10 take politics and mathematics
>
> 5 take all 3 subjects

21. How many students in the report do not take politics, biology, or mathematics?

(A) 0
(B) 30
(C) 60
(D) 100

22. If a student in the report is chosen at random, what is the probability that he studies mathematics but neither politics nor biology?

(A) $\dfrac{1}{24}$

(B) $\dfrac{1}{18}$

(C) $\dfrac{1}{6}$

(D) $\dfrac{5}{24}$

Answers and Explanations*

1. **(C)** We can show how to fill the 4 "slots" in the license plate schematically by

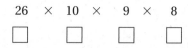

$$26 \quad \times \quad 10 \quad \times \quad 9 \quad \times \quad 8$$

where the number above a position indicates how many ways it may be filled. Note that a digit may *not* be repeated.

2. **(B)** Here we have

$$26 \quad \times \quad 25 \quad \times \quad 9 \quad \times \quad 9$$

The letter may not be repeated, but any of the 9 nonzero digits may be.

3. **(15)** $_6C_4$ or its equal, $_6C_2$, which is $\dfrac{(6 \cdot 5)}{(1 \cdot 2)}$.

4. **(C)** $_5C_3 \times \, _4C_2$, or $\dfrac{5 \cdot 4}{1 \cdot 2} \times \dfrac{4 \cdot 3}{1 \cdot 2}$, since $_5C_3 = \, _5C_2$.

5. **(26)** $_5C_2 + \, _5C_3 + \, _5C_4 + \, _5C_5 = 26$.

6. **(D)** The first may be answered in 2 ways, after which the second may be answered in 2 ways, after which the third and so on. This yields $2 \times 2 \times 2 \times \cdots \times 2$, where there are 10 twos, or 2^{10}. Note for just 3 T-F questions that there are 8 different ways of answering them. List them.

7. $\left(\dfrac{1}{6}\right)$ There are 6 possible outcomes, of which obtaining 5 is 1 outcome.

8. **(8)** A tree diagram may be useful:

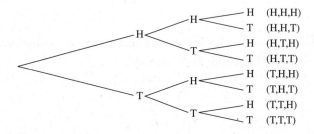

There are 8 possible outcomes. Note that the answer is obtainable immediately from

$$2 \quad \times \quad 2 \quad \times \quad 2$$

where there are 2 outcomes on the first toss; for each of these there are 2 on the second; and for each of the first four there are 2 outcomes on the third.

In some explanations of the Practice Sets we verify that incorrect answers are indeed incorrect—even though we have recommended that you not do this when taking the examination. Our intention here is to review and reinforce the mathematics, when time restrictions are not a factor.

9. $\left(\dfrac{1}{4}\right)$ The probability that the coin shows heads is $\dfrac{1}{2}$ and that the die shows an even number $\dfrac{1}{2}$. The answer is the product since the events are independent.

10. **(A)** Draw a Venn diagram. Since $14 + 14 + 19$, or 47, students failed one or both exams, it follows that $100 - 47$ passed both.

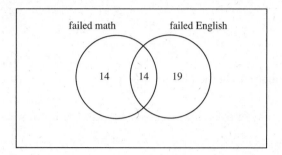

11. **(C)** $P(\text{failed both if failed math}) = \dfrac{P(\text{failed both})}{P(\text{failed math})} = \dfrac{{}^{14}/100}{{}^{28}/100} = \dfrac{1}{2}$

12. **(–4.99)** If you played this lottery 1,000 times, you would expect to lose 999 times and win once. Therefore, you would lose $999 \times 10 = \$9{,}990$ and would win $5,000. This is a net loss of $4,990, which spread over all 1,000 plays produces an expected value of –$4.99.

13. **(C)** The "favorable" draws are 1 and 6, 2 and 5, or 3 and 4. The desired probability is therefore
$$\frac{3}{{}_6C_2} = \frac{3}{\dfrac{6\cdot 5}{1\cdot 2}} = \frac{1}{5}$$

14. **(B)** The probability that no ball drawn is green is
$$\frac{{}_6C_2}{{}_9C_2} = \frac{5\cdot 4}{9\cdot 8} = \frac{5}{19}$$

Therefore, the probability that at least 1 green ball is drawn equals $1-\dfrac{5}{18}$, or $\dfrac{13}{18}$.

15. **(D)** $\dfrac{750}{500{,}000} = 0.0015$.

16. **(C)** If the two A's were distinguishable (perhaps subscripted), there would be $5!$ permutations. We divide by 2 to eliminate identical pairs of permutations.

17. **(D)** If M is the set of males and B is the set of blue-eyed people, then we want
$$\frac{P(M\cup B)}{\text{number in the class}} = \frac{6+3+7}{20} = \frac{4}{5}.$$

18. **(A)** $\dfrac{{}_3C_1}{8} \times \dfrac{{}_2C_1}{6} \times \dfrac{3}{8} \times \dfrac{1}{3} = \dfrac{1}{8}.$

19. **(D)** There are 6×6 or 36 possible outcomes when the pair of cubes is cast. A sum that exceeds 9 can be obtained in the following 6 ways:

CUBE I	CUBE II
4	6
5	6
5	5
6	6
6	5
6	4

Therefore the probability of the event is $\dfrac{6}{36} = \dfrac{1}{6}$.

20. **(C)** The 2 events, day of the week selected and whether it rains, are independent. The desired product is $\dfrac{1}{7} \times \dfrac{9}{10}$.

21. **(C)** A Venn diagram helps.

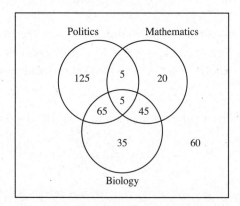

22. **(B)** Since 20 students out of 360 take mathematics but neither politics nor biology, the answer is $\dfrac{20}{360}$ or $\dfrac{1}{18}$.

Data Analysis and Statistics

The subtopics include data interpretation and representation using tables, bar graphs, line graphs, circle graphs, pie charts, scatterplots, and histograms; numerical summaries of data including mean (average), median, mode, and range; and conceptual questions about the standard deviation and normal distribution.

EXAMPLES

Answer questions 1 and 2 below using the following bar graph, which shows the number of students who ordered each lunch option one day at a certain elementary school.

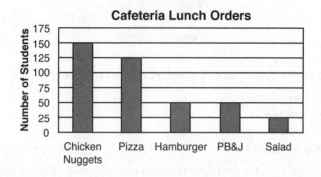

1. What percent of students ordered a hamburger?

   (A) 12.5%
   (B) 33.3%
   (C) 50.0%
   (D) 80.0%

   Explanation: The height of the bars tells how many students placed each order. Count the totals for each order; the total comes to 400 students. Fifty students ordered a hamburger, so 50 ÷ 400 = 0.125 → 12.5%. The correct answer is A.

2. How many more students ordered chicken nuggets than ordered a salad?

   Explanation: 150 students ordered chicken nuggets and 25 students ordered a salad. The correct answer is 125.

The pie chart below shows the favorite movie genre of the students in a large college class. Use this chart to answer questions 3 and 4.

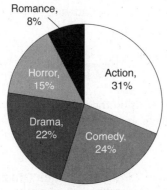

Favorite Genre

3. Which of the following pairs of genres represents the largest group of students?

   (A) action and romance
   (B) drama and horror
   (C) drama and comedy
   (D) comedy and romance

   Explanation: Add the percentages for each pair of genres. Drama and comedy together represent 46% of students, the largest of any other pair. The correct answer is C.

4. If half the students who picked drama changed their minds and chose horror instead, what would the percentage of students who like horror now be?

   (A) 18.5%
   (B) 26%
   (C) 29.5%
   (D) Impossible to calculate without knowing how many students were surveyed.

   Explanation: Half of the students who liked drama is 11% of the class. If they switched to horror, the percentage who liked horror would now be 26%. The correct answer is B.

5. If every value in a set of numbers is multiplied by 10, what happens to the median and the range?

   (A) Both the median and the range are multiplied by 10
   (B) The median is multiplied by 10, but the range does not change.
   (C) The range is multiplied by 10, but the median does not change.
   (D) Neither the median nor the range changes.

   Explanation: If each value in the set becomes 10 times as large, then the median (the middle value) must become 10 times as large. Since the minimum and maximum values will become 10 times as large, the difference between them (the range) will also become 10 times as large. The correct answer is A.

6. If Marcus got a 75, 82, and 88 on his first three tests, what grade must he get on his fourth in order to have an average of an 85?

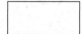

Explanation: In order for Marcus to have an average of 85 points across four tests, he needs a total of 85 × 4 = 340 points. On his first three tests, he currently has 245 points total. He needs to get a 95 on the fourth test to meet his goal.

7. Which of these sets of numbers has the same standard deviation as the set {2, 4, 6, 8, 10, 12}?

   (A)   {1, 3, 5, 7, 9, 11}
   (B)   {2, 3, 4, 10, 11, 12}
   (C)   {10, 20, 30, 40, 50, 60}
   (D)   {98.0, 98.2, 98.4, 98.6, 98.8, 99}

Explanation: The standard deviation measures the amount of spread in the set as determined by how far the values tend to be from the average. The values in set A are spaced two units apart, as are the values in the given set, and thus the spread is exactly the same. The correct answer is A.

   Note that even though set B has the same *range* as the given set, many values are farther from the average. Because the values in set C are 10 times as large, the standard deviation would be 10 times that of the original set. Set D would have a much smaller standard deviation, because those values are much closer together.

1. Which of the following accurately describes the relationship between the variables graphed in the scatterplot?

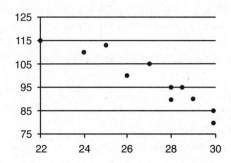

(A) strong and positive
(B) strong and negative
(C) weak and positive
(D) weak and negative

Frozen Foods sells ice cream, frozen yogurt, and other cold treats. The owner kept track of sales of a particular flavor over the past week and created the following line graph. Use it to answer questions 2 and 3.

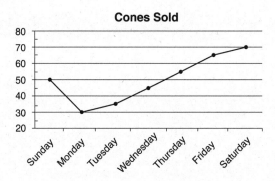

2. How many more cones were sold on Saturday than were sold on Sunday?

(A) 20
(B) 30
(C) 40
(D) 70

3. At what rate were sales increasing over the period of Tuesday to Friday?

(A) 5 cones per day
(B) 10 cones per day
(C) 35 cones per day
(D) 65 cones per day

4. What is the difference between the mean and the median of the following set of data: {55, 64, 43, 95, 63}

(A) 1
(B) 21
(C) 63
(D) 64

5. Assume that x = the standard deviation of the set of numbers {5, 10, 15, 20, 25}.
Check the boxes of each of the following that also has a standard deviation of x.

Set	Has a standard deviation equal to x
{5, 6, 15, 21, 25}	
{10, 20, 30, 40, 50}	
{10, 15, 20, 25, 30}	
{−25, −20, −15, −10, −5}	

6. If the average of the set of numbers {3, 5, 6, 11, x} is 7, then the median is

(A) 5
(B) 5.5
(C) 6
(D) 7

7. After getting the lowest test score in the class, one student points out to the teacher that there was a grading mistake on his test. The teacher agrees and raises that student's score. The student is happier because now he has a passing grade, even though it's still the lowest score in the class. Although one score has changed, which of these statistics remains the same for the class?

(A) mean
(B) median
(C) range
(D) standard deviation

8. Consider these three sets of numbers:

R = {10, 10, 20, 30, 30}
S = {40, 45, 50, 55, 60}
T = {70, 80, 80, 80, 90}

Rank them in order of their standard deviation, from smallest to largest.

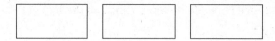

9. Which of the following is true for the data set {6, 9, 10, 17, 11, 14, 9, 12}?

(A) mode > median
(B) mean = median
(C) median > mean
(D) mean > median

Answers and Explanations*

1. **(B)** The dots of the scatterplot are all relatively close together in a linear pattern, indicating a strong relationship between the variables graphed. Because the y-values decrease as the x-values increase, the relationship is negative.

2. **(A)** 70 cones were sold on Saturday and 50 cones were sold on Sunday. 70 – 50 = 20.

3. **(B)** Each day from Tuesday to Friday, the number of cones sold increased by 10 cones per day.

4. **(A)** The mean is equal to (55 + 64 + 43 + 95 + 63) ÷ 5 = 64. Sorting the numbers in order puts 63 in the middle, making it the median. 64 – 63 = 1.

5.

Set	Has a standard deviation equal to x
{5, 6, 15, 21, 25}	
{10, 20, 30, 40, 50}	
{10, 15, 20, 25, 30}	✔
{−25, −20, −15, −10, −5}	✔

The first set has the same range and mean as the given set, but numbers are generally farther away from the mean. The values of the second set are 10 times the values in the original set, so the standard deviation will be 10 times as large. The third set is just the original set increased by 5, leaving the standard deviation unchanged, and the fourth set is the negatives of the original set and so the amount of deviation is unchanged.

In some explanations of the Practice Sets we verify that incorrect answers are indeed incorrect—even though we have recommended that you not do this when taking the examination. Our intention here is to review and reinforce the mathematics, when time restrictions are not a factor.

6. **(C)** $(3 + 5 + 6 + 11 + x) \div 5 = 7 \rightarrow (25 + x) \div 5 = 7 \rightarrow x = 10$. The median of the set $\{3, 5, 6, 10, 11\}$ is 6.

7. **(B)** Only the smallest value changed, so the median (the middle value) remains the same. Note that the mean increases, while both the range and the standard deviation decrease.

8. **T S R** Standard deviation measures how far the values spread away from the mean. Note that all three sets have the same range. Set T has the smallest standard deviation because three of its values are at the mean of 80. Set R has the largest standard deviation because four of its values are very far from the mean of 20.

9. **(D)** mode = 9, median = 10.5, mean = 11

Financial Mathematics

The subtopics include percent change, markups, discounts, taxes, profit and loss, simple and compound interest calculations, continuous interest, effective interest rate, effective annual yield or annual percentage rate (APR), and present and future value. See page 305 for a list of important formulas to be used in this section.

EXAMPLES

1. What percent of 108 is 13.5?

   (A) 8%
   (B) 12.5%
   (C) 13.5%
   (D) 94.5%

   Explanation: Divide $13.5 \div 108 = 0.125 \rightarrow 12.5\%$. The correct answer is B.

2. 25% of 148 is what number?

   (A) 5.92
   (B) 37
   (C) 123
   (D) 3,700

   Explanation: Convert 25% to a decimal and multiply: $148 \times 0.25 = 37$. The correct answer is B.

3. If Sofiya leaves a 20% tip on a dinner bill that costs $24.20, how much did she pay in total?

   (A) $4.84
   (B) $19.36
   (C) $29.04
   (D) $44.20

   Explanation: 20% of 24.20 is 4.84. When Sofiya pays for both the meal and the tip, she pays a total of $29.04. The correct answer is C.

---

4. Rashawn bought a CD that cost $18.99 and paid $20.51 including sales tax. Approximately what was the percent of the sales tax?

(A) 2%
(B) 3%
(C) 5%
(D) 8%

Explanation: Rashawn paid $1.52 in sales tax. This corresponds to $1.52 \div 18.99 \approx 0.08$. The correct answer is D.

5. If Julie deposited a $1,000 check she got from her grandparents when she graduated high school into an account that earns 3% annual interest, compounded quarterly, and made no further withdrawals or deposits to the account, approximately how much money would be in the account 6 years later?

(A) $1,046
(B) $1,194
(C) $1,196
(D) $1,720

Explanation: Use the formula $A = P\left(1+\dfrac{r}{n}\right)^{nt}$ with $P = 1,000$, $r = 0.03$, $n = 4$, and $t = 6$.

6. Michael and Trevor both invest $15,000 into accounts earning 5% annual interest. Michael's account earns simple interest, and Trevor's account is compounded continuously. If neither of the two make any further deposits or withdrawals from the account over 10 years, who will have more and how much more will they have?

(A) Michael will have $2230.82 more than Trevor
(B) Trevor will have $297.40 more than Michael
(C) Trevor will have $296.55 more than Michael
(D) They will have the same amount of money after 10 years.

Explanation: The amount of money Michael will end with is found using the formula $A = P(1 + r)^t$, and Trevor's using the formula $A = Pe^{rt}$ where $P = 15,000$, $r = 0.05$, and $t = 10$. Michael will end with approximately $24,433.42, and Trevor will end the 10 years with approximately $24,730.82. The correct answer is B.

7. Which of the following is closest to the APR of an account with an annual interest rate of 2.6%, compounded weekly?

(A) 2.60%
(B) 2.63%
(C) 2.96%
(D) 11.6%

Explanation: Use the formula $APR = \left(1+\dfrac{r}{n}\right)^{n} - 1$ with $r = 0.026$ and $n = 52$. The correct answer is B.

1. A cell phone manufacturer produces a phone that costs $126 per unit. Sellers mark up the price by 75% but after poor sales, later change the markup to only 50%. For what two prices was the phone sold?

    (A) $220.50 and $189
    (B) $220.50 and $110.25
    (C) $225 and $200
    (D) $225 and $175

2. If an artist can sell a project for $35 when it cost $15 in materials to produce, what is her approximate percentage profit?

    (A) 20%
    (B) 33%
    (C) 43%
    (D) 133%

3. In 2014, approximately 19,750,000 people lived in New York State, and 8,491,000 lived in New York City. Approximately what percentage of the state's population lived in the city?

    (A) 2.3%
    (B) 4.3%
    (C) 43.0%
    (D) 57.0%

4. The price of gas at your local station was $3.65 per gallon last weekend, but you notice it has gone down 3% since then. What is the current price of gas?

    (A) $3.54
    (B) $3.55
    (C) $3.62
    (D) $3.76

5. Ben invested a certain amount of money into an account earning an annual interest rate of 1.5% compounded monthly and made no other deposits or withdrawals for 5 years. At the end of the 5 years, he had $3,988. Which of the following is the closest to the amount of money he initially invested?

    (A) $3,538
    (B) $3,700
    (C) $3,702
    (D) $3,963

6. If $5,000 is invested at an annual interest rate of 7% compounded weekly and no other withdrawals or deposits are made, what is the smallest whole number of years before the investment will be worth $100,000?

$$\boxed{}$$

7. If an initial investment of $13,500 into an account with annual interest rate of 3.2% is worth $18,583.31 after 10 years, how frequently was the account compounded?

   (A) quarterly
   (B) monthly
   (C) weekly
   (D) continuously

8. The APR on a certain account is 5.25%. If the account is compounded daily, what is the annual interest rate?

   (A) 5.11%
   (B) 5.12%
   (C) 5.13%
   (D) 5.14%

9. Which of the following compounding frequencies will yield the largest final investment?

   (A) annually
   (B) quarterly
   (C) continuously
   (D) cannot be determined without more information

10. A painting is valued at $175,000 and is estimated to increase in value by 2% every year. Approximately how much will it be worth in 30 years?

    (A) $280,000
    (B) $317,000
    (C) $319,000
    (D) $5,355,000

11. A college graduate is offered a part-time job at a salary of $20,000. He is promised a 5% raise every year. His salary in the third year can be expressed as:

    (A) $20,000(0.05)
    (B) $20,000(1.05)
    (C) $20,000(1.05)^2$
    (D) $20,000(1.05)^3$

Answers and Explanations*

1. **(A)** 75% of $126 is $94.50. 50% of $126 is $63.

2. **(D)** The artist is making a $20 profit. $20 \div 15 \approx 1.33 \rightarrow 133\%$

3. **(C)** $8{,}491{,}000 \div 1{,}975{,}000 \approx 0.43$

4. **(A)** 3% of 3.65 is 0.1095. $3.65 - 0.1095 = 3.5405$

5. **(B)** Use the equation $A = P\left(1+\dfrac{r}{n}\right)^{nt}$ with $A = 3{,}988$, $r = 0.015$, $n = 12$, and $t = 5$.

6. **(10)** Use the formula $A = P\left(1+\dfrac{r}{n}\right)^{nt}$ with $P = 5{,}000$, $r = 0.07$, and $n = 52$. Experiment with different values of t until you find that the value surpasses $100,000 after 10 years.

7. **(B)** Use the formula $A = P\left(1+\dfrac{r}{n}\right)^{nt}$ with $P = 13{,}500$, $r = 0.032$, and $t = 10$. Experiment with the different values of n until you find the correct one.

8. **(B)** Use the formula $APR = \left(1+\dfrac{r}{n}\right)^{n} - 1$ with $n = 365$ and experiment with the different values of r until you find the correct one.

9. **(D)** While option C would be the correct answer in many, perhaps most, circumstances, particularly low values of P, r, or t could result in the same value for the frequencies listed (consider, for example, $P = 1$, $r = 0.001$, and $t = 1$).

10. **(B)** Use the formula $A = P(1 + r)^{t}$ with $P = 175{,}000$, $r = 0.02$, and $t = 30$.

11. **(C)** The grad's salary (in dollars) each year is as follows:
    1st year: $20,000
    2nd year: $20,000 + (0.05)(20,000) = $20,000(1.05)
    3rd year: (2nd year amount)(1.05) = $20,000(1.05)(1.05) = $20,000(1.05)^2

In some explanations of the Practice Sets we verify that incorrect answers are indeed incorrect—even though we have recommended that you not do this when taking the examination. Our intention here is to review and reinforce the mathematics, when time restrictions are not a factor.

GEOMETRY

The subtopics include properties of triangles and quadrilaterals, including perimeter, area, similarity, and the Pythagorean theorem; properties of circles, including circumference, area, central angles, inscribed angles, and sectors; and parallel and perpendicular lines. See page 307 for a number of formulas that could be useful for questions on this topic.

EXAMPLES

1. Which of the following is false?

   (A) All rectangles are parallelograms.
   (B) All trapezoids are quadrilaterals.
   (C) All squares are rhombuses.
   (D) All rhombuses are rectangles.

   Explanation: Quadrilaterals (four-sided figures) can be sorted into the following hierarchy:

   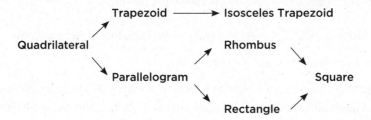

   All of the statements above are true except for the last one. The correct answer is D.

Base your answers to questions 2–4 on the following diagram.

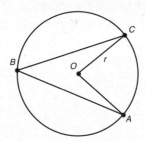

2. If the measure of arc *AC* = 50°, what is the measure of ∠*AOC* ?

   (A) 25°
   (B) 50°
   (C) 100°
   (D) Impossible to tell without knowing the radius of the circle.

   Explanation: A central angle is one with its vertex at the center of a circle, such as ∠*AOC*. Central angles always have a measure equal to the arc along the edge of the circle that they create. The correct answer is B.

3. If the measure of arc $AC = 80°$, what is the measure of $\angle ABC$?

   (A) 40°
   (B) 80°
   (C) 160°
   (D) Impossible to tell without knowing the radius of the circle.

   Explanation: An inscribed angle is one with its vertex on the edge of a circle, such as $\angle ABC$. Inscribed angles always have a measure equal to half the arc along the edge of the circle that they create. The correct answer is A.

4. If the measure of $\angle AOC = 72°$ and the radius of the circle is 15 cm, what is the area of the sector of the circle formed by $\angle AOC$?

   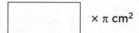 $\times \pi \text{ cm}^2$

   Explanation: An angle measuring 72° is $\frac{1}{5}$ th the measure all the way around the circle $\left(\frac{72}{360}\right)$. Therefore, the area of the sector (wedge) defined by the angle is $\frac{1}{5}$ th the area of the circle.

   $$A = \frac{1}{5}\pi r^2 = \frac{1}{5} \times 15^2 \times \pi = 45\pi.$$

   The correct answer is 45.

5. What is the slope of a line parallel to the line given by the equation $5x + 2y = 4$?

   (A) $-\frac{5}{2}$

   (B) $\frac{5}{2}$

   (C) $\frac{2}{5}$

   (D) $-\frac{2}{5}$

   Explanation: Parallel lines have the same slope. The slope of the given line is $-\frac{5}{2}$. The correct answer is A.

6. What is the slope of a line perpendicular to the line given by the equation $5x + 2y = 4$?

   (A) $-\frac{5}{2}$

   (B) $\frac{5}{2}$

   (C) $\frac{2}{5}$

   (D) $-\frac{2}{5}$

   Explanation: Perpendicular lines have slopes that multiply to –1 (they are negative reciprocals). The correct answer is C.

1. What is the perimeter of a right triangle with two shorter sides measuring 5 inches and 12 inches?

   (A) 13 inches
   (B) 30 inches
   (C) 31 inches
   (D) 34 inches

2. Rectangle *ABCD* and *WXYZ* are similar to each other. Segment *AB* is 2 inches long, segment *BC* is 10 inches long, and segment *XY* is 15 inches long. How long is segment *WX*?

   (A) 3 inches
   (B) 7 inches
   (C) 12 inches
   (D) 75 inches

3. The one base of a trapezoid measures 3.5 cm and the height is 4 cm. If the area of the trapezoid is 28 cm^2, how long is the other base of the trapezoid?

   (A) 2 cm
   (B) 3.5 cm
   (C) 10.5 cm
   (D) 20.5 cm

4. What is the area of a circle with a circumference of 16π?

   (A) 4π
   (B) 16π
   (C) 64π
   (D) 256π

5. Let l be the line defined by the equation $4y - 2x = 8$. For the lines defined by the equations below, check whether they are parallel to l, perpendicular to l, or neither of these things.

Equation	Parallel to l	Perpendicular to l	Neither
$y = \frac{1}{2}x + 5$			
$4y + 2x = 10$			
$y = \frac{1}{2}x + 4$			
$2y + 4x = -6$			

6. Angle DUR is inscribed in circle O as shown.

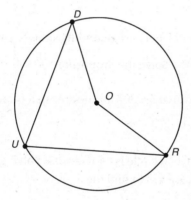

If the measure of $\angle DUR = 74°$, what is the measure of $\angle DOR$?

(A) 148°

(B) 74°

(C) 37°

(D) Impossible to tell based on the given information.

7. One slice of a pizza cut into 6 equally sized pieces has an area of 24π in^2. What is the diameter of the pizza?

(A) 8 in

(B) 12 in

(C) 24 in

(D) 144 in

8. If the length of all sides of a cube are doubled, then the volume of the cube is multiplied by

(A) 2
(B) 3
(C) 6
(D) 8

9. A rectangular garden has an area of 168 square feet. If its length exceeds its width by 2 feet, what is the perimeter of the garden?

(A) 54 ft
(B) 52 ft
(C) 50 ft
(D) 48 ft

Answers and Explanations*

1. **(B)** Use the Pythagorean theorem to find the length of the third side: 13 inches. $5 + 12 + 13 = 30$.

2. **(A)** Draw a diagram and label corresponding sides to show that BC and XY correspond to each other. Solve the proportion $\frac{10}{15} = \frac{2}{x}$.

3. **(C)** Use the formula from page 307 for the area of a trapezoid to get $28 = \frac{1}{2} \cdot 4 \cdot (3.5 + x)$ and solve.

4. **(C)** The circumference of a circle is equal to $2\pi r$. Solving $16\pi = 2\pi r$ gives $r = 8$. Use this in the formula $A = \pi r^2$ to find the area.

5.

Equation	Parallel to l	Perpendicular to l	Neither
$y = \frac{1}{2}x + 5$	✔		
$4y + 2x = 10$			✔
$y = \frac{1}{2}x + 4$			✔
$2y + 4x = -6$		✔	

Note that the third equation is equivalent to the original question, meaning it represents the exact same line.

6. **(A)** $\angle DUR$ is inscribed in circle O and therefore has a measure half that of arc DR, to which $\angle DOR$ is equal.

*In some explanations of the Practice Sets we verify that incorrect answers are indeed incorrect—even though we have recommended that you not do this when taking the examination. Our intention here is to review and reinforce the mathematics, when time restrictions are not a factor.

7. **(C)** The whole pizza has an area of 144π in^2. $144\pi = \pi r^2 \rightarrow r = 12 \rightarrow d = 24$.

8. **(D)** Let the length original be x, then the volume is x^3. After the sides are doubled, the new volume is $(2x)^3 = 8x^3$, 8 times the original volume.

9. **(B)** If l represents the length, then the width is $(l - 2)$ and the area is $l(l - 2)$. Solve the equation $l^2 - 2l = 168$, noting that $l^2 - 2l = 168 = (l - 14)(l + 12)$, which equals 0 if $l = 14$. Hence, the perimeter is $2(14) + 2(14 - 2) = 52$ feet.

LOGIC AND SETS

The subtopics include logical operations and statements, including conditional statements, conjunctions, disjunctions, negations, hypotheses, logical conclusions, converses, inverses, counterexamples, contrapositives, logical equivalences; set relationships, including subsets, disjoint sets, equality of sets, and Venn diagrams; and operations on sets, including union, intersection, complement, and Cartesian product.

EXAMPLES

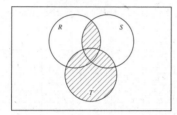

1. The Venn diagram above is for the set

   (A) $R \cap (S \cup T)$
   (B) $(R \cap S) \cup T$
   (C) $(R \cup S) \cap T$
   (D) $R \cap S \cup T$

   Explanation: The shaded area consists of elements that are either in both R and S, i.e., in $R \cap S$, or in T. The correct answer is B.

2. If $R = \{0,1\}$ and $S = \{2,3,4\}$, then $R \cup S$ equals

   (A) $\{0\}$
   (B) $\{2,3,4\}$
   (C) $\{1,2,3,4\}$
   (D) $\{0,1,2,3,4\}$

   Explanation: $R \cup S$ denotes the *union* of sets R and S; it consists of *all* the elements in set R or in set S or in both. The correct answer is D.

3. If set A = {a, e, i, o, u} and set B = {$red, white, blue$}, how many elements are in the set A × B?

   (A) 8
   (B) 15
   (C) The set A × B cannot be formed because A and B are not sets of numerical values.
   (D) The set A × B cannot be formed because sets A and B do not have the same number of values.

Explanation: A × B denotes the Cartesian product of the two sets, consisting of all possible ordered pairs (x,y) where $x \in$ A and $y \in$ B. Elements of A × B therefore include (a,red), $(a,white)$, $(a,blue)$, (b,red), and so on. Since each of the five elements of set A may be paired with each of the three elements of set B, there are $5 \times 3 = 15$ ordered pairs in A × B. The correct answer is B.

4. The converse of the statement $p \to q$ is

   (A) $p \to \sim q$
   (B) $q \to p$
   (C) $\sim q \to \sim p$
   (D) $\sim p \to \sim q$

   Explanation: $p \to q$ denotes "if p then q"; its converse is "if q then p," i.e., $q \to p$. The correct answer is B.

5. Which of the following is false?

   (A) If p is false, then $p \to q$ is true.
   (B) If p and q are both false, then $p \leftrightarrow q$ is true.
   (C) If q is true, then $p \land q$ is true.
   (D) If p is true, then $p \lor q$ is true.

   Explanation: Here are the truth tables for the most common logical connectives:

p	$\land$	q	p	$\lor$	q	p	$\to$	q	p	$\leftrightarrow$	q
T	T	T	T	T	T	T	T	T	T	T	T
T	F	F	T	T	F	T	F	F	T	F	F
F	F	T	F	T	T	F	T	T	F	F	T
F	F	F	F	F	F	F	T	F	F	T	F

   Use the tables to verify (A), (B), and (D). Note that for $p \land q$ to be true, both p and q must be true. The correct answer is C.

6. The statement $p \to q$ may be translated as

   (A) q only if p
   (B) p is necessary for q
   (C) p is sufficient for q
   (D) p is necessary and sufficient for q

   Explanation: See the third truth table in Example 5. Note that $p \to q$ is true *except* when p is true and q is false. The statement $p \to q$ is called the *conditional* and may be translated by any of the following:

   > if p then q
   > p only if q
   > p is sufficient for q
   > q is necessary for p
   > p implies q

   The correct answer is C.

   The fourth table in Example 5 is for the *biconditional* $p \leftrightarrow q$ and can be translated

   > p if and only if q (p if q)
   > p is necessary and sufficient for q

   The biconditional is true when p and q have the same values and false when they have opposite values.

7. Suppose the statement "If it rains on Tuesday, then the sun will shine on Wednesday" is true. Which of these statements must also be true?

(A) If it doesn't rain on Tuesday, then the sun won't shine on Wednesday.
(B) If the sun doesn't shine on Wednesday, then it didn't rain on Tuesday.
(C) If the sun shines on Wednesday, then it rained on Tuesday.
(D) It rains on Tuesday, and the sun shines on Wednesday.

Explanation: Let R represent "It rains on Tuesday" and S represent "The sun shines on Wednesday"; then the original statement is the conditional $R \rightarrow S$.

- Choice A is the inverse $\sim R \rightarrow \sim S$. The inverse of a true statement need not be true. Consider the true statement "If a figure is a square, then it has four sides." The inverse "If a figure is not a square, then it does not have four sides" is false; a trapezoid is not a square, but it does have four sides.
- Choice B is the contrapositive $\sim S \rightarrow \sim R$. The contrapositive of a true statement is always true. It is true that "If a figure does not have 4 sides, then it is not a square." The correct answer is B.
- Choice C is the converse $S \rightarrow R$. The converse of a true statement need not be true. A trapezoid serves as a counterexample to the converse "If a figure has four sides, then it is a square."
- Choice D is the conjunction $R \wedge S$, asserting that it does rain on Tuesday. The original statement is conditional, indicating a conclusion that can be reached *if* it rains on Tuesday. That does not mean it *must* rain on Tuesday.

Note that $R \rightarrow S$ is also equivalent to $\sim R \vee S$, "It doesn't rain on Tuesday, or the sun shines on Wednesday." In our other example, "If a figure is a square, then it has four sides" is equivalent to "A figure is not a square, or the figure has four sides." That's true of all figures.

8. Which statement is the negation of "If a dog barks, then it will not bite"?

(A) If a dog barks, then it will bite.
(B) If a dog does not bark, then it will bite.
(C) A dog either barks or bites.
(D) A dog barks, and it does bite.

Explanation: The conditional $p \rightarrow q$ is false if p is true and q is false, so the negation of $p \rightarrow q$ is $p \wedge \sim q$. The correct answer is D.

The negation of a statement fully contradicts the original statement; it is true whenever the original statement is false, and false whenever the original statement is true. Note these negations of common forms of statements:

Statement	Negation	Example
$p \vee q$	$\sim p \wedge \sim q$	I bike or I jog. *Negation*: I don't bike and I don't jog.
$p \wedge q$	$\sim p \vee \sim q$	The house has a pool and a garage. *Negation*: The house has no pool or no garage.
$p \rightarrow q$	$p \wedge \sim q$	If it's Monday, then I go to work. *Negation*: It's Monday, and I don't go to work.
All A are B.	Some A are not B.	All drivers wear seat belts. *Negation*: Some drivers don't wear seat belts.
Some A are B.	No A are B.	Some apples are ripe. *Negation*: No apple is ripe.
No A are B.	Some A are B.	No lights are on. *Negation*: Some lights are on.

1. If $R = \{0,2,4\}$ and $S = \{0\}$, then $R \cap S =$

   (A) $\{0,2,4\}$
   (B) $\{2,4\}$
   (C) $\{0\}$
   (D) $\emptyset$

2. If $R = \{a,b\}$, $S = \{b,c\}$, and $T = \{a,c\}$, then $R \cap (S \cap T)$ equals

   (A) $\emptyset$
   (B) $\{a,b,c\}$
   (C) $\{a,b\}$
   (D) $\{c\}$

3. Which of the following is not a subset of $\{p,q,s,v,w\}$?

   (A) $\{p,q,s,v,w\}$
   (B) $\emptyset$
   (C) $\{p\}$
   (D) $\{p,q,t\}$

4. If $U = \{a,b,c\}$ and $V = \{d\}$, then $U \times V =$

   (A) $\{a,b,c,d\}$
   (B) $\emptyset$
   (C) $\{(a,d)(b,d)(c,d)\}$
   (D) $\{(d,a)(d,b)(d,c)\}$

5. If $R = \{x : 1 < x < 5\}$, then the number of integers in R is

6. $R = \{x : x \geq 0\}$ and $S = \{x : x \leq 3\}$. The number of integers in $R \cup S$ is

   (A) none
   (B) 2
   (C) 4
   (D) infinite

7. Which of the following is a Venn diagram for $(R \cup S) \cap T$?

(A)
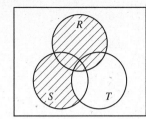

(B)
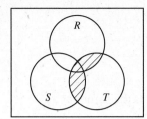

(C)
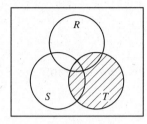

(D)
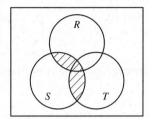

8. $V = \{a,b,c,d\}$ and $W = \{b,d,f\}$. Check the appropriate box to indicate whether each statement is true or false.

Statement	True	False
$W \subset V$		
$\{b,f\}$ is a subset of $V \cap W$		
$\{a,c\}$ belongs to $V \times W$		
$\{a,c,f\}$ is a subset of $V \cup W$		

9. If $R = \{x : x > 1\}$ and $S = \{x : x \leq 2\}$, then which of the following is false?

(A) $R \cap S$ contains two integers
(B) $1 \notin R$
(C) $R \cap S = \{x : 1 < x \leq 2\}$
(D) $1 \in S$

10. If $R = \{a,b\}$ and $S = \{a,c\}$, then the number of ordered pairs in $R \times S$ is

11. The number of subsets of {a,b,c} is

    (A) 8
    (B) 6
    (C) 5
    (D) 3

12. $R \cap (S \cup T)$ yeilds the same set as

    (A) $(R \cap S) \cup T$
    (B) $(R \cap S) \cup (R \cap T)$
    (C) $(R \cup S) \cup (R \cup T)$
    (D) $(R \cup S) \cap T$

13. Which of the following is a false statement about the Venn diagram?

    (A) $S \subset R$
    (B) $R \cap S = S$
    (C) $(R \cap S) \subset R$
    (D) $R \cap S = \emptyset$

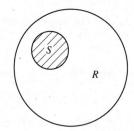

14. If $P = \{x | x \geq 1\}$ and $Q = \{x | x < 7\}$ then the number of integers in $P \cup Q$ is

    (A) none
    (B) 6
    (C) 7
    (D) infinite

15. If p denotes "He is a professor" and q denotes "He is absent-minded," then the statement "It is not true that he is an absent-minded professor" can be written symbolically as

    (A) $p \wedge q$
    (B) $\sim(p \vee q)$
    (C) $\sim p \wedge q$
    (D) $\sim(p \wedge q)$

16. Let p be "Mary is smart" and q be "Mary is conscientious." Then $p \rightarrow q$ may be translated as

    (A) If Mary is conscientious, then she is smart.
    (B) If Mary is smart, then she is conscientious.
    (C) Mary is smart but not conscientious.
    (D) Mary is both smart and conscientious.

17. Which of the following is the negation of "If p, then not q"?

    (A) p and q
    (B) If not p then q
    (C) If q then not p.
    (D) q and not p

18. Which of the following statements is *not* equivalent to "All mathematicians are clever"?

    (A) If a man is a mathematician, then he's clever.
    (B) If a man is not clever, then he's not a mathematician.
    (C) If a man is clever, then he's a mathematician.
    (D) A man is a mathematician only if he is clever.

19. The negation of the statement "If stock prices are rising, then food prices are high" is

    (A) If stocks are not rising, then food prices are not high.
    (B) If food prices are not high, then stocks are not rising.
    (C) If stocks are falling, then food prices are low.
    (D) Stocks are rising but prices are not high.

20. Let p be "A triangle is isosceles" and q be "A triangle is equilaterial." Symbolically, the statement "In order for a triangle to be equilateral it must be isosceles" is

    (A) $p \leftrightarrow q$
    (B) $p \rightarrow q$
    (C) $q \leftrightarrow p$
    (D) $q \rightarrow p$

21. Which of the following is false?

    (A) $2 + 1 = 4$ if and only if $(-1)^2 = -1$.
    (B) $3 + 2 = 5$ if and only if $(-x)^2 = x^2$.
    (C) $1 + 1 = 3$ if $4 - 4 = 0$.
    (D) $x^2 = 4$ if and only if $x = 2$ or $x = -2$.

22. If a statement is true so is its

    (A) converse
    (B) contrapositive
    (C) inverse
    (D) negation

23. Consider the set of true implications: "If Carl enjoys a subject, then he studies it. If he studies a subject, then he does not fail it." Which of the following is a valid conclusion?

   (A) Since Carl failed history he did not enjoy it.
   (B) If Carl does not enjoy history, then he fails it.
   (C) If Carl does not study a subject, then he does not pass it.
   (D) Carl did not fail mathematics; therefore he enjoyed it.

24. The converse of the statement "If dentists have no cavities, then they use Screen toothpaste" is

   (A) If dentists have cavities, then they do not use Screen.
   (B) If dentists do not use Screen, then they have cavities.
   (C) If dentists use Screen, then they have no cavities.
   (D) Dentists must use Screen if they are to have no cavities.

25. To disprove the statement "$x^2 > 0$ for all real x," which value of x may be offered as a counterexample?

   (A) $x = -2$
   (B) $x = -1$
   (C) $x = 0$
   (D) $x = 1$

26. The negation of the statement "Some students have part-time jobs" is

   (A) All students have part-time jobs.
   (B) Some students do not have part-time jobs.
   (C) Only one student has a part-time job.
   (D) No student has a part-time job.

Answers and Explanations*

1. **(C)** $R \cap S$ is the *intersection* of sets R and S; it consists of the elements that are in both R and S.

2. **(A)** $S \cap T = \{c\}$; $R \cap (S \cap T) = \emptyset$ When the intersection of two sets is the empty (or null) set $\emptyset$, then the sets are said to be *disjoint*. Disjoint sets have *no* elements in common.

3. **(D)** Any element in a subset of a set must be an element of the set. Remember that the null set $\emptyset$ is a subset of every set.

4. **(C)** $U \times V$ is the set of ordered pairs whose first element is an element of U and whose second is an element of V. $U \times V$ is called the *Cartesian product* of U and V.

5. **(3)** The integers are 2, 3, 4.

6. **(D)** Think of a number line:

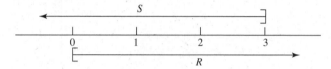

$R \cup S$ is the whole number line.

7. **(B)** Often it helps to label the disjoint, exhaustive sets as shown:

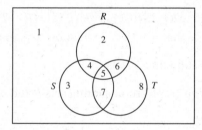

R consists of regions 2, 4, 5, 6
S consists of regions 3, 4, 5, 7
T consists of regions 5, 6, 7, 8
$(R \cup S) \cap T$ consists of $(2, 3, 4, 5, 6, 7) \cap (5, 6, 7, 8) = 5, 6, 7$.

8.

Statement	True	False
$W \subset V$		✔
$\{b,f\}$ is a subset of $V \cap W$		✔
$\{a,c\}$ belongs to $V \times W$		✔
$\{a,c,f\}$ is a subset of $V \cup W$	✔	

Note that $V \cap W = \{b,d\}$, that $\{a,c\} \notin V \times W$, that $V \cup W = \{a,b,c,d,f\}$.

In some explanations of the Practice Sets we verify that incorrect answers are indeed incorrect—even though we have recommended that you not do this when taking the examination. Our intention here is to review and reinforce the mathematics, when time restrictions are not a factor.

9. **(A)**

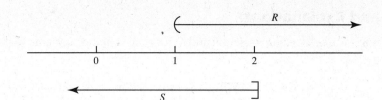

The only integer in $R \cap S$ is 2. *(Note that "$\in$" denotes "is an element of," "$\notin$" denotes "is not an element of," some specified set.)*

10. **(4)** $R \times S = \{(a,a), (a,c), (b,a), (b,c)\}$.

11. **(A)** The subsets of $\{a,b,c\}$ are $\emptyset$, $\{a\}$, $\{b\}$, $\{c\}$, $\{a,b\}$, $\{a,c\}$, $\{b,c\}$, and $\{a,b,c\}$.

12. **(B)** A Venn diagram helps.

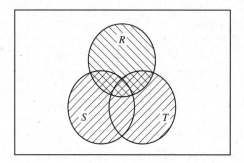

The crosshatched region is $R \cap (S \cup T)$ or $(R \cap S) \cup (R \cap T)$. See also the explanation to question 8 above. Note that $R \cap (S \cup T)$ includes regions 4, 5, 6.

13. **(D)** Note that $R \cap S = S$, and that $S \neq \emptyset$.

14. **(D)** Here are number line graphs representing sets P and Q.

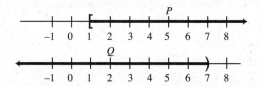

Note that the *union* of P and Q contains the entire set of integers.

15. **(D)** $p \wedge q$ denotes "He is an absent-minded professor."

16. **(B)** A translation of $p \rightarrow q$ is "if p then q."

17. **(A)** "If p then not q" can be written $p \rightarrow \sim q$. This is equivalent to $\sim p \vee \sim q$. The negation is $\sim(\sim p \vee \sim q) = p \wedge q$.

18. **(C)** A Venn diagram for the given statement shows mathematicians as a subset of clever men. Note that some clever men may not be mathematicians.

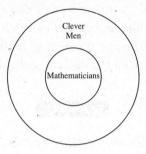

19. **(D)** The negation of "if p then q" is "p and not q."

20. **(D)** A restatement is "If a triangle is equilateral, then it is isosceles."

21. **(B)** "p if and only if q" or simply "p iff q" is called the biconditional and denoted by $p \leftrightarrow q$. It is true when p and q have the same truth values (both true or both false) and is false otherwise.

22. **(B)** A statement and its contrapositive are equivalent.

23. **(A)** Use contrapositives to work "backward." Since Carl failed history, he did not study it. Since he did not study history, he therefore did not enjoy it.

24. **(C)** The converse of "if r then s" is "if s then r."

25. **(C)** If $x \neq 0$, then $x^2 > 0$. But if $x = 0$, then $x^2 = 0$.

26. **(D)** Since "some" means "at least one," the negation of "some" is "none."

NUMBERS

The subtopics are properties of numbers and their operations, including integers and rational, irrational, and real numbers (including recognizing rational and irrational numbers); elemental number theory (including factors and divisibility), primes and composites, odd and even integers, and the fundamental theorem of arithmetic; measurements, including unit conversion, scientific notation, and numerical precision; and absolute value.

EXAMPLES

1. If a and b are real numbers, then $(a)[b + c] = (ab) + (ac)$ because

   (A) addition is commutative
   (B) multiplication is commutative
   (C) the real numbers are closed under multiplication
   (D) multiplication is distributive over addition

   Explanation: This is referred to briefly as the *distributive property*.

2. If $x^2 - x \geq 0$, then which of the following statements is true?

   (A) x must be positive.
   (B) x must be negative.
   (C) x must be greater than 1.
   (D) $x \neq 0$ or $x \geq 1$.

   Explanation: Since $x^2 - x = 0$ when $x = 0$, we can eliminate (A) and (B) immediately. Since $x^2 - x \geq 0$ for any negative x, (C) is false. Darken oval (D) immediately. Note that you need not justify choice (D), since it is the only alternative left. For completeness, we add here that (D) is true since $x^2 - x = x(x - 1)$, which equals 0 if $x = 0$ or 1, and is positive if x is negative or greater than 1.

3. What are the solutions to the equation $|x - 5| = 4$?

   (A) −1 and 9
   (B) 1 and 9
   (C) 9 only
   (D) −1 only

   Explanation: The absolute value of a quantity is that quantity's distance from zero. The statement $|x - 5| = 4$ means that the expression $x - 5$ is four units away from zero, in either direction. This equation can be used to create two new equations: $x - 5 = 4$ or $x - 5 = -4$, which produce the solutions 1 and 9. The correct answer is B.

4. Most weather forecasters aren't 100% certain of the predictions they make and use an interval of temperatures they are satisfactorily confident in. One forecaster announces a predicted high temperature of 65°. If he is confident in that prediction to within 2.5°, which of the following could be used to represent all predictions, x, he is confident are the potential high temperatures?

   (A) $|65 - x| \leq 2.5$
   (B) $|65 - x| > 2.5$
   (C) $|x - 65| \leq 2.5$
   (D) $|x - 65| > 2.5$

Explanation: If the forecaster is confident in his prediction to within 2.5°, this means he is confident the high temperature will be between 62.5° and 67.5°. Solving the absolute value inequalities above results in only A matching this interval. The correct answer is A.

5. Which of the following is equivalent to the expression $\dfrac{(2.0\times10^3)(3.5\times10^{-5})}{5\times10^{-4}}$?

(A) 1.4×10^{-11}
(B) 1.4×10^{-6}
(C) 1.4×10^{2}
(D) $1.4 \times 10^{3.75}$

Explanation: Note that the only difference between answer choices is the exponent on the 10. When multiplying powers of the same base, the exponents add. When dividing, exponents subtract. 3 + –5 – (–4) = 2. The correct answer is C.

DIRECTIONS: You will have access to an online scientific calculator during this test.

For multiple-choice questions, select the *best* of the four choices, then fill in the corresponding oval on the answer sheet. For the other questions, write your answer in the box.

Notes:

1. If the domain of a function f is not specified in a question, assume that it is the set of all real numbers for which $f(x)$ is defined.
2. Figures are drawn to scale and lie in a plane, *unless* otherwise specified.

---

1. Which of the following is *not* a prime number?

(A) 2
(B) 17
(C) 27
(D) 37

2. Which of the following statements is false?

(A) If $ab > 0$, then a and b are both positive.
(B) $a < 0 \rightarrow -a > 0$.
(C) If $a > b$, then $-a < -b$.
(D) If $0 < a < 1$, then $a^2 < a$.

3. Which of the following provide a counterexample to the false statement "If $a > b$, then $a^2 > b^2$"?

(A) $a = 2, b = 1$
(B) $a = 1, b = 0$
(C) $a = -2, b = -1$
(D) $a = 1, b = -1$

4. Which number is irrational?

  (A) $\sqrt[3]{-27}$

  (B) $\sqrt[3]{9}$

  (C) $\sqrt[4]{81}$

  (D) $\sqrt{16}$

5. There 16 cups in a gallon and 60 minutes in an hour. If a bathtub is filling at a rate of 2.2 gallons per minute, at what rate is it filling in cups per hour?

6. Which of the following statements about the real number system is false?

  (A) The real numbers are closed under addition and multiplication.
  (B) Subtraction of reals is commutative.
  (C) Every number except 0 has a multiplicative inverse.
  (D) The square of every nonzero number is positive.

7. The inequality $|12 - x| \le 0.001$ is used to indicate the precision of a particular manufactured ruler in number of inches, x. Which of the following would not be an acceptable precise measurement of a ruler manufactured under this guideline?

  (A) 12.0005
  (B) 19.9996
  (C) 12.001
  (D) 19.998

8. If $|a - 2| = a - 2$, then it is false that

  (A) $a > 0$
  (B) $a = 2$
  (C) $a > 2$
  (D) $a < 2$

9. Which of the following numbers is rational?

  (A) $\sqrt{2}$

  (B) $\sqrt{3}$

  (C) $\sqrt{4}$

  (D) $\sqrt{5}$

10. The prime factorization of 300 is

    (A) $3 \cdot 10^2$
    (B) $2 \cdot 3^2 \cdot 5^2$
    (C) $2 \cdot 3 \cdot 5^2$
    (D) $2^2 \cdot 3 \cdot 5^2$

11. Which of the following expressions cannot be evaluated?

    (A) $0 \cdot 1$
    (B) $\dfrac{0}{1}$
    (C) 1^0
    (D) $\dfrac{1}{0}$

12. Which statement is false?

    (A) There is a rational number between every pair of rationals.
    (B) There is an irrational between every pair of rationals.
    (C) There is a rational number between every pair of irrationals.
    (D) The sum of two irrational numbers is always irrational.

13. The repeating decimal 0.444 . . . equals the fraction

$$\frac{\boxed{}}{\boxed{}}$$

14. If $R = \{x : x$ is an integer$\}$ and $S = \{x : x$ is a positive real number$\}$, then $R \cap S$ equals

    (A) $\{x : x$ is a positive integer$\}$
    (B) the empty set
    (C) R
    (D) S

15. Which of the following is equivalent to the number 0.00244×10^5?

    (A) 2.444×10^2
    (B) 2.444×10^3
    (C) 2.444×10^8
    (D) 0.0000000244

16. Given that a and b are positive integers with a odd and b even, check (✔) the appropriate boxes to indicate whether each of the following numbers is even or odd.

Number	Even	Odd
$3a + b$		
$a^2 + 3b$		
$ab + 2a$		
b^a		

This number line with points q and t as shown is for questions 17 and 18.

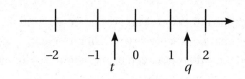

17. Which statement is false?

   (A) $q + t > 0$
   (B) $q - t > 0$
   (C) $q^2 > 1$
   (D) $t > -t$

18. If the expression $(3.7 \times 10^{10})(4.9 \times 10^{-4})$ is evaluated and written in scientific notation, what will be the exponent of the 10?

   (A) -40
   (B) -39
   (C) 6
   (D) 7

19. Which set is not empty?

   (A) $\{x : x + 2 = 2\}$
   (B) $\{x : |x| = -1\}$
   (C) $\{x : x \text{ is real and } x^2 + 1 = 0\}$
   (D) $\{x : x \neq x\}$

20. The set of different factors of 135 is

   (A) $\{3,5\}$
   (B) $\{3,7\}$
   (C) $\{5,7\}$
   (D) $\{7,9\}$

21. If p denotes "$x \leq 1$" and q denotes "$x > -2$," then the set that satisfies $p \wedge q$ is

  (A) $-2 < x \leq 1$
  (B) $1 \leq x$ or $x > -2$
  (C) $x < -2$ and $x \geq 1$
  (D) $-2 \leq x < 1$

22. To disprove the statement "If x is irrational, then x^2 is rational," choose x to be

  (A) $\sqrt{2}$
  (B) $\sqrt{9}$
  (C) π
  (D) 7

23. If p is divisible by 2 and q is divisible by 5, which of the following must be divisible by 10?

  (A) $pq + 15$
  (B) $5p + 2q$
  (C) $5(p + q)$
  (D) $p + q + 10$

Answers and Explanations*

1. **(27)** A prime number is an integer greater than 1 that has only itself and 1 as factors; $27 = 3 \cdot 9$.

2. **(A)** If a and b are both negative, then ab is positive. Verify the truth of (B), (C), and (D).

3. **(D)** $1 > -1$, but $(1)^2 = (-1)^2$. (C) is not a counterexample because $-2 \geq -1$.

4. **(B)** Note that $\sqrt[3]{27} = -3$, $\sqrt[4]{81} = 3$, and $\sqrt{16} = 4$.

5. **(2,112)** Use the conversion $\dfrac{2.2 \text{ gallons}}{1 \text{ minute}} \cdot \dfrac{16 \text{ cups}}{1 \text{ gallon}} \cdot \dfrac{60 \text{ minutes}}{1 \text{ hour}}$.

6. **(B)** A counterexample to statement (B): $5 - 3 \neq 3 - 5$.

7. **(D)** The inequality equation produces the solution set $19.999 \leq x \leq 2.001$. Only option D is outside of this interval.

8. **(D)** $|a - 2| = a - 2$ if $a - 2 \geq 0$, i.e., if $a > 2$ or $a = 2$. If $a \geq 2$, certainly $a > 0$.

9. **(C)** $\sqrt{4} = 2$.

10. **(D)** No other product given equals 300!

11. **(D)** Division by 0 is impossible.

12. **(D)** $\sqrt{2} + (3 - \sqrt{2}) = 3$ is a counterexample to statement (D). (A), (B), and (C) are true.

In some explanations of the Practice Sets we verify that incorrect answers are indeed incorrect—even though we have recommended that you not do this when taking the examination. Our intention here is to review and reinforce the mathematics, when time restrictions are not a factor.

13. $\left(\dfrac{4}{9}\right)$ Let $r = 0.444\ldots$ (where the three dots indicate an infinite number of 4's).

Then $\qquad 10r = 4.44\ldots$

$\qquad\qquad 9r = 4$

and $r = \dfrac{4}{9}$. The technique shown here will work for all repeating decimals.

14. **(A)** The intersection of two sets contains those elements that are in both sets.

15. **(A)** $0.00244 \times 10^5 = 244 = 2.44 \times 10^2$

16.

Number	Even	Odd
$3a + b$		✔
$a^2 + 3b$		✔
$ab + 2a$	✔	
b^a	✔	

Try $a = 3$ and $b = 2$.

17. **(D)** Since $t < 0$, $-t > 0$.

18. **(D)** $(3.7 \times 10^{10})(4.9 \times 10^{-4}) = 18{,}130{,}000 = 1.813 \times 10^7$.

19. **(A)** $\{x : x + 2 = 2\} = \{0\}$. None of the other sets contain any elements.

20. **(A)** Note that $135 = 3 \cdot 45 = 3 \cdot 3 \cdot 15 = 3 \cdot 3 \cdot 3 \cdot 5$ or $3^3 \cdot 5$.

21. **(A)** $(x \le 1) \wedge (x > -2)$ is true when both inequalities are satisfied. Thus, x must both exceed -2 and be less than or equal to 1.

22. **(C)** π is irrational, but so is π^2.

23. **(B)** Find p and q that satisfy the given conditions but for which the expressions in (A), (C), and (D) are not divisble by 10, for example, $p = 2$ and $q = 5$.

ANSWER SHEET
Sample Examination 1

COLLEGE MATHEMATICS

1. ☐

2. Ⓐ Ⓑ Ⓒ Ⓓ

3. ☐

4. Ⓐ Ⓑ Ⓒ Ⓓ

5. Ⓐ Ⓑ Ⓒ Ⓓ

6. ☐

7. Ⓐ Ⓑ Ⓒ Ⓓ

8. Ⓐ Ⓑ Ⓒ Ⓓ

9. Ⓐ Ⓑ Ⓒ Ⓓ

10.

Number(s)	Rational	Irrational
$\sqrt[3]{-125}$		
$\dfrac{5}{\sqrt{9}}$		
$\sqrt{18}$		

11. Ⓐ Ⓑ Ⓒ Ⓓ

12. Ⓐ Ⓑ Ⓒ Ⓓ

13. Ⓐ Ⓑ Ⓒ Ⓓ

14. Ⓐ Ⓑ Ⓒ Ⓓ

15. Ⓐ Ⓑ Ⓒ Ⓓ

16. Ⓐ Ⓑ Ⓒ Ⓓ

17. Ⓐ Ⓑ Ⓒ Ⓓ

18. Ⓐ Ⓑ Ⓒ Ⓓ

19. Ⓐ Ⓑ Ⓒ Ⓓ

20. Ⓐ Ⓑ Ⓒ Ⓓ

21. Ⓐ Ⓑ Ⓒ Ⓓ

22. Ⓐ Ⓑ Ⓒ Ⓓ

23. Ⓐ Ⓑ Ⓒ Ⓓ

24. Ⓐ Ⓑ Ⓒ Ⓓ

25. Ⓐ Ⓑ Ⓒ Ⓓ

26. Ⓐ Ⓑ Ⓒ Ⓓ

27. Ⓐ Ⓑ Ⓒ Ⓓ

28. ☐

29. Ⓐ Ⓑ Ⓒ Ⓓ

30.

Number	Prime	Composite
4		
5		
25		
39		

31. Ⓐ Ⓑ Ⓒ Ⓓ

32. Ⓐ Ⓑ Ⓒ Ⓓ

33. Ⓐ Ⓑ Ⓒ Ⓓ

34. Ⓐ Ⓑ Ⓒ Ⓓ

35. Ⓐ Ⓑ Ⓒ Ⓓ

36. Ⓐ Ⓑ Ⓒ Ⓓ

37. ☐

38. Ⓐ Ⓑ Ⓒ Ⓓ

39. Ⓐ Ⓑ Ⓒ Ⓓ

40. Ⓐ Ⓑ Ⓒ Ⓓ

41. Ⓐ Ⓑ Ⓒ Ⓓ

42. Ⓐ Ⓑ Ⓒ Ⓓ

43. Ⓐ Ⓑ Ⓒ Ⓓ

44. Ⓐ Ⓑ Ⓒ Ⓓ

45. Ⓐ Ⓑ Ⓒ Ⓓ

46. Ⓐ Ⓑ Ⓒ Ⓓ

47. Ⓐ Ⓑ Ⓒ Ⓓ

48. ☐ / ☐

49. Ⓐ Ⓑ Ⓒ Ⓓ

50. Ⓐ Ⓑ Ⓒ Ⓓ

51. Ⓐ Ⓑ Ⓒ Ⓓ

52. Ⓐ Ⓑ Ⓒ Ⓓ

53. Ⓐ Ⓑ Ⓒ Ⓓ

54. Ⓐ Ⓑ Ⓒ Ⓓ

55. Ⓐ Ⓑ Ⓒ Ⓓ

56. Ⓐ Ⓑ Ⓒ Ⓓ

57. ☐

58. Ⓐ Ⓑ Ⓒ Ⓓ

59. Ⓐ Ⓑ Ⓒ Ⓓ

60. Ⓐ Ⓑ Ⓒ Ⓓ

Sample College Mathematics Examinations

11

This chapter has two sample CLEP College Mathematics Examinations. Each is followed by an answer key, a scoring chart, and answer explanations. The examination consists of 60 questions for which 90 minutes are allowed. Most questions are of the multiple-choice type; for others you may be asked to enter a checkmark (✔) or a numerical answer in a box.

It is very important that you not spend too much time on any one question. It is probably best to answer first those questions that you are pretty sure about, returning after you've gone through the entire section to those questions that need more thought or work. Keep track of the time so you can pace yourself, remembering that it is not expected that anyone taking the test will answer every question.

For a reminder about the major topics that are covered in each part and the approximate number of questions for each topic, see pages 301–302.

It will be helpful at this point to reread the tips on pages 310–311. Here, again, are some reminders and additional tips:

1. Read the test directions carefully and study any illustrative examples.
2. Pay attention to any notes about figures, which are intended to provide information useful in answering the questions and are drawn as accurately as possible except when specifically noted otherwise.
3. Answer the easy questions first; you will have a chance to go back to the others.
4. Remember the College Board's "rights-only" policy on grading. Your score will be based *only* on the number of questions you answer correctly.
5. Because there is no penalty for incorrect or omitted answers, you should try to answer every question even if you have to guess.
6. When practicing, it is sometimes worthwhile to verify that choices not selected are truly incorrect. However, when taking the actual examination it would be needlessly time-consuming (and therefore foolish) to do that. When you decide on the answer to a particular question, type it in and move on immediately to the next question.
7. Work steadily, trying not to be careless.
8. Pace yourself but try to take a breather from time to time.
9. Keep cool. Remember that practically no one answers every question.

SAMPLE MATHEMATICS EXAMINATION 1

Number of Questions: 60

TIME LIMIT: 90 MINUTES

DIRECTIONS: You will have access to an online scientific calculator during this test.

For multiple-choice questions, select the *best* of the four choices, then fill in the corresponding oval on the answer sheet. For the other questions, write your answer in the box.

Notes:

1. If the domain of a function *f* is not specified in a question, assume that it is the set of all real numbers for which *f(x)* is defined.
2. Figures are drawn to scale and lie in a plane, *unless* otherwise specified.

---

1. If $g(x) = 2 - x^3$, then $g(-1) =$

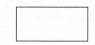

2. The negation of the statement "He is tall, or he is handsome" is

   (A) He is tall and handsome
   (B) He is not tall or he is not handsome
   (C) He is neither tall nor handsome
   (D) He is tall but he is not handsome

3. The Early Bird dinner menu lists 2 salads, 6 entrees, and 3 desserts. If a guest may choose 1 of each course, how many different dinners are available?

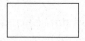

4. If *m* and *n* are positive integers, then which of the following *cannot* be an integer?

   (A) $\dfrac{1}{m+n}$

   (B) $\sqrt{m+n}$

   (C) $\dfrac{m+n}{m-n}$

   (D) $\dfrac{m}{n}$

5. A circle with a circumference of 36π cm would have an area of which of the following?

   (A) 18π cm^2
   (B) 36π cm^2
   (C) 324π cm^2
   (D) $1{,}296\pi$ cm^2

6. If students must answer 3 of 6 questions on a test, how many different choices do they have?

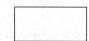

7. Mr. Bockton noticed that his receipt after a family dinner in a restaurant came to $90.10 after tax. If the before tax total was $85, what is the percent tax in Mr. Bockton's area?

   (A) 5.1%
   (B) 5.7%
   (C) 6.0%
   (D) 94.3%

8. The temperature of a fluid in a lab (in degrees Celsius) is a linear function of the time. Initially, at noon, the temperature was –4°C and at 2 P.M. it was –1°C. What was the temperature at 3 P.M.?

   (A) –2°C
   (B) 0°C
   (C) 0.5°C
   (D) 1.5°C

9. If the operation @ is defined by

   $m@n = \dfrac{3m}{n+4}$, for what value of x does

   $12@x = 4$?

   (A) 5
   (B) 8
   (C) 9
   (D) 13

10. Indicate whether each number is rational or irrational by checking the appropriate box.

Number(s)	Rational	Irrational
$\sqrt[3]{-125}$		
$\dfrac{5}{\sqrt{9}}$		
$\sqrt{18}$		

11. According to the local weather stations in cities X and Y, the probability that it will snow today in X is 0.2 and in Y is 0.4. Based on these predictions and assuming these events are independent, the probability that it will snow today in both cities is

   (A) 0.08
   (B) 0.48
   (C) 0.8
   (D) 0.92

12. Given the predictions in question 11, the probability that it will not snow today in either city X or city Y is

   (A) 0.08
   (B) 0.48
   (C) 0.52
   (D) 0.92

13. A car travels a scenic route at an average rate of 30 mph and returns along the same route at an average rate of 60 mph. Its average speed for the trip is

   (A) 40 mph
   (B) 45 mph
   (C) 50 mph
   (D) 55 mph

14. If $R = \{a,b,c,w\}$ and $S = \{a,c,d,w\}$, then $R \cap S$ equals

   (A) $\{a,b,c,d,w\}$
   (B) $\{a\}$
   (C) $\{a,c\}$
   (D) $\{a,c,w\}$

15. The bar graph below shows the high and low temperatures in a particular town over the course of a week.

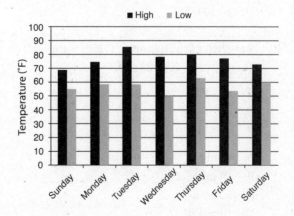

On which day was the highest low temperature?

   (A) Sunday
   (B) Tuesday
   (C) Wednesday
   (D) Thursday

16. Let p denote "Warren wears braces" and let q denote "Warren wears glasses." Then the statement "Warren wears neither braces nor glasses" is written symbolically as

    (A) $\sim p \vee \sim q$
    (B) $\sim p \vee q$
    (C) $\sim p \wedge \sim q$
    (D) $\sim p \wedge q$

17. The negation of "Every college graduate has studied geometry" is

    (A) Some college graduates have not studied geometry
    (B) No college graduate has studied geometry
    (C) Geometry is not necessary for graduation from college
    (D) If a person has studied geometry, then he is not a college graduate

18. If there are 5,280 feet in a mile, approximately 30.5 centimeters in a foot, and 100 cm in a meter, approximately how many meters are in a mile?

    (A) 1.7
    (B) 1,610.4
    (C) 17,311.5
    (D) 16,104,000

19. For which of the following values is the inequality $|x + 2| > 12$ *false*?

    I. $x = -15$
    II. $x = -14$
    III. $x = -13$

    (A) I only
    (B) III only
    (C) I and II
    (D) II and III

20. Jamie has two sets of data: Set A has a mean of 10 and a standard deviation of 2 while Set B has a mean of 20 and a standard deviation of 4. What could Jamie do to the data in set A so that it has the same mean and standard deviation as the data in Set B?

    (A) Double all the values
    (B) Increase the values by 10
    (C) Double all the values and then increase them by 10
    (D) Increase all the values by 10 and then double them

21. If $f(x) = 2x^2 - 3x + 2$, then $f(-x) =$

    (A) $2x^2 + 3x + 2$
    (B) $-2x^2 + 3x - 2$
    (C) $-2x^2 + 3x + 2$
    (D) $-f(x)$

22. If the population of a city decreases by 1.5% each year, what will its population be in 10 years if it started at 15,000, rounded to the nearest whole person?

    (A) 2,953
    (B) 12,750
    (C) 12,896
    (D) 17,408

23. The histograms below show the distributions of pizza prices (in $) found in four U.S. cities. In which is the standard deviation the greatest?

(A)
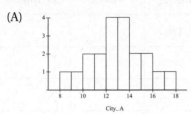
City_A

(B)
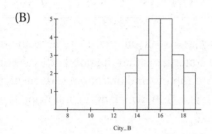
City_B

(C)
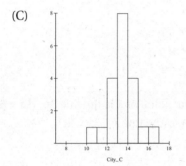
City_C

(D)
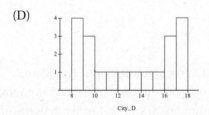
City_D

24. If a fair, 6-sided cube numbered 1 through 6 is tossed twice in succession, the probability of getting 4 on the first roll or 5 on the second is

(A) $\dfrac{1}{36}$

(B) $\dfrac{7}{36}$

(C) $\dfrac{11}{36}$

(D) $\dfrac{1}{3}$

25. A simple closed curve is one that starts and stops at the same point without passing through any point twice. Which of the following is a simple closed curve?

(A)
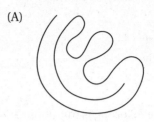

(B)
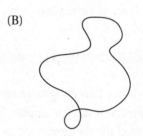

(C)
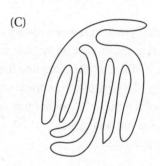

(D)
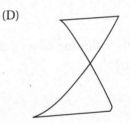

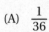

26. If an account with a 17% annual interest rate has an effective annual yield of 18.5%, how often over the course of the year is the interest compounded?

    (A) twice
    (B) quarterly
    (C) monthly
    (D) weekly

27. Which of the following is true about a rectangle that is *not* necessarily true about a parallelogram?

    (A) A rectangle has two pairs of parallel sides.
    (B) A rectangle has four congruent sides.
    (C) A rectangle has four right angles.
    (D) The angles of the rectangle add to 360°.

28. Alyssa's overall grade in her economics class is based on five test grades. So far, she has gotten a 74, 85, 67, and 89 on the first four tests. If her goal is to finish the course with an average of at least an 80, what must she get on the fifth and final test?

29. Which one of the following tables defines a function $y = f(x)$?

    (A)
x	1	1	2
y	3	4	5

    (B)
x	0	0	1
y	–1	1	2

    (C)
x	–1	0	1	1
y	0	1	2	3

    (D)
x	1	2	3	4
y	2	2	2	2

30. Indicate whether each number is prime or composite by checking the appropriate box.

Number	Prime	Composite
4		
5		
25		
39		

31. Let $f(x) = x + 2$ and $g(x) = x^2$; let p and q be the statements that the point (x,y) lies on the graph of f and on that of g, respectively. If $(x,y) = (1,3)$, which of the following is false?

    (A) $\sim q$
    (B) $p \vee q$
    (C) $p \wedge q$
    (D) $p \wedge \sim q$

32. For what value of k is the line $3y - kx = 6$ parallel to the line $y + 3x = 9$?

    (A) 9
    (B) 3
    (C) –3
    (D) –9

33. If $1,000 is deposited into an account earning 5% interest annually, compounded continuously, and no further deposits or withdrawals are made, how much will the account have increased by after 10 years, rounded to the nearest cent?

    (A) $648.66
    (B) $648.72
    (C) $1,648.66
    (D) $1,648.72

34. Which of the following sets has a standard deviation that is different from the other three?

(A) {0, 2, 6, 8, 10}
(B) {2, 4, 8, 10, 12}
(C) {27, 29, 33, 35, 37}
(D) {0, 4, 12, 16, 20}

35. If $4^m = 6$ and $4^n = 9$, then 4^{2m-n} equals

(A) 3
(B) 4
(C) 27
(D) 324

36. If $f(x) = \dfrac{x}{x^2 - 1}$, then the domain of f is

(A) the real numbers
(B) $x \neq 1$
(C) $x \neq 1, -1$
(D) $x \neq 0, 1, -1$

37. If 2 positive numbers are in the ratio of 6 to 11 and differ by 15, then the smaller number is

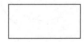

38. A registrar's records show that of 300 transfer students, 150 students signed up for a psychology course, 190 signed up for a computer course, and 70 signed up for both. The probability that a transfer student did not sign up for either psychology or computers is

(A) $\dfrac{1}{10}$

(B) $\dfrac{1}{2}$

(C) $\dfrac{19}{30}$

(D) $\dfrac{9}{10}$

39. How many subsets does the set $\{a, b, c\}$ have?

(A) 3
(B) 4
(C) 7
(D) 8

40. Which statement is equivalent to the statement "If she has invested wisely, then she is rich"?

(A) If she is not rich, then she has not invested wisely
(B) If she is rich, then she has invested wisely
(C) To be rich, you must invest wisely
(D) If she has not invested wisely, then she is not rich

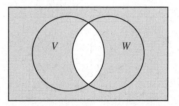

41. If $\overline{P}$ denotes the complement of Set P, then the shaded set in the Venn diagram above is

(A) $\overline{V \cup W}$
(B) $\overline{V \cap W}$
(C) $\overline{V} \cap \overline{W}$
(D) $\overline{V} \cup \overline{W}$

42. 30% of the boys in a school have brown hair, 20% have blue eyes, and 15% have both brown hair and blue eyes. If a boy chosen at random has brown hair, what is the probability that he also has blue eyes?

(A) $\dfrac{3}{20}$

(B) $\dfrac{3}{8}$

(C) $\dfrac{1}{2}$

(D) $\dfrac{3}{4}$

43. The graph of $\begin{cases} y \geq 1-x \\ x^2+y^2 \leq 4 \\ x \geq 0, y \geq 0 \end{cases}$ is

(A)

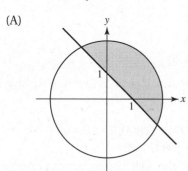

(B)

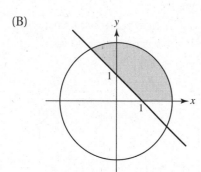

(C)

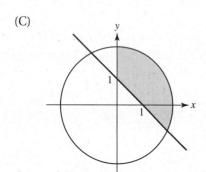

(D)

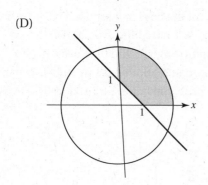

44. Which Venn diagram is *incorrect* if the following statements are true: $P \subset Q$; $P \cap R = \varnothing$?

(A)

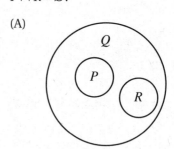

(B)

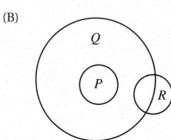

(C)

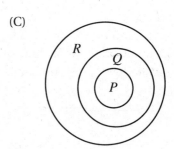

(D)

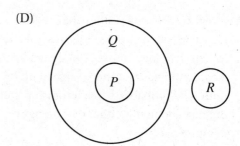

45. The solution set of {x : x is a real number
and $x^3 - x^2 - 2x = 0$} is

(A) {0,1,2}
(B) {0,–1,2}
(C) {–1,2}
(D) {0,1,–2}

46. How long is the arc *AB* indicated in the
circle below, measured in degrees?

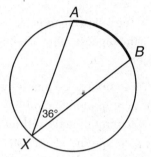

(A) 18°
(B) 36°
(C) 72°
(D) Impossible to know without the radius
of the circle

47. If two lines *m* and *n* are both perpendicular
to a third line *l* on a Euclidean plane, what
must be true about *m* and *n*?

(A) Lines *m* and *n* are perpendicular to
each other.
(B) Lines *m* and *n* are parallel to each
other.
(C) Lines *m* and *n* will move farther apart
from each other.
(D) Nothing can be concluded about lines
m and *n* based on this information.

48. There are 5 identical black socks and
5 identical brown ones in a drawer. If
you reach in and choose 2 socks without
looking, what fraction is the probability that
you will get a matching pair?

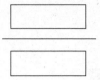

49. Ken put some money into a college savings
account when his son was born and made
no further deposits or withdrawals for
18 years. The account earned 3% interest
compounded yearly, and after 18 years the
account totaled $19,578. How much did
Ken put into the account when his son was
born, rounded to the nearest dollar?

(A) $11,409
(B) $11,417
(C) $11,500
(D) $11,700

50. A counterexample to the claim that if
$(a^2 > b^2)$, then $(a > b)$ is

(A) $a = 3, b = 2$
(B) $a = -2, b = -1$
(C) $a = 1, b = 0$
(D) $a = \dfrac{1}{2}, b = \dfrac{1}{3}$

51. If $f(x) = x + \dfrac{4}{x}$ and $g(x) = \sqrt{x+4}$, then

$f(g(0))$ is

(A) 2
(B) 3
(C) 4
(D) undefined

52. Which of the following statements is true about the data represented by this histogram?

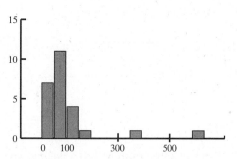

(A) The mean and the median are approximately equal.
(B) The mean is greater than the median.
(C) The median is greater than the mean.
(D) The relative sizes of the mean and median cannot be determined from the graph.

53. $(x-1)(3-x)^2 > 0$ if and only if

(A) $x > 1$
(B) $1 < x < 3$
(C) $x < 1$
(D) $x > 1, x \neq 3$

54. To resize a photo for publishing in a newspaper, the editor shrinks the length and width of the photo by 25%. By what percentage has the area decreased?

(A) 12.50%
(B) 25.00%
(C) 43.75%
(D) 50.00%

55. A student received quiz grades of 10, 7, 7, 10, 6, 9, 8, 7 in a language class. Her median score was

(A) 7
(B) $7\frac{1}{2}$
(C) 8
(D) $8\frac{1}{2}$

56. Which of the following interest rates would produce the highest value of a one year investment?

(A) 2.5% compounded quarterly
(B) 2.6% compounded monthly
(C) 2.4% compounded continuously
(D) 2.7% compounded annually

57. Every week, Devin withdraws $150 from her checking account for that week's expenses. Her job automatically deposits her $850 paycheck into her checking account every other week. At the end of every month, Devin transfers half of what's currently in her checking account into her savings. Assuming exactly four weeks per month, how much money would she have in her checking account at the end of three months if her starting balance was $450?

58. A store is offering two discounts: a flat 35% reduction, or a pair of coupons for 15% and 20% off. Which is the better option, assuming both coupons must be used together?

(A) The flat reduction is better.
(B) The pair of coupons are better.
(C) Both options are equally beneficial.
(D) The better option is dependent on the cost of the item purchased.

59. Triangles *ABC* and *DEF* are similar to each other, with angle *A* congruent to angle *D* and angle *B* congruent to angle *E*. Side *AB* is 9 cm long, side *BC* is 6 cm long, and side *EF* is 18 cm long. How long is side *DE*?

(A) 3 cm

(B) 9 cm

(C) 12 cm

(D) 27 cm

60. The prime factors of 96 are

(A) 2 and 3

(B) 6 and 8

(C) 2, 3, and 4

(D) 8 and 12

If there is still time remaining, you may review your answers.

ANSWER KEY
Sample Examination 1

COLLEGE MATHEMATICS

1. **3**
2. **C**
3. **36**
4. **A**
5. **C**
6. **20**
7. **C**
8. **C**
9. **A**
10.

✔	
✔	
	✔

11. **A**
12. **B**
13. **A**
14. **D**
15. **D**
16. **C**
17. **A**
18. **B**
19. **D**
20. **A**
21. **A**
22. **C**
23. **D**
24. **C**
25. **C**
26. **D**
27. **C**
28. **85**
29. **D**
30.

	✔
✔	
	✔
	✔

31. **C**
32. **D**
33. **B**
34. **D**
35. **B**
36. **C**
37. **18**
38. **A**
39. **D**
40. **A**
41. **B**
42. **C**
43. **D**
44. **C**
45. **B**
46. **C**
47. **B**
48. **$\frac{4}{9}$**
49. **C**
50. **B**
51. **C**
52. **B**
53. **D**
54. **D**
55. **B**
56. **D**
57. **1,018.75**
58. **A**
59. **D**
60. **A**

SCORING CHART

After you have scored your Sample Examination 1, enter the results in the chart below; then transfer your score to the Progress Chart on page 12.

Total Test	Number Right	Number Wrong	Number Omitted
60			

ANSWER EXPLANATIONS

1. **(3)** $g(-1) = 2 - (-1)^3 = 3$.

2. **(C)** The negation of statement $p \vee q$ is $\sim p \wedge \sim q$. Verify with truth tables if necessary.

3. **(36)** The answer is the product $2 \times 6 \times 3$.

4. **(A)** $\dfrac{1}{m+n}$ is a fraction for all positive integral m and n. (If, for example, $m = 6$ and $n = 3$, then (B), (C), and (D) are all integers.)

5. **(C)** For a circle, $C = 2\pi r$ and $A = \pi r^2$. Based on the information given, $r = 18$ cm.

6. **(20)** They have $_6C_3$ choices; $_6C_3$ equals $\dfrac{6 \cdot 5 \cdot 4}{3 \cdot 2 \cdot 1}$.

7. **(C)** Divide the amount of tax by the original before tax total: $5.10 \div 85 = 0.06$.

8. **(C)** Let $f(t) = at + b$, where $f(t)$ denotes the temperature at time t. We are given that $f(0) = -4$ and $f(2) = -1$. These yield $f(t) = \dfrac{3}{2}t - 4$, hence $f(3) = \dfrac{1}{2}$.

9. **(A)** $12@x = \dfrac{3 \cdot 12}{x+4}$; if $\dfrac{36}{x+4} = 4$, then $x + 4 = 9$.

10.

Number(s)	Rational	Irrational
$\sqrt[3]{-125}$	✔	
$\dfrac{5}{\sqrt{9}}$	✔	
$\sqrt{18}$		✔

Note: $\sqrt[3]{-125} = -5$; $\dfrac{5}{\sqrt{9}} = \dfrac{5}{3}$; but $\sqrt{18} = 3\sqrt{2}$, which is irrational.

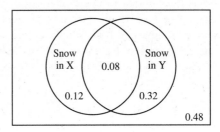

11. **(A)** The relevant probabilities for questions 11 and 12 are shown in the Venn diagram above.

12. **(B)** (1) Pr of snow in X = 0.2
     (2) Pr of snow in Y = 0.4
     (3) Pr of snow in both cities = (1) × (2) = 0.08
     (4) Pr of snow in X only = (1) − (3) = 0.12
     (5) Pr of snow in Y only = (2) − (3) = 0.32
     (6) Pr of snow in neither city =
     1 − (3) − (4) − (5) =
     1 − 0.08 − 0.12 − 0.32 = 0.48

13. **(A)** The distance along the route is irrelevant here, so choose a convenient distance, say 60 miles. Then it took 60 ÷ 30 = 2 hours going, and 60 ÷ 60 = 1 hour on the way back. The total journey of 120 miles took 3 hours to complete, hence the average speed was 120 ÷ 3 = 40 miles per hour. (Try letting the distance be d miles and note that you get the same average speed.)

14. **(D)** $R \cap S$ contains elements both in R and in S.

15. **(D)** Note that the low temperature bars for answers (A), (B), and (C) are all lower than for option (D).

16. **(C)** A restatement is "He does not wear braces and he does not wear glasses."

17. **(A)** The negation of "p is true for all" is "p is false for some."

18. **(B)** Multiply 5,280 by 30.5 to get centimeters per mile and divide by 100 to get meters per mile.

19. **(D)** Evaluate the inequality for the three given values.

20. **(A)** Option (B) will produce a mean of 20 but leave the standard deviation unchanged, (C) will produce a mean of 30, (D) will produce a mean of 40.

21. **(A)** $f(-x) = 2(-x)^2 - 3(-x) + 2 = 2x^2 + 3x + 2$.

22. **(C)** Use the formula $A = P(1 - r)^t$ with $P = 15{,}000$, $r = 0.015$, and $t = 10$. Note that (D) has a higher population than the original one, so shows a 1.5% *increase* over 10 years.

23. **(D)** Standard deviation measures how far each value is from the mean. More values are farther from average in City D than in any of the others.

24. **(C)** The probability that one event *or* another occurs is the sum of the probabilities of the two events minus the probability that they both occur. Since the successive tosses are independent, the probability that they both happen is the product of their probabilities.

   Hence the answer is $\dfrac{1}{6} + \dfrac{1}{6} - \dfrac{1}{36} = \dfrac{11}{36}$.

25. **(C)** Choice (A) starts and stops at different points. Each curve in (B) and (D) goes through one point twice.

26. **(D)** Use the formula $APR = \left(1 + \dfrac{r}{n}\right)^n - 1$ with $r = 0.17$, and test the provided values for n.

27. **(C)** A rectangle is a special case of a parallelogram where all four angles are right angles.

28. **(85)** Alyssa needs $80 \times 5 = 400$ points total on her five tests, and currently has 315 on the four she has already taken.

29. **(D)** Remember that if f is a function from a set X into a set Y, each element of X must correspond to a *unique* element in Y. In (A), (B), and (C) there are *two* different images of a single element in the domain.

30.

Number	Prime	Composite
4		✔
5	✔	
25		✔
39		✔

   A prime number has only 1 and itself as factors. Since $4 = 2 \cdot 2$, $25 = 5 \cdot 5$, and $39 = 3 \cdot 13$, then 4, 25, and 39 are composite numbers.

31. **(C)** The point (1,3) lies on the graph of f but not on the graph of g. So p is true, q false. Only $p \wedge q$ is false.

32. **(D)** The slope of $y + 3x = 9$ or $y = -3x + 9$ is -3. Therefore $\dfrac{k}{3}$ must equal -3.

33. **(B)** Use the formula $A = Pe^{rt}$ with $P = 1{,}000$, $r = 0.05$, and $t = 10$. Note that the question asks for the amount of increase not the final amount.

34. **(D)** The numbers in this set are twice those of (A) and so will have a standard deviation twice as big.

35. **(B)** $4^{2m-n} = (4^m)^2 \div 4^n = 6^2 \div 9 = 4$.

36. **(C)** The denominator of f equals 0 at 1 and -1. Every other real is in f's domain.

37. **(18)** Let the numbers be $6x$ and $11x$. Then $5x = 15$ and $x = 3$. So the smaller number is 18.

38. **(A)** Draw a Venn diagram. Since 30 students $(300 - 80 - 70 - 120)$ did not sign up for either course, the required probability is $\dfrac{30}{100}$ or $\dfrac{1}{10}$.

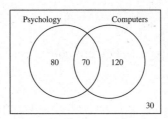

39. **(D)** The subsets are $\varnothing$, $\{a\}$, $\{b\}$, $\{c\}$, $\{a,b\}$, $\{a,c\}$, $\{b,c\}$, and $\{a,b,c\}$. The number of subsets of an n-element set is 2^n.

40. **(A)** The contrapositive of $p \to q$ is $\sim q \to \sim p$.

41. **(B)** The unshaded region is $V \cap W$. The complement is the shaded region.

42. **(C)** The probability equals $\dfrac{0.15}{0.30} = \dfrac{1}{2}$.

43. **(D)** The inequalities $x \geq 0$, $y \geq 0$ restrict the graph to the first quadrant.

44. **(C)** Verify that the given statements are illustrated correctly in (A), (B), and (D). Note, however, that (C) is incorrect because in (C), $P \subset R$, contradicting the statement given that $P \cap R = \varnothing$.

45. **(B)** $x^3 - x^2 - 2x = x(x^2 - x - 2) = x(x+1)(x-2)$.

46. **(C)** Note that arcs subtended by inscribed angles are always twice the measure of the angle.

47. **(B)** Lines that are perpendicular to the same line on the Euclidean plane are necessarily parallel to each other. Draw a picture to help you understand this.

48. $\left(\dfrac{4}{9}\right)$ You may initially choose any sock from the set of 10, but then, to obtain a matching pair, there are only 4 choices among the remaining 9 socks. The probability is therefore $\dfrac{10}{10} \cdot \dfrac{4}{9}$ or $\dfrac{4}{9}$.

49. **(C)** Use the formula $A = P\left(1 + \dfrac{r}{n}\right)^{nt}$ with $A = 19{,}578$, $r = 0.03$, and $n = 1$, and then solve for P.

50. **(B)** A counterexample cites values of a and b that satisfy the hypothesis but not the conclusion. Although $(-2)^2 > (-1)^2$, $-2 \not> -1$.

51. **(C)** Since $g(0) = \sqrt{4} = 2, f(g(0)) = f(2) = 2 + \dfrac{4}{2} = 4$.

52. **(B)** Most of these data lie between 0 and 150, but there are 2 unusually large values. The mean, based on the sum of the data, will be affected by these large values, whereas the median, representing the middle entry in an ordered list of the data, will not.

53. **(D)** $(x - 1)(3 - x)^2 > 0$ if and only if $x - 1 > 0$ and $3 - x \neq 0$; i.e., if and only if $x > 1$, $x \neq 3$.

54. **(D)** Since the actual values of the dimensions are irrelevant, use convenient values such as a 16 cm by 16 cm square. Decrease both length and width by 25% and compare the new area to the old one.

55. **(B)** The median score of the arranged grades 6, 7, 7, 7, 8, 9, 10, 10 is halfway between the two middle grades, 7 and 8.

56. **(D)** The initial principal is irrelevant, so make up a value and test it with the formula $A = P\left(1 + \dfrac{r}{n}\right)^{nt}$ and then given values of r and n ($t = 1$).

57. **(1,018.75)** Carefully increase and decrease the starting balance according to the specifications:
    Week 1—Subtract $150.
    Week 2—Add $700.
    Week 3—Subtract $150.
    Week 4—Add $700; then divide in half.
    Repeat this cycle three times.

58. **(A)** Using a cost of $100, the 35% off option reduces the cost to $65, while the two coupons reduce it to $68. A similar tendency will be observed with any starting cost.

59. **(D)** The sides of triangle DEF are all three times the length of the corresponding sides of triangle ABC. Drawing a diagram is beneficial here.

60. **(A)** $96 = 32 \times 3 = 2^5 \cdot 3$; the prime factors are 2 and 3.

ANSWER SHEET
Sample Examination 2

COLLEGE MATHEMATICS

1. Ⓐ Ⓑ Ⓒ Ⓓ
2. Ⓐ Ⓑ Ⓒ Ⓓ
3. Ⓐ Ⓑ Ⓒ Ⓓ

4. [ ]

5. Ⓐ Ⓑ Ⓒ Ⓓ
6. Ⓐ Ⓑ Ⓒ Ⓓ

7. [ ]

8. Ⓐ Ⓑ Ⓒ Ⓓ
9. Ⓐ Ⓑ Ⓒ Ⓓ
10. Ⓐ Ⓑ Ⓒ Ⓓ
11. Ⓐ Ⓑ Ⓒ Ⓓ
12. Ⓐ Ⓑ Ⓒ Ⓓ
13. Ⓐ Ⓑ Ⓒ Ⓓ
14. Ⓐ Ⓑ Ⓒ Ⓓ
15. Ⓐ Ⓑ Ⓒ Ⓓ

16.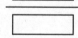

17.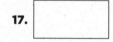

18. Ⓐ Ⓑ Ⓒ Ⓓ
19. Ⓐ Ⓑ Ⓒ Ⓓ
20. Ⓐ Ⓑ Ⓒ Ⓓ
21. Ⓐ Ⓑ Ⓒ Ⓓ

22. [ ]

23. Ⓐ Ⓑ Ⓒ Ⓓ
24. Ⓐ Ⓑ Ⓒ Ⓓ
25. Ⓐ Ⓑ Ⓒ Ⓓ
26. Ⓐ Ⓑ Ⓒ Ⓓ
27. Ⓐ Ⓑ Ⓒ Ⓓ

28.

Statement	True	False
$-q < -r$		
$pq < pr$		
$p(q - r) > 0$		
$q + p > r + p$		

29. Ⓐ Ⓑ Ⓒ Ⓓ

30. Ⓐ Ⓑ Ⓒ Ⓓ
31. Ⓐ Ⓑ Ⓒ Ⓓ
32. Ⓐ Ⓑ Ⓒ Ⓓ
33. Ⓐ Ⓑ Ⓒ Ⓓ
34. Ⓐ Ⓑ Ⓒ Ⓓ
35. Ⓐ Ⓑ Ⓒ Ⓓ
36. Ⓐ Ⓑ Ⓒ Ⓓ

37. [ ]

38. Ⓐ Ⓑ Ⓒ Ⓓ
39. Ⓐ Ⓑ Ⓒ Ⓓ

40. [ ]

41. Ⓐ Ⓑ Ⓒ Ⓓ
42. Ⓐ Ⓑ Ⓒ Ⓓ
43. Ⓐ Ⓑ Ⓒ Ⓓ
44. Ⓐ Ⓑ Ⓒ Ⓓ
45. Ⓐ Ⓑ Ⓒ Ⓓ
46. Ⓐ Ⓑ Ⓒ Ⓓ

47.

Number	Even	Odd
$m + n^2$		
$-m + 2n$		
$2m^2 + n^2$		
$2m + 3n$		

48. [ ]

49. Ⓐ Ⓑ Ⓒ Ⓓ
50. Ⓐ Ⓑ Ⓒ Ⓓ
51. Ⓐ Ⓑ Ⓒ Ⓓ
52. Ⓐ Ⓑ Ⓒ Ⓓ
53. Ⓐ Ⓑ Ⓒ Ⓓ

54. [ ]

55. Ⓐ Ⓑ Ⓒ Ⓓ
56. Ⓐ Ⓑ Ⓒ Ⓓ
57. Ⓐ Ⓑ Ⓒ Ⓓ
58. Ⓐ Ⓑ Ⓒ Ⓓ
59. Ⓐ Ⓑ Ⓒ Ⓓ
60. Ⓐ Ⓑ Ⓒ Ⓓ

SAMPLE MATHEMATICS EXAMINATION 2

Number of Questions: 60

TIME LIMIT: 90 MINUTES

> **DIRECTIONS:** You will have access to an online scientific calculator during this test.
>
> For multiple-choice questions, select the *best* of the four choices, then fill in the corresponding oval on the answer sheet. For the other questions, write your answer in the box.
>
> **Notes:**
>
> 1. If the domain of a function *f* is not specified in a question, assume that it is the set of all real numbers for which *f(x)* is defined.
> 2. Figures are drawn to scale and lie in a plane, *unless* otherwise specified.

1. The packaging on a particular brand of snack nuts indicates that one serving contains 29% of the daily recommended intake (DRI) of total fat. If the serving contains 19 grams of fat, approximately how many grams is the DRI of total fat?

   (A) 5.5
   (B) 24.5
   (C) 46.5
   (D) 65.5

2. The same brand of snack nuts mentioned in question 1 also indicates that one serving contains 30% of the daily recommended intake (DRI) of copper. If the DRI for copper is 0.8 mg, approximately how many milligrams of copper is in one serving of nuts?

   (A) 0.24
   (B) 0.56
   (C) 1.9
   (D) 2.7

3. The domain of the function $y = \dfrac{4}{(x-1)^2}$ is

   (A) all real numbers
   (B) all reals except $x = \pm 1$
   (C) all reals except $x = 1$
   (D) all positive numbers except $x = 1$

4. If you can choose to answer 4 essay questions out of 6, how many choices do you have?

5. The contrapositive of "If a triangle is equilateral, then it is isosceles" is

   (A) If a triangle is not equilateral, then it is not isosceles
   (B) If a triangle is isosceles, then it is equilateral
   (C) Some isosceles triangles are not equilateral
   (D) If a triangle is not isosceles, then it is not equilateral

6. Bag I contains 3 nickels and 2 dimes; Bag II contains 1 nickel and 5 dimes. If 1 coin is drawn from each bag, what is the probability that one is a nickel and the other is a dime?

   (A) $\dfrac{17}{30}$

   (B) $\dfrac{1}{2}$

   (C) $\dfrac{1}{28}$

   (D) $\dfrac{1}{30}$

7. If $(2 \times 10^3)^2 \times 5$ is multiplied out, then the number of zeros following the digit 2 is

8. If Z, Q, R denote, respectively, the sets of integers, of rationals, and of reals, then each point of the Cartesian plane corresponds to an element of

(A) $R \times R$
(B) $Q \times Q$
(C) $Z \times Z$
(D) R

9. If $P = \{x : x^2 - 2x - 3 = 0\}$ and $Q = \{x : x^2 + x = 0\}$, then $P \cap Q$ equals

(A) $\varnothing$
(B) $\{0, -1, 3\}$
(C) $\{1\}$
(D) $\{-1\}$

10. The negation of $s \to t$ is

(A) $s \wedge {\sim}t$
(B) ${\sim}s \to t$
(C) ${\sim}s \wedge {\sim}t$
(D) $t \to {\sim}s$

11. Which of the following histograms is most likely to have a mean that is greater than the median?

(A)

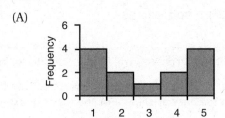

(B)

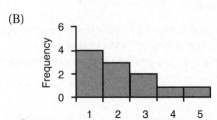

(C)

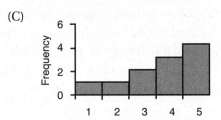

(D)

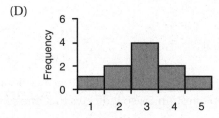

12. Which statement about real numbers is false?

(A) If $a \neq 0$, then $a^2 > 0$.
(B) If $a > 0$, then $\dfrac{1}{a} > 0$.
(C) If $a > b > 0$, then $a^2 > b^2$.
(D) If $a < b$, then $a^2 < b^2$.

13. Evaluate $\||3| - |{-5}|\|$.

(A) -8
(B) -2
(C) 2
(D) 8

14. Bathroom tiles 1 inch on a side are available in sheets of 10 by 12 tiles. How many sheets are needed to cover a wall 5 ft by 8 ft?

(A) 30
(B) 40
(C) 44
(D) 48

(The dotted line segment and dotted curve indicate that the boundaries of the region are excluded.)

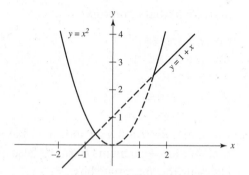

15. Points in the region enclosed by the parabola and line, shown in the diagram, satisfy the inequalities

(A) $y < 1 + x, y < x^2$
(B) $y > x^2, y < 1 + x$
(C) $y > 1 + x, y < x$
(D) $y > x^2, y > 1 + x$

16. A fair, 6-sided cube labeled 1 to 6 is tossed. What fraction (in lowest terms) represents the probability that it shows a number greater than or equal to 2?

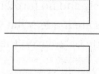

17. For the data 3, 3, 7, 11, 11, 13, 15 the median minus the mean is equal to

18. The central angle in the diagram below measures 24°. What is the area of the shaded region?

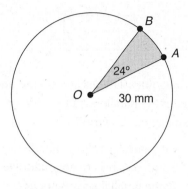

Note: picture is not to scale

(A) 1.6π in^2
(B) 30π in^2
(C) 60π in^2
(D) 900π in^2

19. If $f(x) = 2x + 1$ and $g(x) = x^2 - 3$, then $g(f(x)) =$

(A) $4x^2 + 4x - 2$
(B) $2x^2 - 5$
(C) $4x^2 + 2x - 2$
(D) $2x^2 - 2$

20. Which equation has no rational solution?

(A) $x^2 - 1 = 0$
(B) $x^2 - 2 = 0$
(C) $x^2 - 4x + 4 = 0$
(D) $x^2 - x - 2 = 0$

21. The negation of the statement "Some mathematicians are teachers" is

(A) No mathematicians are teachers.
(B) Some mathematicians are not teachers.
(C) Some teachers are not mathematicians.
(D) All mathematicians are teachers.

22. In how many ways can a group of 12 faculty members choose from among themselves a chairperson and an assistant chairperson?

23. If some quadrilaterals are squares and all squares are parallelograms, which of the following *must* be true?

   (A) All quadrilaterals are parallelograms.
   (B) Some squares are not quadrilaterals.
   (C) Some parallelograms are not quadrilaterals.
   (D) Some quadrilaterals are parallelograms.

24. Ryan and Colin are discussing investment accounts. Ryan states that an account with 1.7% annual interest compounded quarterly will have a higher effective annual yield, while Colin believes that an account with 1.6% annual interest compounded weekly will be better. Who is correct?

   (A) Ryan
   (B) Colin
   (C) Both accounts will produce the same effective annual yield.
   (D) It is unknown whether Ryan or Colin is correct without knowing how much money is invested.

25. Elaine's teacher scaled her class's most recent 20-point quiz by doubling all of their scores and then adding 10. If the mean and standard deviation before the scaling were 15 and 3, respectively, what are they now?

   (A) mean = 30, standard deviation = 6
   (B) mean = 40, standard deviation = 16
   (C) mean = 30, standard deviation = 16
   (D) mean = 40, standard deviation = 6

26. If $a > 0$ and $a^x = 0.6$, then $a^{-2x} =$

   (A) -1.2
   (B) -0.36
   (C) $-\dfrac{1}{0.36}$
   (D) $\dfrac{1}{0.36}$

27. If the lines given by the equations $ax - 2y = 4$ and $bx + 3y = 5$ are perpendicular to each other, which of the following values of a and b would *not* work?

   (A) $a = 1; b = 6$
   (B) $a = -6; b = -1$
   (C) $a = 2; b = -3$
   (D) $a = -3; b = -2$

28. Given that $p < 0$ and $q > r$, indicate whether each of these statements is true or false by checking the approriate box.

Statement	True	False
$-q < -r$		
$pq < pr$		
$p(q - r) > 0$		
$q + p > r + p$		

29. If $3,000 is invested into an account that pays 3.5% interest compounded continuously and no further withdrawals or deposits are made, what will the approximate balance on the account be in 5 years?

   (A) $3,525.00
   (B) $3,563.06
   (C) $3,573.71
   (D) $3,573.74

30. Which number is *not* a prime factor of 84?

(A) 2

(B) 3

(C) 6

(D) 7

31. To ensure a reasonable profit, a store owner will generally mark up the price of a product they obtain from a wholesaler. One owner marks up the cost of a $25 train set by 75%. At what price does she sell the train set in her store?

(A) $18.75

(B) $31.25

(C) $43.75

(D) $100

32. If $g(x) = \frac{\sqrt{x-3}}{x}$, then $g(4) =$

(A) $\frac{1}{2}$

(B) $\frac{1}{4}$

(C) $-\frac{1}{4}$

(D) $\pm\frac{1}{4}$

33. Which function has a graph symmetric to the *y*-axis?

(A) $y = |x|$

(B) $y = 2x$

(C) $y = \frac{1}{x}$

(D) $y = x^2 + x$

34. If set $R = \{a,b\}$, set $S = \{1,2\}$, and set $T = \{2,3\}$, then the number of elements in $R \times (S \cap T)$ is

(A) 2

(B) 4

(C) 6

(D) 8

35. If Set $A = \{1, 2, 3, 4, 5\}$; Set $B = \{2, 3, 5, 7, 11\}$; and Set $C = \{2, 4, 6, 8\}$, then $A \cap (B \cup C) =$ which of the following?

(A) $\{1, 2, 3, 4, 5\}$

(B) $\{2, 3, 4, 5\}$

(C) $\{2\}$

(D) $\{1, 2, 3, 4, 5, 6, 7, 8, 11\}$

36. The table below shows the enrollment in different major programs of study at a certain college.

Major	Gender	
	Male	Female
Math	75	49
Literature	53	48
Psychology	37	82
Chemistry	44	61
American History	33	35
Medicine	22	27

Based on this table, which of the following statements is *false*?

(A) More people major in psychology than any other program.

(B) Men are more likely to major in math than they are to major in psychology.

(C) Women are less likely to major in chemistry than men are to major in medicine.

(D) Medicine is the least popular major among both men and women.

37. An average of 60 in five tests is considered passing. If a student's average on the first four tests is 55, what grade must he get on the fifth test to pass?

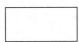

38. In a certain city's mayoral election, 15,400 residents voted. In the next election, 1.8% more residents voted than in the first election. In the third and most recent election, 1.8% fewer residents voted than in the second election. How many city residents voted in the most recent election?

(A) 15,123
(B) 15,395
(C) 15,400
(D) 15,677

39. In how many ways can 3 French and 4 German books be arranged on a shelf so that books in the same language are together, if all the books are different?

(A) 24
(B) 72
(C) 144
(D) 288

40. If g is a linear function such that $g(1) = 3$ and $g(-1) = 9$, then $g(2)$ equals

41. $(2+\sqrt{3})(3-\sqrt{3})$ equals

(A) $3-\sqrt{3}$
(B) 3
(C) $3+\sqrt{3}$
(D) $6+\sqrt{3}$

42. If $R = \{x : x > 2\}$ and $S = \{x : x < 13\}$, then the number of primes in $R \cap S$ is

(A) 3
(B) 4
(C) 5
(D) infinite

43. If a circle's circumference is doubled, by what factor is the area of the circle changed?

(A) The area is doubled.
(B) The area is quadrupled.
(C) The area is halved.
(D) The area is quartered.

44. For which of these changes to a set of data would the standard deviation remain the same?

(A) Convert heights from inches to centimeters by multiplying each value by 2.54.
(B) Add 2 inches to each inseam measurement as extra fabric for the cuff.
(C) Use the formula $F = \frac{9}{5} C + 32$ to convert temperatures from Celsius to Fahrenheit.
(D) None of these. The standard deviation would change in each of (A), (B), and (C).

45. Which statement about primes is false?

(A) Every odd prime is of the form $2^n - 1$, where n is an integer.

(B) If a product mn of 2 positive integers is divisible by a prime p, then either m or n is divisible by p.

(C) Every positive integer can be uniquely expressed as a product of primes, except perhaps for the order in which the factors occur.

(D) There are an infinite number of primes.

46. Jordan invests in an account that pays 5.5% interest compounded quarterly. He makes no additional withdrawals or deposits apart from the initial investment, and after 5 years he has $2,168.21 in the account. Which of the following is the closest to Jordan's initial investment?

(A) $1,576
(B) $1,626
(C) $1,650
(D) $2,025

47. If m and n are odd integers, indicate whether each of the following is even or odd by checking the appropriate box.

Number	Even	Odd
$m + n^2$		
$-m + 2n$		
$2m^2 + n^2$		
$2m + 3n$		

48. If a divided by 4 leaves a remainder of 2, and b divided by 4 leaves a remainder of 3, then when $a + b$ is divided by 4 the remainder is

49. What is the equation of a line parallel to the line $5x - 2y = 4$ that passes through the point (5,1)?

(A) $y = \frac{2}{5}x - 1$

(B) $y = \frac{2}{5}x + 1$

(C) $y = -\frac{2}{5}x - 1$

(D) $y = -\frac{2}{5}x + 3$

50. One mile is approximately equal to 1,610 meters, and there are 60 seconds in a minute and 60 minutes in an hour. A car traveling at 30 miles per hour is moving at what speed measured in meters per second?

(A) 5.2
(B) 13.4
(C) 17.4
(D) 67.1

51. Which of the following expressions should be used to calculate the value of a $1,000 investment into an account earning 4% interest compounded monthly over the course of 10 years?

(A) $1,000\left(1+\dfrac{0.04}{12}\right)^{12}$

(B) $1,000\left(1+\dfrac{0.04}{10}\right)^{10}$

(C) $1,000\left(1+\dfrac{0.04}{12}\right)^{120}$

(D) $1,000\left(1+\dfrac{0.04}{10}\right)^{120}$

52. Which statement about the intersection of a cubic curve and a line is false?

(A) They need have no intersection.
(B) They intersect at least once.
(C) They may intersect twice.
(D) They cannot intersect more than three times.

53. Suppose 3 of a dozen apples are bruised and 2 are chosen at random from the dozen. The probability that both are bruised is

(A) $\dfrac{1}{22}$

(B) $\dfrac{1}{11}$

(C) $\dfrac{1}{6}$

(D) $\dfrac{1}{4}$

54. If 60% of a population reads the *Journal*, 45% reads the *Moon*, and 30% reads both papers, what percent of the population reads neither paper?

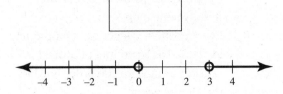

55. The graph above represents which set?

(A) $\{x : x < 0 \text{ or } x > 3\}$
(B) $\{x : 0 < x < 3\}$
(C) $\{x : x \leq 0 \text{ or } x \geq 3\}$
(D) $\{x : 0 > x > 3\}$

56. What is the perimeter of a right triangle with an area of 96, with one leg equaling 12?

(A) 16
(B) 20
(C) 48
(D) 96

57. If Z is the set of integers, Q the set of rationals, and R the set of reals, then

(A) $Q \subset Z \subset R$
(B) $R \subset Q \subset Z$
(C) $Z \subset Q \subset R$
(D) $Z \subset R \subset Q$

58. Tess opens two bank accounts with $5,000 each, one offering a simple interest rate of 2% annually, the other compounding continuously, also at 2%. She makes no further withdrawals or deposits into either account for 5 years. Approximately how much more money will be in the account that is compounding continuously?

(A) $5.44
(B) $5.45
(C) $25.84
(D) $25.85

59. A counterexample to the statement "If $ax^2 + bx + c = 0$ has 2 real unequal roots, then $b^2 - 4ac > 3$" is

(A) $x^2 - 3x + 2 = 0$
(B) $x^2 - x + 1 = 0$
(C) $x^2 - 2x + 1 = 0$
(D) $x^2 - 4x + 3 = 0$

60. Which graph below is not that of a function $y = f(x)$?

(A)

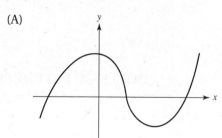

(B)

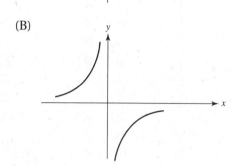

(C)

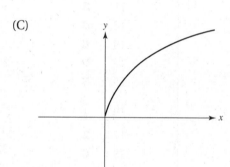

(D)

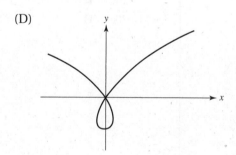

STOP

If there is still time remaining, you may review your answers.

ANSWER KEY
Sample Examination 2

COLLEGE MATHEMATICS

1. **D**	21. **A**	35. **B**	49. **A**
2. **A**	22. **132**	36. **A**	50. **B**
3. **C**	23. **D**	37. **80**	51. **C**
4. **15**	24. **A**	38. **B**	52. **A**
5. **D**	25. **D**	39. **D**	53. **A**
6. **A**	26. **D**	40. **0**	54. **25**
7. **7**	27. **C**	41. **C**	55. **A**
8. **A**	28.	42. **B**	56. **C**
9. **D**		43. **B**	57. **C**
10. **A**		44. **B**	58. **B**
11. **B**		45. **A**	59. **A**
12. **D**		46. **C**	60. **D**
13. **C**		47.	
14. **D**			
15. **B**			
16. $\frac{5}{6}$	29. **D**		
17. **2**	30. **C**		
18. **C**	31. **C**		
19. **A**	32. **B**		
20. **B**	33. **A**		
	34. **A**	48. **1**	

28.

✔	
✔	
	✔
✔	

47.

✔	
	✔
	✔
	✔

SCORING CHART

After you have scored your Sample Examination 2, enter the results in the chart below; then transfer your score to the Progress Chart on page 12.

Total Test	Number Right	Number Wrong	Number Omitted
60			

ANSWER EXPLANATIONS

1. **(D)** 29% of the total DRI is equal to 19 grams. Solve the equation $0.29x = 19$.

2. **(A)** Multiply 0.3×0.8.

3. **(C)** The function $y = \dfrac{4}{(x-1)^2}$ is defined for every real number except 1 (where the denominator is equal to zero).

4. **(15)** You have $_6C_4$, which equals $_6C_2$ choices; $_6C_2 = \dfrac{6 \cdot 5}{1 \cdot 2} = 15$.

5. **(D)** The contrapositive of $p \to q$ is $\sim q \to \sim p$.

6. **(A)** The "favorable" draws are a nickel from bag I and a dime from bag II or a nickel from bag II and a dime from bag I. The probability is, therefore, $\dfrac{3}{5} \cdot \dfrac{5}{6} + \dfrac{1}{6} \cdot \dfrac{2}{5} = \dfrac{17}{30}$.

7. **(7)** Note that $(2 \times 10^3)^2 \times 5 = 4 \times 10^6 \times 5 = 20 \times 10^6$ or 2×10^7.

8. **(A)** If R is the set of reals, then each point in the plane is of the form (x,y) where $(x,y) \in R \times R$.

9. **(D)** $P = \{3,-1\}$; $Q = \{0,-1\}$.

10. **(A)** "$s \to t$" is symbolic for "if s then t." The negation is "s but not t" or $s \wedge \sim t$.

11. **(B)** Note that more than half of the data displayed is weighted to the left side of the histogram, lowering the median with respect to the mean.

12. **(D)** Note that if $a = -2$, $b = -1$, then $a < b$ but $a^2 > b^2$.

13. **(C)** $|3| - |-5| = 3 - 5 = -2$. $|-2| = 2$.

14. **(D)** We divide the area of the wall, in square inches, by the area of a sheet of tiles, in square inches: $\dfrac{5 \times 12 \times 8 \times 12}{10 \times 12} = 48$ sheets.

15. **(B)** The area enclosed by the dotted line segment and dotted arc of the parabola is both above the parabola (that is, $y > x^2$) and below the line (that is, $y < 1 + x$).

16. $\left(\dfrac{5}{6}\right)$ There are 5 out of 6 ways to get a 2 or more when tossing a die.

17. **(2)** The median or middle number is 11; the mean is

$$\frac{3+3+7+11+11+13+15}{7} = \frac{63}{7} = 9.$$

18. **(C)** The shaded region represents 24/360 = 1/15th of the whole circle, which has an area of 900π in^2.

19. **(A)** $g(f(x)) = (2x+1)^2 - 3 = 4x^2 + 4x + 1 - 3 = 4x^2 + 4x - 2.$

20. **(B)** $x^2 - 2 = 0$ has roots $\pm\sqrt{2}$. Both roots are irrational. Verify that the roots in (A), (C), and (D) are rational.

21. **(A)** The negation of $\exists_x P_x$ (there is a mathematician who is a teacher) is $\forall_x \sim P_x$ (no mathematician is a teacher—literally, "all mathematicians are not teachers").

22. **(132)** The answer is 12×11.

23. **(D)** See the tree of quadrilaterals on page 344 in the Geometry section of Background and Practice Questions.

24. **(A)** Investigate using the formula $APR = \left(1 + \dfrac{r}{n}\right)^n - 1$ with $r = 0.017$ and $n = 4$ for Ryan and $r = 0.016$ and $n = 52$ for Colin.

25. **(D)** The mean is impacted by both changes to the scores, but the standard deviation is only impacted by the doubling.

26. **(D)** Let $a = 0.6$ and $x = 1$.

27. **(C)** For the two lines to be perpendicular, $\dfrac{a}{2} \times \dfrac{-b}{3} = -1 \rightarrow ab = 6$.

28.

Statement	True	False
$-q < -r$	✔	
$pq < pr$	✔	
$p(q - r) > 0$		✔
$q + p > r + p$	✔	

Since $p < 0$ and $q - r > 0$, the product $p(q - r)$ is negative.

29. **(D)** Use the formula $A = Pe^{rt}$ with $P = 3,000$, $r = 0.035$, and $t = 5$.

30. **(C)** Since $84 = 4 \cdot 21 = 2^2 \cdot 3 \cdot 7$, the prime factors are 2, 3, and 7; 6 is not a prime number.

31. **(C)** Find 75% of $25 and add it on to that original cost: $25 + 25 \times 0.75 = 43.75$.

32. **(B)** $g(4) = \dfrac{\sqrt{4-3}}{4} = \dfrac{\sqrt{1}}{4} = \dfrac{1}{4}$. The square root of a positive number is positive, by definition.

33. **(A)** Remember that |x| is positive or zero for all *x*. Its graph is at the right. Can you sketch the graphs in (B), (C), and (D)?

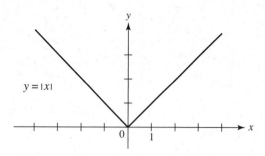

$y = |x|$

34. **(A)** $S \cap T = \{2\}$. Since there are two elements in *R* and one in $S \cap T$, the Cartesian product $R \times (S \cap T)$ has 2×1 or 2 elements.

35. **(B)** $A \cap (B \cup C)$ refers to every element of *A* that can also be found in either *B* or *C*.

36. **(A)** Carefully read all four statements. While 119 students major in psychology, 124 students major in math.

37. **(80)** His total score on the first four tests is 4×55 or 220. If *x* is the score needed on the fifth test in order to average 60 on all 5, then $\dfrac{220+x}{5}$ must equal 60. So $x = 80$.

38. **(B)** Find 1.8% of 15,400 and add it on, then find 1.8% of that result and subtract it.

39. **(D)** The 3 French books can be arranged in 3! ways, the 4 German books in 4! ways, and the 2 sets in 2! ways. Multiply ($3! \times 4! \times 2!$).

40. **(0)** Let $g(x) = ax + b$. Since $g(1) = 3$, we have $a + b = 3$; since $g(-1) = 9$, we have $-a + b = 9$. So $2b = 12$, $b = 6$, and $a = -3$. Then $g(x) = -3x + 6$ and $g(2) = 0$.

41. **(C)** $(2+\sqrt{3})(3-\sqrt{3}) = 6 + 3\sqrt{3} - 2\sqrt{3} - 3 = 3 + \sqrt{3}$.

42. **(B)** $R \cap S = \{x : 2 < x < 13\}$. The primes in this set are 3, 5, 7, 11.

43. **(B)** Make up a convenient value for the original circumference, 4π for example, and explore the effects doubling the circumference has on the radius of the circle, and therefore the area.

44. **(B)** Adding the same amount to each value does not change the difference between values, so the standard deviation remains the same.

45. **(A)** 5 is a prime, for example, but there is no positive integer *n* such that $5 = 2^n - 1$.

46. **(C)** Test each possible value for *P* in the formula $A = P\left(1 + \dfrac{r}{n}\right)^{nt}$ with $r = 0.055$, $n = 4$, and $t = 5$, or plug in 2,168.21 for *A* and solve for *P*.

47.

Number	Even	Odd
$m + n^2$	✔	
$-m + 2n$		✔
$2m^2 + n^2$		✔
$2m + 3n$		✔

$m + n^2$ is the sum of two odds. Each of the other sums is odd, because each adds an even integer to an odd integer.

48. **(1)** Since there are integers p and q such that $a = 4p + 2$ and $b = 4q + 3$, $a + b = 4(p + q) + 5 = 4(p + q + 1) + 1 = 4m + 1$, where m is an integer.

49. **(A)** If the lines are parallel, the second will have a slope of $\frac{2}{5}$. Solve the equation $1 = \frac{2}{5}(5) + b$ to find the appropriate y-intercept.

50. **(B)** Divide 30 by 60 twice to convert to miles per second; then multiply by 1,610 to convert to meters per second.

51. **(C)** Use the formula $A = P\left(1 + \frac{r}{n}\right)^{nt}$ with $n = 12$ and $t = 10$.

52. **(A)** Every cubic curve and every line intersect at least once and at most three times. Draw several sketches to illustrate this statement.

53. **(A)** The probability is $\dfrac{_3C_2}{_{12}C_2} = \dfrac{3 \cdot 2}{2 \cdot 1} \div \dfrac{12 \cdot 11}{2 \cdot 1}$ or just $\dfrac{3 \cdot 2}{12 \cdot 11}$.

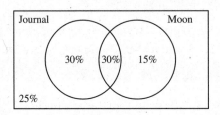

54. **(25)** Use a Venn diagram to show the percentages of people who read the papers. Subtract from 100 to get the percentage that reads neither paper.

55. **(A)** The hollow circles at 0 and 3 signify *exclusion* of these points.

56. **(C)** In a right triangle, the two legs are the base and height for the area formula $A = \frac{1}{2}bh$. Use the Pythagorean theorem to find the hypotenuse of the triangle; then add the three sides together for the perimeter.

57. **(C)** Every integer is a rational number; every rational number is a real number.

58. **(B)** Use the formula $A = P(1 + r)^t$ for the simple interest account and $A = Pe^{rt}$ for the continuously compounding account, with $P = 5,000$, $r = 0.02$, and $t = 5$.

59. **(A)** $x^2 - 3x + 2 = (x - 1)(x - 2)$, which is zero for $x = 1, 2$. But $b^2 - 4ac = (-3)^2 - 4(2) = 1$, which is not greater than 3.

60. **(D)** For some x-values there is more than one y-value in the graph in (D).

The Social Sciences–History Examination

ANSWER SHEET
Trial Test

SOCIAL SCIENCES-HISTORY

1. Ⓐ Ⓑ Ⓒ Ⓓ Ⓔ	33. Ⓐ Ⓑ Ⓒ Ⓓ Ⓔ	65. Ⓐ Ⓑ Ⓒ Ⓓ Ⓔ	97. Ⓐ Ⓑ Ⓒ Ⓓ Ⓔ
2. Ⓐ Ⓑ Ⓒ Ⓓ Ⓔ	34. Ⓐ Ⓑ Ⓒ Ⓓ Ⓔ	66. Ⓐ Ⓑ Ⓒ Ⓓ Ⓔ	98. Ⓐ Ⓑ Ⓒ Ⓓ Ⓔ
3. Ⓐ Ⓑ Ⓒ Ⓓ Ⓔ	35. Ⓐ Ⓑ Ⓒ Ⓓ Ⓔ	67. Ⓐ Ⓑ Ⓒ Ⓓ Ⓔ	99. Ⓐ Ⓑ Ⓒ Ⓓ Ⓔ
4. Ⓐ Ⓑ Ⓒ Ⓓ Ⓔ	36. Ⓐ Ⓑ Ⓒ Ⓓ Ⓔ	68. Ⓐ Ⓑ Ⓒ Ⓓ Ⓔ	100. Ⓐ Ⓑ Ⓒ Ⓓ Ⓔ
5. Ⓐ Ⓑ Ⓒ Ⓓ Ⓔ	37. Ⓐ Ⓑ Ⓒ Ⓓ Ⓔ	69. Ⓐ Ⓑ Ⓒ Ⓓ Ⓔ	101. Ⓐ Ⓑ Ⓒ Ⓓ Ⓔ
6. Ⓐ Ⓑ Ⓒ Ⓓ Ⓔ	38. Ⓐ Ⓑ Ⓒ Ⓓ Ⓔ	70. Ⓐ Ⓑ Ⓒ Ⓓ Ⓔ	102. Ⓐ Ⓑ Ⓒ Ⓓ Ⓔ
7. Ⓐ Ⓑ Ⓒ Ⓓ Ⓔ	39. Ⓐ Ⓑ Ⓒ Ⓓ Ⓔ	71. Ⓐ Ⓑ Ⓒ Ⓓ Ⓔ	103. Ⓐ Ⓑ Ⓒ Ⓓ Ⓔ
8. Ⓐ Ⓑ Ⓒ Ⓓ Ⓔ	40. Ⓐ Ⓑ Ⓒ Ⓓ Ⓔ	72. Ⓐ Ⓑ Ⓒ Ⓓ Ⓔ	104. Ⓐ Ⓑ Ⓒ Ⓓ Ⓔ
9. Ⓐ Ⓑ Ⓒ Ⓓ Ⓔ	41. Ⓐ Ⓑ Ⓒ Ⓓ Ⓔ	73. Ⓐ Ⓑ Ⓒ Ⓓ Ⓔ	105. Ⓐ Ⓑ Ⓒ Ⓓ Ⓔ
10. Ⓐ Ⓑ Ⓒ Ⓓ Ⓔ	42. Ⓐ Ⓑ Ⓒ Ⓓ Ⓔ	74. Ⓐ Ⓑ Ⓒ Ⓓ Ⓔ	106. Ⓐ Ⓑ Ⓒ Ⓓ Ⓔ
11. Ⓐ Ⓑ Ⓒ Ⓓ Ⓔ	43. Ⓐ Ⓑ Ⓒ Ⓓ Ⓔ	75. Ⓐ Ⓑ Ⓒ Ⓓ Ⓔ	107. Ⓐ Ⓑ Ⓒ Ⓓ Ⓔ
12. Ⓐ Ⓑ Ⓒ Ⓓ Ⓔ	44. Ⓐ Ⓑ Ⓒ Ⓓ Ⓔ	76. Ⓐ Ⓑ Ⓒ Ⓓ Ⓔ	108. Ⓐ Ⓑ Ⓒ Ⓓ Ⓔ
13. Ⓐ Ⓑ Ⓒ Ⓓ Ⓔ	45. Ⓐ Ⓑ Ⓒ Ⓓ Ⓔ	77. Ⓐ Ⓑ Ⓒ Ⓓ Ⓔ	109. Ⓐ Ⓑ Ⓒ Ⓓ Ⓔ
14. Ⓐ Ⓑ Ⓒ Ⓓ Ⓔ	46. Ⓐ Ⓑ Ⓒ Ⓓ Ⓔ	78. Ⓐ Ⓑ Ⓒ Ⓓ Ⓔ	110. Ⓐ Ⓑ Ⓒ Ⓓ Ⓔ
15. Ⓐ Ⓑ Ⓒ Ⓓ Ⓔ	47. Ⓐ Ⓑ Ⓒ Ⓓ Ⓔ	79. Ⓐ Ⓑ Ⓒ Ⓓ Ⓔ	111. Ⓐ Ⓑ Ⓒ Ⓓ Ⓔ
16. Ⓐ Ⓑ Ⓒ Ⓓ Ⓔ	48. Ⓐ Ⓑ Ⓒ Ⓓ Ⓔ	80. Ⓐ Ⓑ Ⓒ Ⓓ Ⓔ	112. Ⓐ Ⓑ Ⓒ Ⓓ Ⓔ
17. Ⓐ Ⓑ Ⓒ Ⓓ Ⓔ	49. Ⓐ Ⓑ Ⓒ Ⓓ Ⓔ	81. Ⓐ Ⓑ Ⓒ Ⓓ Ⓔ	113. Ⓐ Ⓑ Ⓒ Ⓓ Ⓔ
18. Ⓐ Ⓑ Ⓒ Ⓓ Ⓔ	50. Ⓐ Ⓑ Ⓒ Ⓓ Ⓔ	82. Ⓐ Ⓑ Ⓒ Ⓓ Ⓔ	114. Ⓐ Ⓑ Ⓒ Ⓓ Ⓔ
19. Ⓐ Ⓑ Ⓒ Ⓓ Ⓔ	51. Ⓐ Ⓑ Ⓒ Ⓓ Ⓔ	83. Ⓐ Ⓑ Ⓒ Ⓓ Ⓔ	115. Ⓐ Ⓑ Ⓒ Ⓓ Ⓔ
20. Ⓐ Ⓑ Ⓒ Ⓓ Ⓔ	52. Ⓐ Ⓑ Ⓒ Ⓓ Ⓔ	84. Ⓐ Ⓑ Ⓒ Ⓓ Ⓔ	116. Ⓐ Ⓑ Ⓒ Ⓓ Ⓔ
21. Ⓐ Ⓑ Ⓒ Ⓓ Ⓔ	53. Ⓐ Ⓑ Ⓒ Ⓓ Ⓔ	85. Ⓐ Ⓑ Ⓒ Ⓓ Ⓔ	117. Ⓐ Ⓑ Ⓒ Ⓓ Ⓔ
22. Ⓐ Ⓑ Ⓒ Ⓓ Ⓔ	54. Ⓐ Ⓑ Ⓒ Ⓓ Ⓔ	86. Ⓐ Ⓑ Ⓒ Ⓓ Ⓔ	118. Ⓐ Ⓑ Ⓒ Ⓓ Ⓔ
23. Ⓐ Ⓑ Ⓒ Ⓓ Ⓔ	55. Ⓐ Ⓑ Ⓒ Ⓓ Ⓔ	87. Ⓐ Ⓑ Ⓒ Ⓓ Ⓔ	119. Ⓐ Ⓑ Ⓒ Ⓓ Ⓔ
24. Ⓐ Ⓑ Ⓒ Ⓓ Ⓔ	56. Ⓐ Ⓑ Ⓒ Ⓓ Ⓔ	88. Ⓐ Ⓑ Ⓒ Ⓓ Ⓔ	120. Ⓐ Ⓑ Ⓒ Ⓓ Ⓔ
25. Ⓐ Ⓑ Ⓒ Ⓓ Ⓔ	57. Ⓐ Ⓑ Ⓒ Ⓓ Ⓔ	89. Ⓐ Ⓑ Ⓒ Ⓓ Ⓔ	121. Ⓐ Ⓑ Ⓒ Ⓓ Ⓔ
26. Ⓐ Ⓑ Ⓒ Ⓓ Ⓔ	58. Ⓐ Ⓑ Ⓒ Ⓓ Ⓔ	90. Ⓐ Ⓑ Ⓒ Ⓓ Ⓔ	122. Ⓐ Ⓑ Ⓒ Ⓓ Ⓔ
27. Ⓐ Ⓑ Ⓒ Ⓓ Ⓔ	59. Ⓐ Ⓑ Ⓒ Ⓓ Ⓔ	91. Ⓐ Ⓑ Ⓒ Ⓓ Ⓔ	123. Ⓐ Ⓑ Ⓒ Ⓓ Ⓔ
28. Ⓐ Ⓑ Ⓒ Ⓓ Ⓔ	60. Ⓐ Ⓑ Ⓒ Ⓓ Ⓔ	92. Ⓐ Ⓑ Ⓒ Ⓓ Ⓔ	124. Ⓐ Ⓑ Ⓒ Ⓓ Ⓔ
29. Ⓐ Ⓑ Ⓒ Ⓓ Ⓔ	61. Ⓐ Ⓑ Ⓒ Ⓓ Ⓔ	93. Ⓐ Ⓑ Ⓒ Ⓓ Ⓔ	125. Ⓐ Ⓑ Ⓒ Ⓓ Ⓔ
30. Ⓐ Ⓑ Ⓒ Ⓓ Ⓔ	62. Ⓐ Ⓑ Ⓒ Ⓓ Ⓔ	94. Ⓐ Ⓑ Ⓒ Ⓓ Ⓔ	
31. Ⓐ Ⓑ Ⓒ Ⓓ Ⓔ	63. Ⓐ Ⓑ Ⓒ Ⓓ Ⓔ	95. Ⓐ Ⓑ Ⓒ Ⓓ Ⓔ	
32. Ⓐ Ⓑ Ⓒ Ⓓ Ⓔ	64. Ⓐ Ⓑ Ⓒ Ⓓ Ⓔ	96. Ⓐ Ⓑ Ⓒ Ⓓ Ⓔ	

Trial Test

12

This chapter contains a Trial Test in Social Sciences and History. Take this Trial Test to learn what the actual exam is like, and to determine how you might score on the exam before any practice or review.

The CLEP General Exam in Social Sciences and History measures your knowledge of these areas, including government and political science, geography, economics, psychology, sociology, anthropology, and history (including United States history, Western civilization, and world history).

Number of Questions: 125

TIME LIMIT: 90 MINUTES

DIRECTIONS: Each of the questions or incomplete statements below is followed by five suggested answers or completions. Select the one that is best in each case.

1. Membership in the House of Representatives is determined by

   (A) the overall population of the state
   (B) population, but subject to a definite maximum number of members from any one state
   (C) the state as a unit regardless of population
   (D) the number of qualified voters of the state
   (E) all states having the same number of representatives regardless of the size of the state

2. The most important U.S. Supreme Court case affecting membership in the House of Representatives was

   (A) *Brown* v. *Board of Education*
   (B) *Baker* v. *Carr*
   (C) *Jones* v. *Clinton*
   (D) *Schenck* v. *United States*
   (E) *Roe* v. *Wade*

3. In the 19th century, United States Senators were elected by

   (A) popular election
   (B) the state legislatures
   (C) the electoral college
   (D) state conventions
   (E) officials selected from each county in the state

4. The amendment that changed how senators were elected is the

   (A) Thirteenth Amendment
   (B) Fourteenth Amendment
   (C) Fifteenth Amendment
   (D) Seventeenth Amendment
   (E) Nineteenth Amendment

5. The period of Japanese history from 1861 to 1945 was marked by

   (A) Japanese isolationism
   (B) the Meiji Restoration and the return to emperor rule
   (C) westernization and modernization
   (D) choices B and C only
   (E) choices A, B, and C

6. Ten men produce 1,000 bushels of tomatoes on ten acres. If ten additional men are hired, the production on the same acreage rises to 1,700 bushels. This phenomenon relates to which one of the following economic concepts?

   (A) Law of diminishing marginal utility
   (B) Supply and demand
   (C) Marginal propensity to consume
   (D) Gross national product
   (E) Law of diminishing returns

7. To the Marxist, profits or surplus value are

   (A) essential to the health of any economy
   (B) payments to the businessman for his labor
   (C) controlled and kept by the capitalists, the bourgeoisie
   (D) the key to a rising standard of living
   (E) constantly increasing in a capitalist society

8. Which of the following can be used to illustrate the cultural impact of China on Japan?

    I. Social and political status of the Samurai class
    II. The Confucian ethical code
    III. Artistic styles in painting, sculpture, and ceramics
    IV. Buddhist religious teaching
    V. Characters used in the written language

    (A) I and II only
    (B) III, IV, and V only
    (C) I, II, III, and IV only
    (D) II, III, IV, and V only
    (E) I, II, III, IV, and V

9. Apes and other higher primates cannot be taught to use highly complex language because

    (A) they are without the biological apparatus of speech
    (B) they are without the ability to learn from communications directed toward them
    (C) they have little mental ability to store or transmit highly abstract ideas
    (D) all of the above
    (E) none of the above

10. The culture concept in social science implies that

    (A) the biological evolution of man is the most important reason for his advances in the past few centuries
    (B) the moral aspects of a thinking, cultured society and people must enlighten its institutions
    (C) the most important lessons for man are to be found in the cultured societies of Europe
    (D) the reason for differences between our own and other societies is that we, as members of our society, learn different things from those that others learn
    (E) art and music are more important than technology in building cultivated tastes

11. The U.S. Supreme Court case *Brown* v. *Board of Education of Topeka, Kansas* (1954) made a landmark decision over the issue of

    (A) desegregation
    (B) legalized abortion
    (C) religion and the first amendment
    (D) violating the system of checks and balances
    (E) balloting of presidential elections

12. The most advanced primate next to humans are

(A) baboons
(B) chimpanzees
(C) orangutans
(D) lemurs
(E) monkeys

13. Which of the following American political figures was unpopular with the democratic followers of Jefferson because of a treaty he had negotiated in 1794 with England?

(A) Hamilton Fish
(B) John Jay
(C) John Quincy Adams
(D) James Madison
(E) Patrick Henry

14. As a result of strong nationalistic movements, which two countries became unified and centralized nations during the 19th century?

(A) France and Great Britain
(B) France and Spain
(C) Czechoslovakia and Finland
(D) Germany and Portugal
(E) Italy and Germany

15. Germany violated the neutrality of which of the following nations in both the First and Second World Wars?

(A) Netherlands
(B) Norway
(C) Switzerland
(D) Belgium
(E) France

16. The United States Senate has the power to

Choice 1: approve treaties
Choice 2: approve appointments of federal judges
Choice 3: impeach public officials

(A) Choice 1 only
(B) Choices 1 and 2 only
(C) Choices 2 and 3 only
(D) Choice 3 only
(E) All three choices

17. A man who lived in a certain country from 1860 to 1960 would have lived through military rule, constitutional monarchy, imperialist expansion, foreign occupation, extraordinary economic development, and a democratic political order that was quickly followed by a long-lasting communist government. The above description best fits which of the countries below?

   (A) Thailand
   (B) China
   (C) Japan
   (D) Egypt
   (E) Brazil

18. The belief that one's culture is the best, better than anyone else's is known as:

   (A) cultural isolation
   (B) cultural universals
   (C) ethnocentrism
   (D) assimilation
   (E) cultural diffusion

19. This totalitarian communist state has been conducting nuclear tests and has come under strong criticism from the United States and the United Nations.

   (A) China
   (B) North Korea
   (C) Iraq
   (D) Hong Kong
   (E) Cuba

20. Anthropologists such as Mary, Louis, and Richard Leakey have provided humankind with a better picture of the evolution of the human race by excavating and reconstructing previous sites of human occupation. This type of anthropology is known as the study of

   (A) cultural anthropology
   (B) physical anthropology
   (C) linguistics
   (D) primatology
   (E) archeology

21. The legal basis for the separation of church and state in the United States is found in the

   (A) First Amendment
   (B) Fifth Amendment
   (C) Tenth Amendment
   (D) The Articles of Confederation
   (E) The Declaration of Independence

22. The American economy is

   (A) pure laissez-faire
   (B) more planned than laissez-faire
   (C) more laissez-faire than planned
   (D) centrally directed as under socialism
   (E) dominated by traditional custom

23. The most recently created cabinet post in the U.S. Executive Branch is the Department of

   (A) Veterans Affairs
   (B) Housing
   (C) Terrorism
   (D) Women's Affairs
   (E) Homeland Security

24. "The community is a fictitious body . . . the sum of the several members who compose it." This individualist viewpoint is the basic premise of

   (A) François Quesnay
   (B) Thomas Aquinas
   (C) William Petty
   (D) Jeremy Bentham
   (E) August Comte

25. More characteristic of class than caste is

   (A) vertical mobility
   (B) endogamy
   (C) distinguishing attire
   (D) occupational prohibitions
   (E) prestige differences

26. Both the revolution in Russia in 1917 and the revolution in China in 1949 would have surprised Marx and Engels in that they both were

   (A) highly industrialized capitalistic nations
   (B) followed by democratic elections
   (C) violent proletariat revolutions
   (D) led by the upper landowners that wanted change
   (E) predominantly agrarian-based countries at the time of the revolution

27. The sociological term that reflects such events as the Tiananmen Square incident, the Amritsar Massacre, and the antiwar protests of the 1960s, is

   (A) collective behavior
   (B) primary groups
   (C) civil disobedience
   (D) passive resistance
   (E) rebellion

28. These three concepts—the Common Market, the Eurodollar, and NATO—indicate that European nations

   (A) are growing further apart, both economically and politically
   (B) are joining together in a common bond of economic and political unity
   (C) have developed a strong military alliance system to reduce the threat from communist Russia
   (D) rely heavily on the United States for economic and political aid
   (E) are becoming economically and politically isolated from the Western world

29. Both Presidents George H. Bush and George W. Bush were involved in the eventual defeat of what dictatorial government?

   (A) Afghanistan
   (B) Cuba
   (C) Iraq
   (D) North Korea
   (E) Libya

30. The only remaining communist Cold War nation still existing in the western hemisphere today is

   (A) Mexico
   (B) Brazil
   (C) South Korea
   (D) Dominican Republic
   (E) Cuba

31. During the second term of President George W. Bush, his administration was most criticized for its

   (A) support of the right-to-life movement
   (B) invasion of Afghanistan
   (C) failure to prevent the 9–11 disaster
   (D) decision to continue to maintain military forces in Iraq
   (E) friendly relations with communist China

32. Carthage was established as a colony of the

   (A) Greeks
   (B) Phoenicians
   (C) Romans
   (D) Hittites
   (E) Egyptians

33. In the United States at present, the kinship system

    (A) really does not exist
    (B) is formal, highly elaborated, and closely relevant to all the experiences of the family members
    (C) appears only in times of family crises
    (D) puts strong emphasis on the immediate conjugal family
    (E) emphasizes the role of the patriarch

34. Max Weber pointed out that the bureaucratization of society is usually accompanied by

    (A) raising specific educational standards for officeholders
    (B) the decline of the role of "experts"
    (C) greater publicity given to public affairs
    (D) a decline in the role played by intellectuals in public affairs
    (E) a more humane order brought about by efficiency

35. Which of the following developments of the first half of the 20th century seem most clearly to have been forecast in 19th-century Marxian writings?

    (A) The increasing number of people in advanced societies who consider themselves proletarians
    (B) The spread of ownership through the device of corporate stock
    (C) The spread of communism among nonindustrialized peoples
    (D) The rise of wage standards
    (E) Crises of trade and unemployment

36. In the early 1800s, the Industrial Revolution in England and the United States resulted in poor labor conditions for men, women, and children in both factories and mines. By the late 1800s, these conditions had significantly improved. This was because of

    (A) the success of labor unions and pro labor legislation
    (B) the popular growth of communism as an economic system
    (C) capitalists by and large supporting better conditions for the workers
    (D) governments playing a "laissez-faire" policy toward big business
    (E) capitalism being rapidly replaced by socialistic economies

37. The Kentucky and Virginia Resolutions of 1798–1799 were invoked in order to prove the

    (A) right of social revolution
    (B) right of a state to secede when it feels wronged
    (C) right of a state to be the judge of constitutionality
    (D) right to refuse the authority of the Bank of the United States
    (E) right to treat Indians with a strong hand

Questions 38 and 39 refer to a similar time period in history.

38. This location was the site of ancient Mesopotamia and was also called the the cradle of civilization. In order to visit this famous historical site today, one would visit the modern nation of

    (A) Iran
    (B) Turkey
    (C) Pakistan
    (D) Egypt
    (E) Iraq

39. The site referred to in question 38 was located around the rich fertile river valley called the

    (A) Indus River Valley
    (B) Yellow River Valley
    (C) Nile River Valley
    (D) Tigris-Euphrates River Valley
    (E) Congo River Valley

---

40. Which of the following ideas would Edmund Burke have rejected?

    (A) The specific is to be preferred over the abstract.
    (B) Society can be safely based on reason alone.
    (C) Lawless action is generally destructive.
    (D) It is often an easy jump from democracy to tyranny.
    (E) Society and government are best when the role of human wisdom and human custom are given due respect.

41. Socrates was condemned to death because he

    (A) taught young men to question accepted ideas and practices
    (B) was the teacher of Alexander
    (C) accepted a bribe from the Persians
    (D) denied that there were any fixed standards of good
    (E) taught the Greeks that they were inferior

42. The Edict of Nantes

    (A) outlawed Roman Catholicism in France
    (B) outlawed Protestantism in France
    (C) permitted a limited toleration to Protestants in France
    (D) established freedom of religion in France
    (E) established the doctrine of the trinity in France

43. The patriotic Greek of the 5th century B.C. was primarily loyal to

    (A) the Greek nation
    (B) his emperor
    (C) his religion, which was thought to have no connection with political affairs
    (D) his city-state
    (E) his race

44. The chief object of Spartan education was to develop

    (A) a cultured and artistic citizenry
    (B) good soldiers who were obedient citizens
    (C) an able body of tradesmen
    (D) a select group of priests
    (E) expert technicians

45. "People in the same trade seldom meet together but the conversation ends in a conspiracy against the public, or in some diversion to raise prices." This would most likely be found in the writings of

    (A) John Law
    (B) Adam Smith
    (C) William Petty
    (D) Thomas Mun
    (E) Emile Durkheim

46. The birthplace of democracy was

    (A) Nero's Rome
    (B) Sparta
    (C) Colonial America
    (D) Pericles' Athens
    (E) Confucius' China

47. "Human history is the chronology of the inevitable conflict between two opposing economic classes." This statement was made by

    (A) John Locke
    (B) Emile Durkheim
    (C) Karl Marx
    (D) Adam Smith
    (E) Francois Quesnay

48. Physicist is to engineer as sociologist is to

    (A) psychologist
    (B) theologian
    (C) social reformer
    (D) historian
    (E) social philosopher

49. The American psychologist B.F. Skinner is most closely associated with

    (A) Sociobiology
    (B) intelligence testing
    (C) Behaviorism
    (D) humanistic psychology
    (E) brain research

50. As a culture becomes more complex it tends to have within it fewer

    (A) alternatives
    (B) specialties
    (C) universals
    (D) exigencies
    (E) institutions

51. Which one of the following arguments did Malthus try to prove?

    (A) Developments in technology are unlikely to relieve, permanently, the pressure of population on the means of subsistence.
    (B) Poverty is primarily the result of employers' greed.
    (C) Population pressure forces national governments into colonization and imperialistic schemes, which is only proper.
    (D) Intelligent government action, such as subsidies to mothers and taxes on bachelors, can alleviate the effects of the laws of population.
    (E) Poverty is particular to capitalism.

52. United States reaction to the Iraqi invasion of Kuwait in 1990 ultimately resulted in

    (A) the assassination of Saddam Hussein
    (B) United States boycott of oil from Iraq
    (C) United States boycott of oil from Kuwait
    (D) full action of an international military force
    (E) United States position of neutrality in the affair

53. Emile Durkheim described a type of suicide resulting from excessive social integration and called it

    (A) egoistic
    (B) alienative
    (C) altruistic
    (D) anomic
    (E) rational

54. The development of agriculture nearly 12,000–15,000 years ago was a major event in human history in that it enabled humankind to

Choice 1: settle permanently in one place
Choice 2: store surplus food for the winter months
Choice 3: end malnutrition and famine

(A) Choice 1 only
(B) Choice 1 and 2 only
(C) Choices 2 and 3 only
(D) Choice 3 only
(E) All three choices

55. Which of the following usually includes all the others?

(A) Institutions
(B) Folkways
(C) Laws
(D) Social symbols
(E) Mores

56. The German Imperial constitution of 1871

(A) gave Prussia a preferred position in the German union
(B) was a generally democratic instrument
(C) declared the equality of all member states
(D) declared the ruler of Austria to be emperor
(E) was similar to the British constitution

57. William the Conqueror and the Battle of Hastings of 1066 both played a major role in the development and early history of which of the following nation states?

(A) Prussia
(B) Germany
(C) Spain
(D) England
(E) France

58. England and Japan are similar in that they both

(A) are rich in natural resources
(B) became imperialistic nations by the late 19th century
(C) were isolated from the civilized world
(D) were easily conquered
(E) saw little benefit in global trade

59. The period of the "Roman peace" (Pax Romana) was

(A) during the first two hundred years of the Empire
(B) between the reign of Diocletian and 476 A.D.
(C) between the last Punic War and the reign of Diocletian
(D) between the foundation of the Republic and the first Punic War
(E) during the reign of Charlemagne

60. The Punic Wars were between Rome and

(A) Macedonia
(B) Carthage
(C) Persia
(D) Athens
(E) Israel

61. The caliphs were

(A) the political successors of Mohammed
(B) prophets of Islam through whom further revelation of God's will was made known
(C) peoples from Central Asia who adopted the Islamic faith
(D) a family of Moslem rulers who lived in Spain
(E) foot soldiers in the armies of Islam

62. The geographical nature of ancient China is such that its mountains, deserts, and plateaus

(A) have encouraged isolationism and unity among the Chinese people
(B) made China far more difficult to conquer
(C) made successful farming highly possible
(D) allow for a great deal of cultural diffusion
(E) have welcomed foreigners, making the Chinese culture very diverse

63. The enlightened despots of the 18th century were so styled because they

(A) saw how important it was to give important concessions to the common people
(B) were enlightened enough to maintain the monarchic form of government in an age when the people increasingly demanded representation
(C) were able to expand their domains
(D) possessed a high degree of learning and a deep belief in religion
(E) possessed a desire to improve the lot of their subjects and to improve their own education

64. According to Marx and Lenin, the state, in the high stage of communism, will wither away because

    (A) universal coercion will reign over the earth and make national states unnecessary
    (B) the bourgeoisie and proletariat will be able to live in peace without need for the state to mediate between them
    (C) the Communist Party will have consolidated its position to such an extent and rendered the masses so docile that they will no longer need the state
    (D) when there is only one social class, the state, defined as an instrument of class domination, will no longer serve any function and hence will disappear
    (E) the triumphant dialectical process of history will prove statehood to be only a penultimate truth, hence ultimately false in the presence of the final political form, the super-state

65. The Augustinian system of theology held that "Human nature is hopelessly depraved. . . . Only those mortals can be saved whom God for reasons of His own has predestined to inherit eternal life." Which of the following best represents the attitude of the Protestant leaders of the Reformation?

    (A) They knew nothing of Augustine and were ignorant of this idea.
    (B) They strongly opposed this idea since they believed that it would discourage men from doing good works in the hope of winning salvation.
    (C) The idea became very important in the Protestant position.
    (D) They refused to consider the idea, since they thought that Roman Catholic Church fathers such as St. Augustine had no claim to authority.
    (E) They considered it an idea from pagan Rome and without proper Christian charity.

66. The argument most used to support the congressional committee system is that it

    (A) makes sure that minority groups get a fair hearing
    (B) increases congressional control of the executive department
    (C) reduces the cost of lawmaking
    (D) makes possible more careful consideration of bills
    (E) makes sure that presidential wishes will prevail

67. The "heroic age," "time of troubles," "stability," and "decline" are historical concepts found in the historical writings of

    (A) Marx
    (B) Sorokin
    (C) Toynbee
    (D) Becker
    (E) Kant

68. The "id," "ego," and "superego" are all associated with

(A) Albert Einstein
(B) Sigmund Freud
(C) Lewis P. Lipsitt
(D) Harry Harlow
(E) Kenneth B. Clark

69. Which country had more of its citizens and soldiers killed in World War II than did the other countries?

(A) The United States
(B) Great Britain
(C) Italy
(D) France
(E) USSR

70. Which of the following countries was not in the League of Nations in 1935?

(A) The United States
(B) USSR
(C) The United Kingdom
(D) France
(E) Yugoslavia

71. The tearing down of the Berlin Wall in 1989 led to the reunification of which nation?

(A) Germany
(B) Scotland
(C) Berlin
(D) England
(E) USSR

72. What Supreme Court decision established the guidelines for the legalization of abortion in the United States?

(A) *Griswald* v. *Connecticut*
(B) *Miranda* v. *Arizona*
(C) *Dred Scott* v. *Sanford*
(D) *Roe* v. *Wade*
(E) *Brown* v. *Board of Education*

73. The Soviet Union break-up in 1989 was as result of the

(A) economic problems coupled with an atmosphere of liberal reform
(B) horrors of the Stalin era
(C) successful war effort in Afghanistan
(D) assassination of Mikhail Gorbachev
(E) liberal reform that was being initiated in communist China

74. "He (Napoleon) would have liked to establish a colonial empire, but he knew the British fleet ruled the seas, and so, to prevent this vast region from falling to the British, he sold it to the Americans." What was the region called?

(A) Louisiana
(B) Florida
(C) Alaska
(D) Hawaii
(E) California

75. The Erie Canal connected

(A) the Susquehanna and the Potomac
(B) the Hudson and the Delaware
(C) Lake Erie and Niagara
(D) the Hudson and Lake Erie
(E) Lake Huron and the Ohio

76. Note the following events:

■ Louisiana and Gadsden purchases
■ "54 40 or Fight"
■ Mexican War

All of the events listed above are associated with

(A) the Proclamation of Neutrality
(B) the Monroe Doctrine
(C) Manifest Destiny
(D) late-19th-century imperialism
(E) the American Civil War

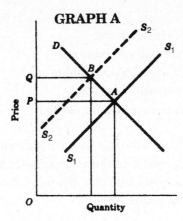

GRAPH A

77. The line $S_2 S_2$ compared to the line $S_1 S_1$ indicates

   (A) an increase in demand
   (B) an increase in supply
   (C) an increase in monopoly
   (D) a decrease in supply
   (E) a decrease in demand

78. The shift from line $S_1 S_1$ to $S_2 S_2$ in Graph A could have occurred because of a

   (A) good year in salt production
   (B) bad year, in that few people desired to purchase "old masters"
   (C) discovery of a new diamond field in Africa
   (D) freeze in the orange groves of Florida
   (E) famine reducing the number of subsistence farmers in a small area of the economy

---

79. Which of the following statements comes closest to the true Malthusian idea?

   (A) "Population increases rapidly while agriculture lags behind."
   (B) "It is the constant tendency in all animated life to increase beyond the nourishment prepared for it."
   (C) "No progress is possible because of the basic sex drive, which increases population at a geometric rate."
   (D) "Nations which are over-populated must be allowed to expand or send their inhabitants abroad."
   (E) "Things can be produced more cheaply if more is produced."

80. Which practice is most compatible with the supposedly rational nature of "the economic man"?

(A) Installment buying at high interest
(B) Borrowing from small loan companies
(C) Reading a consumer research publication
(D) Asking a salesman's advice
(E) Buying more than was on your shopping list

81. During the 1800s, immigrants from this foreign nation initially entered our nation to help meet the demanding need for railroad laborers. Denied entrance into the United States after 1882, it was not until 1943 that they were allowed to become naturalized citizens. These foreign immigrants were

(A) Italians
(B) Latinos
(C) Chinese
(D) Arabs
(E) Japanese

82. Little Italy and Chinatown in New York City are both examples of

(A) ethnocentricity
(B) cooperatives
(C) cultural universals
(D) subcultures
(E) communal living

83. Under the British Parliamentary Act of 1911, the House of Lords

(A) lost all power in legislation
(B) could delay enactment of an ordinary bill for only two years
(C) was abolished
(D) was transformed into a house appointed for life terms
(E) became finally dominant over the House of Commons

84. Besides Israel, which Middle Eastern nation has also been a close ally to the United States?

(A) Turkey
(B) Iran
(C) Libya
(D) Syria
(E) Lebanon

85. *Anthropomorphism* is a religious concept meaning

(A) belief in animal gods
(B) belief in a god who died and lived again
(C) rituals in common usage
(D) attribution of human characteristics to a god or gods
(E) holding ancestors worthy of worship

86. The behavior expected of any particular group member is his

(A) role
(B) status
(C) performance
(D) culture
(E) ideology

87. This political-economic theory is characterized by accumulating wealth (gold and silver) through colonies, an extensive merchant marine, and a favorable balance of trade. This economic concept practiced extensively in Europe during the 16th to 18th centuries was called

(A) utopian socialism
(B) marxism
(C) capitalism
(D) social darwinism
(E) mercantilism

88. It was at this time that women participated in the war effort by providing a much needed addition to the industrial labor force. This vital role of the female laborer was to define an entirely new role for women in our society. During which war did women first make their appearance as industrial laborers?

(A) The Civil War
(B) The Spanish American War
(C) World War I
(D) World War II
(E) The Vietnam Conflict

89. From 1845 to 1855 a considerable number of the immigrants to the United States came from

(A) China
(B) Ireland
(C) Greece
(D) Russia
(E) Spain

90. As a result of the Congress of Vienna in 1815, Germany

    (A) consisted of thirty-eight states loosely joined in the German Confederation
    (B) was established as a unified state
    (C) existed only as the Holy Roman Empire
    (D) was all included within the bounds of Prussia
    (E) formed a part of the Austrian Empire

91. Under the British system of government, the monarch normally selects a prime minister who commands the support of the

    (A) retiring prime minister
    (B) majority party and with the concurrence of the minority party in the House of Commons
    (C) majority party in the House of Commons
    (D) majority party in the House of Commons and the House of Lords
    (E) commonwealth nations

92. Which country was the moving spirit in organizing the various coalitions against Napoleon?

    (A) Russia
    (B) Austria
    (C) Britain
    (D) Prussia
    (E) Sweden

93. The doctrine of "Manifest Destiny" was most closely associated with which of the following wars involving the United States?

    (A) Civil War
    (B) War of 1812
    (C) World War I
    (D) World War II
    (E) Spanish-American War

94. "Non-slaveholders of the South: farmers, mechanics and working men, we take this occasion to assure you that the slaveholders, the arrogant demagogues whom you have elected to offices of power and profit, have hoodwinked you, trifled with you, and used you as mere tools for the consummation of their wicked designs." These words reflect the viewpoint of this abolitionist newspaper publisher.

    (A) Henry Clay
    (B) Stephen A. Douglas
    (C) William Lloyd Garrison
    (D) George Fitzhugh
    (E) John C. Calhoun

95. "The great object of Jacobinism, both in its political and moral revolution, is to destroy every trace of civilization in the world and force mankind back into a savage state." The Era of the Jacobins, the Committee of Public Safety, and Robespierre are all associated with

(A) the Declaration of the Rights of Man, 1789
(B) the National Assembly, 1789–1791
(C) the Reign of Terror, 1793–1794
(D) the rise of Napoleon, 1799
(E) the Stalin purges, 1935–1936

96. "Men, consciously or unconsciously, derive their moral ideas in the last resort from the practical relations on which their class position is based—from the economic relations in which they carry on production and exchange." Which of the following said this?

(A) Freud
(B) Goethe
(C) Kant
(D) Engels
(E) Hegel

97. The popular election of U.S. Senators was provided for in the

(A) Constitution
(B) Articles of Confederation
(C) Bill of Rights
(D) Declaration of Independence
(E) Seventeenth Amendment

98. The person most responsible for German unification was

(A) Hitler
(B) Bismarck
(C) Von Moltke
(D) Heine
(E) Brandt

99. William G. Sumner thought the "social question" (existence of social problems) to be the result of the fact that

(A) all men are not equally equipped for the onerous struggle against nature
(B) the virtuous are not ordinarily successful
(C) political equality is absent
(D) equality before the law is unattainable
(E) man knows too little about his society

100. It is difficult for an addict to avoid taking drugs after he has been released from treatment because

(A) he generally returns to his old circle of drug-using friends
(B) psycho-physiological dependence on drugs, once established, can never be completely eliminated
(C) people around him generally expect him to become re-addicted
(D) Choices A and C only
(E) Choices A, B, and C

101. The terms *anticlerical* and *worldliness* mean hostility toward the

(A) business class
(B) government officials
(C) white-collar workers
(D) church
(E) retail trade

102. Nelson Mandela, F.W. de Klerk, and Bishop Desmond Tutu all are a part of the fight for racial equality in the nation of

(A) Southern Rhodesia
(B) Kenya
(C) India
(D) Nigeria
(E) South Africa

103. The Supreme Court has been referred to as a "continuous constitutional convention." The reason for this may be found in the fact that the Supreme Court

(A) is in session all the time
(B) changes and enlarges the Constitution by its practice of interpreting the Constitution through its opinions
(C) is given the right to sit as a constitutional assembly, and to propose, but not ratify or accept, constitutional amendments
(D) must rule on any proposed amendment regarding its constitutionality
(E) convokes conventions of high judges which test the Constitution

104. During the 1920s and '30s, Japanese history was marked by the

(A) growth of democracy
(B) introduction of industrial development
(C) return to an isolationist policy
(D) rise of imperialistic aggression in Asia
(E) fall of Japan to the Allies

105. Identify the correct chronological order for the origins of the following religions:

    (A) Buddhism, Christianity, Islam
    (B) Confucianism, Islam, Christianity
    (C) Christianity, Zen Buddhism, Confucianism
    (D) Islam, Christianity, Buddhism
    (E) Buddhism, Islam, Confucianism

106. Sadly, the Cold War led to the rise of a number of nations that were split into two, a communist nation and a democratic nation. The only former united nation still existing today with both a communist government and a democratic government is

    (A) Germany
    (B) Viet Nam
    (C) Korea
    (D) the USSR
    (E) Cambodia

107. With the leadership of Nkrumah shortly after the Second World War, this British colony was the first African territory to achieve independence and did so in a somewhat smooth and nonviolent manner. This nation was

    (A) Nigeria
    (B) Ghana
    (C) Ethiopia
    (D) Kenya
    (E) Angola

108. In 2011, the population of the United States reached

    (A) 250 million people
    (B) 280 million people
    (C) 310 million people
    (D) 330 million people
    (E) 410 million people

109. In 1298 A.D., he wrote a book that described Cathay and its people. He mentioned strange customs such as the use of paper money, and he told of the wars that Kublai Khan fought with the Japanese. His book inspired later explorers such as Christopher Columbus. Who was the author of this travel book?

    (A) Dante
    (B) Aquinas
    (C) Marco Polo
    (D) Roger Bacon
    (E) Cicero

110. In 1791, the French Constituent Assembly presented France with its first written constitution. This declared France to be

    (A) a limited constitutional monarchy
    (B) an absolute monarchy
    (C) a democracy
    (D) a republic
    (E) a military dictatorship

111. The modern name for what was formerly referred to as Persia is

    (A) Iraq
    (B) Kuwait
    (C) Yemen
    (D) Iran
    (E) Pakistan

112. A general meaning of the term Freudian slip is

    (A) fear of going out in public
    (B) sexual desires toward one's mother
    (C) fear of heights
    (D) an allergic reaction
    (E) the wants and needs of one's subconscious are accidentally expressed

113. This type of sociological study intensely examines many characteristics of one unit (usually a person or people, work group, a community) over a long period of time. This type of investigated behavior study is known as

    (A) the experiment
    (B) the sample survey
    (C) the case study
    (D) the observation
    (E) the control factor

114. If a president were to be impeached, the trial would be in the

    (A) Supreme Court
    (B) Senate
    (C) United States Court of Appeals
    (D) United States District Court
    (E) House of Representatives

115. Religion, rules of conduct, norms, language, and family are all key elements of

   (A) culture
   (B) ethnocentrism
   (C) diversity
   (D) stratification
   (E) domestication

116. Today, the tendency of most American families is toward

   (A) matriarchy
   (B) patriarchy
   (C) elaboration in symbolism supporting the authority of extended kin
   (D) equality of power of husband and wife
   (E) emphasis on the traditional

117. A caste system of social stratification is extremely difficult to maintain in

   (A) an urban society
   (B) a village or rural society
   (C) a highly religious society
   (D) an economically poor society
   (E) a paternalistic society

118. The geographical crossroads of the three monotheistic religions, Judaism, Christianity, and Islam is

   (A) China
   (B) the Western Hemisphere
   (C) Mecca and Medina
   (D) India
   (E) the Middle East

119. The Japanese rulers suppressed Christianity in the 17th century because they

   (A) thought it would divide their people and bring them under the influence of foreign powers
   (B) feared that the peaceful teaching of Christianity would discourage warlike virtues
   (C) believed that Buddhism was the true faith and that all other religions were necessarily false
   (D) said that it was a "white man's" religion
   (E) believed that only God was divine and no man could be

120. Family, religion, and norms are all examples of cultural universals. A cultural universal is

    (A) found only in the Western world
    (B) found predominantly among Asian nations
    (C) when two cultures meet and assimilate into one new culture
    (D) a cultural trait that is common to all societies
    (E) the result of cultural diffusion

121. The writings and viewpoints of Alexis de Tocqueville and Karl Marx would agree that

    (A) the tyranny of the majority was the ominous threat of the future
    (B) organized religion is an important factor in the preserving of liberty
    (C) religion is a good way to calm an oppressed people
    (D) most controversy in modern society would be over property rights and accumulating wealth
    (E) societies with conflicting economic interests can, through compromise and proper institutions, achieve a long life

122. Negative reaction to British rule surfaced in 1857 when rumor had it that rifles were being greased with a mixture of beef and pork fat. This event eventually led to a British colonial rebellion in India called

    (A) Blood Sunday
    (B) the Taiping Rebellion
    (C) the Sepoy Mutiny
    (D) the Gandhi Salt March
    (E) the Tiananmen Square Massacre

123. As the Age of Metternich progressed (1815–1848), which nation came more and more into conflict with Austria and Metternich's political philosophy?

    (A) France
    (B) Russia
    (C) Spain
    (D) England
    (E) Prussia

124. The Twenty-Seventh Amendment to the U.S. Constitution concerns

(A) equal rights for all citizens, regardless of age, race, background, or sexual orientation
(B) Congress's authority to raise its own pay
(C) the voting rights of mentally disabled citizens
(D) the existence of business monopolies
(E) Medicare and/or Medicaid being denied to AIDS patients

125. The fall of the Berlin Wall and the collapse of the Soviet Union is best associated with what time period or event below?

(A) September 11, 2001
(B) the end of Saddam Hussein in Iraq
(C) 1989–1991
(D) the unification of Viet Nam
(E) the Cuban Missile Crisis of 1962

If there is still time remaining, you may review your answers.

ANSWER KEY
Trial Test

SOCIAL SCIENCES–HISTORY

1.	A	33.	D	65.	C	97.	E
2.	B	34.	A	66.	D	98.	B
3.	B	35.	E	67.	C	99.	A
4.	D	36.	A	68.	B	100.	D
5.	D	37.	C	69.	E	101.	D
6.	E	38.	E	70.	A	102.	E
7.	C	39.	D	71.	A	103.	B
8.	D	40.	B	72.	D	104.	D
9.	C	41.	A	73.	A	105.	A
10.	D	42.	C	74.	A	106.	C
11.	A	43.	D	75.	D	107.	B
12.	B	44.	B	76.	C	108.	C
13.	B	45.	B	77.	D	109.	C
14.	E	46.	D	78.	D	110.	A
15.	D	47.	C	79.	B	111.	D
16.	B	48.	C	80.	C	112.	E
17.	B	49.	C	81.	C	113.	C
18.	C	50.	C	82.	D	114.	B
19.	B	51.	A	83.	B	115.	A
20.	E	52.	D	84.	A	116.	D
21.	A	53.	C	85.	D	117.	A
22.	C	54.	B	86.	A	118.	E
23.	E	55.	A	87.	E	119.	A
24.	D	56.	A	88.	D	120.	D
25.	A	57.	D	89.	B	121.	D
26.	E	58.	B	90.	A	122.	C
27.	A	59.	A	91.	C	123.	D
28.	B	60.	B	92.	C	124.	B
29.	C	61.	A	93.	E	125.	C
30.	E	62.	A	94.	C		
31.	D	63.	E	95.	C		
32.	B	64.	D	96.	D		

SCORING CHART

After you have scored your Trial Examination, enter the results in the chart below, then transfer your score to the Progress Chart on page 12. As you complete the Sample Examinations later in this part of the book, you should be able to achieve increasingly higher scores.

Total Test	Number Right	Number Wrong	Number Omitted
125			

ANSWER EXPLANATIONS

1. **(A)** The distribution of members in the House of Representatives is determined on the basis of population. The Constitution in Article I, Section 2, Clause 3 provides: "Representatives shall be apportioned among the several states which may be included within this Union according to their respective numbers."

2. **(B)** The case of *Baker* v. *Carr*, decided in 1962, held that federal courts could take jurisdiction of challenges to the apportionment formulas from states for membership in the House of Representatives. The decision was a marked change from past decisions, wherein courts held that such cases were "political" in nature and should be resolved by legislatures instead of by courts.

3. **(B)** In the 19th century, United States Senators were elected by the state legislatures. Article I, Section 3, Clause 1 of the original Constitution reads: "The Senate of the United States shall be composed of two Senators from each state, chosen by the legislature thereof."

4. **(D)** The amendment providing for popular election of United States Senators was 17, ratified in 1913. The ratification reflected the populist spirit, which sought to make the selection of Senators more democratic, thereby removing power of selection from the state legislatures. The power of the state legislatures was described in the original Constitution of 1787.

5. **(D)** With the end of the Tokogawa Shogunate also came the end of its anti-Western and pro-isolationist policies. The restoration of the Meiji rule, a period of Japanese modernization, westernization, and aggressive foreign policy, became the direction of the new government. As a result, Japan entered the late 19th and early 20th century as a world power. Eventually Japan joined with Mussolini and Hitler in a military fascist imperialistic pact.

6. **(E)** The law of diminishing returns states that an input of production (such as labor) and the output it helps to produce tend to diminish as more units of the input factor are applied to the same number of the other factors of production (land and capital).

7. **(C)** Marx says surplus value or profits are controlled and kept by the capitalists. The proletariat or workers sees nothing more than subsistent-level salary.

8. **(D)** Japanese culture and values were strongly influenced both by Chinese Confucianism and Buddhism (Ch'an Buddhism, for example, was transmuted into

Zen in Japan). Artistic styles, often transmitted through Korea, frequently reflected Japanese adaptations of Chinese sources. Chinese ideographs were adopted as Japan's first written language. However, the exalted social and political status of the Samurai class as warrior scholars had no equivalent in Ancient China, where soldiers and warlords were held in low esteem by the mandarin scholar gentry.

9. **(C)** Apes and other primates cannot be taught to use highly complex language because they have little mental ability to store or transmit highly abstract ideas. Some higher primates have been shown to possess potential for learning from communications directed toward them.

10. **(D)** The culture concept in social science implies that the reason for differences between our own and other societies is that we, as members of our society, learn different things from those that others learn. This is the sense in which sociologists use the term *culture*.

11. **(A)** *Brown* v. *Board of Education of Topeka, Kansas*, in 1954, was a landmark decision in that it was the most important pro–civil rights decision in ending segregation in U.S. public schools. As a result of this decision, the process of desegregation of public schools, particularly in the South, was put into play.

12. **(B)** Both the chimpanzee and the gorilla are, next to man, the most advanced form of primate. The size of the chimpanzee brain is one-third that of man's brain today, which was the actual size of man's brain two million years ago when Australopithecus traveled as one of the earliest stages of human evolution.

13. **(B)** John Jay was unpopular with the Democratic followers of Jefferson. In 1794, Jay negotiated a treaty with England. The treaty helped keep America out of the war in Europe between France and England. The Jeffersonians thought that the treaty was favorable to England. They favored France in the European war.

14. **(E)** The unification of Italy, called Risorgimento, was achieved under the leadership of Count Camillo Cavour. Victor Emmanuel II was proclaimed king of a united Italy in 1861. German unification was accomplished mainly through the efforts of Otto von Bismarck. King William I of Prussia was proclaimed emperor of a united Germany in 1871.

15. **(D)** German armies attacked neutral Belgium in 1914 at the beginning of World War I and again in May 1940, early in World War II. Switzerland remained independent in both wars. The neutrality of the Netherlands and of Norway was not violated in World War I. France was aligned against Germany in both wars.

16. **(B)** According to our Constitution, the Senate has the power to approved treaties by a 2/3 vote as well as approve the appointment of federal judges by a majority vote. As for removing a President from office, it is the job of the House to bring charges of impeachment. It is the function of the Senate to sit as the judge and jury thus it is the courtroom for the trial.

17. **(B)** At the beginning of this hundred-year period (1860), China was an absolute monarchy ruled by an emperor. After the Revolution of 1912, China became a republic. In the interim, much of Chinese territory was under foreign occupation. In 1948, Chiang Kai-shek became president under a democratic constitution. One year later, commu-

nist forces under Mao Tsetung drove his armies off the mainland and established the Communist People's Republic of China.

18. **(C)** Ethnocentricity is the belief that one culture is superior to another. It is the arrogant attitude that all cultures periodically express. The Yankees are the best; America is the best nation in the world. The danger of this practice is that we can become prejudiced and subjective toward other cultures. An example of this is Kipling's poem "White Man's Burden" and the attitude that the civilized Western nations (Caucasians) were superior to the Asian and African cultures.

19. **(B)** Serious nuclear testing is being conducted by communist North Korea. One of the few communist countries that still remains after the end of the Cold War, North Korea continues to stress the global community as well as the United Nations with their bold attempt to test nuclear weapons.

20. **(E)** While the Leakey family were also physical anthropologists finding numerous remains of human skulls and body parts, the question really deals with the digging up and excavating of human remains. This is known as the study of archeology.

21. **(A)** The First Amendment states: "Congress shall make no law respecting an establishment of religion, or prohibiting the free exercise thereof . . . . " This is the legal basis for the separation of church and state in the U.S.

22. **(C)** The American economy is described as a "free enterprise" system. This would be completely laissez-faire except that there is planning under such agencies as the Federal Reserve System, as well as in committees of Congress and in the various executive departments.

23. **(E)** As a result of September 11th, 2001, and the attack on the World Trade Center, President Bush initiated the creation of a new cabinet post called Homeland Security. This was in response to terrorism and terrorists attacks on the United States.

24. **(D)** Jeremy Bentham (1748–1832), English social philosopher, was the leader of a group called the Utilitarians. He held that each person guides his or her conduct entirely by self-interest.

25. **(A)** In a class system, movement from one class to another (vertical mobility) is possible. In a caste system, endogamy (marriage restrictions), distinguishing attire, occupational prohibitions, and prestige differences tend to prevail.

26. **(E)** Had Karl Marx lived at the time of either the Russian Revolution (1917) or the Chinese Revolution (1949), he would have been dismayed at what would emerge in nonindustrial/agrarian-typed economies. The subsequent revolutions that followed including that of Cuba, Korea, and Viet Nam further support that communism seems to thrive best in agriculture-based societies.

27. **(A)** Collective behavior is a sociological behavior that men and women experience when they are in groups. When collective behavior occurs, individuals that join the group experience intense emotional contagion and are more than willing to follow the direction of the group. Civil rights protests and antiwar protests in the 1960s are both excellent examples of collective behavior.

28. **(B)** With the end of World War II and the rise of communist Eastern Europe, most democratic European nations became members of the common market and NATO as the free nations of Western Europe took steps to develop closer bonds. The goal here was to develop closer ties both politically and economically. Thus, NATO was created along with the development of the European Economic Community or Common Market. Today both organizations have continued to grow, and in particular, the EC (European Community) has become a powerful economic force in world trade.

29. **(C)** Both President George H. Bush and President George W. Bush were involved in the defeat of Iraq in two separate wars. In 1991, Kuwait was invaded by Iraq, but within a short time, a coalition army (Desert Storm) freed Kuwait. Despite a civil war that followed the removal of Iraq's forces from Kuwait, Saddam Hussein remained in power. It was not until the invasion of Iraq by President George W. Bush in 2002 that dictator Saddam Hussein was removed from power.

30. **(E)** The only remaining communist Cold War nation still existing in the Western Hemisphere today is Cuba. The failing health of Cuban leader Fidel Castro who took power in a communist revolution in 1959 leads many Westerners to hope for new and more positive future for the Cuban people.

31. **(D)** The successful invasion of Iraq and the subsequent removal of Saddam Hussein from power was followed by a far less successful occupation by U.S. military forces. Continued terrorism and guerilla warfare continued throughout the second administration of George Bush. The congressional and gubernatorial elections of November 2006 left a mandate for a definite change in Iraq. The Republican Party and the Bush administration lost control of Congress in the 2006 election representing a mandate to bring our troops home.

32. **(B)** Carthage was established as a colony in North Africa by the Phoenicians about 875 B.C. It was situated opposite Sicily near present-day Tunis.

33. **(D)** In the United States at present, the kinship system puts strong emphasis on the immediate conjugal family, that is, the family consisting of husband, wife, and children.

34. **(A)** Max Weber (1864–1920), German sociologist, described the ideal type of bureaucratic structure in his *Essays in Sociology*. He noted that raising specific standards for officeholders went hand in hand with the bureaucratization of society. To Weber, the bureaucratic society, despite its faults, represented an advance over its predecessors.

35. **(E)** In his writings, particularly in his major work entitled *Das Kapital*, which was published in three volumes between 1867 and 1894, Karl Marx predicted the downfall of capitalism because of its inherent contradictions. This included, in his view, both mass unemployment and wars among the capitalist nations for control of resources and trade.

36. **(A)** The early years of the Industrial Revolution witnessed harsh labor conditions in the mines and factories. Although utopian socialism and scientific socialism offered some possible solutions, it was, in the end, labor unions and legislation that brought better working conditions for the newly rising working class. England and the United States were the first two industrial nations of the world and were also democratic.

Thus, it was the very nature of capitalistic democracy that gave rise to the pro labor legislation and the growth of labor unions; these two factors brought relief to the labor force and continued to provide more and more rights and protection for the working class.

37. **(C)** The Kentucky and Virginia Resolutions of 1798–1799 were drafted by Jefferson and Madison. They were passed by the legislatures of Kentucky and Virginia. They declared the Alien and Sedition Acts, passed by Congress in 1798, to be unconstitutional.

38. **(E)** Ancient Mesopotamia was the site of "the cradle of civilization." Man's earliest known cities and thus civilizations emerged in this area. This included such cultures as the Hittites, Sumerians, Babylonians, and many others.

39. **(D)** The area bordered by the Tigris and Euphrates rivers was known as Mesopotamia, "the land between the two rivers." The area is in present-day Iraq.

40. **(B)** Edmund Burke (1729–1797), English statesman and political philosopher, would have rejected the idea that society can be safely based on reason alone. Burke emphasized the need for gradual and orderly change and the significance of historical antecedents in sound social and political development.

41. **(A)** Socrates was condemned to death as a threat to Athens because he taught young men to question accepted ideas. The story of his accusation, trial, and conviction is related by Plato in his dialogue *Apology*. The last hours of Socrates' life are described by Plato in the dialogue *Phaedo*.

42. **(C)** The Edict of Nantes was issued by King Henry IV of France in 1598 after a series of bloody wars between Protestants and Catholics. It allowed Protestantism in towns where it was the chief form of worship but barred it from Paris and its surroundings.

43. **(D)** In the 5th century B.C., Greece consisted of a number of city-states, that is, cities and their surroundings. Each citizen was loyal to his city-state such as Athens, Sparta, and Thebes, not to Greece. The cities often fought against each other.

44. **(B)** Sparta was one of the leading city-states in ancient Greece. It was famous for its army. Sons of the ruling class were trained to be soldiers. Only these warriors, called Spartiates, had legal and civil rights.

45. **(B)** Adam Smith (1723–1790) is best known for his classic work *An Inquiry into the Nature and Causes of the Wealth of Nations* (1776). He showed great insight into the operation of economic forces, including the tendency of tradesmen to seek control of the market.

46. **(D)** The birthplace of democracy was first developed and practiced in Athens by Pericles. The foundations to Roman democracy, English democracy and even American democracy can be said to have been inspired by the famous leader of Athens, Pericles.

47. **(C)** Karl Marx (1818–1883) predicted increasing tension between the capitalist class and the working class.

48. **(C)** The physicist does research and develops the theoretical basis for the science of physics. The engineer makes practical applications of the physicist's findings. The

sociologist does research and develops the theoretical basis for the social science of sociology. The social reformer puts the theories of the sociologist into practice.

49. **(C)** Behaviorism is the theory that psychology is fundamentally a study of observed human behavior, as opposed to internal states and consciousness.

50. **(C)** Primitive cultures are relatively monolithic. Virtually all behavior is prescribed and universally practiced. More complex cultures accommodate numerous variations in behavior. Hence, they tend to have fewer universals.

51. **(A)** Thomas R. Malthus (1766–1834) wrote the famous *Essay on Population* (1798). He opposed an increase in wages, arguing that it only encouraged larger families. His thesis was that population increased much faster than the food supply. This would not be relieved by developments in technology.

52. **(D)** Led by U.S. forces, Italy, Britain, France, and Saudi Arabia pushed Saddam Hussein's Iraqi invasion forces out of Kuwait in Operation Desert Storm.

53. **(C)** Emile Durkheim (1858–1917), French sociologist, wrote a book entitled *Suicide* in 1897. He analyzed the psychological bases of social behavior. He used the term *altruistic* to describe a type of suicide resulting from excessive social integration.

54. **(B)** The development of agriculture, also known as the Neolithic Revolution, first occurred about 12,000 B.C. It was a major event in human history in that it enabled humankind to settle permanently in one place, end a nomadic lifestyle, and be able to store surplus food for the tough winter months. Even the success of the Industrial Revolution continued to provide a better standard of living and a far better food supply. Yet, this did not end world malnutrition and famine. This economic and social factor has unfortunately continued to the present day.

55. **(A)** In sociology, each of the following is classified as an institution: folkways, laws, social symbols, and mores.

56. **(A)** The German Imperial constitution of 1871 went into effect after the defeat of France in the Franco-Prussian War. Prussia became the dominant state under the constitution. The king of Prussia became Emperor Wilhelm I of Germany.

57. **(D)** William I (the Conqueror) of England is also known in history as Duke William II of Normandy. His army crossed the English Channel and defeated the English at the Battle of Hastings in 1066 A.D. He ruled England as William I until his death in 1087.

58. **(B)** During the late 1800s/early 1900s, these two island nations turned to the sea for imperialistic expansion. This need for colonies was spurred on by the expanding demands of industrial society. Britain expanded its empire by becoming heavily involved in Africa. Japan, under the Meiji Restoration, began an aggressive program of modernization so that it too would have its "place in the sun." Japan built a powerful navy and quickly began to expand its empire in southeast Asia.

59. **(A)** The period of the "Roman Peace" (*Pax Romana*) was during the first two hundred years of the Roman Empire. The Empire lasted for five hundred years, from about 31 B.C. to 476 A.D. All the lands around the Mediterranean were part of the Empire. The power and efficiency of the Roman legions kept peace throughout the Empire.

60. **(B)** The Punic Wars (264 B.C.–146 B.C.) were fought between Rome and Carthage. Carthage was founded, as a colony, by the Phoenicians. The Latin word for Phoenicia is *Punicus.*

61. **(A)** In the Islamic religion, the caliph is the religious head of the government as the agent of God. When Mohammed, the Prophet, died, Abu Bakr was chosen as first caliph. Later, Islam split, and different caliphs claimed to be God's agent.

62. **(A)** The geographical nature of China has always encouraged cultural isolation. Until recently, China's mountains to the west and south (Himalayas), its plateaus to the north, its deserts to the northwest, and the Pacific Ocean to the east have provided it with a geographical wall that isolated it from other societies (the Great Wall was added to complete the wall of isolation to the northeast). As a result, despite its size, China developed as one distinct culture.

63. **(E)** The enlightened despots of the 18th century—Joseph II of Austria, Catherine II of Russia, and Frederick II of Prussia—wished to improve both the lot of their impoverished subjects and their own education.

64. **(D)** Marxism sees history in terms of class struggle with the state as an instrument of the dominant class. In the current (final) stage the bourgeoisie is destroyed by the proletariat. With only one class in society, the state will have no function and will disappear.

65. **(C)** Augustine (354–430) taught that divine grace, not human effort, was the source of salvation. This doctrine, called predestination, was a key tenet of the theology of John Calvin (1509–1564) and other leaders of the Protestant Reformation.

66. **(D)** Under the committee system, all bills introduced in the Senate or House of Representatives are referred to the committee in that chamber that is charged with consideration of the particular subject of the bill. Members of each committee specialize in that committee's particular area of legislation so that bills receive special analysis before they are reported to the House or Senate.

67. **(C)** Arnold J. Toynbee, English historian, wrote the scholarly twelve-volume *A Study of History* (1933–1961). He described twenty-one historic civilizations. In his study he found that each undergoes a "heroic age," a "time of trouble," "a period of stability," and a final "decline."

68. **(B)** Sigmund Freud is the founder of psychoanalysis. In 1900, he wrote his book *The Interpretation of Dreams* in which he stressed the role of dreams and the unconscious. One of his most famous concepts was his division of the "self" into the "id, the ego and the superego." His idea and terminology became part of everyday American culture and language.

69. **(E)** The USSR suffered more than 7 million military deaths in World War II. Vast areas of the Soviet Union were overrun by the German armies. Leningrad survived a terrible siege. In addition to the military losses, the USSR lost 13 million civilians in the war for a total of 20 million, by far the heaviest losses of all nations in the conflict.

70. **(A)** Even though President Woodrow Wilson was the architect of the League, the Senate of the United States refused to approve U.S. membership. So the United States did not join the League of Nations.

71. **(A)** East and West Germany were reunited for the first time since World War II after the Berlin Wall was torn down, symbolizing the collapse of Communism in East Germany.

72. **(D)** The *Roe* v. *Wade* decision of 1973 permitted an abortion during the first trimester.

73. **(A)** The Soviet Union break-up in 1989 was larger a result of the economic problems coupled with an atmosphere of liberal reform that was initiated by Mikhail Gorbachev and his programs of glasnost and perestroika. The failure to win in Afghanistan led to further political unrest.

74. **(A)** The region was called Louisiana. This vast territory between the Mississippi River and the Rocky Mountains was sold to the United States in 1803 by Napoleon for $15,000,000. Thirteen states or parts of states were later carved out of this purchase.

75. **(D)** The Erie Canal extended from Albany on the Hudson River westward to Buffalo on Lake Erie. It was formally opened in October 1825.

76. **(C)** Manifest Destiny was a concept developed during the early to mid-1800s in America. It was a belief that America had the natural right to expand its borders west to the Pacific Ocean, north to Canada, and south to Mexico.

77. **(D)** In the graph, the line S_1S_1, moves to S_2S_2 because of an additional cost to the producer. This additional cost causes a decrease in supply represented by movement of the supply curve from S_1S_1 to S_2S_2.

78. **(D)** The shift from S_1S_1 to S_2S_2 which represents a decrease in supply (question 77 above) could have been caused by a freeze in the orange groves in Florida. It could also be caused by a voluntary decrease resulting, for example, from the imposition of a new tax on the producer.

79. **(B)** The concept "It is the constant tendency in all animated life to increase beyond the nourishment prepared for it" is the basic premise of *An Essay on the Principles of Population* (1798). Malthus believed that this tendency would be counteracted by war, famine, disease, or birth control, which he called "moral restraint."

80. **(C)** If "economic man" were to act according to supposedly rational nature, he might well subscribe to a consumer research publication, but he would definitely not act as described in any of the other four choices.

81. **(C)** The Chinese Exclusion Act of 1882 was extended and made permanent in 1902. Chinese immigration to the United States was prohibited, and Chinese could not become naturalized citizens. The law was changed in 1943 to allow Chinese in the United States to become naturalized citizens.

82. **(D)** Subcultures are "cultures within a culture." Within the mother culture, offshoots sometimes develop. The hippies of the 1960s, Chinatown, Little Italy, and the Amish are all subcultures. They have their own unique style of living yet also adhere to some of the traits of mother culture America.

83. **(B)** Prime Minister Herbert Asquith forced the House of Lords to give up its veto power by voting for the Parliament Act of 1911. The House of Lords could still hold up an ordinary bill for two years but no longer.

84. **(A)** Since the end of World War II, Israel and Turkey have been close allies to the United States. Israel has been a symbol of democracy in an otherwise unfriendly Islamic region and Turkey was a key ally during the era of the Cold War.

85. **(D)** The word *anthropomorphic* comes from the Greek, meaning human form. Anthropomorphism as a religious concept means giving human form or characteristics to a god or goddess. This was a key aspect of the religion of the ancient Greeks.

86. **(A)** The term *role* is used in sociology to mean the way a person is expected to behave in a particular group, i.e., family, work group, school, church, or club. Roles are more formalized in primitive societies than they are, for example, in Europe and America.

87. **(E)** During the first wave of exploration and colonialism (1500s–1700s), mercantilism emerged as both a political and economic theory for the European world. It is characterized by the accumulation of wealth (gold and silver), the building of colonial empires, the creation of extensive merchant marines, and the goal of maintaining a favorable balance of trade.

88. **(D)** It was during World War II that women emerged as an important part of the American labor force. Women participated in the war effort by working in defense industries. This entirely new role for women provided the initiative to break the pattern of the traditional role of the female. Some say it may be considered the beginning of the women's lib movement.

89. **(B)** The decade, 1845–1855, marked a mass migration of Irish immigrants to the United States. This was a direct result of the potato famine taking place in Ireland at that time. Prejudice toward these new Catholic Americans resulted in the origins of the KKK.

90. **(A)** The Congress of Vienna (1814–1815) reorganized Europe after the Napoleonic Wars. The Holy Roman Empire ceased to exist. Thirty-eight states were loosely joined in the German Confederation.

91. **(C)** Under the parliamentary system of government developed by the British, the prime minister is the leader of the majority in the House of Commons. The appointment of the prime minister by the monarch is a mere formality.

92. **(C)** Britain was the moving spirit in organizing the various coalitions against Napoleon. The Quadruple Alliance of 1814, consisting of Russia, Prussia, Austria, and Britain, was organized by Viscount Castlereagh, the British foreign minister. Their combined armies, led by the British duke of Wellington, defeated Napoleon at the Battle of Waterloo in Belgium (1815).

93. **(E)** "Manifest Destiny" was the belief of American expansionists that it was the obvious fate of the United States to spread its system of democracy. The term was used to justify the annexation of Texas, the acquisition of the Oregon territory, the purchase of Alaska, and, finally, the involvement in the Spanish-American War.

94. **(C)** William Lloyd Garrison (1805–1879) was a militant abolitionist. He was publisher of the Boston abolitionist newspaper, *The Liberator*. In the first issue (Jan. 1, 1831), he announced his intention to fight against slavery and said: "I will not retreat a single inch—AND I WILL BE HEARD."

95. **(C)** When the radicals (Jacobins led by Danton and Robespierre) of the French Revolution got control of the National Assembly, in 1793, they launched the Reign of Terror. The Grand Terror, as it was also called, was done to eliminate any opposition to the so-called new democracy. It began with the execution of both the king and queen and continued for nearly a year until the Jacobin radicals were removed from power.

96. **(D)** These were the ideas of Friedrich Engels (1820–1895). He was co-author, with Karl Marx, of the *Communist Manifesto* (1848). He collaborated with Marx in the latter's great work, the three-volume *Das Kapital*.

97. **(E)** The Seventeenth Amendment to the U.S. Constitution, adopted in 1913, reads: "The Senate of the United States shall be composed of two Senators from each state, elected by the people thereof." The words "elected by the people thereof" replaced the words "chosen by the legislature thereof" in the original Constitution.

98. **(B)** Bismarck was the chief "architect" of German unification. His use of a "blood and iron" policy led to three wars, the Danish War (1864), the Austro-Prussian War (1866), and the Franco-Prussian War (1870–1871). Consequently, Austria and France no longer remained as obstacles to the German states becoming a united nation in 1871.

99. **(A)** The idea that social problems derive from the fact that all men are not equipped for the onerous struggle against nature was developed by the pioneer American sociologist William Graham Sumner (1840–1910). His classic work, *Folkways*, was published in 1907.

100. **(D)** Addicts usually return to their old circle of friends who expect them to become readdicted, but psycho-physiological dependence on drugs can be completely eliminated as evidenced by the fact that drug treatment centers have on their staffs former drug addicts who have been cured.

101. **(D)** The term *anticlerical* means hostility toward the church. The word *cleric* is derived from the Latin *clericus*, meaning a member of the clergy.

102. **(E)** Bishop Desmond Tutu and Nelson Mandela were black nationalists that played a key role in the liberation of white-controlled South Africa. From the 1980s and into the 1990s, Mandela and F.W. de Klerk, worked together in the transformation of the republic into a politically shared government of both white and black leaders; apartheid officially ended in the mid 1990s.

103. **(B)** The U.S. Supreme Court interprets the Constitution in difficult cases. Its decisions are given in the form of "opinions," both majority and dissenting. These opinions often have the effect of changing or enlarging the Constitution. Hence, the court may be considered a continuous constitutional convention.

104. **(D)** Immediately after World War I, Japan stepped up its imperialistic policies. Its navy became one of the three largest in the world, and with it, Japan began the conquest of other Asian cultures, including Manchuria and shortly thereafter, mainland China.

105. **(A)** Buddhism developed as a response to Hinduism and spread from India to China in the 3rd century B.C. Several centuries later, Christianity emerged in the Middle East, and was later followed by Islam in the 7th century A.D.

106. **(C)** Sadly, the Cold War led to a number of nations that were split into two, a communist nation and a democratic nation. The only former nation still existing today with both a communist government in the north and a democratic government in the south is that of Korea. Currently, communist North Korea continues to create world tension with their persistence to conduct nuclear tests.

107. **(B)** It was with the end of World War II that Ghana began the African movement toward a national independence. Great Britain spearheaded a peaceful transition of Ghana from a colony to a nation-state in 1957. Shortly thereafter, many other African nations also began to achieve their independence.

108. **(C)** In February 2011, the U.S. Census Bureau estimated the population of the United States to be 310 million people.

109. **(C)** Marco Polo, 13th-century merchant and traveler, was born in Venice. He traveled overland to China and reached Peking in 1275. He remained there twenty years. On his return to Venice he wrote an account of his travels and of Kublai Khan, China's ruler.

110. **(A)** The first written constitution, presented in France in 1791 by the Constituent Assembly, vested sovereign power in the Legislative Assembly. The king was given only a suspensive veto power by which legislation desired by the Assembly could be postponed.

111. **(D)** The modern name for what was formerly referred to as Persia is Iran. After World War I, Turkey, and to a lesser extent its neighbor Persia, experienced revolutions. In 1935, to emphasize its break with the past, Persia took the name of Iran.

112. **(E)** A Freudian slip deals with the innermost subconscious thoughts that surface often when one least expects it.

113. **(C)** A case study is like an ongoing diary that records details of specific individuals or groups over a long period of time. A common tool to the sociologists, it examines closely the behavior of that group or individual. Many case studies are used in education to better understand student behavior.

114. **(B)** If a president were to be impeached, the trial would be in the Senate. Article I, Section 3, Clause 6 provides: "The Senate shall have the sole power to try all impeachments."

115. **(A)** Religion, rules of conduct, norms, language, and family are just some of the key elements of culture. All societies have what is known as cultural universals, which are the basic ingredients common to all cultures throughout the world.

116. **(D)** American culture is in flux and is moving toward equality of power of husband and wife. It is moving away from emphasis on the traditional, away from patriarchy, but not toward matriarchy.

117. **(A)** A caste system of social stratification requires that each individual be easily identified by caste and that he or she remain for life within the caste of birth. In an urban society, individuals tend to become anonymous, intermarry more readily, and thus destroy caste structure.

118. **(E)** The crossroads of the three monotheistic religions is the Middle East. The holy cities of Jerusalem, Bethlehem, Canaan, Mecca, and Medina are all in the Middle East.

The birthplace of Christ and Mohammed as well as the Jewish promised land are all, in fact, in close Middle Eastern proximity.

119. **(A)** Christianity had been brought to Japan in 1549 by St. Francis Xavier. For a century, it prospered. Then, in the 17th century, it was violently suppressed. Japan's rulers chose isolation for two centuries. They feared that Christianity, a foreign influence, would be harmful to Japan.

120. **(D)** When introducing the term *culture*, we often refer to cultural universals, which are those traits that are similar to all cultures in the world. Several examples are family, religion, norms (folkways/mores), and government.

121. **(D)** Alexis de Tocqueville (1805–1859), French writer, traveled in America during the 1830s. In his *Democracy in America* (1835) he described, with approval, the political and economic growth he saw. He would agree with the economist Karl Marx that most controversy in modern society would be over property rights, a key tenet of Marxian economics.

122. **(C)** The Sepoy Mutiny in India resulted in changing the power from the hands of trading companies directly to the British government. Some historians feel that it gave the British an excuse to take over India, which became known as the "jewel of the British crown," Britain's richest possession. Sepoy were Indian soldiers fighting in the British army, but when their religious beliefs came into question, they revolted.

123. **(D)** England was one of the four powerful nations at the Congress of Vienna. Although all four nations agreed to prevent future "Napoleons" (thus maintaining a European balance of power), each and every decision made by the Metternich System and the Quadruple Alliance was against the very principles of England's belief in democracy, nationalism, and liberalism. Eventually England withdrew from the Quadruple Alliance.

124. **(B)** The Twenty-Seventh Amendment placed restrictions on Congress's authority to raise its own pay.

125. **(C)** The fall of the Berlin Wall in 1989 and the collapse of the Soviet Union in 1991 marked the end to the Cold War. The Cold War began with the split of Germany into two parts, communist East Germany and democratic West Germany. It ended with the collapse of the Berlin Wall in December of 1989 and the dissolving of the Soviet Union by 1991 into many new republics.

Background and Practice Questions

13

DESCRIPTION OF THE SOCIAL SCIENCES AND HISTORY EXAMINATION

The CLEP General Examination in Social Sciences and History measures your general knowledge of history, sociology, economics, psychology, anthropology, geography, and political science. It covers material that is generally taught in lower-division college courses for non-social science majors. The exam is given in two parts, each consisting of approximately 60 questions and each requiring 45 minutes to complete. See the following chart for approximate percentages of examination items:

Social Sciences and History Exam

	Content and Item Types	Time/Number of Questions
40%	History 17% United States History 15% Western Civilization 8% World History	120 questions 90 minutes
13%	Government/Political Science	
10%	Sociology	
10%	Economics	
10%	Psychology	
11%	Geography	
6%	Anthropology	

The questions on this exam include aspects of the social sciences that may not have been covered in courses you have taken in school. Your ability to answer these questions will depend on the extent to which you have maintained a general interest in these subjects and kept current by reading widely and following current events.

If you want to do well on this test, you should have a very clear sense of chronological relations in history, as well as an understanding of the issues and ideas which have been current in different historical eras. You should have some idea of the relative significance of various ideologies, scientific concepts, and historical events. If you have, on your own or during the course work, read widely in history and sociology (including the history of economic and sociological theories) you will be able to answer a large number of the questions without difficulty. Technical concepts and terms from contemporary economics, social psychology, and political science are tested in a large number of questions. However, if you have an acquaintance with the material emphasized in introductions to these subjects, you are well prepared to answer the questions.

There are a number of accomplishments which the questions endeavor to test. Some questions require mere factual recall. Others ask you to go beyond factual recall to the deduction of a correct answer from the information given in the question and from your own knowledge. Still others are designed to test your ability to apply conceptual principles or theories to particular problems. Many of the questions will demand much of you. You will be asked to judge, to weigh, to rank, to discriminate, and to compare and contrast facts and ideas.

THE KINDS OF QUESTIONS THAT APPEAR ON THE EXAMINATION

Simple Recall

To give you an idea of the various types of questions you will face, we will give some examples here and, where necessary, explain the process by which the right answer is derived. Simple recall questions are straightforward and require no explanation.

EXAMPLES

1. When did the British Navy defeat the Spanish Armada?

   (A) 1066
   (B) 1588
   (C) 1648
   (D) 1688
   (E) 1750

   Answer: (B)

2. What was the name of the treaty ending the Thirty Years' War?

   (A) Treaty of Ghent
   (B) Treaty of Paris
   (C) Treaty of Burgundy
   (D) Treaty of Westphalia
   (E) Treaty of London

   Answer: (D)

3. Where did General Grant accept the surrender of General Lee in 1865?

   (A) Richmond
   (B) Vicksburg
   (C) Gettysburg
   (D) Appomattox
   (E) Atlanta

   Answer: (D)

4. Who was the prime minister of Great Britain during the negotiations leading to the Treaty of Versailles in 1919?

   (A) Winston Churchill
   (B) William Pitt
   (C) Stanley Baldwin
   (D) Lloyd George
   (E) Clement Attlee

   Answer: (D)

Recall of Multiple Facts

A number of questions will test your ability to recall a number of related facts. An example of this type follows:

EXAMPLE

1. You are in a small country which now is landlocked. In the 19th century, its major city was the capital of an empire with a vast polyglot population. In which of the following countries are you?

   (A) Bolivia
   (B) Switzerland
   (C) Paraguay
   (D) Austria
   (E) France

   Explanation: Austria (D) is the answer, but you must know a number of facts to deduce this answer. France's major city was the capital of a vast polyglot empire in the 19th century. But France is not landlocked. Bolivia, Switzerland, and Paraguay are all landlocked, but their major cities were not centers of large empires in the 19th century. Only Austria fits all the conditions. It is now landlocked after losing vast holdings at Versailles. Its capital city, Vienna, was the center of the vast polyglot Austrian Empire during the 19th century.

Source of Concepts

Another type of question tests your ability to attach major concepts to their original authors.

EXAMPLE

1. Who held that the division of labor was the key to economic progress and that freedom in trade broadened markets, which in turn led to more division of labor and thus economic progress?

   (A) Toynbee
   (B) Marx
   (C) Adam Smith
   (D) Thomas Aquinas
   (E) Aristotle

   Explanation: The interests of all the writers except Adam Smith were centered on issues quite otherwise than the effect of free trade on economic progress. Thus, Adam Smith (C) is the answer.

Application of Principles

Another type of question attempts to examine your facility in applying certain social science principles.

EXAMPLE

1. The marginal propensity to consume in a population is 0.50. Investment expenditures increase by one billion dollars. Everything else being equal, you would expect national income to increase by about how many billion dollars?

   (A) 1
   (B) 2
   (C) 5
   (D) 50
   (E) 500

   Explanation: The student who is acquainted with the "multiplier" concept and the fact that it is tied to the marginal propensity to consume by the formula $M = \dfrac{1}{1 - MPC}$ would know that two billion dollars is the answer. He would be applying certain principles from economics to get the answer.

Major Themes of Movements

Yet another type of question deals with the central themes which characterize various schools or traditions of thought.

EXAMPLE

1. History moves in a path which ends only when world-wide stateless communism reigns. The struggle of economic classes is the engine of movement. This view-point is characteristic of

   (A) Transcendentalism
   (B) Dialectical Idealism
   (C) Freudianism
   (D) Scholasticism
   (E) Dialectical Materialism

   Explanation: (E) The student who knows both that Marxism uses dialectical processes and that Marx thought material conditions the basis of change would see that only the term Dialectical Materialism could fit the ideas in the above viewpoint.

HISTORICAL TIME LINE

The time line that follows will give you an overview of important events in history and the sequence in which they occurred. Keep in mind that no list of this sort is exhaustive; do not use the time line alone as the sole source of review for the history portion of the test. Use it as a brief, introductory review, possibly to help you pinpoint the events and historical periods you need to spend most of your study time on. A day or two before the exam, look at the time line again to stimulate your memory and put your mind into the proper historical gear.

Ancient World	
c. 3500 B.C.	Sumerian civilization (Mesopotamia)
c. 3100 B.C.	Upper and Lower Egypt united under King Menes (First Dynasty)
c. 3000–1550 B.C.	Indus Valley culture
c. 2700–2200 B.C.	Egyptian Old Kingdom
c. 2500–1400 B.C.	Minoan civilization (Crete)
c. 1800 B.C	Hammurabi's code of laws (Babylonia)
c. 1800–1100 B.C.	Shang (Yin) Dynasty (China)
c. 1375 B.C.	Akhnaton and Egyptian monotheism
c. 1250 B.C.	Moses and Hebrew law
1194–1184 B.C.	Trojan Wars
c. 1122–256 B.C.	Chou Dynasty in China
1025–930 B.C.	Hebrew monarchy
c. 800 B.C.	Homer's epics
c. 753 B.C.	Founding of Rome
745–612 B.C.	Assyrian Empire
c. 630–553 B.C.	Zoroaster (Persia)
c. 604 B.C.	Birth of Lao Tzu (Chinese Taoism)
594–3 B.C.	Solon's laws (Athens)
563–483 B.C.	Buddha (India)
551–479 B.C.	Confucius (China)
509 B.C.	Roman Republic established
490–449 B.C.	Greek (Delian League)—Persian Wars
431–404 B.C.	Peloponnesian Wars
399 B.C.	Death of Socrates
334–323 B.C.	Conquests by Alexander (the Great) of Macedonia
c. 320 B.C.	Gupta Empire founded India begins a golden age
c. 273–232 B.C.	Reign of Ashoka (India)
264–146 B.C.	Rome's intermittent Punic Wars
221–210 B.C.	Shih Huang-ti (China's "First Emperor"); The Great Wall
202 B.C.	Han Dynasty established (China)
105 B.C.	Chinese invent paper
44 B.C.	Assassination of Julius Caesar
27 B.C.	Augustus Caesar becomes first Roman emperor
c. 6 B.C.	Birth of Jesus

Ancient World	
c. 30 A.D.	The Crucifixion
70	Roman forces capture Jerusalem
c. 200	Rise of power of the Papacy
331	Founding ofConstantinople
c. 400	Peak of Mayan civilization
400–1240	Ghana controls Nigertrade (Africa)
440	Invasion of Europe by the Huns
476	Germanic "barbarians" take Rome

Medieval World	
496	King Clovis of the Franks converted to Christianity
527–565	Justinian I rules Byzantine Empire, codifies Roman Law
570	Birth of Muhammad
c. 600	Buddhism reaches Japan
622	The Hejira (Muhammad's flight from Mecca [Makkah])
711	Arab invasion of Spain from Africa
732	Battle of Tours (Charles Martel leads Franks in victory over invading Arabs)
800	Charlemagne crowned Emperor
936–973	Otto I Holy Roman Emperor
c. 1000	Vikings reach North America
1006	Muslim invasion of India
1066	Norman conquest of England (Battle of Hastings)
1095	Start of the First Crusade
c. 1150	Building of Angkor Wat (Khmers)
1192	Yoritomo becomes first shogun to rule Japan
c. 1200–1500	Aztec Empire (Mexico)
1211–23	Conquests of Ghengis Khan
1215	Magna Carta (England)
c. 1279	Kublai Khan leads Mongols in completing conquest of China
1337–1453	Hundred Years War (Europe)
1348–50	Black Death (Europe)
1450	Gutenberg's movable type perfected
1450	The Renaissance begins in Europe
1453	Constantinople falls to the Turks
1469	Birth of Nanak, founder of Sikhism (India)

	United States		World
1492	Columbus' first voyage to America	1492	"Reconquest" of Spain by Christians
		1492–1517	Columbus' 4 voyages
		1517	Luther's "95 Theses" (beginning of the Reformation)
		1519–22	Magellan circles the globe
		1519	Cortes conquers the Aztecs (Mexico)
		1533	Pizarro invades Peru
		1536	Henry VIII establishes Anglican Church
		1556–1605	Akbar rules Mughal India
		1571	Turkish fleet defeated at Lepanto
		1588	Defeat of Spanish Armada by Royal Navy of England
		1592	Hideyoshi, Japanese unifier, invades Korea
		1500s/1600s	Columbian Exchange takes place between the Old and New Worlds
1607	Founding of Jamestown, Virginia	1603–1867	Tokugawa Shogunate in Japan
		1608	French establish Quebec City
1619	Virginia establishes House of Burgesses (first legislature)	1611	King James version of the Bible
1619	First black indentured servants (slaves) arrive in Virginia	1618–1648	Thirty Years War (Europe)
1620	Puritan Separatists (Pilgrims) arrive at Plymouth		
1620	Mayflower Compact		
1636	Harvard founded		
1643	New England Confederation organized	1642–49	English Civil War ("Great Migration" to America)
1647	Public schools founded (Massachusetts)	1644	Manchu dynasty founded (China)
1651	First English Navigation Act passed	1651	Dutch settlers in South Africa
1676	Bacon's Rebellion (Virginia)		
1676	King Philip's War (New England)		
		1688	Glorious Revolution (England)
		1688	Bill of Rights (England)
1692	Salem witchcraft trials		
1735	John Peter Zenger trial (free press)		

	United States		World
1754–63	French and Indian War (New France ceded to England)	1751 1756–63 1759	Diderot's *Encyclopedia* (France) Seven Years' War (Europe) Watt's steam engine
1765	Stamp Act (repealed in 1766)		
1774 1774 1775–83 1776 1778	"Intolerable Acts" closed Boston Harbor First Continental Congress meets The American Revolution Declaration of Independence Alliance with France	1776 1776	Adam Smith's *Wealth of Nations* The Enlightenment period begins in Europe
1781 1783 1787 1787 1787 1789	Articles of Confederation ratified Treaty of Paris officially ends Revolutionary War Shays' Rebellion (Massachusetts) Northwest Ordinance Constitutional Convention opens Washington becomes first president	1785–86 1789 1789–91	French economic crisis French Revolution begins National Assembly
1790 1791 1793 1793 1794 1798–99 1798 1798	Slater's first textile mill for spinning cotton Bill of Rights ratified Cotton gin perfected Proclamation of Neutrality Whiskey Rebellion Undeclared naval war with France Alien and Sedition Acts Kentucky and Virginia Resolutions	1791–94 1794 1794 1795–99	National Convention Reign of Terror ends in France Mackenzie reaches the Pacific (Canada) Directory rules France
1803 1803 1804–06 1807 1808	Louisiana Purchase doubles size of U.S. *Marbury* v. *Madison* (Marshall Supreme Court establishes precedent for judicial review of laws of Congress) Lewis and Clark expedition Embargo Act Importation of slaves outlawed	1804–14 1809–26	Napoleon is Emperor of France Wars of Latin-American Independence
1812–15 1816 1816	Second war with England (War of 1812) Protective tariff Second Bank of the U.S. chartered	1812 1815 1815 1815–48	Napolean fails to defeat Russia Battle of Waterloo (Napoleon is defeated) Congress of Vienna meets Age of Metternich

	United States		World
1820	Missouri Compromise		
1823	Monroe Doctrine		
1825	Erie Canal opens		
1827	Baltimore and Ohio Railroad chartered		
		1830	Revolutions in Europe
1831	Nat Turner slave rebellion		
1832–33	Nullification crisis (tariff)	1832	English (political) Reform Act
1835	Indian removal ("Trail of Tears")		
1836	Republic of Texas established		
1837	Panic of 1837	1837	Rebellion in Canada
		1839–42	Opium Wars (China)
		1845–47	Potato famine in Ireland, heavy Irish Immigration
1846–48	Mexican War	1846	Repeal of English Corn Laws
1847	Mormons reach Utah		
1848	Gold discovered in California	1848	Revolutions in Europe
1848	Women's Rights Convention (New York)	1848	Marx's *Communist Manifesto*
1850	Compromise Bills		
1854	Kansas-Nebraska Act (slavery)	1854–56	Crimean War
1854	Republican Party founded	1854	Perry arrives in Japan
		1857–58	Sepoy "Mutiny" in India
			John Stuart Mill's *On Liberty*
1859	Drake's oil well (first commercially productive oil well)	1859	Darwin's *The Origin of Species*
1859	John Brown's raid on Harpers Ferry		
1860	Election of Abraham Lincoln		
1861–65	Civil War	1861	Emancipation of Serfs (Russia)
1862	Homestead Act; Landgrant Act	1861–66	Maximillian in Mexico
1863	Emancipation Proclamation		
		1864	Taiping Rebellion in China
1865	Lincoln assassinated		
1865–70	Civil War Amendments (13th–15th)		
1865–76	Southern "Reconstruction"		
1867	U.S. buys Alaska from Russia	1867	Dominion of Canada established (British North America Act)
		1867	Marx's Das Kapital
1868	Impeachment of Andrew Jackson	1868	Meiji Restoration (Japan)
1869	First transcontinental railroad	1869	Suez Canal opened
		1870	Italian unification completed
		1871	Franco-Prussian War
		1871	German unification completed
1876	Bell invents telephone		
1876	Hayes-Tilden disputed election		
1877	Edison invents phonograph	1877	Queen Victoria as "Empress of India"
1879	Edison invents electric light		
1879	Standard Oil Trust organized		

United States		World	
1882	Chinese Exclusion Act	1882	British invade and occupy Egypt
1883	Civil Service reform (Pendleton Act)		
		1884	Berlin Conference (on partitioning Africa)
		1885	Indian Congress Party formed
1886	Haymarket riot in Chicago (labor)		
1886	American Federation of Labor founded		
1887	Interstate Commerce Commission		
1887	Dawes Act (Native Americans)		
1889	First Pan American Conference	1889	Japanese Constitution
1890	Sherman Antitrust Act		
1890	Battle of Wounded Knee (last major conflict between Indians and U.S. troops)		
1890	"Closing" of the frontier		
		1894	First Sino-Japanese War
1896	Marconi's wireless telegraph		
1898	Spanish-American War		
1898	Philippine "Insurrection"		
1899	"Open Door" policy in China	1899–1902	Boer War (South Africa)
		1899	Boxer Rebellion (China)
		1900	Freud's Interpretation of Dreams
1903	Wright Brothers flight		
		1904–05	Russo-Japanese War (Japan defeats Russia)
		1905	Revolution in Russia
		1905	Einstein's theory of relativity
1908	"Model T" Ford auto		
1909	Perry claims to reach North Pole		
		1910	Revolution in Mexico
		1911	Chinese Republic (Sun Yat-sen)
1914	Panama Canal opened	1914–18	World War I (The Great War)
1914	Federal Trade Commission created		
1917	U.S. enters the war	1917	Russian Revolution
1919	Senate rejects Treaty of Versailles		
1919–20	"Great Red Scare"		
1920	Women's suffrage amendment (19th)	1920	Founding of League of Nations
1921	Washington Disarmament Conference		
1921 & 24	Restrictive immigration laws		
		1922	Fascist dictatorship in Italy (Mussolini)
		1924	Death of Lenin; Stalin in power
1927	Lindbergh's solo flight to Paris		
1929	Stock market crash; Great Depression		

United States		World	
		1930	Gandhi's Salt March (India)
		1931	Japan invades Manchuria, second Sino-Japanese War
1933	Roosevelt's "100 Days"; New Deal; "Good Neighbor" policy	1933	Hitler in power (Germany)
		1934–35	Long March (China)
1935–37	Neutrality Acts passed to avoid entrance in World War II (Policy of Isolationism)	1935	Italy attacks Ethiopia
		1936–39	Spanish Civil War
		1937	Japan at war with China
		1938	Munich Conference
		1939–45	World War II
		1939–45	The Holocaust
1941	Japanese attack Pearl Harbor	1941	Germany attacks Russia
1941	The computer perfected	1941	Japanese victories in the Pacific
		1944	"D Day" landings in France
1945	Atomic bombing of Hiroshima and Nagasaki	1945	United Nations organized
		1945	Winston Churchill makes his famous Iron Curtain speech
		1946	Nuremberg war crimes trials
		1946–55	Juan Peron (Argentina)
1947	Truman Doctrine ("Cold War" begins)	1947	Independence for India and Pakistan
1947	Marshall Plan for Europe		
1948	Organization of American States created	1948	Assassination of Gandhi (India)
1948	Television mass-marketing begins	1948	Creation of nation of Israel
		1948–49	Berlin blockade and airlift, First Arab-Israeli War
		1949	NATO established
		1949	Communist victory in China
1950	U.S. enters Korean War		
1953	DNA structure discovered by Watson		
1954	School desegregation decision; integration crises	1954	Battle of Dien Bien Phu (Indo-China)
		1954	Geneva Treaty
		1954	SEATO Alliance formed
1956	Interstate highway system begun	1956	Hungarian Revolution
		1956	Suez crisis, Second Arab-Israeli War
		1957	Russians launch *Sputnik* I, the first space satellite
		1957	Independence for Ghana (Africa)
		1957	European Common Market established
		1959	Castro takes control of Cuba. First communist government in western hemisphere.

United States		World	
1961	Bay of Pigs Invasion of Cuba fails	1961	Berlin Wall constructed
1961	Peace Corps; Alliance for Progress		
1962	Cuban Missile Crisis		
1963	John F. Kennedy assassinated		
1964	U.S. military buildup in Vietnam	1964	Vietnam Conflict escalates
1964	Johnson's "Great Society" and "War on Poverty"		
1966–68	Urban riots	1966–76	Cultural Revolution in China
		1967	Arab-Israeli Six Day War (Third Arab-Israel War)
1968	Assassinations of Martin Luther King, Jr. and Robert Kennedy	1968	"Prague Spring" (Czechoslovakia Uprising)
		1968	Tet Offensive
1969	Men land on the moon		
1969	Anti-Vietnam War demonstrations		
1970	Invasion of Cambodia by Nixon		
1972	Nixon visit to China		
1972	SALT Treaty with USSR		
1972	Watergate break-in		
1973	OPEC oil boycott	1973	Yom Kippur War (Fourth Arab-Israeli War)
1973	U.S. withdrawal in Vietnam		
		1973	Coup unseats Allende in Chile
1974	Nixon resigns; pardoned by Ford		
		1975	Communist victory in Vietnam
1978	Panama Canal retrocession treaty		
1979	Three Mile Island, Pennsylvania, nuclear accident	1979	Revolution in Iran topples Shah
		1979	USSR invades Afghanistan
1979–81	Hostages seized in Iran	1979	Sandinistas oust Somoza (Nicaragua)
1980s	AIDS epidemic; rising drug problem	1980	Iran-Iraq War begins
1981	"Supply side" economics; tax cuts; debt increase; trade imbalances	1981	Assassination of Egyptian President Anwar Sadat
		1981	Solidarity Movement (Poland)
1983	U.S. aid to Nicaraguan contras	1983	Anti-Apartheid movement (South Africa)
1983	Invasion of Grenada		
1984	Geraldine Ferraro, first woman vice-presidential candidate	1984	Assassination of Indian Prime Minister Indira Gandhi
		1984	Famines in Africa
		1985	Gorbachev made Communist Party Secretary (USSR)
1986	Iran-Contra Scandal	1986	Marcos overthrown (Philippines)
		1986	Chernobyl nuclear accident (USSR)
1987	INF Treaty (armaments)	1987	Glasnost and Perestroika (USSR)
		1987	Meech Lake Agreement on French culture in Quebec
		1988	Riots in Israeli-occupied areas; start of Intifada
1989	Exxon Valdez oil spill (Alaska) environmental concerns	1989	Student demonstrations in China suppressed; Tiananmen Square Massacre
1989	George H. Bush becomes 41st U.S. president	1989	Nationalist movements in USSR and Eastern Europe
1989	Congress passes Savings and Loan bailout plans	1989	Emperor Hirohito of Japan dead at 87
		1989	Berlin wall dismantled

	United States		World
1990	U.S. forces invade Panama Drexel Burnham Lambert investment house declares bankruptcy Clean Air Act of 1977 revised and updated	1990	Lech Walesa wins Poland's runoff presidential election Nelson Mandela freed Iraq invades Kuwait East and West Germany become unified into one nation
1991	Civil Rights Act passed (job-bias bill) U.S. Supreme Court Justice Thurgood Marshall resigns Law professor Anita Hill accuses Judge Clarence Thomas of sexual harassment Judge Clarence Thomas becomes 106th Justice of the Supreme Court Major earthquake inSan Francisco U.S. space shuttle *Atlantis* completes successful mission *Rust* v. *Sullivan* case bars federally funded clinics from providing information about abortions Coalition forces attack and defeat Iraq	1991	Access to understanding the Dead Sea Scrolls opened Warsaw Pact disbands Persian Gulf War—Iraq defeated South African Parliament repeals apartheid laws Coup d'etat against Gorbachev; Boris Yeltsin elected president of Russia Soviet Union breakup after Gorbachev resignation; Commonwealth of Independent States formed Warsaw Pact dissolved New Soviet ruling council recognizes independence of Lithuania, Estonia, and Latvia
1992	Gov. Bill Clinton (Democrat) elected 42nd president of the U.S.	1992	"Ethnic cleansing" in former Yugloslavia
1993	NAFTA (North American Free Trade Agreement) approved between U.S., Canada, and Mexico Clinton proposes health care reform bill; Hillary Rodham Clinton leads committee Flooding in Midwest destroys farms and homes, changing landscape	1993	Bush and Yeltsin sign START 2 Treaty to reduce nuclear weapons Civil strife in Bosnia Czechoslovakia divides into two separate nations of the Czech Republic and Slovakia Oslo Agreement between Israel and the Palestinians Israeli Prime Minister Yitzhak Rabin and Palestine Liberation Organization Chairman Yasir Arafat win Nobel Peace Prize
1994	Brady Bill (gun control) passed in Congress and signed by President Bill Clinton 50th anniversary of D-Day (invasion of Europe on June 6, 1944 Republicans win control of Congress for the first time since 1954 Whitewater Affair investigation begins Stephen Breyer replaces Harry Blackmun on the Supreme Court Congress approves U.S. involvement in GATT (General Agreement on Tariffs and Trade)	1994	First multiracial "free" elections in South Africa—Nelson Mandela becomes president The "chunnel" links England and France under the English Channel Palestinian autonomy achieved on the Gaza Nelson Mandela inaugurated as president of South Africa. Civil War breaks out in Rwanda Israel and Jordan sign a peace treaty

	United States		World
1995	Federal government shuts down twice because of failure to pass a funding bill Congress approves major overhaul of welfare programs Bombing of Oklahoma City federal building United States establishes diplomatic relations with Vietnam	1995	Largest gathering ever of world leaders at fiftieth anniversary of United Nations Ebola virus epidemic in Zaire Assassination of Israeli Prime Minister Yitzhak Rabin Presidents of Bosnia-Herzogovina, Serbia, and Croatia sign a treaty to end Bosnian civil war
1996	President Clinton signs into law the most sweeping overhaul of welfare programs in sixty years Olympic Games in Atlanta	1996	Boris Yeltsin wins election to become president of Russia Benjamin Netanyahu wins election to become prime minister of Israel Swiss Parliament agrees to search for missing assets of Holocaust survivors Kofi Annan of Ghana becomes U.N. Secretary-General
1997	President and Congress agree on a plan to balance the federal budget in six years Fund-raising controversy over alleged improprieties in 1996 Democratic campaign Record number of mergers and acquisitions Supreme Court overturns Communications Decency Act that attempted to regulate pornography on the Internet	1997	Several Asian economies begin to falter (e.g., Indonesia, South Korea, Thailand) Diana, Princess of Wales, dies in a car accident China regains sovereignty over Hong Kong Zairian leader Mobutu Sese Soko steps down after a rebel-lion and dies in exile
1998	Stock market breaks the 9,000 mark for the first time President Clinton accused in White House scandal; Clinton denies affair with intern, Monica Lewinsky Life sentence to Terry Nichols, convicted in Oklahoma City bombing Starr report released outlining case of impeachment proceedings against President Clinton House impeaches President Clinton of perjury and obstruction of justice	1998	Iraq objects to weapons inspections Tentative agreement is reached to end strife in Northern Ireland Elections in India result in Atal Bihar Vajpayee becoming prime minister Serbia clashes with the ethnic Albanians in Kosovo; renewed attacks on Kosovo rebels Good Friday Accord reached in Northern Ireland. Irish Parliament backs peace agreement. Europe agrees on the Euro dollar India, then Pakistan, conducts several atomic bomb tests; world protest and disapproval immediately follow Iraq ends cooperation with UN military armed inspectors Agreement between Netanyahu and Arafat moves Middle East peace talks forward

United States		World	
1999	United States opens impeachment charges of President Clinton Columbine High School incidentresults in the death of twelve students and one teacher John F. Kennedy Jr., wife Carolyn, and sister-in-law Lauren lost at sea in a plane crash The United States turns over the Panama Canal to Panama	1999	War erupts in Kosovo as President Milosevic of Yugoslavia massacres and deports thousands of ethnic Albanians Czech Republic, Poland, and Hungary (once part of the Soviet communist bloc) join NATO Boris Yeltsin, Russian president, survives impeachment hearings; cabinet reshuffled Serbs sign agreement to pull troops out of Kosovo after three months of NATO attacks end Nelson Mandela, first black president in South African history, steps down; he is succeeded by Thabo Mbeki Massive 7.4 earthquake in Turkey leaves over 15,000 people dead Barak of Israel and PLO's Arafat announce peace accord Russia sends ground troops to Chechnya as conflict with Islamic militants intensifies The world awaits the consequences of the Y2K bug
2000	Beginning of stock plunge signaling end of Internet stock boom U.S. Navy resumes shelling exercise of the military training site located on Puerto Rico's Vieques Islands Six-year Whitewater investigation of the Clintons ends without indictments U.S. historic presidential election between Bush and Gore is one of the closest in U.S. history. After Florida Supreme Court rules election recount in Florida, U.S. Supreme Court overrides this decision and recount is halted, sealing Bush election victory.	2000	Reformists win control of Iranian parliament for the first time since the Islamic Revolution of 1979 British restore parliamentary powers to Northern Ireland after Sinn Fein agrees to disarm Presidents of North and South Korea sign peace accord and end a half century of antagonism Vicente Fox Quesada elected president of Mexico, ending 71 years of one-party rule by the PRI party Nationwide uprising overthrows Yugoslavian president Milosevic

	United States		World
2001	In his final days as president, Clinton issues controversial pardons including Marc Rich, billionaire fugitive financier George Bush sworn in as 43rd president Balance of U.S. Senate shifts as Jim Jeffords changes his party affiliation from Republican to Independent Execution of Oklahoma City bomber Timothy McVeigh On September 11th, terrorist attacks on the United States hit New York City's World Trade Center and the Pentagon in Washington D.C. Osama Bin Laden and the al-Qaeda terrorists are identified as the parties responsible for the attacks Anthrax scare rivets our nation—several deaths recorded Enron Corporation, one of the world's largest energy companies, files bankruptcy President George W. Bush State of Union labels Iran, Iraq, and North Korea as "axis of evil" and states war on nations that develop weapons of mass destruction U.S. troops attack and quickly defeat Taliban forces in Afghanistan. Taliban government collapses on 12/9	2001	Laurent Kabila, Congo president, assassinated; son Joseph takes over amid continuing civil war Right-wing leader Ariel Sharon elected as Israel's Prime Minister during worst Israeli-Palestinian violence in years British livestock epidemic, "foot and mouth disease," reaches crisis levels NATO ends guerilla warfare in Macedonia Former Yugoslavian president Slobodan Milosevic is delivered to the UN tribunal in the Hague to await war-crime trial Irish Republican Army announces dismantling of its weapons arsenal, marking a dramatic leap forward in the peace process UN-sponsored summit in Bonn, Germany results in Hamid Karzai selected as head of a new transition government in Afghanistan Taliban government collapses after two months of U.S. bombing First ever "same sex marriages" approved in the Netherlands Official end of the Soviet Union 9–11: Terrorists destroy World Trade Center. UN Security Council passes resolution for Iraq attack. Pakistan fights Taliban troops on border. Al Qaeda connected (Bin Laden sighted in the hills of Pakistan) to both Taliban and Bin Laden Ahmed Shah Massoud (pro West supporter) assassinated by Bin Laden and the Taliban two days before 9–11
2002	Enron Scandal impacts Wall Street Bush states, "Iraq trained Al Qaeda terrorist; weapons of mass destruction exist in Iraq" Elections result in Republicans controlling both Houses of Congress New cabinet department of Homeland Security created	2002	Iraq War begins with "coalition forces" (not UN) Milosevic trials begins on human rights violations East Timor becomes 191st member of the UN UN weapon inspections begin in Iraq; Operation "Iraqi Freedom" begins Air strikes begin over Baghdad

United States		World	
2003	Secretary of State tells UN "Saddam Hussein is hiding weapons of mass destruction"; Al-samoud missiles found Invasion of Iraq highly successful; supported by the American people California elected Arnold Schwarzengger as governor Bob Hopes dies at 100 Space shuttle *Columbia* explodes— all seven astronauts killed	2003	UN Security Council members— France, Germany, and Russia—say they will veto in the Security Council any act of war on Iraq Coalition forces invade Iraq—a quick victory: Protest for civil rights occur in Hong Kong China launches first manned mission into space Chechnya tensions increase and violence occurs in this small Russian province Final flight for the Concord
2004	Exploration Rover lands on Mars Controversy begins on Guantanamo detainees; human rights treatment by the U.S. questioned by the UN U.S. forces encounter on-going terrorism in Iraq U.S. occupation of Fallujah begins in Iraq 135,000 troops maintained in Iraq Four hurricanes devastate Florida and other parts of the southern United States	2004	South Korea becomes most wired internet nation in the world Nuclear hardware sent from Pakistan to Iran, North Korea, and Libya Al Qaeda terrorists hit subways in Madrid Israel announces planned withdrawal from 17 settlements in Gaza and West Bank Historic Olympic Games end in Athens UN calls for all Syrian foreign troops to leave Lebanon; PLO leader Arafat dies in November Massive Asian earthquake hits Southeast Asia—death toll reaches 185,000 people! 10 new nations join the EC—Poland, Malta, Estonia, Lituania, Latavia, Czech Republic, Slovakia, Slovenia, Hungary, and Cyprus
2005	U.S. occupation of Fallujah, Iraq begins U.S. says Americans forces to be in Iraq at least 18–24 months longer Hurricane Katrina hits the southeastern part of the U.S. (New Orleans, Georgia, and Louisiana hit bad—3000+ dead) 80% of New Orleans is flooded by Katrina	2005	First elections of representatives for 275-member legislature takes place in Iraq Pope John Paul II dies Tensions supporting greater democracy occurs in Kyrgyzstan ("Tulip Revolution"), Georgia, and Ukraine Mahmoud leader replaces Arafat as Palestinian authority president Saddam Hussein trial begins Israel informs that all settlers will leave the West Bank and the Gaza Strip 11 million people approve first parliamentary election in Iraq

	United States		World
2006	U.S. population hits 300 million President Bush announces that it will take 18 more months before troops can be withdrawn November elections result in the Republicans losing both houses of Congress U.S. Congress approves the Secure Fence Act of 700 miles of fence on the Mexican border	2006	Hamas gains majority of legislature in Palestine World population hits 6.5 billion Montenegro becomes 192nd nation in the UN Iran confirms the production of uranium First democratic elections since 1955 in the Democratic Republic of the Congo Iraq and Syria renew diplomatic relations
2007	Nancy Pelosi becomes the first female Speaker of the U.S. House of Representatives 33 students and professors are killed at Virginia Tech in the worst mass shooting in U.S. history	2007	North Korea agrees to dismantle its nuclear facilities Anti-government protests crushed in Myanmar Former Pakistani prime minister Benazir Bhutto is killed at a campaign rally
2008	Lehman Brothers, a major U.S. investment bank, files for bankruptcy as the world financial crisis becomes acute Senator Barack Obama is elected as the 44th U.S. President	2008	Cuban president Fidel Castro steps down after 49 years in power In Zimbabwe, President Robert Mugabe and opposition leader Morgan Tsvangirai agree to a power-sharing deal Summer Olympics take place in Beijing, China
2009	Barack Obama ia inaugurated, becoming the first African-American President of the United States Tea Party protests begin across the U.S., calling for greater individual freedom and smaller government The U.S. Congress enacts a $787 billion economic stimulus plan Entertainer Michael Jackson dies, sparking mourning across the nation	2009	Iranian President Mahmoud Ahmadinejad wins re-election in a landslide President Barack Obama announces that the U.S., China, Brazil, India, and South Africa have reached an agreement to fight global warming
2010	Major health care reform legislation is signed into law by President Barack Obama President Barack Obama announces revised U.S. nuclear strategy, limiting the use of nuclear weapons U.S. Supreme Court rules that the right to bear arms applies to local and state governments President Barack Obama announces an end to U.S. combat missions in Iraq	2010	A 7.0 magnitude earthquake kills 230,000 people in Haiti North Korea artillery shells Yeonpyeong Island in South Korea The website Wikileaks releases thousands of classified U.S. documents

United States		World	
2011	President Obama and Congress agree to a deal to prevent national default, raising the debt ceiling and cutting spending Occupy Wall Street protest expands from New York to other major cities	2011	Al Qaeda founder Osama bin Laden is shot and killed in a covert operation ordered by U.S. President Barack Obama. Massive earthquake in Japan causes widespread damage and loss of life. The earthquake triggers a tsunami that results in meltdowns at several of Japan's nuclear power plants.
2012	Hurricane Sandy hits East coast, killing 132 people. It's the second deadliest hurricane in U.S. history, behind Katrina President Obama is re-elected, defeating Republican Mitt Romney Gunman kills 26 people, including 20 children, in a Connecticut elementary school	2012	Summer Olympics in London Gunmen storm the American consulate in Benghazi, Libya, killing U.S. ambassador Christopher Stevens In Pakistan, Taliban member shoots 14-year-old Malala Yousafzai, an outspoken critic of the Taliban, in the head and neck
2013	In response to recent massacres, President Obama introduces proposals to tighten gun-control laws Edward Snowden, a former CIA employee, admits he was the source of leaks about top-secret surveillance activities of the National Security Agency U.S. Supreme Court rules that the Defense of Marriage Act, which defines marriage as between a man and a woman, is unconstitutional	2013	Pope Benedict XVI announces his retirement Cardinal Jorge Mario Bergoglio of Argentina becomes the Catholic Church's 266th pope, taking the name Francis The military deposes Egyptian president Mohammed Morsi Nelson Mandela dies at age 95
2014	Police killing of teenager Michael Brown in Missouri causes outrage U.S. and China agree on Climate Change	2014	Russia dispatches troops to Crimea Members of ISIS (Islamic State of Iraq and Syria) take control of Mosul, in northern Iraq Ebola outbreak in west Africa U.S. launches airstrikes on ISIS
2015	Cuba and the U.S. reestablish full diplomatic relations	2015	17 people killed in terrorist attack on French satirical magazine

STUDY SOURCES

For review, you might consult the following books. Note that to prepare for this exam, you will need to use several books since no single book covers all the topics on the test.

General

Frazee, Charles A. *World History the Easy Way.* 2 vols. Hauppauge, NY: Barron's Educational Series, Inc., 1997.

Hunt, Elgin F., and David C. Colander. *Social Science: An Introduction to the Study of Society.* 9th ed. New York: Allyn & Bacon, Inc., 1995.

American History

Brinkley, Alan, Richard Current et al. *American History: A Survey, Vol. 3.* 9th ed. New York: McGraw-Hill, Inc., 1995.

Kellogg, William. *E-Z American History.* 4th ed. Hauppauge, NY: Barron's Educational Series, Inc., 2010.

Norton, Mary Beth et al. *A People and a Nation: A History of the United States.* 4 volumes. 4th ed. Boston: Houghton Mifflin Co., 1994.

Western Civilization

Kagan, Donald, and Steven Ozment. *Western Heritage.* 6th ed. New York: Macmillan, 1997.

African/Asian Civilizations

Fairbank, John K., Edwin O. Reischauer, and Albert M. Craig. *East Asia: Tradition and Transformation.* 3rd ed. Boston: Houghton Mifflin Co., 1989.

Martin, Phyllis M., and Patrick O'Meara, eds. *Africa.* 3rd ed. Bloomington: Indiana University Press, 1995.

Economics

Heilbroner, Robert. *The Worldly Philosophers.* 6th ed. New York: Simon & Schuster, 1987.

Heilbroner, Robert, and Lester Thurow. *Economics Explained.* New York: Simon & Schuster, 1994.

Sociology

Turner, Jonathan H. *Sociology: The Science of Human Organization.* Chicago: Nelson-Hall, 1986.

Political Science

Lawson, Kay. *The Human Polity: An Introduction to Political Science.* 2nd ed. Boston: Houghton Mifflin Co., 1988.

Lose, Richard, ed. *Corwin on the Constitution,* Vol. 1. Ithaca, NY: Cornell University Press, 1981; Vol. 2 1987; Vol. 3 1988.

Anthropo-Geography

De Blij, Harm J. *Human Geography: Culture, Society and Space.* 5th ed. New York: John Wiley and Sons, 1995.

SOCIAL SCIENCE GLOSSARY

accommodation   An adaptation or adjustment.

amendment   A change in the United States Constitution.

Anglican   Pertaining to the Church of England or churches following its doctrines and form, such as the Episcopal churches in Ireland or Scotland.

anomie   Lacking purpose, identity, or ethical values in a person or society; rootlessness.

Aquinas, Thomas (1225–1274)   Italian scholastic philosopher, influenced by the ideas of Aristotle. Wrote *Summa Theologica*, summarizing Christian doctrine and denying any conflict between reason and religious faith.

average revenue   Total sales value divided by the number of units sold and equal, therefore, to average price.

Bacon, Roger (1561–1626)   English philosopher, essayist, and statesman.

Baker **v.** *Carr*   A 1962 Supreme Court decision that ordered state legislatures to apportion representation so that the votes of all citizens would carry equal weight; thus redistricting had to occur where urban areas would have a larger part of representation than rural areas, in proportion to the population of that area.

Baldwin, Stanley (1867–1947)   British statesman and prime minister 1923–29; 1935–37.

Bao Dai   Chief of state in the Vietnam Republic; leader of the noncommunist Vietnam Nationalists in the late 1940s. He and the French recognized the independence of Vietnam in 1949.

Baptist   A member of a Protestant denomination holding that baptism should be given only to adult believers and by immersion in water rather than sprinkling.

Beard, Charles A.   Columbia University history professor whose *An Economic Interpretation of the Constitution* (1913) and *Economic Origins of Jeffersonian Democracy* (1915) set forth the thesis that the founding fathers were primarily motivated by their personal economic interests.

Bellamy, Edward   Social reformer whose utopian novel, *Looking Backward: 2000–1887*, criticized 19th-century capitalism and advocated a cooperative state.

Bentham, Jeremy   English philosopher whose *Introduction to the Principles of Morals and Legislation* explained the philosophy of utilitarianism.

bicameralism   A two-house legislature; example—the Senate and the House of Representatives in the Congress (legislative branch) of the United States federal government.

Bossuet, Jacques (1627–1704)   An early French Enlightenment historian.

bourgeoisie   The middle class in society.

bureaucracy   A social structure built on a hierarchy for administering large organizations in a rational, efficient, and often impersonal manner.

Calhoun, John C.   Senator from South Carolina who used the concept of states' rights and nullification to voice disagreement with the Tariff of 1828.

caste   A social group, characteristic of India, based upon birth and religion, determining the occupation and class of people; usually unchanging.

Cicero, M. Tullius   Roman orator who wrote on philosophy, rhetoric, and politics and passed on much of Greek thought to the Middle Ages.

CIO   See **Congress of Industrial Organizations (CIO)**.

Clay, Henry   Virginia statesman, senator, considered the "Great Compromiser" for his work on the Missouri Compromise of 1820 and the Compromise of 1850. He suggested an American system to stimulate industry, fund internal improvements, and establish a national bank.

Clemenceau, Georges   French statesman, one of the Big Four at Versailles in 1919, who, after World War I, negotiated the peace with Germany.

Clemens, Samuel   The author Mark Twain, who wrote of Americans in the mid-1800s with stories such as *Huckleberry Finn* and *Tom Sawyer*. He helped coin the expression "Gilded Age" to describe his disenchantment with the materialism of the industrial age.

Cleveland, Grover   The 22nd and 24th president of the United States. His honest administration repudiated Tammany Hall. He insisted on sound money, reducing the Wilson Tariff, and authorized an income tax during his administration.

commonwealth   The whole body of people in a state; the body politic; a nation or state in which there is self-government; any of the dominions in the British Commonwealth of Nations, especially Australia.

Comte, Auguste   French philosopher who founded the philosophy known as positivism.

Condorcet, Marie-Jean (1743–1794) French philosopher who provided a classic exposition of the idea of human progress and the ultimate perfectibility of mankind.

Congress of Industrial Organizations (CIO)   A labor union in the United States formed in 1935.

conjugal family   A family group made up of a husband and wife; to unite or join together as husband and wife.

Connecticut Plan   A compromise proposal providing for a popularly elected House of Representatives, determined by population and three-fifths of its slave population. The Senate would have two senators elected by state legislatures. The proposal was made by Connecticut delegate Roger Sherman at the Consitutional Convention of 1787.

Cooper, James Fenimore   One of the first important American novelists. He wrote the *Leather-Stocking Tales*, a group of novels that highlighted the frontiersman, the Indian, and the clash between civilization and the wilderness.

Dante, Alighieri   Italian poet, considered the greatest literary figure of the Middle Ages, who wrote in Latin and in Italian. Probably his best-known work is *The Divine Comedy*.

deflation   A reduction in available currency and credit that results in a decrease in the general price level.

DeFoe, Daniel   English novelist who wrote *Robinson Crusoe* and *Moll Flanders*, and satirical novels.

deGaulle, Charles   French soldier who headed the French Committee of National Liberation during World War II and became president of France in 1959.

demographic transition   The shift from high birth and death rates through a period of high population growth to a new balance of low birth and death rates.

Dewey, John   Educator and philosopher who initiated the theories and practices of progressive education, by advocating "learning by doing."

Diocletian   Roman emperor who tried to contain the disintegrating Roman Empire by appointing a loyal general to govern the western provinces while he ruled in the East.

dominion   Sovereign or supreme authority; the power of governing and controlling.

Douglas, Stephen A.   Illinois senator who endorsed the doctrine of popular sovereignty as an answer to the slavery issue in the territories.

Duke of Sully   French statesman who served as Henry IV's finance minister. He established government monopolies and a canal system in England.

Durkheim, Emile   The founder of modern sociology who held that secularism, rationalism, and individualism threaten society with disintegration.

Einstein, Albert   Scientist best known for his general theory of relativity, ultimately leading to the development of the first atomic bomb.

endogamy   Of marrying within one's tribe or social group.

ethnocentrism   The tendency to judge other groups and cultures by the norms of one's own and to regard them as inherently inferior.

Faubus, Orval   Governor of Arkansas who ordered the national guard to block Negro students from entering Central High School in Little Rock in 1957.

Fifteenth Amendment   Defines a citizen's right to vote; provided the right to vote for former male slaves after the Civil War. Ratified in 1870.

Fish, Hamilton   Served as a congressman and a senator, and as lieutenant governor and governor of New York. Under President Grant, he served as secretary of state.

Fitzhugh, George   Praised the slave economy and social order of the South as superior to the North in his writings, such as *The Failure of Free Society*.

fixed costs   Costs that do not vary with output, for example, the rent on a factory lease.

Fletcher v. Peck   The first time the Supreme Court, in 1810, invalidated a state law as contrary to the Constitution. The Court decided that the Georgia legislature had violated a contract when it rescinded the sale of tracts of land.

Fourteenth Amendment   As part of the Reconstruction period after the Civil War, it gave blacks the right to vote and extended the Bill of Rights protections to citizens of the states. Key phrases included "nor shall any state deprive any person life, liberty, or property without due process of law, nor deny to any person within its jurisdiction the equal protection of the laws." Ratified in 1868.

Freedmen's Bureau Act   Passed on March 3, 1865, it coordinated many organizations that had been created to deal with problems faced by freed slaves, particularly labor relations.

Freud, Sigmund   The father of psychoanalysis who held that human behavior is governed by inner forces that are hidden from consciousness.

functionalism   Theory and practice of emphasizing the necessity of adapting the structure and design of anything to its function.

Gadsden Purchase   Approved in 1853, James Gadsden, U.S. minister to Mexico, agreed to buy a strip of land south of the Gila River that would provide a route for a southern railroad to California.

Gaitskell, Hugh   British politician who was leader of the Labour party in 1955.

Gandhi, Mahatma Spiritual and political leader of India who never held a political office, yet wielded great power with his people. Followed the philosophy of nonviolent civil disobedience in the struggle to end British rule of India.

Gladstone, William Liberal English leader who promoted land distribution to Irish peasants and won passage of the Reform Bill of 1884.

Goethe, Johann Wolfgang One of the greatest German literary figures of modern times whose greatest masterpiece was *Faust.*

Good Neighbor Policy Policy with Latin America established by Franklin D. Roosevelt during the 1930s, advocating cooperation to solve problems and supporting nonaggression and nonintervention.

Great Compromise Plan discussed at the Constitutional Convention in 1787 regarding a two-house legislature that settled differences between large and small states concerning representation in Congress.

Greeley, Horace (1811–1872) Newspaper editor, established the *New York Tribune* in 1841, emphasized journalism for an emerging literate middle class; opposed any compromise over the issue of slavery.

Grey, Charles A Whig in England who secured the passage of the Reform Bill of 1832.

gross national product Also known as GNP, this figure represents the total of all goods and services produced in a nation in a given year.

habeas corpus The writ of habeas corpus is the right to know the charge for which an accused person is being held in custody. During times of war, for instance, the Civil War, it was suspended for security reasons.

Hammurabi King who formed the Babylonian Empire in the Tigris-Euphrates Valley about 1750 B.C. The Code of Hammurabi is the oldest known legal system.

Hannibal Carthage's great general who led an army from Spain across the Alps and into Italy, yet was unable to seize the city of Rome during the Second Punic War (218–201 B.C.).

Hegel, Georg German philosopher of the Romantic period who held that ideas develop in an evolutionary fashion that involves conflict.

Herodotus Considered the "father of history" (484–424 B.C.) who described the Persian invasions of Greece, embellishing facts with fable and hearsay.

Homer A blind Greek poet, around 750 B.C., known for his epic poems *The Iliad* and *The Odyssey.*

Hughes, Charles Evans (1862–1948) An American jurist and political figure who was the 10th chief justice of the Supreme Court; he supported U.S. involvement in the League of Nations and worked for limiting naval armaments in the 1920s.

Huxley, Thomas British scientist who criticized evolutionary ethics in *Evolution and Ethics.* He held that the struggle in nature held no ethical implications except to show how human beings should not behave.

impeach Part of a process for removal of a public official from office. The House of Representatives first presents and adopts a formal charge against an official, whereupon the Senate acts as a court to consider those charges.

injunction A court order to prevent a strike by union workers.

installment buying Paying for a product through timely payments; for example, using a credit card or repaying an auto loan over a specified period of time.

International Monetary Fund (IMF) Part of the post–World War II economic plan to rebuild European nations.

judicial review The power of the Supreme Court to decide the constitutionality of laws prepared by the legislative and executive branches of the U.S. government; established by the 1803 case of *Marbury* v. *Madison*.

Kant, Immanuel A philosopher who acted as a bridge between 18th- and 19th-century thinking; wrote that a careful examination of the structure of the human mind made it possible to arrive at necessary and universal truths.

Kellogg-Briand Pact Signed by 62 countries in 1928, this agreement renounced the use of war to settle disputes. It was ineffective because there was no way of enforcing decisions.

Keynes, John Maynard An economic philosopher from England, influencing the ideas of President Franklin D. Roosevelt in the 1930s, where government would increase spending, creating a deficit during a depression to bolster the economy; it was called pump priming during the New Deal period.

Koch, Robert Along with others, he detected the bacterial origin of several common diseases, thus making possible effective control of epidemics through public sanitation and quarantine.

LaFollette, Robert United States senator from Wisconsin and a progressive who supported the direct primary, tax reform, and "Wisconsin Idea" for other states to follow when attempting to eliminate corruption in government and provide more service to the people.

laissez-faire A term that may be defined as noninterference and has been used in government and economics during the late 19th and early 20th centuries to mean a minimum amount of government regulation of business.

Law, John Scottish mathematician who put his monetary theories into practice in France as controller general with the Banque Royale and the Compagnie des Indes. He favored replacement of specie coin by paper money.

law of diminishing marginal utility The psychological law that as extra units of a commodity are consumed by an individual, the satisfaction gained from each unit will fall.

Lister, Joseph Paved the way in Britain for the application of antiseptic surgery in the practice of medicine and in public health policy.

Lochner* v. *New York (1905) A case that invalidated a state law limiting working hours in bakeries to ten a day or sixty a week on the grounds that it interfered with the rights of individuals and deprived them of freedom of contract.

Locke, John Instrumental in shaping political thinking during the Enlightenment, his *Two Treatises on Government* was seen as justification for revolutions and as government being derived from the consent of the people. Government should also protect the natural rights of people or be overthrown.

Louis X During his brief reign (1314–1316), the real ruler of France was Louis's uncle, Charles of Valois.

Louis XIII His reign (1610–1643) was marked by the dominance of Cardinal de Richelieu as the king's chief adviser and architect of French absolutism.

Louis XV His reign (1715–1774) was characterized by the reinstitution of the parliament' s power to allow or disallow laws, some financial pruning and planning, royal scandals, and a lack of political leadership.

Louis XVI   His reign began in 1774 and resulted in hampering political and financial reform, which led to the French Revolution and ultimately to the execution of the king in 1793.

Mao Tse-tung (or Zedong)   Leader of the Communists in China who led the "Long March" to protect his people from the Kuomintang and later defeated the Nationalists in 1949 to secure control of Mainland China and establish the People's Republic of China or Red China. Died in 1976.

Marcus Aurelius (121–180 A.D.)   Roman emperor from 161 to 180 A.D.

marginal propensity to consume   The most important variable determining expenditure on consumption is income.

marginal revenue   The increase in the total revenue received by a firm from the sale of one extra unit of its output. For a small firm that cannot influence market prices, the extra revenue gained is equal to the price of the sale.

Marshall, John   As Supreme Court chief justice, he supported a loose interpretation of the Constitution to help increase the power of the federal government. Established the procedure of judicial review with his decision in *Marbury* v. *Madison* (1803).

Marxism   The belief that history can be explained as an economic struggle between classes.

McKinley, William (1843–1901)   The 25th president of the United States who backed high protective tariffs and during whose administration the Spanish-American War (1898) gained territory in America's quest for empire. He was assassinated in Buffalo in 1901.

melioristic   The belief that the world tends to get better and, especially, that it can be made better by human effort; the betterment of society by improving people's health and living conditions.

Mendel, Gregor   Austrian monk whose work on heredity concluded that many traits segregated into dominant and recessive alternatives and that combined traits assorted independently.

Mendès-France, Pierre   French premier from 1954 to 1955 who was opposed to complete independence for any of the French territories in North Africa. He was also instrumental in an agreement on the basic provisions for an Indo-Chinese political settlement involving Vietnam.

mercantilism   The theory and system of political economy where the economy of the colonies should be controlled by and should benefit the mother country; that government must direct economic activity in order to compete for scarce world resources.

Merton, Robert   Sociologist who wrote about "anomie" in *Social Structure and Anomie* regarding alienation when there is a scarcity of socially acceptable institutionalized means to satisfy people's legitimate needs.

Methodist   A member of any branch of a Protestant Christian denomination that developed from the evangelistic teachings and work of John and Charles Wesley, George Whitefield, and others in the early 1700s.

Metternich, Klemens von   The pivotal figure at the Congress of Vienna, this prince of Austria had organized the coalition that defeated Napoleon. He helped institute monarchy in Europe after 1815.

Mills, C. Wright   Sociologist who was the leading advocate of the "power elite" school of thought, arguing that American society is dominated by a power elite that has not seized power, but possesses it by positions of power in formal organizations.

miscegenation   The mixing of the races, especially black and white.

Missouri v. Holland   A 1920 case that upheld a federal statute to enforce a treaty with Great Britain for the mutual protection of migratory birds flying between the United States and British possessions to the north and south.

Montaigne, Michel   French Renaissance writer whose *Essays* expressed skepticism toward accepted beliefs, condemning superstition and intolerance. This collection urged people to live nobly.

Mormon   Member of the religious group called the Church of Jesus Christ of Latter-Day Saints, based on the Book of Mormon, which is said to be a lost section of the Bible.

Mun, Thomas   An English mercantilist and director of the East India Company.

National Industrial Recovery Act (NIRA)   A New Deal act of FDR approved in 1933, setting up a system of industial self-government by drawing up codes of fair trade practices for each industry regarding working conditions and abolishing child labor.

nativism   A sociopolitical policy in the United States that favors the interests of native inhabitants over those of immigrants.

Neutrality Acts   Several acts passed between 1935 and 1937 that limited America's involvement in the growing tensions of Europe.

Newton, Sir Isaac   English mathematician and physicist who formulated the mathematics for the universal law of gravitation and determined the nature of light. His experiments were important to the Scientific Revolution of the late 1600s.

Nietzsche, Friedrich (1844–1900)   German philosopher who condemned Christianity as a slave religion and democracy as the rule of mediocrity. He believed that a small group of "supermen" would eventually dominate the world, and may have influenced the thinking of those who accepted Adolf Hitler's rise in Germany.

norms   Rules or patterns for behavior.

Northwest Ordinance   Approved in 1787 by the Articles of Confederation government, this legislation organized the region north of the Ohio River, including Ohio, Indiana, Illinois, Michigan, and Wisconsin. It provided a plan of government for this territory that would result in three to five states equal to that of the other 13 states. It also banned slavery from the area.

nullification   The political belief that a state has the right to not adhere to the guidelines of a federal law. Expressed in 1798 against the Alien and Sedition Acts in the Kentucky and Virginia Resolutions, and against the Tariff of 1828 with the South Carolina Ordinance of Nullification.

Owen, Robert   A wealthy British cotton manufacturer who created a model industrial community in Scotland at New Lanark. He paid high wages, reduced working hours, provided sanitary factory conditions, built decent homes for workers, established schools for their children, and permitted the workers to share in management and profits. In 1825, a similar venture in New Harmony, Indiana, failed.

parity   Equivalence, maintained by government support of farm-product prices, between farmers' current purchasing power and their purchasing power during a chosen base period.

Pascal, Blaise (1632–1662)   French philosopher and mathematician who worked out a number of theorems dealing with probability.

Pendleton Act   Passed in 1883, it provided that some government workers would be hired based on competitive examinations. It also set up a Civil Service Commission to administer the tests. It forbade government employees from being forced to give money to political parties.

Petty, William (1623–1687)   English political economist.

Pitt, William (1759–1806)   British prime minister who supported moderate reform of Parliament during the 1780s, but by the 1790s he secured parliamentary approval to suspend habeas corpus.

planned economy   An economy where state authorities, rather than market forces, directly determine prices, output, and production.

Platonism   The philosophy of Plato insofar as it asserts ideal forms as an absolute and eternal reality of which the phenomena of the world are an imperfect and transitory reflection.

Populism   Political movement begun by farmers and labor unions in the 1890s. It sought to limit the power of big business and grant individuals more say in the governmental process.

pragmatism   Theory developed by Charles S. Peirce and William James that the meaning of a proposition or course of action lies in its observable consequences and that the sum of these consequences constitutes meaning.

protectorate   The relation of a strong state to a weaker state under its control and protection; a state or territory so controlled and protected; the authority exercised by the controlling state.

Quaker   A member of a religious sect, the Society of Friends, founded by George Fox, an Englishman, about 1650. Friends believe in plainness of dress, manners, and religious worship, and are opposed to military service and the taking of oaths.

Quesnay, François (1694–1774)   French physician and political economist.

recession   A moderate and temporary decline in the economy.

remonetization   The restoration of silver for use as legal tender.

Ricardo, David (1772–1823)   English economist who worked out a theory of rent and wages using Malthusian ideas; made poverty seem inevitable and irremediable. Wages tended to remain at the minimum needed to maintain workers, with increased wages encouraging laborers to increase their families.

Riis, Jacob   An immigrant who became a muckraker photographer and journalist exposing the poorer conditions found in slums and tenements. He wrote *How the Other Half Lives*, and was committed to eliminating slums in New York City.

Rodbertus, Johann Karl   German sociologist who was instrumental in introducing French ideas into Germany.

Rostow, Walter   Educated at Yale and Oxford, this English scholar wrote *Essays on the British Economy of the Nineteenth Century* (1948) and other books postulating that societies passed through five stages of economic development from traditional society to a mature society of high mass consumption.

Saint Simon   One of the 12 Apostles.

Salvation Army   An organization founded in England and the United States as part of the Social Gospel movement during the late 19th-century progressive period. Formed to aid urban poor and immigrants during the industrial period.

samurai   The warrior class in feudal Japan.

Say, Jean-Baptiste (1767–1832)   French economist espousing economic liberalism.

secondary groups   Groups in which interaction between members is more superficial than in a primary group and generally based on utilitarian goals.

Senior, Nassau William (1790–1864)   English utilitarian economist who wrote with references to the struggles of the working classes.

Sherman Antitrust Act   Approved in 1890, this act prohibited monopolies by declaring illegal combinations of business that were "in restraint of trade or commerce."

Sismondi, Jean Simonde de (1773–1842)   Swiss historian who attacked the laissez-faire doctrine of the liberal school and was one of the first to call for state action on behalf of the helpless working class.

Smith, Adam   Scottish economist whose *Wealth of Nations* (1776) expressed the idea of laissez-faire; that is, the government should not interfere in business.

socialism   An economic philosophy or political system in which the community, not private individuals, owns and operates the means of production and distribution. All will share in the work and the profits.

Sorokin, Pitirim   Sociologist who argued that societies are oriented toward either "sensate" or "ideational" values.

Spock, Benjamin   Dr. Spock's book, *Baby and Child Care,* was widely used as a child-centered guide to child rearing, reflecting the 1950s emphasis on family life and featuring the middle-class woman in her role as a mother at home.

subsidy   Monetary assistance by a government to a person, group, or commercial enterprise.

supply and demand   Economic terms referring to the amount of goods available for sale and the interest of the consumer in purchasing them.

Supreme Court-packing bill   A judiciary reorganization bill submitted to Congress by FDR in 1937, proposing an additional member of the Supreme Court for each one over 70 years of age (five in total) as Roosevelt's reaction to the Court's invalidation of several New Deal pieces of legislation.

Taft, William Howard   After easily winning the presidential election in 1908, with the support of progressives and conservatives, he soon found that his only support came from conservatives. He lost a hotly contested three-party election in 1912.

Taft-Hartley Act   Legislation passed in 1947 that was considered an anti-union law prohibiting the closed shop, requiring union leaders to take a non-communist oath, and establishing a 60-day cooling-off period before striking.

Taney, Roger B.   Supreme Court justice most remembered for his decision in the Dred Scott case of 1857. His opinion asserted that Negroes could not be citizens and Congress could not ban slavery in the territories, thus effectively disallowing the 1820 Missouri Compromise.

tariff   A tax or duty imposed by a government on imports or exports.

Thirteenth Amendment   Ratified after the Civil War in 1865, this Reconstruction amendment provided that slavery should end.

Thomas, Norman   A six-time Socialist party candidate for president between 1928 and 1948, championing such reforms as unemployment compensation and old age pensions.

Thoreau, Henry David   Essayist who believed in the right of an individual to disobey an unjust law in a nonviolent manner, that is, through civil disobedience. He believed it was unjust to pay taxes to a nation that permitted slavery. His philosophy was developed during the period of reform movements in the 1840s.

transcendentalism   A philosophy developed in the 1840s stressing intuition, belief in individual human dignity, equality, and social reform.

transfer payments   Grants or other payments not made in return for a productive service, such as pensions, unemployment benefits, or other forms of income support.

Treaty of Greenville   Signed by Little Turtle of the Miami Confederacy, this treaty ended wars with the United States in Ohio and Indiana in the early 1790s.

Turner, Frederick Jackson   Historian from the University of Wisconsin who used the 1890 census in an 1893 paper to explain that the American frontier served as a place where democracy grew with each wave of population movement westward. Pioneers had a chance to build the kind of society they wanted in new communities. The frontier also served as a "safety valve" for problems in the East.

variable costs   Costs that vary directly with the rate of output, such as labor costs, raw material costs, or fuel and power costs.

Veblen, Thorstein   A pessimistic American critic of society and its economic system, whose most important book was *The Theory of the Leisure Class* (1899).

vertical mobility   The ability to move up or down the social class ladder, depending on a person's ability to gain economic status.

WASP   White Anglo-Saxon Protestants, designated by some nativists in America as the original Americans who epitomized American values, as opposed to immigrants, African-Americans, or various religious groups.

Weaver, James B.   Populist candidate for president in 1892 who received 22 electoral votes and over 1 million popular votes.

Weismann, August   German biologist whose theory of the continuity of the germ plasm cast doubt upon the inheritance of acquired characteristics.

welfare state   A social system whereby the state assumes primary responsibility for the economic and social well-being of its citizens.

Wirth, Louis   Sociologist who looked at urbanism and concluded that the many occupations found in cities and the spaces alloted resulted in compartmentalizing the city dweller's life, causing a weakness in social cohesion.

Zeno   Greek philosopher who established the Stoic School, which held that humans must live in harmony within themselves and with nature.

Zorach* v. *Clauson   A 1952 case that upheld New York City public schools' release-time religious education program, which allowed students to secure religious instruction during school hours on premises other than school property.

PRACTICE QUESTIONS ON SOCIAL SCIENCES-HISTORY

Before attempting a whole sample examination over the vast social sciences area, let's look at some other examples, by specific subject. You should become acquainted with the various kinds of information that you will be asked to provide when you take the entire CLEP Exam. Sometimes it is difficult to decide in which subject area a question belongs, and in some cases we have had to arbitrarily assign a question to a particular discipline.

American History

> **DIRECTIONS:** Each of the questions or incomplete statements below is followed by five suggested answers or completions. Select the one that is best in each case.

1. The purpose of the Monroe Doctrine was to

    (A) make the world safe for democracy
    (B) let European nations know that the Western Hemisphere was closed to further colonization
    (C) let the world know that America had become isolationist
    (D) free the slaves so that they could fight on the side of the North during the Civil War
    (E) allow Americans to establish control over Latin American nations

2. "He made the American vernacular the medium of a great literary work. The vigor of his prose comes directly from the speech of the great valley of the Far West." This statement refers to which of the following people?

    (A) Frederick Jackson Turner
    (B) James Fenimore Cooper
    (C) Thomas Jefferson
    (D) John Dewey
    (E) Samuel Clemens

3. During a time in which America followed a cautious policy of economic isolationism, tariffs made up more than 85% of the federal government's revenue. This occurred during the time period

    (A) of the early 1800s
    (B) of the Civil War, 1860–1865
    (C) of the early 1900s
    (D) of World War II
    (E) of the 1950s

4. The following events are associated with which president?

- Opening up the doors and begins trading with communist China
- The invasion of Cambodia during the Viet Nam War
- Watergate scandal

(A) President Dwight Eisenhower
(B) President John F. Kennedy
(C) President Lyndon Johnson
(D) President Richard Nixon
(E) President Ronald Reagan

5. Which sequence of historical events is chronologically correct?

(A) Spanish-American War, War of 1812, World War I, Vietnam War
(B) World War I, World War II, the Spanish-American War, Vietnam War
(C) War of 1812, Spanish-American War, World War II, Vietnam War
(D) Spanish-American War, World War I, Vietnam War, World War II
(E) Vietnam War, World War I, World War II, Spanish-American War

6. Note the following items:

- March on Washington 1963
- "I have a dream."
- Selma demonstration on voting registration

These events are associated with

(A) the Black Panthers
(B) the NAFTA
(C) the PLO
(D) Martin Luther King, Jr.
(E) Governor George Wallace

MAP A

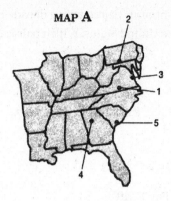

Question 7 pertains to map A.

7. This location was the place of the famous Battle of Gettysburg during the Civil War. This state was located at

   (A) 1
   (B) 2
   (C) 3
   (D) 4
   (E) 5

_____

8. Which development led to the other four?

   (A) The founding of Jamestown colony
   (B) The Spanish introduce the horse to the Americas
   (C) Thousands of Native Americans dying from new diseases
   (D) Columbus lands in Hispaniola in the Caribbean
   (E) Europeans and American Natives exchange tobacco and potatoes

9. Andrew Jackson, the "people's president," was known for

   (A) creating the spoil system in which he gave jobs to loyal supporters
   (B) the establishment of the Republican Party
   (C) legislation creating land grant colleges
   (D) legislation regulating rail transport
   (E) the regular employment of Negroes in government

10. Which of the following sets represent a major civil rights event in the 20th century?

   (A) Congressional Acts declared unconstitutional—President F.D. Roosevelt
   (B) Salt Talks—President Reagan
   (C) Roosevelt's Corollary—Theodore Roosevelt
   (D) Nullification—President Andrew Jackson
   (E) Little Rock, Arkansas—President Eisenhower

11. Each of the following countries is paired with a decade during which large numbers of its citizens migrated to the United States. Which pair is correct?

(A) Sweden—1980s
(B) Germany—1920s
(C) Russia—1790s
(D) Ireland—1845–1855
(E) Italy—1945–1955

12. Note the following headlines:

■ "South Carolina Must Pay Tariff"
■ "National Bank Vetoed"
■ "To the Victors, Go the Spoils"

These headlines are associated with the presidency of

(A) Thomas Jefferson
(B) Andrew Jackson
(C) Abraham Lincoln
(D) Theodore Roosevelt
(E) George Washington

13. "How can an industrialized Northeast, a cotton-growing South, and a small farming West now live side by side in peace in our country?"

This question about the United States might have been asked in

(A) 1780
(B) 1800
(C) 1815
(D) 1850
(E) 1970

14. The geographical distribution of Negroes to more urban communities in the United States changed most in which period?

(A) 1840–1860
(B) 1860–1880
(C) 1880–1900
(D) 1920–1940
(E) 1940–1960

15. Which of the following pairs is correct?

(A) George Washington—Embargo and Non Intercourse Acts
(B) Theodore Roosevelt—Stacking the Supreme Court
(C) Lyndon B. Johnson—Civil Rights Acts of the 1960s
(D) John F. Kennedy—The Watergate Affair
(E) Dwight Eisenhower—The Cuban Missile Crisis

16. The United States' membership in which of the following organizations is most consistent with the Monroe Doctrine?

(A) North Atlantic Treaty Organization

(B) Southeast Asia Treaty Organization

(C) International Monetary Fund

(D) Organization of American States

(E) United Nations Organization

17. "Every state should agree before an action is taken by the federal government." This states' rights sentiment is similar to the ideas expressed by

(A) Jackson

(B) Webster

(C) Hamilton

(D) Adams

(E) Calhoun

18. In which presidential election did traditionally Democratic Georgia, Alabama, and Mississippi vote Republican because of a liberal Democratic ticket?

(A) 1928

(B) 1932

(C) 1956

(D) 1964

(E) 1968

19. In order to avoid involvement in Europe and Asia in the 1930s, the United States relied chiefly upon

(A) collective security

(B) neutrality legislation

(C) the Kellogg-Briand Pact

(D) the League of Nations

(E) the "Good-Neighbor" policy

20. The 2000 election between Bush and Gore was finally solved when the issue of the Florida ballots was solved

(A) by a vote of Congress

(B) by the U.S. Supreme Court in a 5–2 decision

(C) by executive action of President Clinton

(D) with an amendment to the U.S. Constitution

(E) by the Florida Supreme Court

21. Some historians say that this American leader should have stood trial for crimes against humanity for his decision to drop the atomic bomb on the cities of Hiroshima and Nagasaki. This president was

(A) Ulysses Grant
(B) Franklin D. Roosevelt
(C) Harry S. Truman
(D) Richard Nixon
(E) Lyndon Baines Johnson

22. What do former Presidents Andrew Johnson and Bill Clinton have in common?

(A) Impeachment charges were brought against them, but they remained in office
(B) They served only one term
(C) Both were removed from office as a result of scandals
(D) They were strong Republican conservatives on foreign policies issues
(E) They initiated two wars, Johnson the Civil War and Clinton the Persian Gulf War

23. The president connected with the Monica Lewinsky scandal was

(A) Herbert Hoover
(B) Bill Clinton
(C) George Bush
(D) Jimmy Carter
(E) Richard Nixon

24. Which time period most accurately reflects the Cold War?

(A) Churchill's Iron Curtain speech in 1945 to the rise of Boris Yeltsin
(B) The building of the Berlin Wall in 1961 to 1989, when it was removed
(C) World War I to World War II
(D) The entire 20th century
(E) World War I to Desert Storm

25. With the end of the Cold War, a United States proposal to expand a military alliance in the 1990s caused much controversy. The alliance was

(A) SEATO
(B) CENTO
(C) NATO
(D) METO
(E) NAFTA

ANSWERS

1.	**B**	6.	**D**	11.	**D**	16.	**D**	21.	**C**
2.	**E**	7.	**B**	12.	**B**	17.	**E**	22.	**A**
3.	**A**	8.	**D**	13.	**D**	18.	**D**	23.	**B**
4.	**D**	9.	**A**	14.	**E**	19.	**B**	24.	**A**
5.	**C**	10.	**E**	15.	**C**	20.	**B**	25.	**C**

Western Civilization

1. Which of the following was known to man before the Neolithic period?

    (A) Use of fire
    (B) Domestication of animals
    (C) Making pottery
    (D) Practice of agriculture
    (E) Permanent dwellings

2. The center of the civilization that we call Minoan was

    (A) in the islands along the Black Sea
    (B) on the island of Crete
    (C) in the central part of Asia Minor
    (D) on the mainland of Greece
    (E) on the Italian peninsula

3. The decline of power among the Greek city-states can be explained by

    (A) the military power of Persia
    (B) soft living
    (C) rivalry and civil war among the city-states
    (D) the pursuit of philosophy and art to the neglect of political action
    (E) inability to deal with sea power

4. Which civilization accepted monotheistic religious beliefs?

    (A) The Roman Republic
    (B) The Greek city-states
    (C) The Hindus of the Indus River Valley
    (D) The Egyptians
    (E) The Hebrews

5. As contrasted with English colonial administration, which of the following is true concerning Spanish colonial administration in the 17th and 18th centuries?

    (A) The authority of the Spanish king declined.
    (B) Spain did not maintain or enforce a mercantilist policy.
    (C) Spain permitted religious dissenters in its colonies.
    (D) Spain allowed less autonomy in its provinces in the New World.
    (E) Spain imposed less of a tax burden upon its colonies.

6. Which of the following would have been a member of the bourgeoisie in France prior to 1789?

   (A) Landed noble
   (B) Peasant
   (C) Merchant
   (D) Lower-class workman in Paris
   (E) Bishop

7. The art center of the Renaissance world was the city of

   (A) Florence
   (B) Paris
   (C) Moscow
   (D) Granada
   (E) Pompeii

8. The "Donation of Constantine" was a document that supposedly established

   (A) Charlemagne's claim to the throne
   (B) the pope's right to political power in the West
   (C) Christianity as the legal religion within the Roman Empire
   (D) the capital of the Roman Empire at the city of Constantinople
   (E) legitimized transfer of power to Byzantium

9. Because of its extensive colonial empire, this nation was among the most populous on earth. As one of the key nations of the "new imperialistic" age, its language was widely used outside its borders. By 1970 it was not among the top ten countries in population, and its influence was much reduced. To what country are we referring?

   (A) Netherlands
   (B) Russia
   (C) U.S.A.
   (D) Japan
   (E) France

10. Summer, cuneiform, ziggurats, and the first written set of laws are all part of the ancient civilization of

   (A) Rome
   (B) Greece
   (C) Harappa
   (D) Mesopotamia
   (E) Huang He Valley

11. "Some say that there are perhaps two nations in this country and great efforts have been made to erase this fact. There is hope these efforts (such as changing the flag design) may succeed." Twice, in 1980 and again in 1995, a separatist movement by a major province to secede from the nation failed. This nation is

   (A) France
   (B) Sweden
   (C) Denmark
   (D) Switzerland
   (E) Canada

12. In the 16th century, England was under the rule of which Protestant family?

   (A) Tudors
   (B) Stuarts
   (C) Hapsburgs
   (D) Medici
   (E) Windsors

13. The Versailles Peace Treaty resulted in a

   (A) more powerful Germany
   (B) Austria gaining additional land for the role it played in the Allied victory
   (C) financial collapse for Germany by 1923
   (D) the immediate rise of Hitler and the Nazi Party
   (E) Germany restoring the monarchy to the throne

14. The Law of the Twelve Tables, the plebian, the tribunes, and the Assembly of Tribes are all associated with what great civilization?

   (A) Athens
   (B) Egypt
   (C) Roman Republic
   (D) Sparta
   (E) Phoenicians

15. The development of early civilizations usually depended on

   (A) the formation of democratic governments
   (B) a plentiful water supply and fertile land
   (C) a location near large deposits of gold and silver
   (D) the existence of large armies
   (E) strong religious centers

16. Which nation below was unified in the 19th century through "blood, sweat and iron"?

    (A) England
    (B) France
    (C) Italy
    (D) Germany
    (E) Russia

17. Note the following headlines:

    ■ "Auschwitz Commits Genocide"
    ■ "The Final Solution Results in Millions Dead"
    ■ "Chamberlain Saves Czechoslovakia by Giving Up the Sudetenland"

    These headlines are each associated with

    (A) events dealing with Nazi Germany during World War II
    (B) imperialism of the 19th century
    (C) the unification of Germany after World War I
    (D) the invasion of Russia by Napoleon
    (E) Vietnam War during the 1960s and '70s

18. In 1904–05, Japan demonstrated its industrial success by modernizing its armed forces and defeating which nation?

    (A) Britain
    (B) France
    (C) Germany
    (D) Spain
    (E) Russia

19. The Huns were

    (A) one of the German tribes
    (B) Asian invaders attacking the Western Roman Empire
    (C) Moslem invaders of Europe
    (D) the people led by Theodoric who conquered Italy
    (E) Vikings who conquered Normandy

20. "If God shows you a way in which you may lawfully get more than in another way (without wrong to your soul or to any other), if you refuse this and choose the less gainful way, you cross one of the ends of your callings, and you refuse to be God's steward." This strong religious sentiment was most representative of

    (A) Scholasticism
    (B) 16th-century Anglicanism
    (C) 17th-century English Puritanism
    (D) Monastic thought
    (E) Christianity in the 1st century A.D.

21. The conservative Austrian foreign minister who played an important role at the Congress of Vienna 1814–15 was

    (A) Talleyrand
    (B) Metternich
    (C) Castlereagh
    (D) Baron Von Stein
    (E) Hindenburg

22. The journals of early travelers such as Ibn Battuta of Morocco, Zheng He of China, and Mansa Musa of Mali are examples of

    (A) works of fiction intended to describe the adventure of these travelers
    (B) primary sources describing observations of their travels to other cultures
    (C) secondary sources that record the traveler's interpretations of history
    (D) imperialistic expansion by non-Caucasian cultures
    (E) great Asian and African leaders of their people

23. "As to the speeches which were made either before or during the Peloponnesian War, it is hard for me, and for others who reported them to me, to recollect the exact words. I have therefore put into the mouth of each speaker the sentiments proper to the occasion, expressed as I thought he would be likely to express them." This quote deals with what ancient civilization?

    (A) The Roman Republic
    (B) The Hebrews
    (C) The Roman Empire
    (D) The Greek city-states
    (E) The Phoenicians

Base your answer to questions 24 and 25 on the following poem and on your knowledge of social studies.

> "Here is a new city shall be wrought (built) . . . .
> Shall break a window to the West . . .
> Here flags of foreign nations all
> By waters new to them will call."
>   Alexander Pushkin, "The Bronze Horseman"

24. Which Russian ruler's goals are described in the poem?

    (A) Gorbachev
    (B) Peter the Great
    (C) Nicholas II
    (D) Ivan the Terrible
    (E) Catherine the Great

25. Which major Russian policy was developed to implement the plans described in the poem?

   (A) westernization
   (B) isolationism
   (C) appeasement
   (D) status quo
   (E) balance of power

ANSWERS

1. **A**		6. **C**		11. **E**		16. **D**		21. **B**
2. **B**		7. **A**		12. **A**		17. **A**		22. **B**
3. **C**		8. **C**		13. **C**		18. **E**		23. **D**
4. **E**		9. **E**		14. **C**		19. **B**		24. **B**
5. **D**		10. **D**		15. **B**		20. **C**		25. **A**

African/Asian Civilizations

> **DIRECTIONS:** Each of the questions or incomplete statements below is followed by five suggested answers or completions. Select the one that is best in each case.

1. Chinese culture and influence were most significant in shaping the institutions of which of the following countries?

   (A) India, Japan, and Korea
   (B) Indonesia, Thailand, and the Philippines
   (C) Burma, Pakistan, and Bangladesh
   (D) Japan, Korea, and Vietnam
   (E) Japan, Korea, and the Philippines

2. During the late 19th century through most of the 20th century, the British used passes for identification in several colonies. The Indian nationalist leader Mahatma Gandhi responded with a policy of passive resistance. These events would be associated with

   (A) India only
   (B) South Africa only
   (C) India and South Africa
   (D) China
   (E) Japan

3. Today, mainland China

(A) is no longer communist
(B) controls the nationalist island known as Taiwan
(C) has significantly increased human rights for its people since the Tiananmen Square incident
(D) continues to build its economic system around collective farms
(E) took over Hong Kong when the British gave it up in 1997

4. Between 1965 and 1974, which of the following was true concerning Nigeria, Uganda, and Ethiopia?

(A) Independence was shortly followed by military dictatorship.
(B) Democratic governments were organized.
(C) Apartheid became national policy.
(D) They joined the European Common Market.
(E) They became independent nations.

5. The samurai were

(A) Japanese scholars
(B) a people from Central Asia who invaded Japan
(C) a Buddhist sect in Japan
(D) a Japanese warrior class
(E) Japanese industrialists

6. In which African area did the Leakeys do most of their pioneering archaeological work?

(A) the Congo Basin
(B) the Nigerian rain forest
(C) the Valley of the Kings in middle Egypt
(D) the Saharan Desert
(E) Olduvai Gorge

7. The Chinese considered foreigners to be barbarians. This attitude was an example of

(A) cultural diffusion
(B) empathy
(C) interdependence
(D) chauvinism
(E) ethnocentrism

8. Kim Il Sung and Kim Jong Il have held power in

(A) Singapore
(B) Hong Kong
(C) North Korea
(D) South Korea
(E) Taiwan

9. When the British colony of India became independent in 1947, which new nation was split into two parts nearly 3,000 miles apart because of its Muslim belief?

   (A) India
   (B) Sri Lanka
   (C) Kashmir
   (D) Pakistan
   (E) Nepal

10. The collapse of the "bubble economy" was a trend that occurred during the 1990s in the highly capitalistic nation of

    (A) Indonesia
    (B) Taiwan
    (C) Saudi Arabia
    (D) China
    (E) Japan

11. One of the world's greatest supplies of gold and diamonds comes from this African nation:

    (A) Nigeria
    (B) Egypt
    (C) Ethiopia
    (D) Kenya
    (E) South Africa

12. Mansa Musa, Timbuktu, and Mali are all associated with the African civilizations of

    (A) Western Sudan
    (B) Benin
    (C) Zimbabwe
    (D) Kilwa
    (E) Zanzibar

13. Which pair of religions is best associated with both traditional and modern day sub-Saharan Africa?

    (A) Islam and Hinduism
    (B) Animism and Judaism
    (C) Christianity and Islam
    (D) Animism and Islam
    (E) Christianity and Palestinian

14. One similarity between Japanese Shintoism and African animism is the belief that

    (A) everything in nature has a spirit and should be respected
    (B) only one god exists in the universe
    (C) people's moral conduct determines their afterlife
    (D) religious statues should be erected to honor the gods
    (E) reincarnation is based on how good or how bad you are in your current life

15. "take up the White Man's Burden—
Send forth the best ye breed—
Go, bind your son in exile
To serve your captives' need."

Rudyard Kipling, *The Five Nations* (1903)

The words of this poem have been used to support the practice of

(A) isolationism
(B) cultural borrowing
(C) self-determination
(D) imperialism
(E) humanitarianism

16. Sun Yat-sen of China and Mahatma Gandhi of India were similar in that both

(A) rejected violence as a way to aim political power
(B) supported Marxist philosophy to change existing governments
(C) led a successful nationalistic movement in their respective countries
(D) promoted a society ruled by religious leaders
(E) failed to bring about any permanent change

17. Which statement describes India's foreign policy between 1947 and 1990?

(A) It imitated its former mother country, Great Britain.
(B) It supported strong ties with Communist China.
(C) It joined NATO, developing strong ties with the West.
(D) It generally followed a policy of nonalignment.
(E) It maintained a strong and positive relationship with neighboring Pakistan.

18. Examine the following information:

- President Nkrumah
- A Western Sudanic Empire
- The first African colony to become independent after World War II—1957
- Famous for the trans-Saharan gold salt trade

These events are associated with

(A) Ghana
(B) Songhai
(C) Zaire
(D) Rhodesia
(E) Nigeria

19. During the 1960s, the Biafran Civil War tore this western African nation apart. Despite great oil reserves, this nation still struggles from division caused by strong tribal loyalties. This nation is

    (A) the Republic of South Africa
    (B) Ethiopia
    (C) Rwanda
    (D) Tanzania
    (E) Nigeria

20. The Khmer Rouge, Pol Pot, and the Killing Fields are all associated with the

    (A) Viet Nam War
    (B) Cambodian genocide
    (C) Rape of Nanking
    (D) liberation of the Philippines
    (E) boat people of SE Asia

21. The climate most common to sub-Saharan Africa is

    (A) Savanna Grasslands
    (B) Rain Forest
    (C) Desert
    (D) Mediterranean
    (E) Humid Continental

22. This former British colony is rich in farmland. While the equator passes right through the center of this nation, its elevation (the eastern highlands) provides cool temperature and fertile soil. This nation is

    (A) Nigeria
    (B) Kenya
    (C) Egypt
    (D) Rhodesia
    (E) Congo

23. This Asian nation that has the largest number of Islamic followers is

    (A) Pakistan
    (B) India
    (C) Japan
    (D) Korea
    (E) Philippines

24 Since World War II, this Asian country was the best representative of a capitalistic and democratic government in the entire region. This country is

(A) China
(B) Indonesia
(C) Philippines
(D) Japan
(E) Mongolia

25. Which non-Western nation is closest to China in overall population?

(A) Japan
(B) Sri Lanka
(C) Russia
(D) Bangladesh
(E) India

ANSWERS

1. **D**	6. **E**	11. **E**	16. **C**	21. **A**
2. **C**	7. **E**	12. **A**	17. **D**	22. **B**
3. **E**	8. **C**	13. **D**	18. **A**	23. **A**
4. **A**	9. **D**	14. **A**	19. **E**	24. **D**
5. **D**	10. **E**	15. **D**	20. **B**	25. **E**

Economics

> **DIRECTIONS:** Each of the questions or incomplete statements below is followed by five suggested answers or completions. Select the one that is best in each case.

1. The most important factor in creating the world "population explosion" has been

(A) higher fertility
(B) more multiple births
(C) fewer wars
(D) more family sentiment
(E) lower death rates

2. Malthus thought that human population, if unchecked, would tend to grow at

(A) an arithmetic rate
(B) a geometric rate
(C) a constantly slow rate
(D) an undetermined rate
(E) a rate determined by the sex ratio

3. Scarcity of resources in relation to desires or needs occurs

   (A) only under capitalism
   (B) only under socialism
   (C) only during wartime
   (D) in all societies
   (E) in money-using societies

4. The percentage of our workforce in agricultural pursuits in 1800 was about

   (A) 20%
   (B) 33%
   (C) 50%
   (D) 75%
   (E) 95%

5. The main reason for organizing the C.I.O. in the 1930s was to

   (A) organize African-Americans and immigrants who seldom belonged to a labor union
   (B) organize mass-production workers
   (C) escape the high fees of the A.F. of L.
   (D) organize craft workers
   (E) organize white-collar workers

6. Currently in what part of the world is the education of women most behind as to percentage and quality?

   (A) North America
   (B) Europe
   (C) Australia
   (D) Islamic Middle East
   (E) Japan

7. "Like Peter the Great westernized Russia, we rapidly transformed our country from a traditional based economic system into a modern industrial economic system and became a leading colonial power by the end of the 19th century." This quote refers to the industrial and economic growth of

   (A) Mongolia under the Tokugawa Shogunate
   (B) China under the Q'ing Dynasty
   (C) South Africa under the Boers
   (D) India led by the Sepoys
   (E) Japan under the Meiji emperor

8. The English economist John Maynard Keynes is associated with the policy of

   (A) trickle-down
   (B) high tariffs
   (C) priming the pump
   (D) balancing the budget
   (E) collective bargaining

9. Historically, the country considered to be the most deficient in natural resources is

   (A) Brazil
   (B) Canada
   (C) Indonesia
   (D) Japan
   (E) Nigeria

10. If anyone can be said to profit from a depression, the group favored would likely be

    (A) people with secure sources of fixed income, such as government bonds
    (B) people who borrowed money before the depression and must repay during it
    (C) industrial owners producing consumer goods
    (D) assembly-line workers in automobile plants
    (E) low-level local government workers

11. Statistical evidence shows that the typical American family behaves in which of the following ways with respect to spending out of income?

    (A) An increasing proportion of income is spent on consumption as income increases.
    (B) The same proportion of income is spent on consumption at all except very low income levels.
    (C) The same proportion of income is spent on consumption at all income levels.
    (D) A decreasing proportion of income is spent on consumption as income decreases.
    (E) The same proportion of income is spent on consumption at all except very high income levels.

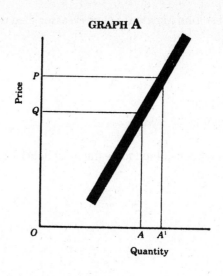

GRAPH **A**

12. The thick black line in Graph A represents

   (A) supply
   (B) cost
   (C) subsidy
   (D) demand
   (E) interest

13. Examine the following economic principles:

   ■ laissez-faire
   ■ free competition
   ■ private ownership
   ■ profit motive

   These philosophical economic principles were first developed and promoted by

   (A) Mao Tse Tung
   (B) Karl Marx and Robert Engel
   (C) Adam Smith
   (D) John Stuart Mill
   (E) Vladimir Lenin

14. "I don't know how old I am. . . . I began to work when I was about 9. I first worked for a man who used to hit me with a belt. . . . I used to sleep in the pits that had no more coal in them; I used to eat whatever I could get; I ate for a long time the candles that I found in the pit."

E. Royston Pike
Adapted from *Hard Times,*
Human Documents of the Industrial Revolution

What was one immediate response to the conditions described in this passage?

(A) Marx wrote the *Communist Manifesto*
(B) Henry Ford developed the assembly line approach to production
(C) Charles Darwin developed the theory and book *On the Origin of Species*
(D) Joseph Stalin instituted the collectivization of Russian land
(E) Europe created the EEC, the European Economic Community

15. The various editions of John Stuart Mill's *Principles of Political Economy* indicate that he

(A) became increasingly conservative and antisocialist as he grew older
(B) made remarkably few changes in the views that he first held as a young Benthamite
(C) completely abandoned the socialist views he had held as a young man
(D) increasingly recognized exceptions to a general policy of a laissez-faire society
(E) became more convinced that economic justice and political monarchy were tied together

16. In Western Europe during the medieval time of the 11th and 12th centuries, the right to coin money was

(A) reserved to the Holy Roman Emperor
(B) held only by kings
(C) a monopoly of the Church
(D) held by a number of nobles, kings, towns, and cities
(E) in the care of the state banks

17. Today the capitalistic countries of the United Kingdom, Canada, and the United States are all mainly

(A) market economy
(B) traditional economy
(C) command economy
(D) mixed economy
(E) communist economy

18. In Western Europe, debate and philosophical conflict over the economic and social value of the private property concept would have been of most concern during what two time periods?

(A) Early Middle Ages and the early Renaissance years
(B) Early 1600s and mid-1600s
(C) Beginning of the 1700s to late 1700s
(D) Mid-1750s and 1800s
(E) 1850s to the late 20th century

19. The Hanseatic League was

(A) a trading organization of the Greek city-states
(B) organized by Marco Polo to help the Italian cities to monopolize and control Middle Eastern and Asian trade
(C) a group of medieval manors united for protection against the invading tribes
(D) an association of northern medieval cities and merchants that bonded to protect their commercial interest including sea piracy
(E) a group of trading nations that crossed Europe into Asia along the secret silk road

20. India's gross national product is about twice that of Sweden. This means

(A) India is more advanced in technology
(B) that the average Indian is twice as well-off as the average Swede
(C) India has sufficient capital
(D) all of these
(E) none of these

21. The Federal Reserve Bank has the power to change

(A) tariffs
(B) insurance premiums
(C) the discount rate
(D) the minimum wage
(E) stock prices

22. Increasingly, the transportation of goods in the United States is moving toward

(A) motor trucks
(B) canal barges
(C) pipelines
(D) railroads
(E) airlines

23. The theory behind what consumers want and how the society meets consumer demands (market price) was first proposed in the late 18th century when he published his book *The Wealth of Nations*. This economist was

(A) John Malthus
(B) Karl Marx
(C) Adam Smith
(D) Robert Owen
(E) Bentham

24. Travel by people between cities in the U.S. is now primarily by

(A) ship
(B) railroad
(C) motor bus
(D) airplane
(E) automobile

25. "In these (economic) structures, people looked to past practices plus cultural and religious beliefs to decide what to produce, how to produce it, how products would be distributed, and even when task should be preformed." What type of economy is the author describing?

(A) Market economy
(B) Traditional economy
(C) Command economy
(D) Mixed economy
(E) Communist economy

26. The Industrial Revolution had its very first start in

(A) the United States
(B) Spain
(C) Japan
(D) England
(E) France

27. In 1933 the purpose of the United States government in devaluing the dollar in terms of gold was to

(A) raise domestic prices and make American goods cheaper abroad
(B) lower domestic prices and make American goods more expensive abroad
(C) establish the gold standard
(D) stop excessive exports of American goods
(E) reduce the ability of the gold-producing USSR to exchange gold for industrial and military goods

28. Note the following economic event and concepts:

- pump priming
- deficit spending
- Black Friday

These are all related to

(A) the birth of communism in Russia in 1917
(B) the collapse of the German economy in 1929
(C) the New Deal and the Great Depression
(D) the recession of the late 1970s
(E) the fall of communism throughout eastern Europe

29. From ancient times to the time of Christopher Columbus, the most important body of water for international trade was the

(A) Mediterranean Sea
(B) Atlantic Ocean
(C) Pacific Ocean
(D) Baltic Sea
(E) Black Sea

30. The economic system inaugurated by Jean Baptiste Colbert, financial minister and economic advisor to Louis XIV, was

(A) capitalism
(B) utopian socialism
(C) scientific socialism
(D) laissez faire
(E) mercantilism

ANSWERS

1. **E**	6. **D**	11. **D**	16. **D**	21. **C**	26. **D**
2. **B**	7. **E**	12. **A**	17. **D**	22. **D**	27. **A**
3. **D**	8. **C**	13. **C**	18. **E**	23. **C**	28. **C**
4. **E**	9. **D**	14. **A**	19. **D**	24. **E**	29. **A**
5. **B**	10. **A**	15. **D**	20. **E**	25. **B**	30. **E**

Sociology

1. "Caste" and "class" are

    (A) both representative of social strata but to different degrees
    (B) sociological and economical concepts that are identical
    (C) not found in our American society but found in the nation of India
    (D) associated strictly with a capitalistic society
    (E) a result of the Industrial Revolution

2. The marriage of one female to more than one male is called

    (A) monogamy
    (B) celibacy
    (C) polyandry
    (D) polygyny
    (E) endogamy

3. Mormons practiced the act of having multiple wives. What level of social behavior would such an act violate in today's American society?

    (A) A folkway
    (B) The mores
    (C) Law
    (D) Polygamy
    (E) None of the above

4. At the very end of the 20th century and the beginning of the 21st century, which immigrant group came under increasing attack due to their illegal alien status?

    (A) African Americans
    (B) Canadians
    (C) Indians
    (D) Philippinos
    (E) Latin American Hispanics

5. The 2000 Census report indicated that

    (A) people were moving more into rural America
    (B) America's senior citizen population was decreasing
    (C) that there was widespread child abuse in the Roman Catholic Church
    (D) the largest number of people lived in America's suburbs
    (E) the percent of career women had continued to increase since the last census

6. Which type of social system accepts that all classes should be equal and eventually all classes would disappear?

   (A) Capitalistic societies
   (B) Communistic societies
   (C) Fascist societies
   (D) Feudalistic societies
   (E) Caste system societies

7. Stratification is most closely related to social

   (A) identification
   (B) differentiation
   (C) amalgamation
   (D) disorganization
   (E) assimilation

8. Which series represents a trend from little to more social mobility?

   (A) Caste, class, estates
   (B) Estates, caste, class
   (C) Caste, estates, class
   (D) Class, caste, estates
   (E) There is an equal amount of social mobility in each.

9. Which of the following statements is correct?

   (A) Mores are more powerful and more important than folkways.
   (B) Form and content of mores are universally identical.
   (C) There is no sanction (punishment) when you violate mores.
   (D) Violation of mores is not necessary for the overall welfare of the society.
   (E) Violating a folkway will result in taboos and positive injunction.

10. The two most significant influences on childhood socialization (ages 3–11) is the school and the

   (A) computer
   (B) peer group
   (C) television
   (D) religious center
   (E) family

11. Harlow's famous experiments with monkeys in the 1940s showed that

   (A) monkeys and humankind are at a very similar level of development
   (B) social isolation from mothers and peers had irreversible effects on the personality of these monkeys
   (C) monkeys can be taught to communicate with humans at least through sign language
   (D) monkeys need a mother to survive his experiment
   (E) social isolation from mother and peers had no effect on the development of these monkeys

12. A subculture is

   (A) totally opposed to the existing values of the society at large
   (B) better known as a religious cult
   (C) an ethnic group that is an outcast of society that lives mainly in rural areas
   (D) willing to be different yet not willing to totally leave the mother culture
   (E) generally very outspoken about political issues

13. "Childhood moves through cognitive stages of development," according to

   (A) Mead
   (B) Skinner
   (C) Erickson
   (D) Piaget
   (E) Freud

14. Which situation is the best example of the concept of "culture shock"?

   (A) The refusal of the Amish to drive motor vehicles
   (B) The hippies' rejection of "The Establishment" in the 1960s
   (C) The difference in life-styles between Eastern and Western American Indian tribal groups
   (D) The playing of international soccer tournaments on United States soil
   (E) The initial reaction of a Peace Corps volunteer upon entering a developing nation

15. A caste society is characterized by the following:

   Choice 1: Intermarriage is forbidden across caste.
   Choice 2: Most statuses are achieved.
   Choice 3: Occupations are specific to special hereditary groups.

   (A) Choice 1 only
   (B) Choice 3 only
   (C) Choices 1 and 3
   (D) Choices 2 and 3
   (E) All three choices

16. A "sect" religion tends to be

   (A) in accord with the values of the society in which it exists
   (B) lenient toward the indifferent
   (C) a reforming element hoping to make the society more livable
   (D) withdrawn from societal norms and extremely pietistic
   (E) the official religion of the state in which it exists

17. A Russian by the name of Pavlov conducted a series of experiments with animals and discovered conditioned reflex. This finding was the basis of which school of thought?

   (A) psychoanalysis
   (B) behaviorism
   (C) relativism
   (D) the new idealism
   (E) Hegelianism

18. If teaching facts are the sole aim of a teacher, she will probably do better if she is

   (A) nondirective
   (B) permissive and informal
   (C) directive and authoritarian
   (D) disorganized
   (E) group oriented

19. Assigning subjects in an experiment to one treatment or another by flipping a coin is an example of

   (A) randomization
   (B) experimentation
   (C) statistics
   (D) field study
   (E) diary record keeping

20. In *Civilization and its Discontents*, Freud expressed his viewpoint concerning the necessity of controlling the antisocial and aggressive propensities of man. Which of the following authors saw similar ideas in 18th- and 19th-century politics?

   (A) Rousseau
   (B) Locke
   (C) Voltaire
   (D) Hobbes
   (E) Montesquieu

21. Opposition that focuses on the opponent, basically, and only secondarily on the reward is most closely associated with social

   (A) accommodation
   (B) stratification
   (C) competition
   (D) conflict
   (E) differentiation

22. Cases where infants were subjected to prolonged isolation show that

    (A) human beings can acquire culture without human contact
    (B) human beings cannot become socialized unless they are brought up among human beings
    (C) mental-physical development does not depend upon human contact
    (D) people are born with most of the traits they exhibit as adults
    (E) language use comes at a certain age, regardless of the social situation

23. When applying Marxian philosophy to sociology, Karl Marx thought that throughout the history of mankind, the economic and social classes

    (A) were in constant conflict with each other
    (B) accepted the fact that some classes should live better than others
    (C) were all equal in society
    (D) lived in a state of constant harmony
    (E) recognized the right of the powerful class to dominate the society

24. The study of cults shows us that it is often accompanied by isolation from the main society. A classical study of cults is Lofland's study of the "Divine Precepts." According to his findings, the individual most predisposed to cult religious conversion would

    (A) be undergoing political stress, be religiously oriented, but be closed to new religious outlooks
    (B) have a religiously oriented problem-solving perspective, know people in the new religious group, and be personally secure
    (C) be personally secure, be religiously oriented, and be open to new religious outlooks
    (D) be undergoing personal stress, have few if any ties with individuals outside of new religious groups, and be open to new religious outlooks
    (E) be very conservative and believe in the status quo

25. A secondary group is characterized by

    (A) impersonal relationships
    (B) strong emotional ties
    (C) permanence over time
    (D) small size and intimacy
    (E) being with you throughout your life

ANSWERS

1. **A**	6. **B**	11. **B**	16. **D**	21. **D**
2. **C**	7. **B**	12. **D**	17. **B**	22. **B**
3. **C**	8. **C**	13. **D**	18. **C**	23. **A**
4. **E**	9. **A**	14. **E**	19. **A**	24. **C**
5. **E**	10. **E**	15. **C**	20. **D**	25. **A**

Political Science

1. To which of the following did the U.S. Supreme Court apply the phrase "separate but equal"?

   (A) The formula for racial segregation (1896)
   (B) The nature of federal-state relations (1828)
   (C) The status of Indian tribal governments (1874)
   (D) The Civil War amendments (1865–1870)
   (E) The legal status of men and women (1913)

2. The law that can be considered the most important impetus to trade union organization was the

   (A) Sherman Act of 1890
   (B) Wagner Act of 1935
   (C) Taft-Hartley Act of 1947
   (D) Social Security Act of 1935
   (E) National Recovery Act of 1933

3. The case of *McCulloch* v. *Maryland* is considered one of the most important cases decided by the U.S. Supreme Court. In its decision, the court announced a major constitutional concept concerning

   (A) separation of church and state
   (B) judicial review
   (C) segregation
   (D) antitrust regulation
   (E) implied powers

4. Which political concept did we derive from English government when the Constitution was put into existence in the late 18th century?

   (A) limited monarchy
   (B) judicial review
   (C) cabinet system
   (D) bicameralism
   (E) direct democracy

5. The calling of the lords to attend the first parliament and then shortly thereafter the request for commoners or bourgeoisie to also attend parliament all originated with the

   (A) Battle of Hastings
   (B) Doomsday Book
   (C) signing of the Magna Carta
   (D) Act of Supremacy
   (E) creation of the Bills of Rights

6. The position of the Chief Justice of the United States Supreme Court is filled by

   (A) seniority
   (B) promotion
   (C) specific appointment
   (D) election
   (E) rotation among justices

7. The principle of judicial review in the Constitution was established in the case of

   (A) *Marbury* v. *Madison*
   (B) *McCulloch* v. *Maryland*
   (C) *Fletcher* v. *Peck*
   (D) *Missouri* v. *Holland*
   (E) *Zorach* v. *Clauson*

8. The body of legal rules based upon reason as applied in past cases going far back in English history is known as

   (A) constitutional law
   (B) statutory law
   (C) common law
   (D) administrative law
   (E) international law

9. The American Bill of Rights was modeled after the Glorious Revolution and the

   (A) Declaration of Independence
   (B) British Bill of Rights
   (C) Magna Carta
   (D) French Declaration of the Rights of Man
   (E) Napoleonic reforms

10. Ambassadors are appointed by the

   (A) president without the approval of Congress under a special provision of the constitution
   (B) president from a list chosen by the merit system
   (C) president with the consent of the Senate
   (D) retiring ambassadors, with the approval of the president, from a list of technically trained individuals
   (E) president from a list of graduates of the Foreign Service Academy

11. Currently Puerto Rico is an illustration of

   (A) a state
   (B) an incorporated territory
   (C) a protectorate
   (D) a commonwealth
   (E) a dominion

12. The armed forces of the United States are under the control of

   (A) the Departments of War and of the Navy
   (B) President
   (C) Congress
   (D) the General Staff
   (E) the Secretary of Defense

13. The policy of imperialism in the United States from 1890 to 1910 was largely the result of

   (A) the theory of isolation
   (B) an attack by Spain on the United States
   (C) demands for commercial expansion
   (D) a widespread desire to become a world power
   (E) missionary zeal

14. In the Constitution, the states were granted the right to

   (A) exercise only the powers given to them by the Constitution
   (B) settle directly their disputes with Mexico or Canada
   (C) establish their own militia without reference to United States Army standards
   (D) exercise all powers not denied by the Constitution
   (E) veto acts of Congress

15. The Senate must ratify or reject all

    (A) treaties with other nations, by a two-thirds vote of the senators present
    (B) appointments of the president by a majority vote
    (C) treaties or agreements between two states
    (D) decisions of the Supreme Court
    (E) appointments of minor officials by the president

16. The work of the Department of Labor in the president's cabinet is, in the main,

    (A) supporting the American Federation of Labor and other labor organizations in their activities
    (B) collecting statistics on labor conditions and making recommendations to the president
    (C) regulating labor conditions in industry by issuing orders modifying wages or hours, or both
    (D) regulating working conditions of government employees
    (E) providing for binding arbitration in industrial disputes

17. The Prohibition Amendment, ratified in 1919, was

    (A) repealed by the Twenty-First Amendment
    (B) modified but not repealed entirely
    (C) repealed by Congress to meet an economic emergency
    (D) acted upon by popular conventions in each state
    (E) a war measure, not intended to be permanent

18. In some states, voters may originate legislation by

    (A) common consent
    (B) initiative petition
    (C) letters to the legislature
    (D) ordinance
    (E) church rules

19. When the government (state or national) takes possession and ownership of private property for public use, it is exercising the right of

    (A) public ownership
    (B) eminent domain
    (C) state confiscation
    (D) public domain
    (E) *ad hoc* rule

20. An American male in 2014 is white, 50 years old, lives in Topeka, Kansas, makes $100,000 a year as an owner of a small business. You would, on the basis of probability, expect him to vote

(A) Democratic
(B) Right to Life
(C) States Rights or American Independent
(D) Republican
(E) Socialist Labor

21. Which of the following do most historians agree is most significant for the continuance of democracy, which is verified in the first ten amendments?

(A) A written constitution
(B) Control of finances by legislatures
(C) Separation of powers
(D) A large number of political parties
(E) Protection of civil liberties for all citizens

22. Which state held the balance in the 2000 election between George Bush and Al Gore?

(A) Washington, D.C.
(B) New York
(C) Florida
(D) California
(E) Texas

23. "The right of citizens of the United States to vote in any primary or other election for President or Vice-President, for electors for elections for President or Vice-President, or for Senator or Representative in Congress shall not be denied or abridged by the United States or any state by reason of failure to pay any poll tax or other tax." The above statement is taken from which of the following amendments to the United States Constitution?

(A) Fifth
(B) Fifteenth
(C) Twentieth
(D) Twenty-Third
(E) Twenty-Fourth

24. Which political philosopher had little impact on the origins of our liberal and democratic government?

(A) Hobbes
(B) Voltaire
(C) Montesquieu
(D) Locke
(E) Jefferson

25. What do Ralph Nader and George Wallace have in common?

    (A) They were both Republicans.
    (B) They defected from the union.
    (C) They were both vice presidents in the 20th century.
    (D) They were both assassinated while in office.
    (E) They both ran for President as third-party candidates.

26. Which is an example of the unwritten Constitution?

    (A) The Congress
    (B) The Supreme Court
    (C) The appellate courts
    (D) The presidential cabinet
    (E) The Bill of Rights

27. Which statement is true concerning the Electoral College system? It was

    (A) part of the original Constitution
    (B) passed as a law by Congress
    (C) modified by the Bill of Rights
    (D) part of English Common Law
    (E) added to the Constitution in the 20th century

28. Consider the following events:

    ■ Lyndon Johnson decided not to seek a second term as president
    ■ Richard Nixon resigned from the office of president
    ■ George H. Bush was defeated by Clinton in his attempt to seek a second term

    What statement below reflects why each of these events happen?

    (A) Political scandals hurt the attempts of these men to be re-elected.
    (B) A long drawn out war made them lose public support.
    (C) As incumbent presidents, they lost the popularity and support of the people.
    (D) They were impeached by the Congress of the United States.
    (E) Their economic programs were largely a failure.

29. This president broke the tradition of the two-term president which led to the ratification of the 22nd Amendment (presidency limited to two terms):

    (A) Ulysses S. Grant
    (B) Teddy Roosevelt
    (C) Woodrow Wilson
    (D) Franklin D. Roosevelt
    (E) Harry S Truman

30. Which statement accurately describes how the Constitution improved the Articles of Confederation?

(A) The power of the president can be checked by the other two branches.

(B) Congress is responsible to the state governments.

(C) States have some power, but most power is given to the national government.

(D) State courts were equal in power and authority to the national courts.

(E) The power of Congress was reduced.

ANSWERS

1. **A**	7. **A**	13. **C**	19. **B**	25. **E**
2. **B**	8. **C**	14. **D**	20. **D**	26. **D**
3. **E**	9. **B**	15. **A**	21. **E**	27. **A**
4. **D**	10. **C**	16. **B**	22. **C**	28. **C**
5. **C**	11. **D**	17. **A**	23. **E**	29. **B**
6. **C**	12. **B**	18. **B**	24. **A**	30. **C**

Anthropology

> **DIRECTIONS:** Each of the questions or incomplete statements below is followed by five suggested answers or completions. Select the one that is best in each case.

1. Which of the following statements about gorillas are true?

(A) They have a structured, hierarchical social organization.

(B) They spend nearly all of their time in the trees.

(C) Their brain size is equal to that of humans.

(D) They are violent killers.

(E) Their behavior is unpredictable.

2. Why are present-day hunting and gathering societies of value to the study of anthropology?

(A) They can learn Western technology so they can raise their standard of living.

(B) They help us to justify the belief in ethnocentrism.

(C) Their social organization is similar to that of other primates such as chimps and gorillas.

(D) These societies may give some indication of how man lived in prehistoric times.

(E) These societies demonstrate that man can live in a desert climate without technology.

3. The best method to test a two-million-year-old Australopithecus is

   (A) carbon 14
   (B) seriation
   (C) dendrochronology
   (D) potassium argon
   (E) fluorine

4. The *Origin of Species* is an important anthropological work because it

   (A) clearly states that man originated from apes
   (B) presents the argument that species have evolved over periods of time
   (C) confirmed the authenticity of Piltdown man
   (D) states that population will increase at a greater rate than the food supply
   (E) states that man was once a chimpanzee

5. The Neolithic period was considered a revolution for humankind because

   (A) armies first developed during this time
   (B) people descended from trees and became bipedal
   (C) it was a change from a hunter-gatherer to a food-producing society
   (D) religion first began
   (E) a nomadic way of life began

6. A student once demonstrated among other fellow students in a cafeteria the eating of a live goldfish. The reaction of his fellow classmates was that of surprise. This is an example of

   (A) cultural assimilation
   (B) ethnocentrism
   (C) cultural diffusion
   (D) cultural universals
   (E) culture shock

7. Dian Fossey did her most famous work studying the behavior of African

   (A) chimpanzees
   (B) orangutans
   (C) gorillas
   (D) monkeys
   (E) lemurs

8. What were the first societies of man characterized by?

   (A) They produced a surplus of food.
   (B) They were chiefly hunters and gatherers.
   (C) They had domesticated plants and animals.
   (D) They lived in large, urban-type communities.
   (E) They lived in trees.

9. The first civilizations found by archaeologists were in

    (A) Olduvai Gorge
    (B) The Tigris-Euphrates river valley
    (C) Mesoamerica
    (D) The Yellow River valley
    (E) Western Europe

10. Which event in human evolution came first?

    (A) Burial of the dead
    (B) Wall and cave paintings
    (C) Monotheistic religion
    (D) The invention of farming
    (E) The use of fire

11. All primates, including man's ancestors, live primarily in

    (A) desert areas
    (B) extremely cold environments
    (C) plateaus
    (D) mountain areas
    (E) rain forests

12. Which period best reflects the Paleolithic Age?

    (A) Two–three million years ago
    (B) 50,000 years ago
    (C) 12,000 B.C.
    (D) Post-Christ
    (E) The age of farming

13. "I depend primarily on fruits, nuts, roots, berries and the like. . . . I'm armed with small spears, throwing clubs, and sticks . . . and my people are restricted to a very low density of population." This quote was by a

    (A) hunter/gatherer
    (B) seminomadic herder
    (C) horticulturalist
    (D) nonnomadic individual
    (E) farmer

14. Which civilization is associated with the correct location?

    (A) Jarmo, Jericho—Mesoamerica
    (B) Tikal, Chichen-Itza—Nile River valley
    (C) Harrappa, Mohenjo Daro—Tigris-Euphrates River valley
    (D) Rome, Greece—Yellow River valley
    (E) Babylon, Sumer—Mesopotamia

15. Stonehenge, in England, was

    (A) built by the ancient Druids
    (B) an archaeological site of a primitive civilization for its time
    (C) a religious center where the stars were worshipped
    (D) built in a similar fashion to the Egyptian pyramids
    (E) an ancient city

16. The Neolithic Age began independently in Southeast Asia and the New World,
    yet cultures of these two areas had no contact with each other. This illustrates the
    concept of

    (A) parallel invention
    (B) culture shock
    (C) ethnocentrism
    (D) cultural diffusion
    (E) cultural assimilation

17. The lowest level or least developed of all the primates are the

    (A) gorillas
    (B) prosimians
    (C) old-world monkeys
    (D) new-world monkeys
    (E) gibbons

18. Which of the following would study and identify skeletal remains?

    (A) Primatologist
    (B) Ethnologist
    (C) Paleontologist
    (D) Archaeologist
    (E) Linguist

19. Mary Leakey and Margaret Mead were cultural anthropologists, which means that they studied

   (A) archaeological fossil sites
   (B) human skulls and bones
   (C) contemporary human social life
   (D) monkeys and apes to understand human behavior
   (E) primitive technological societies such as the Eskimos

20. All of the following made important contributions to anthropology except

   (A) Claude Levi-Strauss
   (B) Richard Feynman
   (C) Edward Sapir
   (D) Franz Boas
   (E) Clifford Geertz

ANSWERS

1.	**A**	6.	**E**	11.	**E**	16.	**A**
2.	**D**	7.	**C**	12.	**A**	17.	**B**
3.	**D**	8.	**B**	13.	**A**	18.	**C**
4.	**B**	9.	**B**	14.	**E**	19.	**E**
5.	**C**	10.	**E**	15.	**C**	20.	**B**

ANSWER SHEET
Sample Examination 1

SOCIAL SCIENCES–HISTORY

1. Ⓐ Ⓑ Ⓒ Ⓓ Ⓔ
2. Ⓐ Ⓑ Ⓒ Ⓓ Ⓔ
3. Ⓐ Ⓑ Ⓒ Ⓓ Ⓔ
4. Ⓐ Ⓑ Ⓒ Ⓓ Ⓔ
5. Ⓐ Ⓑ Ⓒ Ⓓ Ⓔ
6. Ⓐ Ⓑ Ⓒ Ⓓ Ⓔ
7. Ⓐ Ⓑ Ⓒ Ⓓ Ⓔ
8. Ⓐ Ⓑ Ⓒ Ⓓ Ⓔ
9. Ⓐ Ⓑ Ⓒ Ⓓ Ⓔ
10. Ⓐ Ⓑ Ⓒ Ⓓ Ⓔ
11. Ⓐ Ⓑ Ⓒ Ⓓ Ⓔ
12. Ⓐ Ⓑ Ⓒ Ⓓ Ⓔ
13. Ⓐ Ⓑ Ⓒ Ⓓ Ⓔ
14. Ⓐ Ⓑ Ⓒ Ⓓ Ⓔ
15. Ⓐ Ⓑ Ⓒ Ⓓ Ⓔ
16. Ⓐ Ⓑ Ⓒ Ⓓ Ⓔ
17. Ⓐ Ⓑ Ⓒ Ⓓ Ⓔ
18. Ⓐ Ⓑ Ⓒ Ⓓ Ⓔ
19. Ⓐ Ⓑ Ⓒ Ⓓ Ⓔ
20. Ⓐ Ⓑ Ⓒ Ⓓ Ⓔ
21. Ⓐ Ⓑ Ⓒ Ⓓ Ⓔ
22. Ⓐ Ⓑ Ⓒ Ⓓ Ⓔ
23. Ⓐ Ⓑ Ⓒ Ⓓ Ⓔ
24. Ⓐ Ⓑ Ⓒ Ⓓ Ⓔ
25. Ⓐ Ⓑ Ⓒ Ⓓ Ⓔ
26. Ⓐ Ⓑ Ⓒ Ⓓ Ⓔ
27. Ⓐ Ⓑ Ⓒ Ⓓ Ⓔ
28. Ⓐ Ⓑ Ⓒ Ⓓ Ⓔ
29. Ⓐ Ⓑ Ⓒ Ⓓ Ⓔ
30. Ⓐ Ⓑ Ⓒ Ⓓ Ⓔ
31. Ⓐ Ⓑ Ⓒ Ⓓ Ⓔ
32. Ⓐ Ⓑ Ⓒ Ⓓ Ⓔ

33. Ⓐ Ⓑ Ⓒ Ⓓ Ⓔ
34. Ⓐ Ⓑ Ⓒ Ⓓ Ⓔ
35. Ⓐ Ⓑ Ⓒ Ⓓ Ⓔ
36. Ⓐ Ⓑ Ⓒ Ⓓ Ⓔ
37. Ⓐ Ⓑ Ⓒ Ⓓ Ⓔ
38. Ⓐ Ⓑ Ⓒ Ⓓ Ⓔ
39. Ⓐ Ⓑ Ⓒ Ⓓ Ⓔ
40. Ⓐ Ⓑ Ⓒ Ⓓ Ⓔ
41. Ⓐ Ⓑ Ⓒ Ⓓ Ⓔ
42. Ⓐ Ⓑ Ⓒ Ⓓ Ⓔ
43. Ⓐ Ⓑ Ⓒ Ⓓ Ⓔ
44. Ⓐ Ⓑ Ⓒ Ⓓ Ⓔ
45. Ⓐ Ⓑ Ⓒ Ⓓ Ⓔ
46. Ⓐ Ⓑ Ⓒ Ⓓ Ⓔ
47. Ⓐ Ⓑ Ⓒ Ⓓ Ⓔ
48. Ⓐ Ⓑ Ⓒ Ⓓ Ⓔ
49. Ⓐ Ⓑ Ⓒ Ⓓ Ⓔ
50. Ⓐ Ⓑ Ⓒ Ⓓ Ⓔ
51. Ⓐ Ⓑ Ⓒ Ⓓ Ⓔ
52. Ⓐ Ⓑ Ⓒ Ⓓ Ⓔ
53. Ⓐ Ⓑ Ⓒ Ⓓ Ⓔ
54. Ⓐ Ⓑ Ⓒ Ⓓ Ⓔ
55. Ⓐ Ⓑ Ⓒ Ⓓ Ⓔ
56. Ⓐ Ⓑ Ⓒ Ⓓ Ⓔ
57. Ⓐ Ⓑ Ⓒ Ⓓ Ⓔ
58. Ⓐ Ⓑ Ⓒ Ⓓ Ⓔ
59. Ⓐ Ⓑ Ⓒ Ⓓ Ⓔ
60. Ⓐ Ⓑ Ⓒ Ⓓ Ⓔ
61. Ⓐ Ⓑ Ⓒ Ⓓ Ⓔ
62. Ⓐ Ⓑ Ⓒ Ⓓ Ⓔ
63. Ⓐ Ⓑ Ⓒ Ⓓ Ⓔ
64. Ⓐ Ⓑ Ⓒ Ⓓ Ⓔ

65. Ⓐ Ⓑ Ⓒ Ⓓ Ⓔ
66. Ⓐ Ⓑ Ⓒ Ⓓ Ⓔ
67. Ⓐ Ⓑ Ⓒ Ⓓ Ⓔ
68. Ⓐ Ⓑ Ⓒ Ⓓ Ⓔ
69. Ⓐ Ⓑ Ⓒ Ⓓ Ⓔ
70. Ⓐ Ⓑ Ⓒ Ⓓ Ⓔ
71. Ⓐ Ⓑ Ⓒ Ⓓ Ⓔ
72. Ⓐ Ⓑ Ⓒ Ⓓ Ⓔ
73. Ⓐ Ⓑ Ⓒ Ⓓ Ⓔ
74. Ⓐ Ⓑ Ⓒ Ⓓ Ⓔ
75. Ⓐ Ⓑ Ⓒ Ⓓ Ⓔ
76. Ⓐ Ⓑ Ⓒ Ⓓ Ⓔ
77. Ⓐ Ⓑ Ⓒ Ⓓ Ⓔ
78. Ⓐ Ⓑ Ⓒ Ⓓ Ⓔ
79. Ⓐ Ⓑ Ⓒ Ⓓ Ⓔ
80. Ⓐ Ⓑ Ⓒ Ⓓ Ⓔ
81. Ⓐ Ⓑ Ⓒ Ⓓ Ⓔ
82. Ⓐ Ⓑ Ⓒ Ⓓ Ⓔ
83. Ⓐ Ⓑ Ⓒ Ⓓ Ⓔ
84. Ⓐ Ⓑ Ⓒ Ⓓ Ⓔ
85. Ⓐ Ⓑ Ⓒ Ⓓ Ⓔ
86. Ⓐ Ⓑ Ⓒ Ⓓ Ⓔ
87. Ⓐ Ⓑ Ⓒ Ⓓ Ⓔ
88. Ⓐ Ⓑ Ⓒ Ⓓ Ⓔ
89. Ⓐ Ⓑ Ⓒ Ⓓ Ⓔ
90. Ⓐ Ⓑ Ⓒ Ⓓ Ⓔ
91. Ⓐ Ⓑ Ⓒ Ⓓ Ⓔ
92. Ⓐ Ⓑ Ⓒ Ⓓ Ⓔ
93. Ⓐ Ⓑ Ⓒ Ⓓ Ⓔ
94. Ⓐ Ⓑ Ⓒ Ⓓ Ⓔ
95. Ⓐ Ⓑ Ⓒ Ⓓ Ⓔ
96. Ⓐ Ⓑ Ⓒ Ⓓ Ⓔ

97. Ⓐ Ⓑ Ⓒ Ⓓ Ⓔ
98. Ⓐ Ⓑ Ⓒ Ⓓ Ⓔ
99. Ⓐ Ⓑ Ⓒ Ⓓ Ⓔ
100. Ⓐ Ⓑ Ⓒ Ⓓ Ⓔ
101. Ⓐ Ⓑ Ⓒ Ⓓ Ⓔ
102. Ⓐ Ⓑ Ⓒ Ⓓ Ⓔ
103. Ⓐ Ⓑ Ⓒ Ⓓ Ⓔ
104. Ⓐ Ⓑ Ⓒ Ⓓ Ⓔ
105. Ⓐ Ⓑ Ⓒ Ⓓ Ⓔ
106. Ⓐ Ⓑ Ⓒ Ⓓ Ⓔ
107. Ⓐ Ⓑ Ⓒ Ⓓ Ⓔ
108. Ⓐ Ⓑ Ⓒ Ⓓ Ⓔ
109. Ⓐ Ⓑ Ⓒ Ⓓ Ⓔ
110. Ⓐ Ⓑ Ⓒ Ⓓ Ⓔ
111. Ⓐ Ⓑ Ⓒ Ⓓ Ⓔ
112. Ⓐ Ⓑ Ⓒ Ⓓ Ⓔ
113. Ⓐ Ⓑ Ⓒ Ⓓ Ⓔ
114. Ⓐ Ⓑ Ⓒ Ⓓ Ⓔ
115. Ⓐ Ⓑ Ⓒ Ⓓ Ⓔ
116. Ⓐ Ⓑ Ⓒ Ⓓ Ⓔ
117. Ⓐ Ⓑ Ⓒ Ⓓ Ⓔ
118. Ⓐ Ⓑ Ⓒ Ⓓ Ⓔ
119. Ⓐ Ⓑ Ⓒ Ⓓ Ⓔ
120. Ⓐ Ⓑ Ⓒ Ⓓ Ⓔ
121. Ⓐ Ⓑ Ⓒ Ⓓ Ⓔ
122. Ⓐ Ⓑ Ⓒ Ⓓ Ⓔ
123. Ⓐ Ⓑ Ⓒ Ⓓ Ⓔ
124. Ⓐ Ⓑ Ⓒ Ⓓ Ⓔ
125. Ⓐ Ⓑ Ⓒ Ⓓ Ⓔ

Sample Social Sciences–History Examinations

14

This chapter has two sample Social Sciences and History examinations, each followed by an answer key, scoring chart, and answer explanations. After you complete each exam, determine your score and mark it on the Progress Chart on page 12. You will see your score climb as you work through each test and become more familiar with the type of questions asked.

SAMPLE SOCIAL SCIENCES–HISTORY EXAMINATION 1

Number of Questions: 125

TIME LIMIT: 90 MINUTES

> **DIRECTIONS:** Each of the questions or incomplete statements below is followed by five suggested answers or completions. Select the one that is best in each case.

1. What do all of the following time periods have in common?

   - 1919–1921
   - 1946–1948
   - 1973–1978

   (A) postwar inflations
   (B) major depressions
   (C) ages of prosperity
   (D) major foreign wars
   (E) conflicts during the Cold War

2. Which of the following migrations involved the greatest number of people?

   (A) Norsemen into Britain in the 9th and 10th centuries
   (B) English into North America in the 17th century
   (C) Blacks from Africa into the Western Hemisphere in the 17th and 18th centuries
   (D) Spaniards into Mexico in the 16th century
   (E) Asiatics into Hawaii in the 19th century

3. Which of the following societies was a totalitarian-type of government?

(A) Athens
(B) Sparta
(C) The Roman Republic
(D) Asoka's rule
(E) Babylonians under Hammurabi

4. When governments control the major industries such as aircraft, radio and television, this is known as

(A) laissez faire economics
(B) socialism
(C) communism
(D) capitalism
(E) traditional economics

5. Adam Smith contended that

(A) government should run the economy
(B) governments that encourage particular industries with various aids increase real wealth
(C) government should not interfere in the economic affairs of big business
(D) government must do something direct about labor's poverty
(E) government must redirect the activities of most men

6. Who was the African-American woman, born in slavery and later to become the respected editor of a newspaper, who fought hard against the campaign of lynching used in the South during the 1890s?

(A) Harriet Beecher Stowe
(B) Ida B. Wells
(C) Harriet Tubman
(D) Dorothea Dix
(E) Ida Tarbell

7. Based on the United States experience in the Viet Nam War, which conclusion is most accurate?

(A) War is the only way to contain Communism.
(B) Communism is not a very strong force.
(C) Public opinion does not affect national policy.
(D) Superior military technology does not guarantee victory.
(E) Unpopular presidents are frequently impeached.

8. Which of the following movements had a lot in common with Calvin's idea of predestination?

   (A) Populism
   (B) Transcendentalism
   (C) Pragmatism
   (D) Puritanism
   (E) Technocratism

9. "It is a symbol of status. It has altered courting patterns. It has contributed to the increase in obesity and heart disease. It has contributed to a host of services and industries. It has helped the growth of suburbs. It has helped to alter state-federal governmental relations." The problematical "it" in the statement is the

   (A) automobile
   (B) elevator
   (C) refrigerator
   (D) subway
   (E) railroad

10. The Supreme Court decision of *Marbury* v. *Madison* set down the principle of

    (A) states rights
    (B) a two-term president
    (C) checks and balances
    (D) Manifest Destiny
    (E) judicial review

11. The Dred Scott decision, in effect, ruled which of the following unconstitutional?

    (A) Agricultural Adjustment Act
    (B) Sherman Act
    (C) Pure Food and Drug Act
    (D) Missouri Compromise of 1820
    (E) The Second Bank of the United States

12. The following ideas reflect the principles of a 15th- to 17th-century economic system:

    - colonies are needed to supply goods to the mother country
    - a nation's wealth is measured in terms of gold and silver
    - absolute monarchs strongly supported this economic theory

    These principles above reflect the ideas of which economic system?

    (A) Market economy
    (B) Communism
    (C) Socialism
    (D) Mercantilism
    (E) Traditional

13. One of the following countries that had been sending large numbers of immigrants to the United States (in the period from 1890 to the mid-1920s) was given a relatively low quota of immigrants by legislation passed in 1924 in the United States. Which one?

(A) Great Britain
(B) China
(C) Japan
(D) Germany
(E) Italy

14. During the 19th century, which two European countries held colonies in Africa?

(A) France and Switzerland
(B) Germany and Finland
(C) Portugal and Spain
(D) Sweden and Denmark
(E) Switzerland and Italy

15. Which of the following countries lost territory because of the Munich Conference in 1938?

(A) Switzerland
(B) Poland
(C) France
(D) Hungary
(E) Czechoslovakia

16. Which of the following assertions in the 19th century influenced Malthus in his formulation of the theory of natural selection?

(A) "Population decreases while agriculture forges ahead."
(B) "It is the constant tendency in all animated life to increase beyond the nourishment prepared for it."
(C) "No progress is possible because of the basic sex drive which increases population at a geometric rate."
(D) "Nations which are over-populated must be allowed to expand their inhabitants abroad."
(E) "Selection of the race which is most military is inevitable."

17. Which best describes the attitude of Mazzini?

   (A) He strongly believed in the racial superiority of the Italians since they had given the world so much.
   (B) He believed that Italian unity could best be attained under the leadership of a patriotic monarch.
   (C) He believed passionately in Italian unifcation and thus founded Young Italy, a secret society that called for a unified Italy under a representative government.
   (D) He firmly believed in the cosmopolitan ideal of the 18th century, that all men were citizens of the world rather than of a single nation.
   (E) He thought that true leadership in Italy would have to come from within the Roman Catholic Church.

18. The formation of the Triple Entente and the Triple Alliance were attempts to

   (A) encourage war
   (B) end imperialism
   (C) achieve a balance of power
   (D) divide territory in Africa
   (E) create free trade zones

19. Which of the following belongs in a different category from the others?

   (A) Wagner Act
   (B) Norris-LaGuardia Act
   (C) Taft-Hartley Act
   (D) National Industrial Recovery Act
   (E) Hawley-Smoot Act

20. In order to declare a law unconstitutional, the Supreme Court must have

   (A) at least six yes votes
   (B) a majority vote
   (C) a two-thirds vote
   (D) a yea vote that needs to be also approved by the President
   (E) a unanimous vote

21. The Hundred Years War (1337–1453):

   (A) reflected an intermittent war between two rival nations, England and France
   (B) was fought primarily on the seas and not on land
   (C) demonstrated the ineffectiveness of the longbows in ground warfare
   (D) was a sea battle war between England and Spain
   (E) resulted in a defeat for France as she was finally expelled from English territory

22. Which of the following is the best example of a primary group?

    (A) The graduating senior class in a big school
    (B) A neighborhood
    (C) The Congress of the United States
    (D) A girls' basketball team
    (E) Spectators at a baseball game

23. Both the germ theory of disease and the theory that bacteria can cause milk to sour was advanced by

    (A) Galileo
    (B) Weismann
    (C) Pasteur
    (D) Swann
    (E) Mendel

24. The traditional feudal economy of the Middle Ages is best represented by the

    (A) medieval towns
    (B) manor
    (C) craft guilds
    (D) burgesses
    (E) Italian city-states

25. The production possibility curve indicates

    (A) the maximum output series of any two products
    (B) the minimum output series of any two products
    (C) the gains that can be made by mass production in one product area
    (D) the gains in profit from wider markets
    (E) the gains in profit from controlling prices

26. Cavour is to Italian unification as _____ is to German unification.

    (A) Hitler
    (B) Garibaldi
    (C) Luther
    (D) Bismarck
    (E) Kaiser Wilhelm III

27. Utopian socialism was made famous when a model community was set up in New Lanark, Scotland, by

    (A) Louis Blanc
    (B) Karl Marx
    (C) John Stuart Mill
    (D) Robert Owen
    (E) Leo Tolstoy

28. The utilitarian movement in the early years of the Industrial Revolution stressed a belief in "the greater good and happiness for the greater number." This economic belief was initiated by

(A) Adam Smith
(B) David Ricardo
(C) John Stuart Mill
(D) William Godwin
(E) Jeremy Bentham

29. The birth rate in the United States over the last 175 years has

(A) remained fairly static
(B) increased greatly
(C) decreased greatly
(D) tended to fluctuate wildly around a stable average
(E) declined in depressed economy periods only

30. "It has a centralized government with one leader, and a common language, and history." This definition applies to a

(A) clan
(B) tribe
(C) family
(D) nation-state
(E) city-state

31. Which empire had an empire as great if not greater than that of Rome at its height?

(A) The Mongolian Empire. 12th–14th century
(B) William the Conqueror, 11th century
(C) Russia under the Ivans 15th–16th centuries
(D) England under Oliver Cromwell, 17th century
(E) Akbar's Empire, 16th–17th centuries

32. The violation of which of the following norms would result in the least punishment?

(A) adultery
(B) incest
(C) divorce
(D) polygamy
(E) theft

33. Besides immigrants of English origin, the next largest group of immigrants that came to America during colonial times was

(A) South Africans
(B) Italians
(C) Russians
(D) Germans
(E) Irish

34. The American Declaration of Independence states that "men are endowed by their creator with certain inalienable rights." The same idea is also very clearly expressed in the writings of

(A) Bossuet
(B) Duke of Sully
(C) Machiavelli
(D) John Locke
(E) Montaigne

35. Consider the following events:

■ the close of the American frontier
■ the expansion and growth of U.S. naval power
■ Social Darwinism becomes popular in America

What time period would these events parallel?

(A) the Washington presidency
(B) 1845–1855
(C) 1890–1910
(D) 1918–1939
(E) the John F. Kennedy presidency

36. "The value of a commodity is, in itself, of no interest to the capitalist. What alone interests him is the surplus value that dwells in it and is realisable by sale." In which of the following works would this statement occur?

(A) *Wealth of Nations*
(B) *Essay on Population*
(C) *The Protestant Ethic and the Spirit of Capitalism*
(D) *Theory of the Leisure Class*
(E) *Das Kapital*

37. The Boers of South Africa were the descendants of settlers who had come to that land from

(A) England
(B) the Netherlands
(C) Germany
(D) Portugal
(E) Ireland

38. In 1688, the last Stuart king of England was removed from power, and William and Mary took the throne, accepting Parliament as supreme authority over the monarch. This great event became known as

   (A) the Magna Carta
   (B) the Model Parliament
   (C) the Act of Supremacy
   (D) the Glorious Revolution
   (E) the Triennial Act

39. The belief in the "new imperialism" under which most of Africa and Asia was colonized in the late 19th century was based on the theory expressed by

   (A) "White Man's Burden"
   (B) the Puritan ethic
   (C) Stanley and Livingston
   (D) the Malthusian theory
   (E) John Locke

40. Byzantium had a significant impact on the culture and people of

   (A) the Western Roman Empire
   (B) the Mongolian Empire
   (C) Kievan Russia
   (D) the people of Western Europe
   (E) Islamic societies in the Middle East

41. What factor was a major cause of both World War I and World War II?

   (A) Nationalism and national borders
   (B) The failure of the League of Nations
   (C) The rise of totalitarian fascist states
   (D) The spread of Marxian ideas into Europe
   (E) The dropping of atomic bombs

42. The Boxer Rebellion in China was

   (A) an effort to overthrow the rule of the Manchu emperor
   (B) a revolt against the Japanese rule in Korea
   (C) an attack to remove foreigners from China
   (D) the revolution that established the Chinese Republic
   (E) a fight to establish Confucianism

43. If you wanted to visit the oldest sites of the civilization of the Incas, you would go to

   (A) Mexico
   (B) Guatemala
   (C) Cuba
   (D) Peru
   (E) Venezuela

44. Which best describes the following 18th-century rulers: Catherine II of Russia, Frederick II of Prussia, and Joseph II of Austria? They

   (A) made mock of the "divine right" idea of kingship
   (B) went to considerable lengths to avoid war
   (C) wished to introduce various reforms that were supposed to contribute to the welfare of their subjects
   (D) constitutional monarchs
   (E) wished to expand their holdings in South America

45. The "Great Trek" refers to

   (A) the expansion of Canada to the west
   (B) the migration of Europeans to New Zealand
   (C) the movement of Dutch-speaking Boers out of Cape Colony
   (D) the great sheep drives in Australia
   (E) General Custer's march into Montana

Questions 46–49 refer to MAP A. Use this map of Europe and your knowledge of history to answer the questions.

MAP A
EUROPE   1945–1990

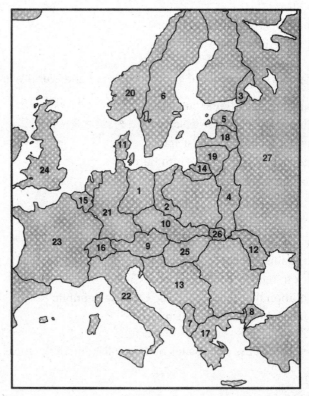

46. Another title or subtitle for this map would be

   (A) Berlin Blockade
   (B) fall of European capitalism
   (C) Arab–Israeli conflict
   (D) Cold War
   (E) rule of Stalin in the USSR

47. This nation was leader of the Warsaw Pact as well as the leader of the communist world. This nation is

   (A) 1
   (B) 2
   (C) 13
   (D) 22
   (E) 27

48. As a result of the "iron curtain" and the post–World War II conflict between Russia and the United States, this nation was split into two. The western part of this nation created a new capital, Bonn. This nation is

   (A) 1
   (B) 2
   (C) 16
   (D) 21
   (E) 23

49. Under the leadership of Tito, this former Communist nation was the only nation to successfully break away from the Soviet Union. Since the early 1990s, it has been split into six smaller nations because of religious and ethnic conflict. This nation is

   (A) 1 and 21
   (B) 10
   (C) 13
   (D) 18 and 19
   (E) 16

50. The best way in economics to define "saving" is to call it

(A) a time deposit
(B) an investment
(C) an act of prudence
(D) refraining from consumption
(E) the building of national solvency

51. *Marginal utility* is a term associated with the law of supply and demand. Thus, a high price for a commodity results from

(A) much labor being required to produce it
(B) a higher desire to purchase the product
(C) its great usefulness to people
(D) its association with an exploitive capitalist system
(E) its not being mass-produced

52. Which order is correct when ranking primates from lowest to highest?

(A) Prosimians, new-world monkeys, old-world monkeys, apes
(B) Lemurs, chimpanzees, baboons, rhesus monkeys
(C) Baboons, orangutans, man, gorillas
(D) Old-world monkeys, new-world monkeys, apes, man
(E) Gibbons, prosimians, gorillas, man

53. Since people interacting take one another into account and modify their behaviors, interaction is

(A) secondary
(B) formal
(C) cohesive
(D) reciprocal
(E) marginal

54. Which document on human rights was written shortly after World War II and was a result of the many human rights violations that people had experienced during both world wars.

(A) The Declaration of the Rights of Man
(B) The UN Declaration of Human Rights
(C) The Johnson Civil Rights Legislation of 1964–1965
(D) The Cambodian Genocide declaration
(E) Gandhi's pledge of civil disobedience

55. Why did the United States become an active party in the Persian Gulf War?

(A) To contain the spread of Communism
(B) To assassinate Saddam Hussein
(C) To protect the U.S. embassy
(D) To protect its interests in oil in the Middle East
(E) To end a civil war taking place there

56. Which of the following is a common trait of a developing nation?

    (A) It is urbanized and industrialized.
    (B) It depends largely on a large farming labor force.
    (C) It has a low infant mortality rate.
    (D) Average life expectancy is about 65–70 years of age.
    (E) Education is a top priority and extensive.

57. The sociologist who analyzed different types of suicide in terms of individuals' attachment or lack of attachment to a group was

    (A) Emile Durkheim
    (B) C. Wright Mills
    (C) Robert Merton
    (D) Louis Wirth
    (E) Pitirim Sorokin

58. The most common way to secure a wife in most simple traditional patrilocal African societies was by

    (A) sororate rules
    (B) purchase
    (C) royal dispensation
    (D) stealing
    (E) capture

59. George Orwell's two books *Animal Farm* and *1984* had one very similar theme or message, which was

    (A) totalitarian states, although dictatorial, do believe in civil liberties
    (B) that communism is the best form of political government
    (C) the general populace supported a powerful secret police that allowed cruel and harsh punishment to be used by the state
    (D) to show readers what a world of horror it would be if communism was allowed to expand at the expense of fundamental human rights
    (E) that the masses support both the government of Big Brother and Napoleon

60. "The young Kaiser William II (1870s–1890s) was jealous of the aged minister who had domineered over Germany so long." Who was the minister?

    (A) Tirpitz
    (B) Dollfuss
    (C) Stein
    (D) Bethman-Hollweg
    (E) Bismarck

61. In European medieval agriculture, the three-field system was a

    (A) means of dividing agricultural land among the three main social classes
    (B) method of rotating crops on the manor
    (C) plan in which both the king and the church received part of the product of the land
    (D) plan to divide manors among various owners
    (E) system of irrigating three or more farms with one canal system

62. When the founding fathers established the electoral college system, they expected that

    (A) mass education would improve the electorate and make direct popular election reasonable
    (B) partisan conflict over the election of a president could be avoided
    (C) a democratic system would evolve whereby the people would select the president according to a weighted formula which equates the popular and electoral votes
    (D) a democratic party system would develop, thus making selection of the president a popular decision
    (E) Washington would serve two terms, after which an amendment would require the election of a president by the House of Representatives

63. Animism is a type of ancient religious belief practiced by traditional

    (A) African tribes and clans
    (B) Middle Eastern civilizations of early Mesopotamia
    (C) Shiite Muslims
    (D) ancient Chinese dynasties
    (E) Aryans that made it a part of Hinduism

64. The philosophical belief that the proletariat communistic revolution would include both city workers and peasants would be opposed only by

    (A) Mao Tse-tung
    (B) Vladimir Lenin
    (C) Joseph Stalin
    (D) Ho Chi Minh
    (E) Karl Marx

65. In the 10th century the ruler of which capital would have called himself "emperor of the Romans"?

    (A) Baghdad
    (B) Cairo
    (C) Kiev
    (D) Constantinople
    (E) London

66. In Cambodia and under the rule of Pol Pot and the Khmer Rouge, the sociological approach to brainwash the masses, feed them little and work them long hours all so that they would be obedient loyal subjects was also a characteristic of America's

(A) Moonie and Jonestown cults
(B) Hippie movement
(C) Yippee movement
(D) Yuppie subculture
(E) Black Muslim cult

67. The 19th-century English reform bills of 1832, 1867, and 1884 all had what in common?

(A) They supported industrial growth for England.
(B) They increased the power of Parliament while decreasing the king's power.
(C) They allowed labor unions to exist and have rights.
(D) They created more and more rights for the masses in the British voting system.
(E) They ended abusive and unfair child labor in the early factories.

68. "Forced by the prospect of having to fight both the British and American fleet as well as the Latin American rebels, the 'Concert of Europe' broke down and Spanish American colonies were allowed to remain republics." This statement refers to what time period below?

(A) 1490s–1500s
(B) 1790s
(C) 1810s–1820s
(D) 1940s
(E) 1850s

69. If greatly diluted amounts of the infection were given in slowly increasing doses, resistance to the disease developed. In 1885, the treatment was tried on a nine-year-old boy bitten by a mad dog. He was cured. Who administered the cure?

(A) Lister
(B) Freud
(C) Pasteur
(D) Spock
(E) Koch

70. Using dogs, the animal physiologist whose discovery of the conditioned reflex showed the exclusion of conscious processes from basic behavior patterns was

(A) Darwin
(B) Rousseau
(C) Freud
(D) Pavlov
(E) Watson

71. The two-income family is associated with a growing solid middle class in which both the husband and wife began to work. This trend became typical

(A) during the colonial period in America
(B) after the Industrial Revolution began in the late 1700s
(C) after World War I
(D) after World War II
(E) during the Kennedy years

72. Which incident below was a major event in the immediate years following World War II ?

(A) Expansion of U.S. holdings in the Pacific
(B) Heavy immigration into the United States from southern Europe
(C) A tendency to feel that the American frontier had finally vanished
(D) A strong movement to end "Jim Crowism" in the United States
(E) Growing sentiment against trusts and monopoly

73. Which of the following civil rights originated with the Justinian Code of Rome?

(A) Freedom of religion
(B) Freedom of speech
(C) Freedom of assembly
(D) The right to vote
(E) The right to trial by jury

74. The political boundaries of states in Africa came about mainly because of

(A) geographic and economic ties between tribes
(B) racial antagonisms
(C) tribal organization and power
(D) 19th-century colonial European power politics
(E) nationalist sentiments in African populations at the end of the 19th century

75. The medieval European intellectual class was drawn almost entirely from

(A) lawyers
(B) the clergy
(C) members of the landed aristocracy
(D) guildsmen
(E) royalty

76. The "sun never set" on this nation and it became the greatest naval power when it defeated the Spanish Armada in 1588. This nation is

(A) France
(B) Germany
(C) Japan
(D) United States
(E) Great Britain

77. At the turn of the 20th century, the two greatest naval powers were

   (A) Great Britain and the United States
   (B) Japan and France
   (C) Germany and Great Britain
   (D) the United States and China
   (E) Russia and Japan

78. The Tudor ruler, King Henry VIII, declared the "Act of Supremacy" in the early 16th century in England. This act created the first state-controlled religion in all Europe. This religion was

   (A) Anglican
   (B) Methodist
   (C) Presbyterian
   (D) Quaker
   (E) Roman Catholic

79. Which famous 20th century leader made these three famous quotes?

   ■ "We stand alone"
   ■ "from Stettin in the Baltic to Trieste in the Adriatic … an iron curtain has been descended across the continent"
   ■ "Never in the field of human conflict was so much owed by so many to so few"

   (A) Woodrow Wilson
   (B) Robert De Gaul
   (C) Winston Churchill
   (D) Harry S Truman
   (E) Theodore Roosevelt

80. The man responsible for gaining independence for Vietnam from French colonial domination was

   (A) Mao Tse-tung
   (B) Mahatma Gandhi
   (C) Ho Chi Minh
   (D) Bao Dai
   (E) Richard Nixon

81. ". . . And yet for the people living in cities, their devalued currency caused by this inflationary period, left this nation crippled with high unemployment and an overall discontented urban population. Most people blamed the Versailles Treaty for their dilemma." This statement would describe

   (A) the United States in 1873
   (B) Germany in 1923
   (C) the United States in 1925
   (D) the United States in 1933
   (E) Great Britain in 1935

82. The growth of the civil rights movement began shortly after World War II and reached its height in the 1960s. The Chief Justice of the Supreme Court during this crucial time period was

(A) Charles Evans Hughes
(B) William Howard Taft
(C) Roger Taney
(D) Earl Warren
(E) John Marshall

83. Which of the following books, cited in the 1954 school segregation case, was authored by Gunnar Myrdal?

(A) *The American Commonwealth*
(B) *America as a Civilization*
(C) *An American Dilemma*
(D) *The Promise of American Life*
(E) *America's Sixty Families*

84. Review the following key events in colonial America:

- The Mayflower Compact
- Virginia House of Burgesses
- Fundamental Orders of Connecticut

What do these events have in common?

(A) They established the right to vote for the American colonist.
(B) They were early steps in the road to American democracy.
(C) These were events after the French and Indian War that led to the Revolution.
(D) These events were all a part of the original colonial settlement in Jamestown.
(E) The British government used these methods to maintain control over its colonies.

85. American marriage and divorce laws

(A) are outlined in the Constitution
(B) vary from state to state
(C) are uniform for the nation
(D) have no effect on marriage and divorces
(E) have not changed over the past 50 years

86. Which group might benefit from inflationary trends?

(A) Old-age pensioners
(B) Bondholders
(C) Land speculators
(D) Salaried workers
(E) Educators

87. Land, labor, and capital are all components of

 (A) the Keynes theory of economics
 (B) the factors of production
 (C) Marxian communistic ideology
 (D) prehistoric agrarian societies
 (E) the traditional economy of the manor

88. Consider the following events:

 ■ The Great Railway Strike 1877
 ■ The Haymarket Affair 1886
 ■ The Homestead Strike

 These events resulted in

 (A) an outpouring of support by the public at large for the labor movement
 (B) the rise of the American communist party
 (C) strong support by big business for labor unions
 (D) the failure of labor to organize against big business
 (E) the federal government supporting big business over labor unions

89. The American family is typically

 (A) matrilocal
 (B) patrilocal
 (C) neolocal
 (D) paleolocal
 (E) rurolocal

90. Urban race riots of the 1960s like the one that occurred in 1965 in Watts, Los Angeles, were characterized by

 (A) emotional contagion and absence or weakness of social norms, two fundamental components of collective behavior
 (B) strict new protest laws that were soon violated by the radical Black Muslim cult
 (C) a time period of American peace in domestic affairs
 (D) Martin Luther King leading the protestors in a violent civil rights demonstration
 (E) whites, blacks, and hippies joining together in a cry to end the Viet Nam conflict

91. Max Weber said that this man's ideas about Christianity contributed in an indirect way to the rise of capitalism. This belief supported a growing middle business class. This individual was

 (A) John Calvin
 (B) Durkheim
 (C) Thomas Aquinas
 (D) Henry VIII
 (E) Augustine

92. Which can be defined as any formal ceremony prescribed by the group as having symbolic significance?

    (A) Mores
    (B) Folkways
    (C) Ritual
    (D) Laws
    (E) None of the above

93. "All persons held as slaves within any State or designated part of a State, the people whereof shall then be in rebellion against the United States shall be then, thenceforward, and forever free." The above statement is taken from the

    (A) Abolitionist papers
    (B) Fifteenth Amendment to the Constitution
    (C) Freedmen's Bureau Act
    (D) Thirteenth Amendment to the Constitution
    (E) Emancipation Proclamation

94. A physical anthropologist made the following observation from the remains of an archaeological dig:

    - bipedal
    - 1400–1600 cc brain capacity
    - foramen magnum in the center of the skull
    - no large canine teeth; arc-shaped jaw

    These physical traits would be that of a

    (A) prosimian
    (B) monkey
    (C) chimpanzee
    (D) gorilla
    (E) human being

95. During the French Revolution, new political terms such as *left vs. right* emerged and they remain with us to this day. A *leftist* would be a

    (A) Nazi
    (B) clergyman
    (C) liberal
    (D) status quo individual
    (E) conservative

96. We sometimes hear a peace described as "carthaginian." Judging from what you know of the conclusion of the Third Punic War, this term means

(A) a soft and lenient peace
(B) an armistice or temporary cessation of the hostilities
(C) a peace so severe that it means virtual destruction of the enemy
(D) a peace that leaves both sides exhausted
(E) the evolution of a group of allies who stand off a common enemy

97. "I proposed never to accept anything for true which I did not clearly know to be such. I think therefore I am." This quote was said by

(A) Pascal
(B) Descartes
(C) Bayle
(D) Locke
(E) Hobbes

98. "The marginal propensity to consume" refers to the

(A) level of income at which consumer spending just equals income
(B) inclination on the part of some to "keep up with the Joneses" in their consumer spending
(C) fraction of extra income that will be spent on consumption
(D) amount a family (or community) will spend on consumption at different levels of income
(E) fact that, at low incomes, families spend more on consumption than the amount of their incomes

99. In the effort to counteract a depression or recession, Federal Reserve Banks might

(A) increase the reserve requirement
(B) decrease the interest rate charged commercial banks
(C) sell government securities to individuals
(D) raise the interest rate charged commercial banks
(E) raise margin requirements on stock purchases

100. The Mullahs are

(A) a Muslim
(B) teachers of Islamic law and dogma
(C) political leaders of the Muslims
(D) a ruling dynasty of Baghdad
(E) followers of Islam who are black

101. A grand jury is

 (A) an organization of outstanding civic leaders
 (B) a group of citizens whose function is to determine the facts in a civil or criminal trial
 (C) the jury used in appellate courts
 (D) a group of citizens responsible for bringing formal charges against a person accused of a serious crime
 (E) a jury that is called in major cases

102. Justices of the Supreme Court who disagree with a decision may prepare a

 (A) concurring opinion
 (B) advisory opinion
 (C) dissenting opinion
 (D) declaratory judgment
 (E) *per curiam* decision

103. The following are examples of one of the several levels of courts in our judiciary system:

 ■ justices are appointed by the President
 ■ it has jurisdiction in disputes between states
 ■ it can overrule an established precedent

 These three examples all apply to

 (A) State Supreme Courts
 (B) The U.S. Supreme Court
 (C) The federal Court of Appeals
 (D) The federal Circuit Courts
 (E) County District Courts

104. The first significant example of colonial unity in America was the

 (A) First Continental Congress
 (B) Albany Congress
 (C) Second Continental Congress
 (D) signing of the Bill of Rights
 (E) Articles of Confederation

105. World War II began

 (A) soon after Hitler became chancellor of Germany
 (B) when Hitler invaded Poland in 1939
 (C) after the bombing attack on Pearl Harbor in 1941
 (D) when the Sudetenland was invaded by the Nazis in 1937
 (E) after a series of German victories had occurred in western and northern Europe

106. Which of the following writers felt that the frontier loosened the bonds of custom, offered new experiences, and had a permanent effect on American institutions?

(A) Henry George
(B) Thorstein Veblen
(C) Charles A. Beard
(D) Allen Nevins
(E) Frederick Jackson Turner

107. The Meiji Restoration in Japan (1867–68) was

(A) an effort to cut all ties with the West and go back to ancient Japanese ways
(B) the beginning of Japan's modernization
(C) the capture of Formosa by Japan
(D) the overthrow of the Japanese emperor
(E) the reestablishment of the power of the shogunate

108. "Inconvenience, suffering, and death are the penalties attached by nature to ignorance, as well as to incompetence. . . . It is impossible in any degree to suspend this discipline by stepping in between ignorance and its consequences, without, to a corresponding degree, suspending the progress. If to be ignorant were as safe as to be wise, no one would become wise." This quotation came from

(A) Nikolai Lenin
(B) Jean Jacques Rousseau
(C) Cardinal Newman
(D) Herbert Spencer
(E) John Locke

109. The Tasadays, the Bushman, the Nuer, the Mbuti, and the Eskimos are all examples of

(A) nonnomadic cultures
(B) traditional nomadic societies
(C) early Neolithic civilizations
(D) remains of man nearly one million years ago
(E) isolated cultures that have been able to maintain their unique identity in the 21st century

110. Which statement is true about bills becoming laws in our American Congress?

(A) Most bills become laws.
(B) All bills cans start off either in the House or in the Senate.
(C) Standing and conference committees are a necessary and integral part of the process.
(D) The Supreme Court can veto a bill passed by both the President and Congress.
(E) There is no floor debate on a bill; all work is done in committees.

111. In Alvin Toffler's book *The Third Wave* (written in the late 1960s), he says that

    (A) the nuclear family will be replaced by the extended family as a result of our industrialized society

    (B) the American family is in a state of crisis as many alternatives become accepted, such as single parents, remarriages, and gay lifestyles

    (C) mothers and religion will become the primary socializing force in America

    (D) fathers will replace mothers in raising children

    (E) the Norman Rockwell model will become the most common family lifestyle

112. The concept of anomie refers to

    (A) folk society

    (B) a highly normative situation

    (C) a condition marked by normlessness

    (D) a highly dense population

    (E) a warring state armed with atomic weapons

113. Ruth Benedict and Margaret Mead are both famous

    (A) cultural anthropologists

    (B) archaeologists

    (C) paleontologists

    (D) sociologists

    (E) historians

114. The Congo territory was developed and exploited during the last half of the 19th century by a private company that was organized by the king of

    (A) Germany

    (B) Italy

    (C) Portugal

    (D) Belgium

    (E) Sweden

115. Genghis Khan was the leader of

    (A) Mongolian nomads of central Asia

    (B) an ancient Chinese dynasty

    (C) a nation of Asian Muslims

    (D) a sea-going people of southeast Asia

    (E) tribes from northern Japan

116. Surplus value, class conflict, and the inevitability of a proletariat revolution each represent the ideas expressed in the book

    (A) *Leviathan,* by Hobbes

    (B) *Wealth of Nations,* by Smith

    (C) *Essay on Population,* by Malthus

    (D) *Communist Manifesto,* by Marx

    (E) *Expansion and Peace,* by Teddy Roosevelt

117. Which of the following is a major advantage of a corporate form of business organization?

    (A) Lower taxes
    (B) The limited liability of the owners
    (C) Fewer regulations to operate under
    (D) Being inexpensive to start
    (E) It has no say from its shareholders

118. Most public utilities are examples of which type of industry?

    (A) Pure competition
    (B) A cartel
    (C) Monopoly
    (D) Oligarchy
    (E) Partnership

119. Which of the following is a disadvantage of organizing a business as a partnership?

    (A) Taxes are higher than on proprietorships.
    (B) It is easier to raise investment capital when the business is a proprietorship.
    (C) If one partner dies, the remaining partner(s) is (are) responsible for continuing the business.
    (D) Each partner is responsible for business actions taken by the other partner(s).
    (E) One partner can terminate the partnership

120. Which of the following men would least likely agree with the other four concerning man's basic nature?

    (A) Thomas Hobbes
    (B) Machiavelli
    (C) Louis XVI
    (D) Bishop Bossuet
    (E) John Locke

121. Which of the following was the only historical event that took place in the 20th century?

    (A) The First Continental Congress meets.
    (B) The Panama Canal is completed.
    (C) Latin American colonies become free as the Monroe Doctrine takes effect.
    (D) Thirteen colonies declare themselves the United States of America.
    (E) The United States enters the Spanish-American War.

122. In his famous book *Leviathan*, he reflects the basic principle that "without a supreme being all would be chaos." This quote was by

    (A) Locke
    (B) Hobbes
    (C) Montesquieu
    (D) Voltaire
    (E) Jefferson

123. If the following historical events below were placed in correct chronological order (with the earliest listed first) that order would be

   I. Stamp Act passed by Parliament
  II. Articles of Confederation are put in place
 III. French and Indian War
 IV. Declaration of Independence adopted

(A) III, II, I, and IV
(B) I, IV, II, III
(C) IV, II, III, I
(D) III, I, IV, II
(E) I, II, III, IV

124. Which sociologist is paired with his contribution in the field of sociology?

(A) Harlow—the Zimbardo experiments on human behavior
(B) Max Weber—study of folkways, norms, and mores
(C) Charles H. Cooley—the nature of primary groups
(D) William G. Sumner—defined the term "cultural universals of all societies"
(E) Emile Durkheim—the bureaucracy, the administrative hierarchy of society

125. Studies of feral children give support to the idea that

(A) man inherits most of his behavior patterns from his parents
(B) we must learn to function in society
(C) even if we are isolated from human society for a long period, we can easily learn to live according to its standards
(D) animals share most of the same qualities as man
(E) early childhood socialization has no effect on the early childhood development of said child

STOP

If there is still time remaining, you may review your answers.

ANSWER KEY
Sample Examination 1

SOCIAL SCIENCES–HISTORY

1.	A	33.	D	65.	D	97.	B
2.	C	34.	D	66.	A	98.	C
3.	B	35.	C	67.	D	99.	B
4.	B	36.	E	68.	C	100.	B
5.	C	37.	B	69.	C	101.	D
6.	B	38.	D	70.	D	102.	C
7.	D	39.	A	71.	D	103.	B
8.	D	40.	C	72.	D	104.	B
9.	A	41.	A	73.	E	105.	B
10.	E	42.	C	74.	D	106.	E
11.	D	43.	D	75.	B	107.	B
12.	D	44.	C	76.	E	108.	D
13.	E	45.	C	77.	C	109.	B
14.	C	46.	D	78.	A	110.	C
15.	E	47.	E	79.	C	111.	B
16.	D	48.	D	80.	C	112.	C
17.	C	49.	C	81.	B	113.	A
18.	C	50.	D	82.	D	114.	D
19.	E	51.	B	83.	C	115.	A
20.	B	52.	A	84.	B	116.	D
21.	A	53.	D	85.	B	117.	B
22.	D	54.	B	86.	C	118.	C
23.	C	55.	D	87.	B	119.	D
24.	B	56.	B	88.	E	120.	E
25.	A	57.	A	89.	C	121.	B
26.	D	58.	B	90.	A	122.	B
27.	D	59.	D	91.	A	123.	D
28.	E	60.	E	92.	C	124.	C
29.	C	61.	B	93.	E	125.	B
30.	D	62.	B	94.	E		
31.	A	63.	A	95.	C		
32.	C	64.	E	96.	C		

SCORING CHART

After you have scored your Sample Examination 1, enter the results in the chart below; then transfer your score to the Progress Chart on page 12.

Total Test	Number Right	Number Wrong	Number Omitted
125			

ANSWER EXPLANATIONS

1. **(A)** Each of the following time periods represent a postwar period (World War I, World War II, and the Viet Nam Conflict) in which inflation surfaced as each of these wars ended. Inflation after a war is rather common in American economics.

2. **(C)** During the 17th and 18th centuries a worldwide slave trade centered in Africa, where blacks were kidnapped by slavers and shipped to the Western Hemisphere, particularly the United States, where they were sold as slaves. Some two million people were involved in this forced migration.

3. **(B)** Ancient Sparta fits the description of a totalitarian state in that it controlled the lives of its people. For example, the state determined whether infants lived or died, how children were to be raised (put in state dormitories from seven on), and that the military was required for all men.

4. **(B)** Socialism is when the state controls the major industries and leaves small businesses to private ownership. Canada is an excellent example of a socialized state in which communications, medicine, and the like are government owned and run.

5. **(C)** Adam Smith (1723–1790), a Scottish economist, wrote *An Inquiry into the Nature and Causes of the Wealth of Nations*, an extremely influential book. In it he developed the theory, usually referred to as "laissez-faire" (let do), that economic forces should be allowed to operate without government interference.

6. **(B)** Ida B. Wells fought for an end to lynching, a terror tactic by whites trying to control black citizens in the south in the 1890s, by using the power of her pen in newspapers published in the United States and in England.

7. **(D)** Guerrilla tactics used by the Vietcong, South Vietnamese supporters of North Vietnam during the 1960s and early 1970s war against the United States, successfully fought the United States with its superior technology and weapons.

8. **(D)** Calvin believed that the fate of the individual was determined by God before birth. This doctrine is called predestination. The Puritans were followers of Calvin. They left England because they did not accept the doctrines of the Church of England.

9. **(A)** The automobile has altered courting patterns, contributed to obesity and heart disease, produced major industries, helped the growth of suburbs and helped to alter state-federal governmental relations. It is also a status symbol. None of the others fit this description.

10. **(E)** It is in the early years of our new nation that the practice of judicial review was established with the *Marbury* v. *Madison* case. Judicial review is the right of the Supreme Court to interpret a law and declare it unconstitutional.

11. **(D)** The Missouri Compromise of 1820 prohibited slavery in the territories north of 36°30′ except Missouri. Dred Scott, a slave, was taken into free territory and claimed his freedom. The Supreme Court ruled that Dred Scott remained a slave even in free territory. Thus, in effect the Court ruled the Missouri Compromise unconstitutional.

12. **(D)** Mercantilism was an economic system in which the monarchs of Europe supported a policy of exploration and colonization to extract as much wealth as possible from its possessions. During the time of absolutism and strong monarchs (15th–17th centuries), mercantilism was the most popular economic system, under which gold and silver was brought back from the New World.

13. **(E)** The immigration law of 1924 limited immigration to the United States from any country to 2 percent of the people of that nationality residing in the United States in 1890. This drastically reduced the numbers admitted from Eastern Europe and Southern Europe (Italy).

14. **(C)** During the mid to late 19th century, the only combination of European powers controlling colonies in Africa was Portugal and Spain. In fact, these two nations were among the last powers to allow colonial rule in Africa to end. Other Western imperialistic powers in Africa were England, France, Belgium, Italy, and Germany. Thus, choice B is the only correct combination.

15. **(E)** Czechoslovakia was forced to yield to Hitler's claim that the Sudetenland should be ceded to Germany because it contained a majority of ethnic Germans. Neville Chamberlain, Prime Minister of Great Britain, returned from Munich saying "I bring you peace in our time."

16. **(D)** Malthus' essay on population warned of the danger of the world becoming overpopulated. Food supply would not keep pace with the growth of population and therefore the world could become overpopulated. This belief helped justify and spread the idea of colonies being good for the mother country. Many European nations sent representatives to new colonies such as Kenya, South Africa, and so on.

17. **(C)** Mazzini was called "the soul of Italian unification." His belief that each nation had a special mission to perform to contribute to the welfare of humanity in general inspired the Italian people and caused them to fight for Italian unification. To help bring about unification, he organized this secret society in the 1830s.

18. **(C)** The Triple Entente consisted of France, Great Britain, and Russia, while the Triple Alliance consisted of Germany, Austria-Hungary, and Italy. These were formed in the early twentieth century, supposedly for defensive purposes. Yet, they really became two armed camps, dividing Europe in a dangerous manner.

19. **(E)** The Hawley-Smoot Act of 1930 was a tariff act. The others related to labor.

20. **(B)** Decisions of the United States Supreme Court are by a simple majority. Since 1869, the Court has consisted of nine judges. If all nine judges participate in a decision, a vote of five or more for or against the appellant determines the case.

21. **(A)** For over a century, the Hundred Years War (1337–1453) was fought between two rival nations, England and France. It was also the war in which Joan of Arc made her heroic appearance as a spark for the French forces. During the battle of Crecy in 1348, the British with their longbow routed the French soldiers. Eventually, the war ended in the French removing England from French soil.

22. **(D)** A primary group is closely knit, small in size, and usually has a long duration of contact. This small and closely knit group usually has intimate feelings for one another like a family. The best example noted is thus a girls' basketball team.

23. **(C)** Pasteur developed the germ theory of disease and showed that innoculation could prevent anthrax and tetanus.

24. **(B)** The self-sufficient manor (manorial system) was characterized by a self-contained community that had all the necessities of life. Trade was generally nonexistent, and, in general, a traditional and isolated lifestyle was common.

25. **(A)** The production possibility curve indicates the maximum output series of any two products. The two products often used as illustrations in economics are guns and butter. The curve shows the maximum output of either.

26. **(D)** Bismarck, the "iron chancellor," was the key to German unification. With his policy of "blood and iron" Bismarck brought unity to Germany by both war (blood) and industrialization (iron).

27. **(D)** Robert Owen was the founder of utopian socialism. He set up communities in both England and, later, the United States (New York). Although his model communities eventually failed, they put into motion the fundamental beliefs of socialism that were modified into present-day economic systems.

28. **(E)** Jeremy Bentham was one of several famous economic philosophers of the Industrial Revolution. Similar to the thinking of John Stuart Mill, his theory of utilitarianism was a 19th-century pre-Marxian belief that stated: "The aim of moral social and political action should be the largest possible balance of pleasure over pain; the greatest good and happiness for the greatest number; the useful is good and what is right should be the usefulness of its consequences."

29. **(C)** The factors responsible for the great decrease in the birth rate in the United States during the past 175 years include (1) decrease in the death rate particularly in childhood, (2) decline in the farm population, and (3) widespread adoption of family planning.

30. **(D)** *Nation-state* is a term that developed during the 13th and 14th centuries. As the Middle Ages came to a slow end, powerful lords, then kings, began to unite their smaller kingdoms into larger states or nations. England and France were two of the first nation-states that developed a feeling of oneness: one nation, one nationality, one common history, one tradition, one religion, and so on.

31. **(A)** It was the Mongolian Empire that extended from the China seas into Eastern Europe and reached as far south as the Black Sea. Long after the collapse of the Western Roman Empire, Genghis Khan had created the largest empire in human history.

32. **(C)** The most mild violation of social norms in our society today is divorce. Adultery, incest, polygamy, and theft are all violations of strict mores that we call laws.

33. **(D)** During colonial times, the greatest number of immigrants came from England. If one was to consider slavery, then Africans would also be right up there with the British. Throughout the colonial period, however, the next largest European immigrant was those of German ancestry.

34. **(D)** John Locke (1632–1704), English philosopher, expressed this idea in his *Two Treatises on Government* (1689). Jefferson had read Locke and may have gotten the idea from him but did not copy it directly when he wrote the Declaration of Independence.

35. **(C)** Both the 1890 census and Frederick Turner essay (1893) on the close of the American frontier led to national support that Manifest Destiny was over. If the American nation was going to expand any further, then it would have to go beyond its borders. This "close of the frontier" theory helped fuel further the growth of our naval power, imperial expansion (Spanish American War), and a new emotional arrogance called social Darwinism.

36. **(E)** Karl Marx (1818–1883), the father of socialism and communism, developed his ideas fully in his major work, *Das Kapital* (*Capital*). One of the ideas is that workers receive in wages only part of what they produce. The rest he called "surplus value."

37. **(B)** The first European settlers in South Africa were farmers from the Netherlands. They were called Boers from the Dutch word "boer" which means farmer.

38. **(D)** The Glorious Revolution in 1688 was a peaceful revolution that brought the fall of the Catholic Stuarts from the throne of England. It also established the supremacy of Parliament, making the king accountable to it. William and Mary of Orange accepted the crown only after they accepted the invitation by Parliament to rule, thus signifying Parliament's supremacy. This marked the evolution of England into a limited monarchy.

39. **(A)** Rudyard Kipling wrote this famous poem to symbolize European, or white men's, domination over African and Asian societies. It stresses the superiority of European over non-Western or inferior societies. It specifically refers to the people in the colonies as "half devil and half child." This poem also justifies social Darwinism, or survival of the fittest.

40. **(C)** The Slavs of southern and Eastern Europe were clearly influenced by the culture and religion of Byzantium. With the city Kiev on the Dnieper River, a great deal of cultural and trading contact began to occur with Byzantium. Vladimir I of Kiev converted to Orthodox Christianity; this was a direct result of Russian contact with Byzantium.

41. **(A)** Nationalism was a major cause of both world wars. Ever since the 19th century and the rapid growth of nationalism, this belief had continued to play a leading role, causing border disputes in the pre–World War I years and leading to the creation of alliance systems that were nationalistic in design. With the rise of fascist dictators in the post–World War I era, nationalism was a force for fascist nations to take over other territories.

42. **(C)** In the spring of 1900, a secret society, which Westerners called "The Boxers," started a rebellion in China against foreigners who were occupying their country. More

than 300 nationals of England, France, the United States, and other countries were killed.

43. **(D)** The pre-Columbian Inca empire had a population of 6,000,000 and territory extending over 650,000 square miles. It was centered in Cuzco, Peru.

44. **(C)** The 18th-century rulers Catherine II of Russia, Frederick II of Prussia, and Joseph II of Austria were inspired by the ideas of the 18th-century Enlightenment. They wished to introduce various reforms, such as liberal land laws, for the welfare of their subjects.

45. **(C)** After the defeat of the Dutch-speaking Boers in South Africa by the British in 1902, the Dutch Boers (farmers) left Cape Colony and made a "Great Trek" north into the interior of the country, where they established new settlements and farms.

46. **(D)** The Cold War began after World War II with the division of Germany into two parts. It was Winston Churchill in his famous speech who first used the term *iron curtain,* which described the separation of free Europe (Western Europe) from Communist Europe (Eastern Europe). The Cold War ended with the fall of the USSR and Berlin Wall in late 1989.

47. **(E)** The USSR represented the leader of the Communist world in the Cold War and as such organized the Communist response to NATO, which was the Warsaw Pact. This, like NATO, was a military alliance of the Communist-bloc countries committed to protecting the Communist world for democracy.

48. **(D)** West Germany was created in 1949 when the Russian-occupied eastern zone of Germany eventually became East Germany with its capital at Berlin. The remaining three occupied zones—England, France, and the United States—combined and thus created democratic West Germany. The new capital of this nation became Bonn. In the 1990s Germany reunited into one nation after the Cold War ended.

49. **(C)** In 1949, Yugoslavia was the only Communist-bloc nation to break away from the Communist hold of the Soviet Union. Other attempts were made by Hungary, Czechoslovakia, and Poland, but all failed to break away from the Soviet grasp.

50. **(D)** The best way in economics to define "saving" is to call it "refraining from consumption." It is in contrast to consuming all that is produced.

51. **(B)** "Marginal utility" in economics refers to the relation between supply and demand in determining the price of a commodity. High price implies big demand and small supply.

52. **(A)** The ranking of primates from lowest to highest (man) is as follows: prosimians, new-world monkeys (rhesus monkeys), old-world monkeys (baboons), gorillas (gibbons, orangutans, chimpanzees, gorillas) and finally, man.

53. **(D)** When people interact they tend to take one another into account and modify their behavior accordingly. This interaction is said to be reciprocal. Efforts to achieve behavior modification has attained importance in contemporary psychology.

54. **(B)** It was the Armenian genocide that took place during World War I and, in particular, the holocaust that occurred during the early 1940s that brought the human rights issue to the forefront in the postwar discussions. In 1948, soon after the UN was orga-

nized, it approved the Universal Declaration of Human Rights. This act set in motion a new modern movement to protect human rights worldwide.

55. **(D)** The Persian Gulf route provides access for oil leaving the Middle East for many industrialized nations.

56. **(B)** A "have not" or "developing" nation is not industrialized or modernized. It depends on traditional agriculture and herding, and thus a large farm labor force is necessary. Most of the population are farmers. Today, more and more of these nations are moving toward an industrialized economy.

57. **(A)** The French sociologist Emile Durkheim (1858–1917) used statistics to support his theories. He analyzed "mechanical" vs. "organic" solidarity. He held that religion and morality originate in the collective mind of society.

58. **(B)** In most patrilocal African societies, the most simple way to secure a wife was by purchase. This was widely accepted. It had no pejorative aspect.

59. **(D)** George Orwell wrote both books in the 1940s, reflecting his fears of a communistic totalitarian world. Thus both are attacks on communism and how a Communist world would result in the lack of any kind of freedom.

60. **(E)** Otto von Bismarck (1815–1898) was premier of Prussia from 1862 to 1890 and Chancellor of Germany from 1871 to 1890. He was called the "Iron Chancellor." The young Kaiser William II was jealous of him and dismissed him in 1890.

61. **(B)** In European Medieval agriculture, the three-field system was a method of rotating crops on the manor. In the absence of artificial fertilizers one of the three fields would lie fallow. The other two would be planted in crops different from the previous year. Exhaustion of the soil was avoided in this way.

62. **(B)** The founding fathers established the electoral college system for choosing a president and vice-president. They provided that the electors be chosen separately in each state and that no Senator or Representative or other United States officer could be an elector. They expected that partisan conflict over the election of a President would thus be avoided.

63. **(A)** Animism is a belief in nature, and therefore nature rules the society. This term was most often used to describe traditional African societies.

64. **(E)** Only Karl Marx said that industrialization must come before communism. Industrialization must make life difficult for the workers, and then they will rise up and create the proletariat revolution. All these other communist leaders recognized the need for the support of a larger peasant class who clearly outnumbered the proletariat force.

65. **(D)** The "Roman Empire" in the east continued to exist with its capital in Constantinople for more than ten centuries (5th to 15th centuries) after the decline and fall of Rome.

66. **(A)** Cults in the United States emerged in the 1960s as an alternative to the deteriorating American family. Several of the more famous cult movements in North America were the Jonestown cult and that of Reverend Moon. The Jonestown cult ended in massive suicide in Guyana.

67. **(D)** All of these reform bills in 19th-century England were a result of the Industrial Revolution changing the economic structure of the British masses. As the middle class and working class became more and more important, new laws protecting their civil liberties evolved, and new rights such as public education surfaced. Eventually both groups had better representation in the British Parliament.

68. **(C)** From the 1810s to 1820s Latin American nations revolted against the Spanish crown. Leaders such as Bolivar, Martin, and Father Hidalgo supported democratic governments in the Americas. In the end, the revolutions were generally successful and the Monroe Doctrine put the final chapter together, making the Western Hemisphere off-limits to further European colonization.

69. **(C)** The cure was administered by Louis Pasteur (1882–1895), the French bacteriologist. He had developed a vaccine that, in accordance with his theory, could conquer the dread disease hydrophobia (rabies).

70. **(D)** Ivan Petrovich Pavlov (1849–1936), the Russian physiologist, demonstrated the working of the conditioned reflex by an experiment on his dog. He rang a bell just before feeding his dog daily. Soon the dog would salivate when the bell rang and prior to (or regardless of) the feeding.

71. **(D)** The great need for laborers in our industries during World War II caused a great demand for the women laborer/worker. The female contribution to the war effort was rewarded with the beginning of the new "liberated" women. This eventually not only resulted in greater economic and social opportunities for women but also helped the growth of a much larger middle class (the two-income family).

72. **(D)** A strong movement to end "Jim Crowism" in the United States (unequal treatment of blacks) dates from World War II. The other events occurred during the last decade of the 19th century or first decade of the 20th century.

73. **(E)** The right to trial by jury is a procedure whereby substantive rights (freedom of speech, press, religion, etc.) may be protected.

74. **(D)** During the 19th century, European powers carved out colonies in Africa by asserting their military power against the Africans and against each other. Most of these colonies gained their independence after World War II.

75. **(B)** The clergy of Medieval Europe had to read and interpret the Bible (often available only in Hebrew, Greek and Aramaic). They also read the commentators (Aquinas) in Latin or in the newly emerging national languages. Thus, as students of religion, philosophy, and literature they were the intellectuals of their time.

76. **(E)** "The sun never sets on the British Empire" was an expression reflecting the vast size of the empire. England had colonies all over the globe, and thus the sun never set on the entire empire at one time. Colonies existed everywhere from the Caribbean to the Middle East to Africa and Asia. As a result, the British maintained one of the largest navies in modern history, and upon defeat of the Spanish Armada it was nicknamed "queen of the seas."

77. **(C)** On the eve of World War I (1913) Great Britain was the greatest naval power in the world. Germany had been building a fleet trying to catch up. The United States was becoming a naval power and had surpassed all but the top two.

78. **(A)** Henry VIII and the Tudor family created the first state-controlled religion in the Western world in 1534. With this "Act of Supremacy," Henry VIII officially broke away from the Church of Rome setting up the new Anglican Church of England.

79. **(C)** Winston Churchill led his country both militarily and psychologically through World War II. At one point, the British stood alone as the only democracy left in Europe after the onslaught of the Nazi war machine. He kept the British people together in both spirit and leadership. After the war, he warned the free world of the dangers of Russian communism and the spread of communistic ideology throughout Eastern Europe.

80. **(C)** Ho Chi Minh led Vietnam in its fight for independence against France. At the Battle of Dien Bien Phu the French army was defeated and driven from Indochina.

81. **(B)** After World War I the German government printed so many marks that by 1923 they were practically worthless. Debtors could easily pay off their debts. People on pensions received money that would buy little or nothing.

82. **(D)** Earl Warren was appointed Chief Justice of the United States Supreme Court in 1953 by President Eisenhower. Under his leadership the Court showed special concern for the civil liberties guaranteed by the Bill of Rights and the Fourteenth Amendment.

83. **(C)** *An American Dilemma*, written by the Swedish sociologist Gunnar Myrdal, was based on a study of the American Negro. It proved that the blacks in America were receiving inferior education and were victims of injustice.

84. **(B)** The Mayflower Compact, the Virginia House of Burgesses, and The Fundamental Orders of Connecticut were all significant steps in the growth of democracy in colonial America. With our democratic British heritage and other key events like the Zenger Trial, the young American nation logically developed into a democratic constitutional government.

85. **(B)** American marriage and divorce laws vary from state to state. Under the Constitution, laws about marriage and divorce are left up to the states, not to the federal government.

86. **(C)** Inflationary trends cause land values to rise rapidly. People on pensions or salaries, or holders of bonds with fixed interest rates, find that their income buys less because of inflation.

87. **(B)** Land, labor, and capital are all components of the factors of production under capitalism. Our capitalistic economy is influence by these components that also have an impact on the four variations of the business cycle.

88. **(E)** The rapid growth of our industrial economy during the second half of the 1800s was followed by an equally and rapidly growing labor movement. When collective behavior failed, workers and unions turned to protests and strikes. Several of the protests turned into violence and riots. The result was support for the business owners over labor by both the government and the public.

89. **(C)** The American family is regarded by sociologists as a new and developing form. Its distinguishing aspect is neither mother, father, ancient nor rural.

90. **(A)** The 1960s was a decade scared with violent protests and riots. Often these events were characterized by urban race riots and antiwar protests. Such was the case in Watts, Los Angeles, when a major race riot occurred in 1965. Sociologists have associated these antiwar protests (like Kent State) and race riots with the fundamental principles of collective behavior. Some of the components of collective behavior are emotional contagion, heightening suggestibility, and absence or weakness of social forms (a liberal society).

91. **(A)** In his *Protestant Ethic and the Spirit of Capitalism* (1920) Max Weber, the German sociologist, developed the idea that John Calvin's teaching about self-denial as a measure of spiritual discipline is closely related to the rise of capitalism.

92. **(C)** Ritual is a formal ceremony prescribed by a group. The form and content of the ceremony are followed exactly on each occasion. The symbolic significance (whether religious or political) is recognized by all members of the participating group.

93. **(E)** These were the words of the Emancipation Proclamation issued by President Abraham Lincoln September 22, 1862, to take effect January 1, 1863.

94. **(E)** All four traits are indicators of the highest level of primate development, that of man. Although apes are partial bipedalist (walk on two feet), their brains are approximately one-third the size of humans' (500–600 cc), their foramen magnum is more to the rear of the skull, and their teeth are more U-shaped. Thus, all four traits fit the description of humans.

95. **(C)** A "leftist" defined by the French Revolution was a liberal, a reformer, and thus someone who wanted change—in fact, quick change. The Jacobins were the true radicals, as they were later called, for they wanted a total end to the monarchy. The "right" were the loyalists or those who were antichange (status quo). Thus they were eventually labeled conservatives.

96. **(C)** At the conclusion of the Third Punic War in 146 B.C., Rome defeated its traditional rival, Carthage, in North Africa. The victor razed Carthage to the ground. This gave rise to the term "a Carthaginian peace."

97. **(B)** René Descartes (1596–1650), French philosopher, mathematician, and scientist, said: "I proposed never to accept anything for true which I do not clearly know to be such." He is best known for his saying: "I think, therefore I am."

98. **(C)** "The marginal propensity to consume" refers, in economics, to the extra amount that people will want to spend on consumption if given an extra dollar of income.

99. **(B)** In an effort to counteract a depression or recession, Federal Reserve Banks might decrease the interest rate charged commercial banks. This would make it easier for banks to lend money to business. This, in turn, would help business to continue to function.

100. **(B)** The Mullahs are Muslim religious teachers trained in traditional Islamic law and doctrine.

101. **(D)** A grand jury is a group of citizens that examines the evidence against a person accused of a serious crime. If the evidence warrants, the grand jury brings formal charges. Then the accused must stand trial.

102. **(C)** Justices of the Supreme Court who disagree with the majority of the Court may prepare a dissenting opinion. In the dissent, the justice states his reason for disagreement.

103. **(B)** The U.S. Supreme Court is the "supreme law of the land." With the addition of judicial review, the highest court makes all final decisions. Possibly the best example was the effect it had on the 2000 presidential election when it ruled in favor of the Bush candidacy in the Florida recount.

104. **(B)** The Albany Congress met in 1754. The Stamp Act Congress met in 1765, the First Continental Congress in 1774, and the Second Continental Congress in 1775. The Articles of Confederation were drawn up in 1778.

105. **(B)** The late 1930s was marked by a policy of appeasement in order to avoid a second world war. The most significant example of appeasement was the Munich Conference in 1938 when the Allies allowed Hitler to occupy the Sudetenland in Czechoslovakia. Shortly thereafter, the Nazis invaded and took over the entire Czech nation. The invasion of Poland in 1939 marked the beginning of World War II and the failure of the Allies' "policy of appeasement."

106. **(E)** The American historian Frederick Jackson Turner (1861–1932) published *The Significance of the Frontier in American History* in 1893. He showed that the frontier exercised the greatest influence on American institutions.

107. **(B)** The Meiji Restoration in Japan (1867–1868) was the beginning of Japan's modernization. The emperor regained power after the Shogunate was overthrown. Then Japan proceeded with modernization along western lines.

108. **(D)** Herbert Spencer (1820–1903), British sociologist, made this statement. He applied the idea of biological evolution to social institutions.

109. **(B)** These primitive technological societies are nearly extinct today but provide us with invaluable insights to how man may have lived thousands of years ago. They were generally hunters and gatherers except for the Nuer, who were herders. These cultures that once existed in the early 20th century were absorbed by the modern shrinking world and are by and large non-existent today.

110. **(C)** Most bills do not become laws. Bills can start off in either house except that money bills must start off in the House of Representatives. Instrumental to the process is the work of standing committees and subcommittees that are used once a bill is introduced. Also, if a bill is on its way to becoming a possible law and the two houses don't agree to the wording, then the bill goes to a conference committee.

111. **(B)** In his book *The Third Wave,* Alvin Toffler discusses the deterioration of the traditional American family (Norman Rockwell type). Such alternative family configurations include single parents, remarriages, group families, and gay families.

112. **(C)** The concept of anomie is used to describe our society where norms of conduct and belief have been weakened or have actually broken down.

113. **(A)** These two famous cultural anthropologists studied the lifestyles of isolated societies that took us back to the early days of the hunter and gatherer. They provide invaluable insights into how humankind may have lived 10,000 years ago.

114. **(D)** The Congo territory was explored and exploited under the leadership of King Leopold II of Belgium. The Congo, in south central Africa, was known as the Belgian Congo until it gained its independence in 1960.

115. **(A)** Genghis Khan was the leader of a nomadic people of Central Asia. Under Genghis Khan's leadership, the Mongols invaded Europe during the 13th century and caused havoc in Poland, Hungary, and much of Russia.

116. **(D)** Marx and Engels developed the idea of scientific socialism that later became known as communism. Basic ideas of this philosophy included surplus value, which is the profit that ends up in the pockets of the capitalist; class conflict, in which the proletariat is in constant battle with the bourgeoisie capitalist; and the inevitability of a proletariat revolution, in which the workers will eventually rise up and overthrow the capitalistic society.

117. **(B)** Limited liability is a major advantage of a corporation in that the corporation can be sued but the individual owners cannot be.

118. **(C)** A public utility is usually a monopoly. The advantage of this is that it is more efficient. Since the breakup of the AT&T phone company, it is easy to comprehend why public utilities should be organized into monopolies.

119. **(D)** One of the major disadvantages of a partnership is that if one partner does something wrong or is corrupt or even inefficient, the other partner(s) is(are) affected. Thus, in a lawsuit, one partner can indeed carry his crime or guilt to his fellow partner or partners.

120. **(E)** John Locke is the true liberal in the group in that he believed in protecting the rights of the individual. Hobbes, Louis XIV, and Bossuet were all supporters of the theory of absolute monarchy and divine right. Machiavelli believed in the power of strong princes that should rule with force. Thus John Locke stands alone as the people's man.

121. **(B)** The only event occurring in the 20th century was the completion of the Panama Canal. The First Continental Congress and the Declaration of Independence by the thirteen colonies occurred in the 18th century. Latin American colonies were freed in the early 19th century, and the Spanish-American War began in 1898.

122. **(B)** In 1651, Thomas Hobbes completed his most famous book, *Leviathan*. This book describes a powerful sea monster in the Bible that is suppose to represent that government (absolute monarchy) must be all-powerful and absolute.

123. **(D)** The French and Indian War—the war between England (and the American colonists) and France (and her Indian allies)—began on the Pennsylvania frontier in 1754. Parliament passed the Stamp Act as a revenue measure in 1765, two years after the war ended. Fifty-five delegates to the First Continental Congress met in Philadelphia beginning September 5, 1774. The Declaration of Independence was adopted by the Second Continental Congress on July 4, 1776. In February 1778, Benjamin Franklin negotiated a treaty of recognition with France and a second treaty creating a formal military alliance.

124. **(C)** Charles H. Cooley was one of the founders of sociology and is particularly known for his work and analysis of primary groups. William G. Sumner is considered the expert on analysis of societies norms. His book *Folkways* discusses the different levels

of intensity that society puts in place to regulate its people (norms = folkways, mores, laws). Emile Durkheim's lifelong interest was the study of suicide and he was one of the first sociologists to use statistical methods of research. Max Weber spent most of his life studying bureaucracy, law, and politics.

125. **(B)** Feral children were kept secluded and isolated by unfit parents. The difficulty to adjust to real life and become socialized shows that socialization is truly a learning process. We are socialized by our environment, which includes our family, friends, and peers. Socialization is critical to the normal development of children. Feral children were denied this right when they grew up in this secluded and isolated environment.

ANSWER SHEET
Sample Examination 2

SOCIAL SCIENCES–HISTORY

1. Ⓐ Ⓑ Ⓒ Ⓓ Ⓔ   33. Ⓐ Ⓑ Ⓒ Ⓓ Ⓔ   65. Ⓐ Ⓑ Ⓒ Ⓓ Ⓔ   97. Ⓐ Ⓑ Ⓒ Ⓓ Ⓔ
2. Ⓐ Ⓑ Ⓒ Ⓓ Ⓔ   34. Ⓐ Ⓑ Ⓒ Ⓓ Ⓔ   66. Ⓐ Ⓑ Ⓒ Ⓓ Ⓔ   98. Ⓐ Ⓑ Ⓒ Ⓓ Ⓔ
3. Ⓐ Ⓑ Ⓒ Ⓓ Ⓔ   35. Ⓐ Ⓑ Ⓒ Ⓓ Ⓔ   67. Ⓐ Ⓑ Ⓒ Ⓓ Ⓔ   99. Ⓐ Ⓑ Ⓒ Ⓓ Ⓔ
4. Ⓐ Ⓑ Ⓒ Ⓓ Ⓔ   36. Ⓐ Ⓑ Ⓒ Ⓓ Ⓔ   68. Ⓐ Ⓑ Ⓒ Ⓓ Ⓔ   100. Ⓐ Ⓑ Ⓒ Ⓓ Ⓔ
5. Ⓐ Ⓑ Ⓒ Ⓓ Ⓔ   37. Ⓐ Ⓑ Ⓒ Ⓓ Ⓔ   69. Ⓐ Ⓑ Ⓒ Ⓓ Ⓔ   101. Ⓐ Ⓑ Ⓒ Ⓓ Ⓔ
6. Ⓐ Ⓑ Ⓒ Ⓓ Ⓔ   38. Ⓐ Ⓑ Ⓒ Ⓓ Ⓔ   70. Ⓐ Ⓑ Ⓒ Ⓓ Ⓔ   102. Ⓐ Ⓑ Ⓒ Ⓓ Ⓔ
7. Ⓐ Ⓑ Ⓒ Ⓓ Ⓔ   39. Ⓐ Ⓑ Ⓒ Ⓓ Ⓔ   71. Ⓐ Ⓑ Ⓒ Ⓓ Ⓔ   103. Ⓐ Ⓑ Ⓒ Ⓓ Ⓔ
8. Ⓐ Ⓑ Ⓒ Ⓓ Ⓔ   40. Ⓐ Ⓑ Ⓒ Ⓓ Ⓔ   72. Ⓐ Ⓑ Ⓒ Ⓓ Ⓔ   104. Ⓐ Ⓑ Ⓒ Ⓓ Ⓔ
9. Ⓐ Ⓑ Ⓒ Ⓓ Ⓔ   41. Ⓐ Ⓑ Ⓒ Ⓓ Ⓔ   73. Ⓐ Ⓑ Ⓒ Ⓓ Ⓔ   105. Ⓐ Ⓑ Ⓒ Ⓓ Ⓔ
10. Ⓐ Ⓑ Ⓒ Ⓓ Ⓔ   42. Ⓐ Ⓑ Ⓒ Ⓓ Ⓔ   74. Ⓐ Ⓑ Ⓒ Ⓓ Ⓔ   106. Ⓐ Ⓑ Ⓒ Ⓓ Ⓔ
11. Ⓐ Ⓑ Ⓒ Ⓓ Ⓔ   43. Ⓐ Ⓑ Ⓒ Ⓓ Ⓔ   75. Ⓐ Ⓑ Ⓒ Ⓓ Ⓔ   107. Ⓐ Ⓑ Ⓒ Ⓓ Ⓔ
12. Ⓐ Ⓑ Ⓒ Ⓓ Ⓔ   44. Ⓐ Ⓑ Ⓒ Ⓓ Ⓔ   76. Ⓐ Ⓑ Ⓒ Ⓓ Ⓔ   108. Ⓐ Ⓑ Ⓒ Ⓓ Ⓔ
13. Ⓐ Ⓑ Ⓒ Ⓓ Ⓔ   45. Ⓐ Ⓑ Ⓒ Ⓓ Ⓔ   77. Ⓐ Ⓑ Ⓒ Ⓓ Ⓔ   109. Ⓐ Ⓑ Ⓒ Ⓓ Ⓔ
14. Ⓐ Ⓑ Ⓒ Ⓓ Ⓔ   46. Ⓐ Ⓑ Ⓒ Ⓓ Ⓔ   78. Ⓐ Ⓑ Ⓒ Ⓓ Ⓔ   110. Ⓐ Ⓑ Ⓒ Ⓓ Ⓔ
15. Ⓐ Ⓑ Ⓒ Ⓓ Ⓔ   47. Ⓐ Ⓑ Ⓒ Ⓓ Ⓔ   79. Ⓐ Ⓑ Ⓒ Ⓓ Ⓔ   111. Ⓐ Ⓑ Ⓒ Ⓓ Ⓔ
16. Ⓐ Ⓑ Ⓒ Ⓓ Ⓔ   48. Ⓐ Ⓑ Ⓒ Ⓓ Ⓔ   80. Ⓐ Ⓑ Ⓒ Ⓓ Ⓔ   112. Ⓐ Ⓑ Ⓒ Ⓓ Ⓔ
17. Ⓐ Ⓑ Ⓒ Ⓓ Ⓔ   49. Ⓐ Ⓑ Ⓒ Ⓓ Ⓔ   81. Ⓐ Ⓑ Ⓒ Ⓓ Ⓔ   113. Ⓐ Ⓑ Ⓒ Ⓓ Ⓔ
18. Ⓐ Ⓑ Ⓒ Ⓓ Ⓔ   50. Ⓐ Ⓑ Ⓒ Ⓓ Ⓔ   82. Ⓐ Ⓑ Ⓒ Ⓓ Ⓔ   114. Ⓐ Ⓑ Ⓒ Ⓓ Ⓔ
19. Ⓐ Ⓑ Ⓒ Ⓓ Ⓔ   51. Ⓐ Ⓑ Ⓒ Ⓓ Ⓔ   83. Ⓐ Ⓑ Ⓒ Ⓓ Ⓔ   115. Ⓐ Ⓑ Ⓒ Ⓓ Ⓔ
20. Ⓐ Ⓑ Ⓒ Ⓓ Ⓔ   52. Ⓐ Ⓑ Ⓒ Ⓓ Ⓔ   84. Ⓐ Ⓑ Ⓒ Ⓓ Ⓔ   116. Ⓐ Ⓑ Ⓒ Ⓓ Ⓔ
21. Ⓐ Ⓑ Ⓒ Ⓓ Ⓔ   53. Ⓐ Ⓑ Ⓒ Ⓓ Ⓔ   85. Ⓐ Ⓑ Ⓒ Ⓓ Ⓔ   117. Ⓐ Ⓑ Ⓒ Ⓓ Ⓔ
22. Ⓐ Ⓑ Ⓒ Ⓓ Ⓔ   54. Ⓐ Ⓑ Ⓒ Ⓓ Ⓔ   86. Ⓐ Ⓑ Ⓒ Ⓓ Ⓔ   118. Ⓐ Ⓑ Ⓒ Ⓓ Ⓔ
23. Ⓐ Ⓑ Ⓒ Ⓓ Ⓔ   55. Ⓐ Ⓑ Ⓒ Ⓓ Ⓔ   87. Ⓐ Ⓑ Ⓒ Ⓓ Ⓔ   119. Ⓐ Ⓑ Ⓒ Ⓓ Ⓔ
24. Ⓐ Ⓑ Ⓒ Ⓓ Ⓔ   56. Ⓐ Ⓑ Ⓒ Ⓓ Ⓔ   88. Ⓐ Ⓑ Ⓒ Ⓓ Ⓔ   120. Ⓐ Ⓑ Ⓒ Ⓓ Ⓔ
25. Ⓐ Ⓑ Ⓒ Ⓓ Ⓔ   57. Ⓐ Ⓑ Ⓒ Ⓓ Ⓔ   89. Ⓐ Ⓑ Ⓒ Ⓓ Ⓔ   121. Ⓐ Ⓑ Ⓒ Ⓓ Ⓔ
26. Ⓐ Ⓑ Ⓒ Ⓓ Ⓔ   58. Ⓐ Ⓑ Ⓒ Ⓓ Ⓔ   90. Ⓐ Ⓑ Ⓒ Ⓓ Ⓔ   122. Ⓐ Ⓑ Ⓒ Ⓓ Ⓔ
27. Ⓐ Ⓑ Ⓒ Ⓓ Ⓔ   59. Ⓐ Ⓑ Ⓒ Ⓓ Ⓔ   91. Ⓐ Ⓑ Ⓒ Ⓓ Ⓔ   123. Ⓐ Ⓑ Ⓒ Ⓓ Ⓔ
28. Ⓐ Ⓑ Ⓒ Ⓓ Ⓔ   60. Ⓐ Ⓑ Ⓒ Ⓓ Ⓔ   92. Ⓐ Ⓑ Ⓒ Ⓓ Ⓔ   124. Ⓐ Ⓑ Ⓒ Ⓓ Ⓔ
29. Ⓐ Ⓑ Ⓒ Ⓓ Ⓔ   61. Ⓐ Ⓑ Ⓒ Ⓓ Ⓔ   93. Ⓐ Ⓑ Ⓒ Ⓓ Ⓔ   125. Ⓐ Ⓑ Ⓒ Ⓓ Ⓔ
30. Ⓐ Ⓑ Ⓒ Ⓓ Ⓔ   62. Ⓐ Ⓑ Ⓒ Ⓓ Ⓔ   94. Ⓐ Ⓑ Ⓒ Ⓓ Ⓔ
31. Ⓐ Ⓑ Ⓒ Ⓓ Ⓔ   63. Ⓐ Ⓑ Ⓒ Ⓓ Ⓔ   95. Ⓐ Ⓑ Ⓒ Ⓓ Ⓔ
32. Ⓐ Ⓑ Ⓒ Ⓓ Ⓔ   64. Ⓐ Ⓑ Ⓒ Ⓓ Ⓔ   96. Ⓐ Ⓑ Ⓒ Ⓓ Ⓔ

SAMPLE SOCIAL SCIENCES–HISTORY EXAMINATION 2

Number of Questions: 125

TIME LIMIT: 90 MINUTES

> **DIRECTIONS:** Each of the questions or incomplete statements below is followed by five suggested answers or completions. Select the one that is best in each case.

MAP A
EUROPE   1945–1990

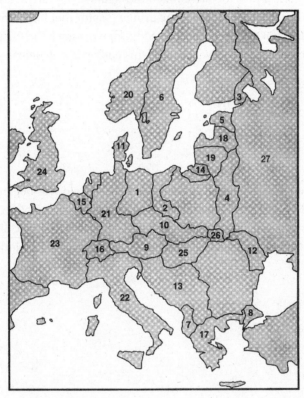

Questions 1–4 refer to Map A.

1. This nation has been the home of the Nazi party since the 1930s. As a fascist nation, it began to invade neighboring nations and actually began World War II when it invaded Poland in 1939.

   (A) 21
   (B) 15
   (C) 24
   (D) 23
   (E) 20

2. It was invaded by Hitler in 1938 when the Nazis took over the Sudetenland region, an area populated with many Germans. Several months later the rest of this nation was successfully taken over by the Nazi army. During the Cold War, this nation attempted to break away from the Soviet-bloc world when its leader, Dubchek, supported a reform movement for civil liberties.

(A) 24
(B) 22
(C) 21
(D) 10
(E) 23

3. A famous general and leader assembled the "grand army" in an attempt to defeat Russia, but the winter of 1812 was the primary factor that led to the grand army's loss. Of the 600,000 soldiers who crossed Europe to attack the Russian Empire, approximately 50,000 returned home in this embarrassing defeat.

(A) 1
(B) 23
(C) 22
(D) 24
(E) 4

4. This nation adapted communism shortly after the Cold War began. However, in 1948, under their leader Tito, this communist nation broke away from "satellites" status and became a trading partner with the United States. After the Cold War ended in the late 20th century, this former communist nation broke into six independent nations. This country is

(A) 10
(B) 13
(C) 17
(D) 22
(E) 24

_____

5. The holding company is possible only because

(A) many stockholders do not permit proxies
(B) some securities do not have voting rights
(C) corporations are permitted to hold stock in other corporations
(D) courts do not enforce the law
(E) stocks can be bought on margin

6. The Securities and Exchange Commission is designed to regulate the securities business for the benefit of

   (A) small business
   (B) the consumer
   (C) the investor
   (D) labor
   (E) the banking system

7. Adolescent-parent tensions have continued to evolve in America because

   (A) there is an increase in the patriarchal nature of the American family
   (B) the youth subculture or generation gap continues to be a part of teen life
   (C) families are getting larger and larger in our society
   (D) single-parent families have become the most common family structure
   (E) religion has failed to bring families closer together

8. The term *secular power* in medieval European history would be used to describe the powers of a

   (A) king or emperor
   (B) pope
   (C) bishop
   (D) church council
   (E) cardinal

9. A campaign speech was made containing a reference to "two chickens in every pot." What event occurred shortly after the speech which made this reference seem ironic?

   (A) Pullman transportation strike in 1894
   (B) Defeat of the Populists in 1896
   (C) Election of Alfred E. Smith in 1928
   (D) Stock market crash in 1929
   (E) Rationing of gasoline after 1941

10. Levittown is a place and a term that describes

   (A) the shantytowns established during the Depression
   (B) the average American town studied by Robert and Helen Merell Lynd
   (C) the new suburbia that emerged in the 1950s
   (D) a utopian society
   (E) the ideal life depicted on television

11. Which law passed by Congress was part of FDR's New Deal legislation?

   (A) Homestead Act
   (B) Pendleton Act
   (C) Social Security Act
   (D) Morrill Act for education
   (E) Pure Food and Drug Act

12. Which of these ancient empires was geographically the largest?

   (A) Egyptian
   (B) Persian
   (C) Assyrian
   (D) Chaldean
   (E) Hittite

13. Which of the following languages has been the spoken and written word for the Roman Catholic Church?

   (A) Arabic
   (B) Sanskrit
   (C) Greek
   (D) Italian
   (E) Latin

14. Monetary policy in the United States is administered by

   (A) Congress
   (B) the President
   (C) the Federal Reserve Board of Governors
   (D) the Department of Commerce
   (E) the Council of Economic Advisors

15. According to Thomas Malthus' "principle of population," the means of subsistence of a population

   (A) can keep pace with a rapidly increasing population if new agricultural technologies are continually adopted
   (B) cannot possibly increase faster than in arithmetical progression
   (C) normally increases in geometrical progression
   (D) is subject to the iron law of marginally increasing returns
   (E) is dependent on the cultural background of the people

16. The belief in reincarnation is an important part of

   (A) Judaism
   (B) Confucius' teachings
   (C) Hinduism
   (D) Zoroastrianism
   (E) Islam

17. The total value (in dollars) of goods and services produced in the American economy during the year is called the

    (A) net national income
    (B) gross private domestic investment
    (C) gross national product
    (D) net producers domestic gain
    (E) net national product

18. In sociology and psychology, *drives* such as thirst, sex, and hunger are

    (A) behavior that must always be suppressed
    (B) factors which incite behavior in the individual
    (C) glands which secrete endocrines
    (D) mysterious forces which induce people to commit crimes
    (E) called norms

Questions 19–22 pertain to this map.

MAP B
SOUTH AND SOUTHEAST ASIA 1947–1954

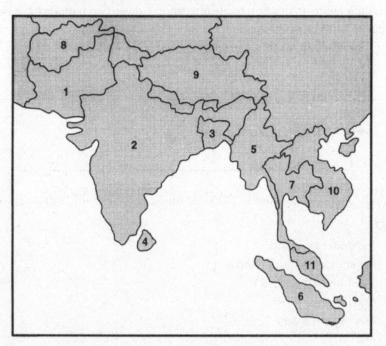

19. This Southeast Asia nation was once a French colony and later, like Korea, was split in two as a result of the Cold War. Today it is once again united under a communist government. This country is

    (A) 5
    (B) 7
    (C) 10
    (D) 11
    (E) 12

20. Which country was ruled until 1959 by a Buddhist religious leader called the Dalai Lama?

(A) 2
(B) 4
(C) 5
(D) 7
(E) 9

21. Nicknamed the "jewel of the British crown," this colony eventually received its independence in 1947 but was split into several new states because of its Hindu majority.

(A) 2
(B) 5
(C) 10
(D) 11
(E) 12

22. In the short history of these two new, independent nations, constant conflict over border disputes and religion have continued to create political and social tension. With their ability to develop nuclear weapons, these two nations have become a global concern in the 21st century.

(A) 2 and 1
(B) 9 and 12
(C) 7 and 10
(D) 1 and 8
(E) 1 and 3

---

23. Both the Peter Zenger case in 1735 and the Schenck case of 1919 dealt with the issue of

(A) freedom of religion
(B) separation of church and state
(C) freedom of the press
(D) due process
(E) blacks' civil rights

24. The United States automobile industry is an example of

(A) monopoly
(B) monopolistic competition
(C) a cartel
(D) holding company
(E) oligarchy

25. In a free market economy, price tends to fall whenever

 (A) the quantity supplied increases more rapidly than the quantity demanded
 (B) the quantity demanded increases more rapidly than the quantity supplied
 (C) supply and demand are equal
 (D) both supply and demand increase
 (E) more of a commodity is produced in a mass production technology

26. Nelson Mandela and F.W. de Klerk served notice that "the moral high ground is no longer big enough for both of them." What happened in South Africa to prompt newspapers to discuss these two men?

 (A) The Nobel Peace Prize was being taken away from them by the Nobel Committee.
 (B) A full-scale campaign for the first national election open to all races took place with Nelson Mandela becoming president.
 (C) The National Party and the African National Congress decided to join as a single party under one of these two dynamic leaders.
 (D) Mr. de Klerk decided to step down as president and allow Mr. Mandela, the "true leader who has freed South Africa," to lead the country for the next four years.
 (E) The two leaders agreed that an international peacekeeping agency was needed to end the moral wrongs of apartheid.

27. Nearly half a million years ago, one of the greatest inventions of all time took place. It enabled humankind to survive a rough, challenging environment. This great invention was

 (A) fire
 (B) agriculture
 (C) wheel
 (D) permanent dwellings
 (E) domesticated animals

28. Which event slowed down the growth and spread of communism?

 (A) The rise of labor unions and pro labor legislation in capitalistic nations
 (B) Lenin's call for a proletariat revolution in Czarist Russia
 (C) Mao Tse Tung agrarian revolution in China
 (D) Labor abuses in the early days of the Industrial Revolution
 (E) The suppression of labor movements in England

29. According to the latest U.S. census report,

 (A) men are living longer than women
 (B) the farm population has shown a surprising growth
 (C) the senior citizen population is growing rapidly
 (D) we have hit zero population growth
 (E) large numbers of people are moving from suburbs to cities

30. Supreme Court justices are

 (A) appointed by the president
 (B) nominated by the Senate and approved by the House
 (C) chosen by electors of the Electoral College
 (D) elected by the populace
 (E) nominated by the president and approved by the Senate

31. In the history of the presidency until 1974, there had never been an instance of

 (A) a vice president becoming president
 (B) a president failing to be elected by the electoral college
 (C) the election of a president by the House of Representatives
 (D) the resignation of a president
 (E) the assassination of a president

32. What do these three amendments have in common?

 ■ Amendment XIII
 ■ Amendment XIV
 ■ Amendment XV

 (A) They all deal with civil rights after the Civil War
 (B) They limit the powers of the presidency
 (C) They are nicknamed the Bill of Rights
 (D) They all deal with the prohibition era
 (E) They increase the power of the federal government

33. "The American expansionists and imperialists of the 1890s appealed to biological evolution and economic and social history (referred to as Social Darwinism) to support their views." Social Darwinism is associated with which of the following American events:

 (A) Entrance into World War I
 (B) Civil War
 (C) Kellogg-Briand Pact
 (D) Spanish American War
 (E) Entrance into World War II

34. The interest which Russia historically manifested in the Dardanelles arose from a desire to have an outlet to the

 (A) Black Sea
 (B) Yellow Sea
 (C) North Sea
 (D) Mediterranean Sea
 (E) Red Sea

35. "L'état, c'est moi." This statement is attributed to

(A) Louis XVI
(B) Louis XV
(C) Louis XIV
(D) Louis XIII
(E) Louis X

36. After the Franco-Prussian War completed the unification of Germany, the German Imperial constitution

(A) made the Prussian king, Kaiser Wilhelm II, the new emperor
(B) was a generally democratic instrument
(C) declared the equality of all member states
(D) declared Metternich the ruler of Austria to be emperor of the Empire
(E) made Roman Catholicism the state religion'

37. In *The Prince*, Machiavelli counsels a ruler that

(A) it is better to be feared than loved
(B) it is better to be loved than feared
(C) he need not worry about arousing the hatred of his subjects
(D) it is best to be both feared and hated
(E) it is better to be truthful with one's subjects

38. The father of anthropology who was the first to prove that man's origin was in sub-Saharan Africa and was known for the discoveries of Zinjanthropus and Australopithecus (discovered in Olduvai Gorge) was

(A) Richard Leakey
(B) George Mendel
(C) Charles Dawson
(D) Louis Leakey
(E) Jacques DePerthes

39. Which pair of words or phrases best describes a cause-and-effect relationship in connection with "the final solution"?

(A) putsch—Nordic supremacy theory
(B) Kristallnacht—rise of the Third Reich
(C) Babi Yar massacre—passage of the Nuremberg Laws
(D) master race theory—genocide
(E) Warsaw Ghetto Uprising—construction of Auschwitz

40. Which Roman emperor ended polytheism by making Christianity the official religion of Rome?

(A) Julius Caesar
(B) Constantine
(C) Octavian
(D) Nero
(E) Marcus Aurelius

41. The most significant agent of childhood socialization is

(A) the peer group
(B) television
(C) religious training
(D) the family
(E) school

42. The Standard Oil trust was originally organized by

(A) Carnegie
(B) Morgan
(C) Vanderbilt
(D) Rockefeller
(E) Gould

43. Which issue in France was significant in the Dreyfus Affair?

(A) Revolutionist
(B) Anti-Semitism
(C) Supremacy of the pope
(D) Reign of terror
(E) Absolutism

44. Bismarck, after 1851, believed that Germany could become strong and united only if

(A) Austria was excluded from German affairs
(B) she became a republic
(C) Austria became the leader
(D) Italy remained divided into small states
(E) colonies could be gained for Germany

45. The Zulus are

(A) Bantus who fought the British in South Africa
(B) the aboriginal peoples of Australia
(C) the French Protestant settlers in South Africa
(D) a people who lived in New Zealand before the coming of the British
(E) a group of Irish revolutionaries

46. A new currency emerged in the mid 1990s in this geographical region that symbolizes both an economic and social bond among their people. This area/region is

   (A) Latin America
   (B) The Caribbean
   (C) Europe
   (D) Southeast Asia
   (E) Russia

47. Which of the following programs of social reform would be, according to the thought of Malthus, based on a correct analysis of the problem of poverty?

   (A) Universal education at public expense
   (B) Guaranteed minimum wage
   (C) Social security
   (D) Consumer subsidies
   (E) Aid to dependent children

48. If people do not consume all their income, but put the unspent amount into a pillow or buy an old security with it, in national income and product terms they are

   (A) saving but not investing
   (B) investing but not saving
   (C) both saving and investing
   (D) neither saving nor investing
   (E) saving, but investing only to the extent that they buy old securities

49. Which of the following is *least* common in our society?

   (A) Group marriage
   (B) Divorce
   (C) Illegitimacy
   (D) Intercourse before marriage
   (E) Homosexuality

50. The student demonstrations for democracy in Tiananmen Square in China were

   (A) violent attacks on government buildings by students
   (B) given relatively little attention from anyone
   (C) allowed to continue peacefully by the government
   (D) attempted to improve academic conditions in school
   (E) suppressed violently by the Chinese government

51. When sociologists talk of "social mobility," they usually have in mind

    (A) horizontal mobility
    (B) interracial marriage
    (C) vertical mobility
    (D) rapid social retrogression
    (E) moral progress

52. The use of canoes and moccasins by the whites are examples of

    (A) parallel inventions
    (B) cultural diffusion
    (C) cultural assimilation
    (D) social mobility
    (E) cultural isolation

53. Which political-economic system practiced the belief that government must be aggressively involved in order to control the success and growth of the economy of a nation?

    (A) Mercantilism
    (B) Capitalism as defined by Adam Smith
    (C) Scientific communism—the fundamental principles of Engel and Marx
    (D) Laissez faire economics
    (E) Manorialism

54. Which of the following was Veblen's attitude toward marginal utility economics? He considered it

    (A) analytically proper
    (B) overly inductive and oriented to biology
    (C) collectivist in its implications
    (D) overly deductive, individualistic, and static
    (E) too strongly oriented to the labor movement

55. In the late 19th century, competitive companies in one field entered into agreements to fix prices. When railroad companies in the 1880s engaged in this kind of activity, they were in fact forming

    (A) pools
    (B) conglomerates
    (C) monopolies
    (D) trusts
    (E) corporations

Questions 56 and 57 refer to the following chart.

U.S. Presidential Elections
1876–1888

Year	Candidates	(Party)	Popular Vote	Electoral Vote
1876	Rutherford B. Hayes	(R)*	4,036,572	185
	Samuel J. Tilden	(D)	4,284,020	184
1880	James A. Garfield	(R)*	4,453,295	214
	Winfield S. Hancock	(D)	4,414,082	155
	James B. Weaver (Greenback-Labor)		308,578	0
1884	Grover Cleveland	(D)*	4,879,507	219
	James G. Blaine	(R)	4,850,293	182
	Benjamin F. Butler (Greenback-Labor)		175,370	0
	John P. St. John (Prohibition)		150,369	0
1888	Benjamin Harrison	(R)*	5,477,129	233
	Grover Cleveland	(D)	5,537,857	168
	Clinton B. Fisk (Prohibition)		249,506	0
	Anson J. Streeter (Union-Labor)		146,935	0

*R = Republican; D = Democrat

56. What would be another appropriate title for the above chart?

(A) The crucial importance of the popular vote in electing the president
(B) The rapid growth of the American electorate
(C) The incumbent's advantage in an election
(D) How the electoral college system operates
(E) The influence of third parties in election outcomes

57. According to the chart, if one favored the direct election of the president by way of the people's vote replacing the electoral vote, one would turn to the election of

(A) 1876
(B) 1880 and 1884
(C) 1884
(D) 1888
(E) 1876 and 1888

58. In 1987, America's Bicentennial observance celebrated the writing of the

    (A) Declaration of Independence
    (B) Monroe Doctrine
    (C) Bill of Rights
    (D) Emancipation Proclamation
    (E) Constitution

59. Which of the following presidents was the only one to serve two full terms?

    (A) President John F. Kennedy
    (B) President Lyndon Baines Johnson
    (C) President Bill Clinton
    (D) President Richard M. Nixon
    (E) President George H. Bush

60. Which is a valid conclusion that can be drawn from the fact that many large cities in the United States still have sections called "Chinatown," "Little Italy," and "Germantown"?

    (A) Racial tension has been fostered by the United States government since the early 1900s.
    (B) Most immigrants are quickly assimilated into the culture of the United States.
    (C) Some sections of large cities are physically isolated from the rest of the city.
    (D) Before becoming citizens, immigrants must live in specified areas of large cities.
    (E) Ethnic goups often try to preserve their cultural heritage.

61. Which would most probably lead to the development of a pluralistic society?

    (A) A policy of open immigration
    (B) A totalitarian form of government
    (C) The requirement that only English be spoken in schools
    (D) The formation of labor unions
    (E) An increased emphasis on social conformity

62. Alexis de Tocqueville's *Democracy in America* had as its basic subject

    (A) American political institutions during the presidency of Andrew Johnson
    (B) modern democracy and an alleged trend toward equality of conditions
    (C) effects of the Industrial Revolution upon America and Europe
    (D) amazing prophecies about the future political development of America and France
    (E) a contrast between English and American democracy

63. What do the following three men all have in common?

- Earl Warren
- John Marshall
- Warren Burger

(A) Presidents
(B) State Governors
(C) U.S. Senators
(D) Astronauts
(E) Supreme Court Chief Justices

64. The Huguenots were

(A) a French family that claimed the throne
(B) a party that opposed the king's powers in England
(C) French Protestants
(D) a fleet that Philip II sent to invade England
(E) members of the First Estate

65. Why do anthropologists study the behavioral traits of higher primates?

(A) To see how advanced these higher primates really are.
(B) It is important to find out why the primates differ so much in their prehensile activities.
(C) Anthropologists need to find out why humans no longer brachiate.
(D) The conditions in which the higher primates live resemble the environmental conditions that existed when human cultures began.
(E) By studying their sexual expression, anthropologists can determine the reasons for human sexual aggression.

66. This great civilization influenced early Russia by diffusing its culture and particularly its religion to Kiev. Once part of the eastern Roman Empire, it was also the home of the great emperor Justinian. The people of this great culture were the

(A) Huns
(B) Mongols
(C) Slavs
(D) Byzantines
(E) Chinese

67. The great expansion of business corporations, monopolies, and holding companies took place

(A) shortly after the Revolutionary War
(B) prior to 1861 and the Civil War
(C) near the end of the 19th century
(D) during the presidency of Franklin D. Roosevelt
(E) after World War II

68. The formation and social behavior of a baboon troop studied by Jane Goodall reflects that baboons are

(A) egalitarian
(B) random and haphazard
(C) rigidly hierarchical and disciplined
(D) a system of concentric circles
(E) low in the order of primate social development

69. He studied the origins and functions of the "self" and laid the foundation of social psychology. This statement refers to

(A) George Herbert Mead
(B) Jean Piaget
(C) William James
(D) John Dewey
(E) Franklin Frazer

70. In an experiment using a control group,

(A) change is induced in the control group only
(B) change is induced in the experimental group only
(C) more change is induced in the control group than in the experimental group
(D) less change is induced in the control group than the experimental group
(E) the control group guarantees the accuracy of the findings

71. In which of the following job categories in the United States has there been an absolute decline over the past thirty years?

(A) Professional
(B) Managerial
(C) Skilled
(D) Service
(E) Farm

72. The great expansion of college-bound students began

(A) at the end of the 19th century
(B) right after World War I
(C) during the time of the New Deal
(D) from the 1960s on
(E) with the onset of the 21st century

73. Louis XIV is best known for

(A) making Calvinism the official state religion for the French people
(B) defeat of the Spanish Armada
(C) defeat of Britain in the Hundred Years War
(D) building the Versailles Palace
(E) being a weak absolute monarch

74. During the Reagan administration, the Iran-Contra Affair reflected U.S. policy toward

(A) Panama
(B) Grenada
(C) Haiti
(D) Brazil
(E) Nicaragua

75. "The government bets you can't live on the land for five years and if you can, you win the land." This statement refers to

(A) the Northwest Ordinance
(B) veterans' preference after World War II
(C) the Homestead Act of 1862
(D) The Morrill Act of 1862
(E) settlement of the Lone Star Republic im the early 1800s

76. The decade of the greatest growth in the American railroad occurred

(A) in the 1790s as the nation was first established
(B) during the Manifest Destiny movement of the 1820s–1850s
(C) during the Civil War years
(D) during the post–Civil War era, as industry rapidly expanded
(E) after America's entrance into World War I in 1917

77. The largest state in area and the smallest in population among the following is

(A) Nevada
(B) Texas
(C) Montana
(D) Maine
(E) Alaska

78. Under which president did the stock market make its greatest advances in the Dow?

(A) President Nixon
(B) President Ford
(C) President Reagan
(D) President Clinton
(E) President George H.W. Bush

79. The greatest number of immigrants arriving to the United States from the late 1800s to the beginning of World War I in 1914 came from

(A) Germany and France
(B) Thailand and India
(C) Brazil and Argentina
(D) Italy and Russia
(E) China and Japan

80. In the famous tale of *A Christmas Carol*, Karl Marx would consider the role played by Ebenezer Scrooge to be that of the

    (A) proletariat
    (B) bourgeoisie
    (C) sharecropper
    (D) blue collar worker
    (E) slave owner

81. This was one of the original thirteen states, it was the home of the first colonial legislature—the House of Burgeses—and it was the site of the first settlement, at Jamestown. The state is

    (A) New York
    (B) Delaware
    (C) Virginia
    (D) Pennsylvania
    (E) North Carolina

82. The most populous state in the United States in 1860 was

    (A) Virginia
    (B) Massachusetts
    (C) Illinois
    (D) South Carolina
    (E) New York

83. The eminent economist who championed the free market, worked for the elimination of conscription and was an important advisor to President Reagan was

    (A) John Maynard Keynes
    (B) Paul Krugman
    (C) Paul Samuelson
    (D) Milton Friedman
    (E) Kenneth Galbraith

84. This great social philosopher is best known for his work with children: "He concluded that there are two major stages in the development of moral judgment in children. The first stage, ages 3–8 are characterized by respect for authority and the morality of constraint and the second stage, ages 9–12, by the gradual ascent of mutual respect and the morality of cooperation."

    (A) Jean Piaget
    (B) Max Weber
    (C) Margaret Mead
    (D) Sigmund Freud
    (E) Ruth Benedict

85. Ascribed status, unlike achieved status, is based on

(A) what you do
(B) who you are
(C) power and prestige
(D) intelligence
(E) your gender

86. During which period was there no margin for saving?

(A) 1929–1931
(B) 1941–1944
(C) 1945–1950
(D) 1965–1970
(E) 1989–1991

87. The opposite of Adam Smith's "invisible hand" would be a "visible hand." Which of the following could be considered the "visible hand"?

(A) God
(B) Competition
(C) Price warfare
(D) Population increase
(E) Government

88. Immigration in the United States almost came to a standstill in

(A) 1845–1855
(B) 1890s
(C) 1900–1910
(D) 1919–1939
(E) 1965–1970s

89. Which is a typical trait of collective behavior that was demonstrated many times in the antiwar protests of the 1960s?

(A) Protestors do not welcome the media.
(B) The group and leaders expect to accomplish very little from their actions.
(C) It is structured and predictable.
(D) Solidarity is commonly exhibited and intensifies as the protest advances.
(E) It occurred in isolated and small populated areas.

90. The increased flow of precious metals from the New World to Europe in the 15th and 16th centuries

(A) caused prices to decrease
(B) caused trade and contact between the two worlds to expand
(C) had no effect on price levels
(D) discouraged speculation
(E) encouraged small-scale agriculture

91. A sociologist's job is often complicated by the nature of the social condition he is studying. Durkheim, in studying deaths from suicide, had such a problem. Which of the following research designs would he have had to employ to make significant generalizations and conclusions?

(A) The case study
(B) The observation method
(C) The survey
(D) The experiment
(E) A diary

92. Which of the following taught the observance of caste rules as a religious obligation?

(A) Islam
(B) Buddhism
(C) Taoism
(D) Hinduism
(E) Judaism

93. "The line of boundary between the territories of the United States and those of Her Britannic Majesty shall be continued westward along the forty-ninth parallel." This provision relates to which of the following?

(A) Gadsden Purchase
(B) Louisiana Purchase
(C) Oregon Territory
(D) Northwest Ordinance
(E) Mexican War

94. Henry VII and Henry VIII were members of which royal family?

(A) Tudors
(B) Stuarts
(C) Romanovs
(D) Hapsburgs
(E) Bourbons

95. In which of the following cities would there be more Mormons in proportion to the population?

(A) Atlanta
(B) Minneapolis
(C) Salt Lake City
(D) New York City
(E) Boston

96. Which of the following smaller states of Europe had only one but nevertheless the largest holding in central Africa before World War I?

(A) Netherlands
(B) Belgium
(C) Denmark
(D) Norway
(E) Switzerland

97. The Roman Empire

(A) was more democratic than the Roman Republic
(B) in 313 A.D., was split into two (east and west) to make it easier to rule
(C) fell in both the east and the west in 476 A.D. to the Mongols
(D) was unable to defeat Hannibal
(E) never accepted Christianity into its society

98. "Implied powers" are the powers of the national government that are necessary to

(A) amend the national Constitution
(B) prevent the state governments from expanding their powers beyond those given to them by the Constitution
(C) allow the national government to do the jobs given to it by the Constitution
(D) allow speedy governmental action in a war
(E) declare emergency powers and temporarily suspend democracy

99. The Supreme Court decision upholding certain tax-supported benefits for parochial school children was an issue dealing with the

(A) "general welfare" clause of the U.S. Constitution
(B) First Amendment
(C) Fourteenth Amendment
(D) Fifth Amendment
(E) Tenth Amendment

100. The Federal Reserve System can control the creation of money by

(A) setting legal reserve requirements, varying the prime rate, and setting quotas on government printing of currency
(B) setting legal reserve requirements, varying the discount rate, and varying the prime rate
(C) setting quotas on bank loans and on the government printing of currency, and by varying the prime rate
(D) setting legal reserve requirements, varying the discount rate, and by open market operations
(E) closing banks and the stock market, varying discount rates, and varying the prime rate

101. Singapore is located

    (A) in China
    (B) near Taiwan
    (C) in the Gulf of Thailand
    (D) in Southeast Asia
    (E) in Southwest Asia

102. The typical American corporation of today is likely to be largely controlled by

    (A) two or three men, who own most of the stock
    (B) a large number of people, each of whom owns a small amount of stock
    (C) managers, who are subject to much pressure from the stockholders
    (D) managers, who are given a very free hand by the stockholders
    (E) a dominant figure who controls the majority of stock

103. Which of these people would have been apt to join one of the craft unions in the American Federation of Labor?

    (A) An automobile assembly line worker in 1937
    (B) A brick mason in 1939
    (C) A department store clerk in 1950
    (D) A nurse in 1965
    (E) A schoolteacher in 1945

104. After he came to power in Turkey, Mustapha Kemal

    (A) attempted to restore traditional Turkish ways
    (B) introduced many modern reforms
    (C) began a war to reconquer the Arab sections of the old Turkish empire
    (D) restored the caliph to power
    (E) tried to reconquer the Balkan peninsula

105. Henry George's "single tax" was to be applied to

    (A) homes
    (B) income
    (C) sales
    (D) land
    (E) imports

106. In the first decade of the 21st century, the greatest number of American women workers were employed in

    (A) social work
    (B) clerical work
    (C) accounting
    (D) real estate
    (E) libraries

107. David Ricardo used Malthusian ideas to indicate the basic wage. To him, the reason this wage always tends toward bare subsistence is that

(A) employers are mean
(B) workers dislike ostentation
(C) society is unfair
(D) workers will always reproduce the labor supply to the maximum
(E) unions are prevented by the state from militant action

108. Consider the following events

- The dividing of Germany into West and East Germany
- The dividing of Vietnam into North and South Vietnam
- The dividing of Korea into North and South Korea

All three events were a result of

(A) World War I
(B) the Vietnam War
(C) the Cold War
(D) the Berlin Wall being created
(E) the Versailles Peace Treaty

109. Which of these peoples were not one of the Germanic tribes?

(A) Visigoths
(B) Vandals
(C) Huns
(D) Lombards
(E) Franks

110. The best source of historical data for an archaeologist would be the discovery of _____, but generally, the archaeologist usually finds only _____ when he make a successful dig.

(A) written remains, written remains
(B) written remains, material remains
(C) written remains, verbal remains
(D) material remains, written remains
(E) written remains, verbal remains

111. The advance of the Islamic religious jihad in the late 8th century was stopped finally by

(A) Charlemagne at the Battle of Tours
(B) the Roman Emperor Octavius and the institution of his policy of Pax Romana
(C) William the Conqueror at the Battle of Hastings
(D) the burning of Rome by the Huns
(E) the joining of two Spanish families of Fernando and Isabel in marriage

112. Which religion was founded in ancient India, spread to China (but didn't take hold), and eventually ended up taking hold in Southeast Asia and Japan?

   (A) Hinduism
   (B) Confucianism
   (C) Shintoism
   (D) Islamic Shiites
   (E) Buddhism

113. A fief was

   (A) a person who swore fealty to a lord
   (B) a grant, usually of land, made in exchange for promised services
   (C) a person bound to the soil
   (D) an oath of loyalty
   (E) a tariff on trade

114. One of the first things the Bolsheviks did in Russia when they came into power in 1917 was to

   (A) have the tsar removed from office
   (B) begin negotiations for peace with the Germans
   (C) make Stalin the head of the state
   (D) drive the Germans completely out of Russian territory
   (E) collectivize the land

115. Stress and strain in adolescence are most characteristic of

   (A) all known societies
   (B) preliterate societies
   (C) peasant societies
   (D) modern industrial societies
   (E) frontier societies

116. Which of the following methods of social science goes deepest into the motivation and problems of people?

   (A) Statistical survey
   (B) Document research
   (C) Interviews
   (D) Case study
   (E) Behavioral model

117. During the constitutional debate in the 1780s, the Federalists

   (A) supported a strong central government to provide order and protection
   (B) emphasized the need for a bill of rights
   (C) were the spokesman for the "common people"
   (D) wanted strong state governments
   (E) feared the abusive power of the new national government

118. Of the following, which is most clearly an example of reducing the domain of ascribed status?

   (A) A young man giving his seat to an older man on a bus that is crowded
   (B) Women who devote their time to their homes and church activities
   (C) Women serving in the armed forces of the United States
   (D) Members of certain racial groups sitting in the back of a bus
   (E) Young people beginning compulsory education at an earlier age

119. Of the following, which stage of human development is closest to modern man, also known as homo sapiens sapiens?

   (A) Neanderthal
   (B) Australopithecus
   (C) Homo Erectus
   (D) Cro-Magnon Man
   (E) Piltdown Man

120. Karl Marx reacted to the capitalist economic system of his time in a famous tract written in 1848. The title of this work was *The Communist Manifesto*. He contended that capitalism was

   (A) an artificial conspiracy imposed on society by greedy people
   (B) a necessary but temporary stage in the evolution of an industrial society
   (C) a retrogressive system that had as its main fault the creation of a proletariat
   (D) going to improve by reforms instituted through state action
   (E) incompatible with Christian morality

121. Consider the following events:

   - A noticeable increase in population occurred with the coming of the Neolithic Age.
   - Man settles down and ideas spread as he begins to make permanent dwellings.
   - Rapid cultural diffusion develops as man begins to establish communities so that he no longer has to be on the move.

   All these events occurred during the:

   (A) Paleolithic Age
   (B) Mesolithic Age
   (C) Neolithic Age
   (D) Industrial Age
   (E) Middle Ages

122. During the Middle Ages, Spain was a mixture of what cultures?

    (A) the Holy Roman emperors and the popes

    (B) Western Christians and the Byzantines

    (C) Christians and Muslims

    (D) the Guelphs and the Ghibellines

    (E) Protestants and Catholics

123. A union shop is a shop

    (A) that has voted to allow union representation

    (B) where the majority of the workers are union members

    (C) designated in right to work as having official union status

    (D) where only union members are allowed to work

    (E) that opposes women in the labor field

124. Judicial self-restraint as applied to the Supreme Court can be described as

    (A) a reluctance on the part of the justices to file a dissenting opinion except in rare cases

    (B) an awareness of the need for dignity and propriety in courtroom proceedings

    (C) a careful consideration of the wisdom and social impact of disputed laws

    (D) a careful consideration of the motives of Congress in enacting the disputed laws

    (E) a proper concern for the role and judgment of the legislative branch of government

125. Which statement is accurate on making a federal law?

    (A) The president's veto cannot be overturned.

    (B) The bill must pass both houses of Congress and be signed by the president.

    (C) A bill cannot be changed from its original form once introduced.

    (D) The bill can be interpreted by the Supreme Court.

    (E) Most bills eventually become laws as little committee work is needed.

If there is still time remaining, you may review your answers.

ANSWER KEY
Sample Examination 2

SOCIAL SCIENCES-HISTORY

1.	A	33.	D	65.	D	97.	B
2.	D	34.	D	66.	D	98.	C
3.	B	35.	C	67.	C	99.	A
4.	B	36.	A	68.	C	100.	B
5.	C	37.	A	69.	A	101.	D
6.	C	38.	D	70.	B	102.	D
7.	B	39.	D	71.	E	103.	B
8.	A	40.	B	72.	D	104.	B
9.	D	41.	D	73.	D	105.	D
10.	C	42.	D	74.	E	106.	B
11.	C	43.	B	75.	C	107.	D
12.	B	44.	A	76.	C	108.	C
13.	E	45.	A	77.	E	109.	C
14.	C	46.	C	78.	D	110.	B
15.	B	47.	A	79.	D	111.	A
16.	C	48.	A	80.	B	112.	E
17.	C	49.	A	81.	C	113.	B
18.	B	50.	E	82.	E	114.	B
19.	C	51.	C	83.	D	115.	D
20.	E	52.	B	84.	A	116.	D
21.	A	53.	A	85.	B	117.	A
22.	A	54.	D	86.	A	118.	C
23.	C	55.	A	87.	E	119.	D
24.	B	56.	D	88.	D	120.	B
25.	A	57.	E	89.	C	121.	C
26.	B	58.	E	90.	B	122.	C
27.	A	59.	C	91.	C	123.	D
28.	A	60.	E	92.	D	124.	E
29.	C	61.	A	93.	C	125.	B
30.	E	62.	B	94.	A		
31.	D	63.	E	95.	C		
32.	A	64.	C	96.	B		

SCORING CHART

After you have scored your Sample Examination 2, enter the results in the chart below; then transfer your score to the Progress Chart on page 12.

Total Test	Number Right	Number Wrong	Number Omitted
120			

ANSWER EXPLANATIONS

1. **(A)** In 1933, the Weimar Republic to the Nazi government and Hitler and his fascist government took over Germany. This new Nazi nation was supposed to last for a thousand years (*Mein Kampf*), but in reality, it lasted only twelve.

2. **(D)** In 1937, Hitler took the German part of Czechoslovakia by force in a quick invasion. Peace efforts were made to avoid a war, and in negotiations with Hitler, Chamberlain of England returned home with the famous "scrap of paper" in which Hitler had agreed to not invade the rest of Czechoslovakia if he was allowed to keep the Sudetenland. Six months later the compromise had failed, for the Nazis had invaded all of Czechoslovakia, taking over the entire country. The stage was set for World War II to begin.

3. **(B)** Napoleon experienced the first failure in his military rule of France when his Grand Army was unable to defeat the Russian army. In 1812, he took the largest army ever assembled across Eastern Europe, but both the cunning Russian military and the winter of 1812 resulted in his first major defeat as ruler of the French people.

4. **(B)** In 1948, under their leader Tito, this communist nation was the only Russian satellite to break away from the Soviet Union. After the death of Tito in the late 1980s, Yugoslavia broke up into six independent nations but not without ethnic and religious tension. During the Cold War, Tito maintained good political and economic relations with the United States.

5. **(C)** A holding company is a corporation that holds stock in another company. This is permitted by law, even though a holding company may not produce any goods or services.

6. **(C)** The Securities and Exchange Commission (SEC) was established by Congress in 1934 under the New Deal to protect investors. The SEC prevents illegal stock market dealing such as prevailed prior to the Great Depression of the 1930s.

7. **(B)** Adolescence is a transition period between childhood and adulthood. This unclear stage leaves the adolescent with some confusion, because the transition is rather sudden and quick. Thus, conflict with parents and society is often common and understandable.

8. **(A)** The term *secular* means worldly or temporal, in contrast to ecclesiastical. In medieval European history, the king or emperor exercised "secular power"; the church exercised ecclesiastical authority.

9. **(D)** In the election of 1928, Republican candidate Herbert Hoover promised two chickens in every pot if he were elected. His election to the presidency was soon followed by the Great Depression of the 1930s, during which there were no chickens in most pots.

10. **(C)** After World War II, William Levitt began mass construction of affordable housing on former potato fields on Long Island, New York. This new suburbia was replicated in Levittown, Pennsylvania.

11. **(C)** The Social Security Act was passed in 1935 under the Democratic administration of Franklin D. Roosevelt. The abolition of slavery came in the Republican administration of Abraham Lincoln; the Pendleton Act in 1883 under Republican President Arthur; the Morrill Act in 1862 under Lincoln; and the Pure Food and Drug Act in 1906 under Republican President Theodore Roosevelt.

12. **(B)** The ancient Persian Empire was the largest. It extended throughout the area we now call the Middle East from Asia Minor in the West to India in the East and from the Caucasus Mountains in the North to the Arabian Sea in the South.

13. **(E)** The official language of the Roman Catholic Church is still Latin. In the past fifty years, however, the vernacular has increasingly been used for actual Mass because it is easier for parishioners to understand and partake in the service.

14. **(C)** Monetary policy in the United States is administered by the Federal Reserve Board of Governors. The seven-member Board of Governors of the Federal Reserve system in Washington exercises control over the nation's money supply and credit conditions. This is referred to as "monetary policy."

15. **(B)** In his "Essay on the Principles of Population," Thomas Malthus argued that population, if left unchecked, increases in geometrical progression, whereas the fastest that the means of subsistence can increase is in arithmetical progression.

16. **(C)** Reincarnation, the return of the soul after death in a new living body, is part of the teaching of Hinduism.

17. **(C)** The total value (in dollars) of all goods and services produced in the American economy during a given year is called the gross national product (GNP) for that year. If we subtract depreciation (the using up of capital equipment), we have net national product (NNP).

18. **(B)** In sociology and psychology, *drives* are factors that incite behavior in the individual. The term *drive* indicates an internal force or push that seeks an outlet. In psychoanalysis, *drive* is regarded as an instinct. Examples are thirst, sex, and hunger.

19. **(C)** Viet Nam, once a French colony, was divided at the 17th parallel, which soon put Viet Nam at the forefront of the Cold War. Shortly after the Geneva Agreement of 1954, a communist North Viet Nam and a democratic South Viet Nam had emerged. What eventually followed was the Viet Nam conflict that ended in the communist takeover of South Viet Nam in 1975.

20. **(E)** Tibet was ruled until 1959 by a Buddhist religious leader called the "Dalai Lama." In 1959, the Dalai Lama fled from Tibet. The country is under control of Communist China.

21. **(A)** The "jewel of the British crown," was the colonial possession of India. After the English lost the thirteen American colonies, this became their greatest possession. When independence came in 1947 through the efforts of Gandhi, the strong religious differences called for the creation of several states, including the division of India and Pakistan into two parts.

22. **(A)** As stated above, these two nations have continued to have strong religious differences into the present. Even Gandhi was unable to bring the two religious groups together, and thus East and West Pakistan (Muslim) and India (Hindu) were created.

23. **(C)** The Peter Zenger case and the Schenck case both dealt with the 1st Amendment, which addresses the freedom of the press.

24. **(B)** Despite foreign competition, the U.S. automobile industry is a monopolistic competition, which means that several key companies control the market. Because we have more than one company, there is competition, but not in the true sense of the word as Adam Smith describes it.

25. **(A)** In a free market economy, price is determined by an equilibrium between supply and demand. When the quantity supplied increases more rapidly than the quantity demanded, the effect is a decline in price.

26. **(B)** All race elections took place for the first time in South Africa, resulting in the election of a black president.

27. **(A)** Approximately 500,000 years ago, humankind invented fire. This great invention provided warmth, enabled human life to cook meat that added protein to the brain, gave humans light at night and thus protection against predators, and finally could be used as a weapon against the human's foes.

28. **(A)** What Marx did not contemplate in his proletariat revolution was that the continual growth of English democracy resulted in both pro labor reform movement and a pro labor legislation (American capitalism followed in a similar reform path).

29. **(C)** For the past decade, the largest growing group of Americans has been senior citizens. With the quality of life in America among the highest in the world, people continue to live longer and longer! Similarly, the senior citizen commands a powerful political vote on the local, state, and national levels.

30. **(E)** The president of the United States nominates the justices of the Supreme Court. After congressional committee discussion, a majority vote of the Senate approves or disapproves of the nominee.

31. **(D)** In the history of the presidency until 1974, there had never been an instance of the resignation of a president. When Richard M. Nixon resigned in 1974, impeachment in the House of Representatives was imminent, and there was every indication that he would be removed by the Senate.

32. **(A)** The American Civil War was followed by a major step toward black equality with the Civil War amendments. Amendments XIII, XIV, and XV abolished slavery, provided citizenship, and instituted voting rights. While civil rights for black Americans was to be a long uphill battle, these amendments were nevertheless a major step in improving their life here in the United States.

33. **(D)** Closely tied to Manifest Destiny, social Darwinism (to Americans) was the idea that the American way of life was superior to other cultures and that therefore the United States was obliged to carry its great society to other peoples. Thus, the belief in American superiority was a form of social Darwinism that first manifested itself in the Spanish American War.

34. **(D)** The Dardanelles are part of the passageway between the Black Sea (dominated by Russia) and the Mediterranean Sea, to which Russia does not have direct access. Hence, Russia has had a historic interest in the Dardanelles.

35. **(C)** Louis XIV of France, who inherited the throne at the age of five in 1643, assumed power in 1661 at the age of 23. He ruled until his death in 1715. He was greatly admired and was called "Le Grand Monarque" or Louis the Great. He is supposed to have said, "L'etat, c'est moi" (I am the state).

36. **(A)** The German Imperial Constitution was adopted after the Franco-Prussian War in 1871. By its terms, King William I of Prussia became Emperor William I of the newly created German Empire.

37. **(A)** Niccolo Machiavelli (1469–1527), Italian political philosopher, is best known for his book, *The Prince*. In it, he counsels a ruler on the best way to acquire and hold political power. In a cynical vein, he advises that it is better to be feared than loved.

38. **(D)** Louis Leakey is not only the father of anthropology but also made it the significant social science that it is today. His revolutionary work in Africa shocked the world when he proved time and time again that man's origin is in the so-called Dark Continent, that of sub-Saharan Africa.

39. **(D)** The "final solution" refers to Hitler's goal of killing all Jews in Europe simply because they were Jewish. The annihilation of a group of people because of its religion is an example of genocide. Hitler's idea of the Germans as a master race required the killing of those whom, like Jews, he considered inferior.

40. **(B)** One of the best known Roman emperors was Constantine the Great. He reorganized provinces within the empire, made strategic economic and political changes, moved the capital to Byzantium, and legalized Christianity. One of his most historical decisions was when he issued the Edict of Milan in 313 A.D. This act ended polytheism by granting freedom of worship to all Christians.

41. **(D)** Despite the changes that the American family has undergone in the last century, it is still the primary socializing agent for children. Even with dual incomes and other changes in the traditional structure, the nuclear family continues to be the primary agent for children.

42. **(D)** The Standard Oil Trust was originally organized in 1882 by John D. Rockefeller. The story is told by Ida Tarbell in *The History of the Standard Oil Company* (1904).

43. **(B)** The Dreyfus Affair began in France in 1894 with the charge that Captain Dreyfus, a Jew, had sold military information to the Germans. He was sentenced to life imprisonment on Devil's Island. Dreyfus protested his innocence. Anti-Semites, and many leaders of the Church lined up against him. His innocence was finally proven, and he was reinstated as a major in the army.

44. **(A)** Otto von Bismarck (1815–1898), leader of German unification, believed Germany could become strong and unified only if Austria were excluded from German affairs. Bismarck was at heart a Prussian. He feared that Austria, if included, would dispute power with Prussia.

45. **(A)** The Zulus were a warlike tribe that fought against the British in South Africa during the wave of 19th-century imperialism. Several impressive battles were fought that surprised the British army. It was only British military technology that eventually led to the defeat of the Zulu warriors.

46. **(C)** Since the end of World War II, moves to coordinate and unite the European community became an on-going process. In the 1950s, the European Coal and Steel Community and Euratom were created. The greatest and most relevant step occurred in 1958 with the creation of the EEC better known as the Common Market (later the EC = European Community). Probably the boldest step toward greater economic unity was the creation of a common currency, the euro (in use since 2000).

47. **(A)** Thomas Malthus (1766–1834), English clergyman and philosopher, was deeply perturbed at the rapid increase in population and the relatively slower increase in the food supply. He foresaw war, plagues, and famine unless population was kept in check. Universal education at public expense offered some hope. The others would only exacerbate the problem.

48. **(A)** If people do not consume all their income, the part not spent is technically saving, no matter what they do with the money. Investing, however, requires that the money be put to work to create new wealth. In national income and product terms, consumption and investment go hand in hand.

49. **(A)** Group marriage, several men and several women living together and cohabiting, is a relatively rare social phenomenon. Each of the other four is far more common in man's various societies.

50. **(E)** The reaction of the Communist Chinese government to these student demonstrations was to quell them.

51. **(C)** When sociologists talk of "social mobility," they usually have in mind vertical mobility, moving from the socioeconomic level into which a person was born into a higher socioeconomic level. In an open society, marked by widespread opportunity, this phenomenon is relatively common.

52. **(B)** America has been called the melting pot of the world. With our diverse ethnic immigrant population, a great deal of cultural diffusion has taken place. Americans love Chinese food, eat many Italian foods, like British music; these are all examples of cultural diffusion. So too is the use of canoes and moccasins by Americans an example of cultural diffusion.

53. **(A)** As the nation-state began to emerge through Europe, so too did these Europeans begin their departure from a traditional economy to a national economy. The new nations of France, England, and Spain employed the use of mercantilism. It meant that the central government would control the economy by setting up colonies to supply the mother country with gold and silver, the mark of economic might for these new nations.

54. **(D)** Thorstein Veblen (1857–1929), American economist and social philosopher, considered marginal utility economics overly deductive, individualistic, and static. Marginal utility economics teaches that the extra utility added by each last unit of a good will be decreasing, although *total* utility will rise with consumption. In his *Theory of the Leisure Class*, Veblen held that, in an affluent society, most goods are useless except for display to establish status.

55. **(A)** With the rise of the giants of industry by the late 1880s, corporations tried to aggressively control production and prices and eliminate the little man. Such was the case of the railroad companies that formed pools in an attempt to fix prices. While these were monopolist steps by big business to end competition, eventually pools were outlawed.

56. **(D)** The chart illustrates how the electoral college system operates. In all four cases, the victor won a majority of the electoral college, but in two of the four elections, the victor did not win a majority of the popular vote. In the electoral college system, a majority of the popular vote is not necessary to win an election (choice A); only a majority of the electoral vote is necessary. Since no incumbents were running in the elections covered, the chart does not illustrate that incumbent's have an advantage (choice C). Nor does the chart present evidence of how third-party candidacies affected the outcome of the elections involved (choice E). Indeed, third-party candidates may have pulled more votes from the winners than from the losers. Only in 1988 is a significant increase in popular vote totals evident (choice B).

57. **(E)** These two elections provide support to those who think we should have the popular vote, not the electoral vote, determine the presidential election.

58. **(E)** The original Constitution was written in 1787 and ratified in 1789. It was eventually to contain twenty-seven changes or amendments. The first ten of these, the Bill of Rights, were added in 1791.

59. **(C)** The only president to serve two full terms was Bill Clinton. President John F. Kennedy was assassinated in his first term, and President Lyndon Baines Johnson chose not to run for a second term with the Viet Nam conflict accelerating. President Richard M. Nixon resigned after Watergate, and President George H. Bush was defeated after one term by Bill Clinton.

60. **(E)** These areas in urban cities contain the most visible signs of ethnicity—restaurants where a group's food is served, churches/religious institutions where the ethnic heritage is evident, stores where ethnic-related products are sold, and streets and homes in which that group's language is heard and spoken.

61. **(A)** Open immigration would enable people from many different areas of the world to migrate to a country. The resulting society would be a pluralistic one because it contained people of various races, languages, and ethnicities or nationalities.

62. **(B)** Alexis de Tocqueville (1805–1859), French writer, traveled throughout the United States in 1831 as an agent of his government. He described his findings in a famous book, *Democracy in America*. In it he wrote: "Nothing struck me more forcibly than the general equality of conditions."

63. **(E)** These three great men all served on the Supreme Court and also rose to the highest position on the Court, that of chief justice. John Marshall was our very first chief justice setting in place the practice of "judicial review." Earl Warren, originally appointed by the conservative President Dwight Eisenhower, became famous throughout the 1960s for his liberal decisions. Warren was followed by Chief Justice Burger who was appointed by President Richard Nixon in the hope to curb the liberal court.

64. **(C)** The Huguenots were French Protestants. They were followers of Calvin and Swiss Protestantism. Persecution in France led many Huguenots to flee to England, Holland, and America.

65. **(D)** The study of the behavior of higher primates is critical in the study of anthropology, for it helps us to better understand how human evolution occurred. Man's ancestors include the ape family, and their behavior has proven to be similar to that of humankind, thanks to the studies of Jane Goodall and Dian Fossey.

66. **(D)** The Byzantine Empire, also known as the Eastern Roman Empire, lasted until 1453 A.D. almost a thousand years longer than the Western Roman Empire. It provided great cultural and religious influence all over Eastern Europe and Asia. This cultural contact between the Byzantine civilization and Russia took place through trade by way of Kiev and other city-states in early Russia.

67. **(C)** The great expansion of business corporations, monopolies, and holding companies took place in the later 1880s. The post-Civil War was followed by rapid industrial expansion and the arrival of the giants of industry. Such giants as Rockefeller (oil), Carnegie (steel), Morgan (banking), and Ford (assembly line, automobile) made their presence in American economics.

68. **(C)** Jane Goodall, a colleague of Louis Leakey, did her greatest work in her study of baboon troops. She proved that there are strong similarities between baboons and humans in terms of social organization and leadership.

69. **(A)** George Herbert Mead (1863–1931), American philosopher and social psychologist, in his *Mind, Self, and Society* (1934), held that the self arises as a result of social experience and that the individual experiences himself indirectly from the standpoint of others of the same group. In Freud's psychology, the id is completely unconscious, as is the self prior to conscious development.

70. **(B)** In an experiment, change is induced in the experimental group only. The control group is used to determine the amount or effect of the change on the experimental group.

71. **(E)** There has been an absolute decline in farm employment during the past thirty years. In 1955, there were 8,381,000 people employed in farming. Thirty-five years later (1990), the number was 3,200,000.

72. **(D)** With the election of President John Kennedy, the 1960s marked the surfacing of an affluent middle class. Sometimes referred to as the "Great Society," the 1960s was marked by a growing move toward civil rights legislation and a more liberal society in general. The growth of the rapidly rising middle class and the "two-income family" resulted in the expansion of college-bound students. This growth of the college experience has continued to the present day.

73. **(D)** Louis XIV, the "Sun King" is known for his construction of the Versailles Palace. This grand effort was a display of his wealth and power. It also kept his strong nobility under his suspicious eyes, for they had to spend a significant amount of time at Versailles. Thus, it helped to secure his absolute power.

74. **(E)** During the civil war in Nicaragua in the 1980s, the Reagan administration helped one faction, the Contras. They were provided with funds to purchase weapons from sales of U.S. arms to Iran.

75. **(C)** The Homestead Act of 1862 granted 160 acres of land free to settlers who would live on the land and farm it for a period of five years.

76. **(C)** Railroad mileage in the U.S. increased from 3,000 in 1840 to 190,000 by 1900. The increase by decades was as follows: 1850, 9,000; 1860, 30,000; 1870, 53,000; 1880, 80,000; 1890, 164,000. Thus, the greatest increase in absolute amount was in the 1880s. The greatest increase in railroad mileage was in the post–Civil War era, from the 1880s to the turn of the 20th century.

77. **(E)** Alaska: area, 589,757 square miles; population, 400,481
Texas: area, 267,338 square miles; population, 14,228,383
Montana: area, 147,138 square miles; population, 786,690
Nevada: area, 110,540 square miles; population, 799,184
Maine: area, 33,215 square miles; population, 1,124,660

78. **(D)** The 1990s saw the greatest economic growth in the history of the American stock market. The greatest rise in the market was under the successful economic period of President Clinton.

79. **(D)** During the years 1885–1914, a torrent of 20 million immigrants arrived in the United States. The rapid expansion of industry from the 1870s on was paralleled with the increased need for blue collar workers. Thus, white unskilled workers from eastern and southern Europe made their way into the United States. The greatest numbers came from Italy and Russia.

80. **(B)** The tale *A Christmas Carol* reflects not only the story of the Christmas spirit but also the story of the proletariat worker and the bourgeoisie capitalist. Karl Marx would thus consider Scrooge to be the cold selfish "bourgeoisie" or capitalist who keeps all the profit or "surplus value" for himself.

81. **(C)** Virginia, a middle colony, was the home of the first pilgrim settlement, Jamestown. It was also the birthplace of the first colonial legislature that eventually became the blueprint of American legislative government.

82. **(E)** The most populous state in the United States in 1860 was New York, with 3,880,735. In 1860, the population of Virginia was 1,596,318; Massachusetts 1,231,066; Illinois 1,711,951; and South Carolina 703,708 (slaves in Virginia and South Carolina were counted as 3/5). West Virginia was still part of Virginia in 1860.

83. **(D)** Friedman extolled the virtues of a free market economic system. He believed strongly in minimal government intervention in both the economic and political sphere. *Capitalism and Freedom* outlines his political and economic philosophy. He said that his role in ending conscription was his proudest achievement. He won the nobel Prize in economic sciences in 1976.

84. **(A)** In preparing for the teaching profession, all future educators get to know the work of Jean Piaget who is best known for his work with children. One of his principal studies concludes that there are two stages of childhood development. The first stage (ages 3–8) is characterized by respect for authority and the second stage (ages 9–12) by the development of mutual respect and cooperation.

85. **(B)** Ascribed status is determined by birth and thus depends on what social scale you are born into.

86. **(A)** As a result of the Great Depression and the stock market crash, which precipitated the worst depression in our history, both savings and income were at an all-time low.

87. **(E)** Adam Smith (1723–1790) wrote a classic analysis of economic forces entitled *An Inquiry into the Nature and Causes of the Wealth of Nations* (1776). He referred to the unimpeded force operating in the marketplace as "the invisible hand." Government intervention in the free market would be the "visible hand."

88. **(D)** Because of our isolationist policy of the post–World War I period, America entered into an anti-immigration age. Thus immigration was at its lowest in American history between the two wars.

89. **(C)** All collective behavior needs unity or solidarity to be effective. Thus, the very term *collective* means to do together. Collective behavior welcomes the media for publicity and is spontaneous and occurs in largely populated areas.

90. **(B)** The increase in precious metals constituted, in effect, an increase in the money supply. Other things being equal, this steady and substantial increase in coinage was certain to cause an increase in trade.

91. **(C)** A survey of the families and friends of victims would be the best way to do research on suicide. Factors underlying the events leading to the suicide could be helpful for researching the reasons why and the different types of suicide.

92. **(D)** Hinduism, the chief religion of India, developed prior to the 6th century B.C. The caste system became an integral part of Hinduism. Each individual is born into a caste. Four major castes, with many subdivisions, were Brahmans (priests), military, farmers and merchants, and laborers. A lowest group, pariahs (untouchables), are without caste.

93. **(C)** The dispute between Britain and the United States over the Oregon Territory was settled by a treaty in 1846. The forty-ninth parallel of north latitude, constituting the then-existing boundary between the U.S. and Canada to the Rockies, was extended to the Pacific.

94. **(A)** Henry VII, Henry VIII, and Queen Elizabeth I were all members of the Tudor family. The reign of each of these leaders helped expand the power of the English nation. Henry VIII is probably most famous for his departure from the Catholic Church when he established the Anglican Church of England. This state-run church was a direct result of Henry's conflict with the Pope and his desire to have many wives.

95. **(C)** The home of the Mormons has always been Salt Lake City.

96. **(B)** Prior to World War I, Belgium was a major imperial power in Africa because of her control of the Congo, a rich territory extending over 331,850 square miles in Central

Africa. The other major imperial powers in Africa prior to 1914 were Britain, France, Germany, Italy, Spain, and Portugal.

97. **(B)** During the 3rd century A.D., the Roman Empire was split into two because it was so large and becoming harder and harder to rule. This was also influenced by the growing number of Germanic and Asian tribes that became more and more of a threat, particularly to the western part of the empire. Eventually, the Huns defeated the western Roman Empire but the east continued to survive for another thousand years.

98. **(C)** The Constitution, in Article I, Section 8, specifically enumerates 17 of the powers of Congress. Then, in clause 18, it gives Congress power "to make all laws which shall be necessary and proper" to do the job given to it by the Constitution. These are called "implied powers."

99. **(A)** The preamble to the Constitution states the reasons for its establishment. One of the reasons is "to promote the general welfare." The Supreme Court looked to this clause in approving public funds for parochial school children.

100. **(B)** In the wake of the rocky stock market of 2001–2002 and the events of September 11, 2001, the Federal Reserve System has stepped in more often to control money by varying discount rates as well as the prime rate.

101. **(D)** The Republic of Singapore is an island country in Southeast Asia. It lies off the southern tip of the Malay Peninsula. Singapore gained independence in 1965 and has become an important economic center.

102. **(D)** In the typical American corporation of today, the managers who control the corporation are given a free hand by the stockholders. Rarely, except for the relatively small corporations, is the majority of the stock held by one or a few individuals.

103. **(B)** The American Federation of Labor was established during the 1880s under the leadership of Samuel Gompers. His purpose was to organize skilled workers into craft unions. Brick masons were organized as one of the constituent unions in the AF of L. The rival union organization, the CIO, organized entire industries such as automotive. It came into being in 1935.

104. **(B)** Mustapha Kemal Ataturk (1880–1938), a Turkish army officer, came into power after World War I. He carried out a revolution in which both the sultanate and the caliphate were abolished and complete separation of church and state instituted in a new Turkish Republic. Universal suffrage, a parliament, a ministry, and a president were established. Women gained a new freedom.

105. **(D)** Henry George (1839–1897), American economist, wrote *Progress and Poverty* (1879). He believed a "single tax" on land would provide for all the necessary costs of government and even leave a surplus.

106. **(B)** The greatest number of American women were employed as clerical workers.

107. **(D)** David Ricardo (1772–1823), British economist, wrote *Principles of Political Economy and Taxation* (1817). He maintained that wages cannot rise above the lowest level necessary for subsistence. Workers reproduce to provide a labor supply that keeps wages at this level. Malthus had previously noted the increase of population in geometric ratio.

108. **(C)** The policy of containment influenced the dividing of nations affected by the Cold War. The dividing of Germany into four zones, then two new countries, began the Cold War in the late 1940s. Subsequent events led to further splits between communism and democracy as the nations of Korea and Vietnam were divided in the 1950s. Today, only Korea is divided, and the fall of the Berlin Wall along with Germany's reunification marked the end of the Cold War.

109. **(C)** The Huns were nomadic horsemen from north central Asia. They occupied China for several centuries. During the 4th century, they invaded the Volga valley of Russia, driving the Visigoths before them. The Visigoths, Vandals, Lombards, and Franks were Germanic peoples.

110. **(B)** The best-case scenario would be to have written records, in fact primary sources, when analyzing and interpreting history. Unfortunately, written records go back only several millennia before Christ, and the period of unwritten human history is far longer. Thus, the next best choice is to rely on material or physical remains left behind. The teeth are the most durable remains an archeologist can find.

111. **(A)** The Islamic invasions of the 7th and 8th centuries into Europe were finally stopped by Charlemagne at the Battle of Tours. The Moors moved through Northern Africa as far east as India and threatened to take over Europe. It was only because of the great Christian leader Charlemagne that the Islamic invasion did not take over all of Europe. His victory at Tours had a lot to do with his being crowned the Holy Roman Emperor in 800 A.D.

112. **(E)** Buddhism originated as an alternative to Hinduism. His ideas were rejected in India and later China but did meet success when his missionary men entered Korea, Japan, and Southeast Asia. Today Buddhism is a major religion in Korea, Japan, Vietnam, and most of eastern Asia.

113. **(B)** A fief in medieval Europe was an estate over which a nobleman exercised control. The grantor would receive a promise of protection or other service in return for the land.

114. **(B)** In November 1917, the Bolsheviks in Russia, led by V. I. Lenin (1870–1914), overthrew the government and came into power. They immediately began negotiations for peace with the Germans. Lenin regarded the war as an imperialist adventure. He thought both sides—the Germans and the Allies—would destroy each other.

115. **(D)** Anthropologists point to excessive stress and strain in adolescence as a characteristic of modern industrial societies. The anthropologist Margaret Mead studied the nonindustrial society of Samoa and reported the relative untroubled adolescence of its members in her *Coming of Age in Samoa* (1928). Her findings have recently been challenged.

116. **(D)** The case study, a method used in the social sciences, delves deeply into the motivation and problems of its subjects.

117. **(A)** During the constitutional debate in the 1780s, the Federalist and Anti-Federalist engaged in a political arena of opposing views on the format of the new centralized government. The Federalists believed in a strong central government and claimed that a bill of rights was unnecessary, while the Anti-Federalists wanted a weak central

government so that it would not threaten the rights of the people or the power of the states. The Federalist papers were instrumental in providing support for the eventual approval of the new Constitution.

118. **(C)** The traditional domain ascribed to women in industrial society is that of home-maker. Women serving in the armed forces of the United States constitute a sharp and symbolic break with this ascribed status.

119. **(D)** The closest to modern-day man is Cro-Magnon man, who lived from about 35,000 to 10,000 years ago. He is the evolutionary ancestor to humankind today. Neanderthal and homo erectus are earlier forms of mankind. Australopithecus, Leakey's great dis-covery, is one of the very earliest forms of human existence. Piltdown man was a 20th-century hoax.

120. **(B)** In *The Communist Manifesto*, Karl Marx (and his co-author Friedrich Engels) con-tended that capitalism was a necessary step in the evolution of society to communism. Marx thought that the inevitable struggle between the capitalists and the proletariat would end in the victory of the latter (communism). Hence, capitalism was a necessary stage in the evolution of society.

121. **(C)** The Neolithic or agricultural age has been one of the most important cultural developments in the history of the human race. With farming, man settled down, built permanent homes, and developed a truly modern society. For the first time he no longer had to hunt for food, and survival was a far greater possibility. The human population began to grow rapidly because of this historic stage.

122. **(C)** The Moors of North Africa converted to Islam in the 8th century and became fanatic Muslims. They crossed into Spain in 711 A.D., overran the country, and spread into France. Christians and Muslims vied for control of Spain from the 11th to the 15th centuries, culminating in 1492 when the Muslims were driven from Spain.

123. **(D)** As unions become stronger and stronger, they attempt to set up union shops in which only union members can belong. This guarantees union solidarity and strength for negotiations.

124. **(E)** Judicial self-restraint as applied to the Supreme Court can be described as a proper concern for the role and judgment of the legislative branch of government. The Court prefers not to overrule an act of Congress if it can see any way of finding the act compatible with the Constitution. The Supreme Court decision in the Florida recount for the 2000 election is an example of judicial self-restraint.

125. **(B)** In order for a bill to become a law, the future law must pass through both houses of Congress and be signed by the president. Changes are very common in this process as committees are the work horse of the legislation process. Few bills become laws and a presidential veto can indeed be overridden by a two-thirds vote of both houses. As for the Supreme Court, it has no say on how a bill becomes a law; it can only interpret a law once it is passed.

The Natural Sciences Examination

ANSWER SHEET
Trial Test

NATURAL SCIENCES

1. Ⓐ Ⓑ Ⓒ Ⓓ Ⓔ	32. Ⓐ Ⓑ Ⓒ Ⓓ Ⓔ	63. Ⓐ Ⓑ Ⓒ Ⓓ Ⓔ	94. Ⓐ Ⓑ Ⓒ Ⓓ Ⓔ
2. Ⓐ Ⓑ Ⓒ Ⓓ Ⓔ	33. Ⓐ Ⓑ Ⓒ Ⓓ Ⓔ	64. Ⓐ Ⓑ Ⓒ Ⓓ Ⓔ	95. Ⓐ Ⓑ Ⓒ Ⓓ Ⓔ
3. Ⓐ Ⓑ Ⓒ Ⓓ Ⓔ	34. Ⓐ Ⓑ Ⓒ Ⓓ Ⓔ	65. Ⓐ Ⓑ Ⓒ Ⓓ Ⓔ	96. Ⓐ Ⓑ Ⓒ Ⓓ Ⓔ
4. Ⓐ Ⓑ Ⓒ Ⓓ Ⓔ	35. Ⓐ Ⓑ Ⓒ Ⓓ Ⓔ	66. Ⓐ Ⓑ Ⓒ Ⓓ Ⓔ	97. Ⓐ Ⓑ Ⓒ Ⓓ Ⓔ
5. Ⓐ Ⓑ Ⓒ Ⓓ Ⓔ	36. Ⓐ Ⓑ Ⓒ Ⓓ Ⓔ	67. Ⓐ Ⓑ Ⓒ Ⓓ Ⓔ	98. Ⓐ Ⓑ Ⓒ Ⓓ Ⓔ
6. Ⓐ Ⓑ Ⓒ Ⓓ Ⓔ	37. Ⓐ Ⓑ Ⓒ Ⓓ Ⓔ	68. Ⓐ Ⓑ Ⓒ Ⓓ Ⓔ	99. Ⓐ Ⓑ Ⓒ Ⓓ Ⓔ
7. Ⓐ Ⓑ Ⓒ Ⓓ Ⓔ	38. Ⓐ Ⓑ Ⓒ Ⓓ Ⓔ	69. Ⓐ Ⓑ Ⓒ Ⓓ Ⓔ	100. Ⓐ Ⓑ Ⓒ Ⓓ Ⓔ
8. Ⓐ Ⓑ Ⓒ Ⓓ Ⓔ	39. Ⓐ Ⓑ Ⓒ Ⓓ Ⓔ	70. Ⓐ Ⓑ Ⓒ Ⓓ Ⓔ	101. Ⓐ Ⓑ Ⓒ Ⓓ Ⓔ
9. Ⓐ Ⓑ Ⓒ Ⓓ Ⓔ	40. Ⓐ Ⓑ Ⓒ Ⓓ Ⓔ	71. Ⓐ Ⓑ Ⓒ Ⓓ Ⓔ	102. Ⓐ Ⓑ Ⓒ Ⓓ Ⓔ
10. Ⓐ Ⓑ Ⓒ Ⓓ Ⓔ	41. Ⓐ Ⓑ Ⓒ Ⓓ Ⓔ	72. Ⓐ Ⓑ Ⓒ Ⓓ Ⓔ	103. Ⓐ Ⓑ Ⓒ Ⓓ Ⓔ
11. Ⓐ Ⓑ Ⓒ Ⓓ Ⓔ	42. Ⓐ Ⓑ Ⓒ Ⓓ Ⓔ	73. Ⓐ Ⓑ Ⓒ Ⓓ Ⓔ	104. Ⓐ Ⓑ Ⓒ Ⓓ Ⓔ
12. Ⓐ Ⓑ Ⓒ Ⓓ Ⓔ	43. Ⓐ Ⓑ Ⓒ Ⓓ Ⓔ	74. Ⓐ Ⓑ Ⓒ Ⓓ Ⓔ	105. Ⓐ Ⓑ Ⓒ Ⓓ Ⓔ
13. Ⓐ Ⓑ Ⓒ Ⓓ Ⓔ	44. Ⓐ Ⓑ Ⓒ Ⓓ Ⓔ	75. Ⓐ Ⓑ Ⓒ Ⓓ Ⓔ	106. Ⓐ Ⓑ Ⓒ Ⓓ Ⓔ
14. Ⓐ Ⓑ Ⓒ Ⓓ Ⓔ	45. Ⓐ Ⓑ Ⓒ Ⓓ Ⓔ	76. Ⓐ Ⓑ Ⓒ Ⓓ Ⓔ	107. Ⓐ Ⓑ Ⓒ Ⓓ Ⓔ
15. Ⓐ Ⓑ Ⓒ Ⓓ Ⓔ	46. Ⓐ Ⓑ Ⓒ Ⓓ Ⓔ	77. Ⓐ Ⓑ Ⓒ Ⓓ Ⓔ	108. Ⓐ Ⓑ Ⓒ Ⓓ Ⓔ
16. Ⓐ Ⓑ Ⓒ Ⓓ Ⓔ	47. Ⓐ Ⓑ Ⓒ Ⓓ Ⓔ	78. Ⓐ Ⓑ Ⓒ Ⓓ Ⓔ	109. Ⓐ Ⓑ Ⓒ Ⓓ Ⓔ
17. Ⓐ Ⓑ Ⓒ Ⓓ Ⓔ	48. Ⓐ Ⓑ Ⓒ Ⓓ Ⓔ	79. Ⓐ Ⓑ Ⓒ Ⓓ Ⓔ	110. Ⓐ Ⓑ Ⓒ Ⓓ Ⓔ
18. Ⓐ Ⓑ Ⓒ Ⓓ Ⓔ	49. Ⓐ Ⓑ Ⓒ Ⓓ Ⓔ	80. Ⓐ Ⓑ Ⓒ Ⓓ Ⓔ	111. Ⓐ Ⓑ Ⓒ Ⓓ Ⓔ
19. Ⓐ Ⓑ Ⓒ Ⓓ Ⓔ	50. Ⓐ Ⓑ Ⓒ Ⓓ Ⓔ	81. Ⓐ Ⓑ Ⓒ Ⓓ Ⓔ	112. Ⓐ Ⓑ Ⓒ Ⓓ Ⓔ
20. Ⓐ Ⓑ Ⓒ Ⓓ Ⓔ	51. Ⓐ Ⓑ Ⓒ Ⓓ Ⓔ	82. Ⓐ Ⓑ Ⓒ Ⓓ Ⓔ	113. Ⓐ Ⓑ Ⓒ Ⓓ Ⓔ
21. Ⓐ Ⓑ Ⓒ Ⓓ Ⓔ	52. Ⓐ Ⓑ Ⓒ Ⓓ Ⓔ	83. Ⓐ Ⓑ Ⓒ Ⓓ Ⓔ	114. Ⓐ Ⓑ Ⓒ Ⓓ Ⓔ
22. Ⓐ Ⓑ Ⓒ Ⓓ Ⓔ	53. Ⓐ Ⓑ Ⓒ Ⓓ Ⓔ	84. Ⓐ Ⓑ Ⓒ Ⓓ Ⓔ	115. Ⓐ Ⓑ Ⓒ Ⓓ Ⓔ
23. Ⓐ Ⓑ Ⓒ Ⓓ Ⓔ	54. Ⓐ Ⓑ Ⓒ Ⓓ Ⓔ	85. Ⓐ Ⓑ Ⓒ Ⓓ Ⓔ	116. Ⓐ Ⓑ Ⓒ Ⓓ Ⓔ
24. Ⓐ Ⓑ Ⓒ Ⓓ Ⓔ	55. Ⓐ Ⓑ Ⓒ Ⓓ Ⓔ	86. Ⓐ Ⓑ Ⓒ Ⓓ Ⓔ	117. Ⓐ Ⓑ Ⓒ Ⓓ Ⓔ
25. Ⓐ Ⓑ Ⓒ Ⓓ Ⓔ	56. Ⓐ Ⓑ Ⓒ Ⓓ Ⓔ	87. Ⓐ Ⓑ Ⓒ Ⓓ Ⓔ	118. Ⓐ Ⓑ Ⓒ Ⓓ Ⓔ
26. Ⓐ Ⓑ Ⓒ Ⓓ Ⓔ	57. Ⓐ Ⓑ Ⓒ Ⓓ Ⓔ	88. Ⓐ Ⓑ Ⓒ Ⓓ Ⓔ	119. Ⓐ Ⓑ Ⓒ Ⓓ Ⓔ
27. Ⓐ Ⓑ Ⓒ Ⓓ Ⓔ	58. Ⓐ Ⓑ Ⓒ Ⓓ Ⓔ	89. Ⓐ Ⓑ Ⓒ Ⓓ Ⓔ	120. Ⓐ Ⓑ Ⓒ Ⓓ Ⓔ
28. Ⓐ Ⓑ Ⓒ Ⓓ Ⓔ	59. Ⓐ Ⓑ Ⓒ Ⓓ Ⓔ	90. Ⓐ Ⓑ Ⓒ Ⓓ Ⓔ	
29. Ⓐ Ⓑ Ⓒ Ⓓ Ⓔ	60. Ⓐ Ⓑ Ⓒ Ⓓ Ⓔ	91. Ⓐ Ⓑ Ⓒ Ⓓ Ⓔ	
30. Ⓐ Ⓑ Ⓒ Ⓓ Ⓔ	61. Ⓐ Ⓑ Ⓒ Ⓓ Ⓔ	92. Ⓐ Ⓑ Ⓒ Ⓓ Ⓔ	
31. Ⓐ Ⓑ Ⓒ Ⓓ Ⓔ	62. Ⓐ Ⓑ Ⓒ Ⓓ Ⓔ	93. Ⓐ Ⓑ Ⓒ Ⓓ Ⓔ	

Trial Test

15

This chapter contains a Trial Test in Natural Sciences. Take this Trial Test to learn what the actual exam is like and to determine how you might score on the exam before any practice or review.

The CLEP Exam in Natural Sciences measures your knowledge of biological and physical sciences, including origin and evolution of life, microbiology, biology, ecology, physics, chemistry, astronomy, geology, and other topics.

Number of Questions: 120

TIME LIMIT: 90 MINUTES

DIRECTIONS: Each of the questions or incomplete statements below is followed by five suggested answers or completions. Select the one that is best in each case.

1. What do malaria, amoebic dysentery, and African sleeping sickness have in common?

   (A) All are found in Africa only.
   (B) All are caused by protozoans.
   (C) Each constitutes a serious disease of the central nervous system.
   (D) None is of great significance to humans.
   (E) All are transmitted by direct contact.

2. Cellular structures responsible for oxidizing food and converting energy to adenosine triphosphate are called

   (A) the Golgi apparatus
   (B) ribosomes
   (C) chromoplasts
   (D) mitochondria
   (E) the endoplasmic reticulum

3. The idea that living things arise from other living things was proven experimentally by

   (A) Lamarck
   (B) Weismann
   (C) Pasteur
   (D) Redi
   (E) Needham

4. The ribosomes associated with the endoplasmic reticulum consist of

   (A) secretory nodes, which control metabolism
   (B) deoxyribose nucleic acid, which synthesizes chromatin
   (C) granular bodies associated with cell division
   (D) ribonucleic acid, which synthesizes protein
   (E) various nucleic acids, each of which is self-perpetuating

5. If a living cell is placed in a hypertonic saline solution,

   (A) the cell will shrink as water migrates out of the cell
   (B) the cell will shrink as salt migrates into the cell
   (C) the cell will maintain its size as salt migrates into the cell and water out of the cell
   (D) the cell will enlarge as water migrates into the cell
   (E) the cell will enlarge as salt migrates out of the cell

6. In typical ecosystems, the producers are

   (A) heterotrophic
   (B) parasitic
   (C) chemotrophic
   (D) photosynthetic
   (E) saprophytic

7. The light reactions of photosynthesis include those in which

   (A) radiant energy is converted into organic materials
   (B) radiant energy is stored
   (C) carbon dioxide is absorbed
   (D) water is split into hydrogen and oxygen
   (E) sugar is formed and oxygen is released

8. The principal water-absorbing structure of a typical root is the

   (A) hair root
   (B) root cap
   (C) endodermis
   (D) root hair cell
   (E) cortex

9. A photosynthetic organism is one which

   (A) obtains energy by the oxidation of inorganic materials
   (B) utilizes solid materials after eating and digesting them
   (C) obtains its nourishment from decaying organic materials
   (D) lives at the expense of other organisms
   (E) uses radiant energy in food synthesis

10. In plants, a growth response to the stimulus of light is called

    (A) geotropism
    (B) phototropism
    (C) thigmotropism
    (D) photoperiodism
    (E) hydrotropism

11. The growing of plants under soilless conditions is called

    (A) aquatics
    (B) hydrology
    (C) hydrotropism
    (D) hydroponics
    (E) hydrotaxis

12. The graph below indicates plant growth in relation to soil pH. A pH reading below 7.0 is acid; a pH reading above 7.0 is alkaline.

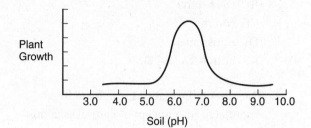

Plant Growth

Soil (pH)

On the basis of the information in the graph, one may conclude that

(A) plant growth causes a shift in soil acidity
(B) most plants grow best in slightly acid soils
(C) no plants can survive in alkaline soils
(D) no plants can survive in acid soils
(E) soil pH has little or no effect on plant growth

13. The enzyme-controlled breakdown of carbohydrates under anaerobic conditions is called

(A) autolysis
(B) decomposition
(C) bacteriophage
(D) fermentation
(E) respiration

14. In plant reproduction, selected cells of the diploid, spore-producing generation undergo

(A) diploidization
(B) oogenesis
(C) spermatogenesis
(D) meiosis
(E) mitosis

15. Structures which are similar because of function are said to be

(A) analogous
(B) homosporous
(C) monoecious
(D) homologous
(E) dioecious

16. In a blood transfusion, an individual with O negative blood may safely

(A) receive blood from any donor and give blood to any recipient
(B) receive blood from any donor with type O positive or negative blood and donate to any recipient
(C) receive blood from only type O negative donors but donate to any recipient
(D) receive blood from only type O negative donors and donate to any recipient with A, B, AB, or O negative (but not positive) blood
(E) receive blood from only type O negative donors but donate to any recipient with either type O negative or O positive blood

17. Many plants produce an orange pigment called carotene which animals convert to

(A) ATP
(B) hemoglobin
(C) vitamin A
(D) phytol
(E) vitamin C

18. Which nerve innervates the semicircular canals?

    (A) Auditory
    (B) Facial
    (C) Trochlear
    (D) Spinal accessory
    (E) Optic

19. The hormone that controls the rate of food conversion to energy is

    (A) insulin
    (B) thyroxin
    (C) adrenalin
    (D) cortisone
    (E) secretin

20. Stimulation by the sympathetic nervous system would result in

    (A) constricted pupils
    (B) dilated arteries
    (C) accelerated heartbeat
    (D) increased peristalsis
    (E) lower blood pressure

21. Progesterone

    (A) constricts blood vessels
    (B) regulates the menstrual cycle
    (C) stimulates production of thyroxin
    (D) regulates rate of basal metabolism
    (E) regulates sodium metabolism

22. The significance of mitosis is that there is

    (A) a quantitative division of the cell
    (B) precise distribution of cell content to the daughter cells
    (C) a qualitative division of cell components
    (D) a reduction of chromosome number
    (E) precise distribution of DNA to each daughter cell

23. Transfer of genetic information from one generation to the next is accomplished by

    (A) RNA only
    (B) DNA only
    (C) codons
    (D) ribosomes
    (E) both RNA and DNA

24. The inherited variations which are so essential to the concept of natural selection have their source in

    (A) acquired characteristics
    (B) nuclear proteins
    (C) mutations
    (D) the environment
    (E) special creation

25. A preformed miniature human within the body of an adult parent was known to the preformationists as a(n)

    (A) homunculus
    (B) epigenesis
    (C) ovist
    (D) cyst
    (E) animalcule

26. Permanent wilting is a plant condition caused by the loss of water from which there is no recovery, i.e., no restoration of turgidity. The data below show the percentages of soil moisture for selected soil types at the time of permanent wilting for the plants indicated.

Soil Moisture % at Time of Permanent Wilting

	Coarse Sand	Fine Clay	Sandy Loam	Loam	Clay Loam
Corn	1.07	3.1	6.5	9.9	15.5
Sorghum	.94	3.6	5.9	10.0	14.1
Oats	1.07	3.5	5.9	11.1	14.8
Pea	1.02	3.3	6.9	12.4	16.6
Tomato	1.11	3.3	6.9	11.7	15.3

On the basis of this information one may conclude that at the time of permanent wilting

(A) sunlight plays a direct role in wilting
(B) water continues to move from particle to particle in the soil
(C) transpiration continues at a reduced rate
(D) soil moisture varies widely for different plants
(E) soil moisture is fairly constant no matter what plant is involved

27. One would expect to observe caribou and lichens in

(A) a tropical rain forest
(B) the arctic tundra
(C) a grassland
(D) a deciduous forest
(E) a coniferous forest

28. Which of the following describes common characteristics of phytoplankton?

(A) plankton are found at all ocean depths.
(B) in the food chain, plankton are producers.
(C) plankton produce carbon dioxide via photosynthesis.
(D) plankton include plant species, but not animal species.
(E) plankton are submicroscopic in size.

29. Marine organisms characteristic of the abyssal zone would be found

(A) in the intertidal zone
(B) on the continental shelf to a depth of 500–600 feet
(C) in light
(D) in the deepest ocean trenches
(E) to a depth of 5,000 feet

30. In studies of predator-prey populations in a hypothetical situation, the data indicated on the graph below illustrate the cyclical population fluctuations of the predators and the prey.

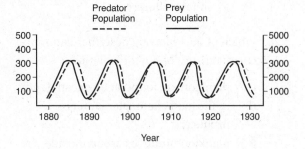

What conclusion may be drawn from these data?

(A) Predators maintain any population above the capacity of a given environment to support it.

(B) Avoidance of predators has no lasting effect on prey population.

(C) Decreases in populations of prey species are followed by decreases in populations of predator species.

(D) Populations of predators are nourished only by surpluses of prey.

(E) Even when exterminating its prey, a predator never exterminates itself.

31. Interrelationships between species are termed *commensalism* when

(A) both species are benefited

(B) mates are defended

(C) one species benefits at the expense of the other

(D) territories are defended

(E) one species benefits and the other is not harmed

32. The Cenozoic Era is best described as the age of

(A) seed plants

(B) mammals

(C) seed plants and mammals

(D) primitive fish

(E) reptiles

33. In the human circulatory system, blood returns to the heart from the lungs through the

(A) superior vena cava

(B) pulmonary veins

(C) inferior vena cava

(D) pulmonary artery

(E) descending aorta

34. Blood is supplied to the muscle wall of the heart by the

(A) hepatic portal vein

(B) coronary arteries

(C) auricular artery

(D) mesenteric artery

(E) coronary veins

35. Hookworm larvae gain access to the body

(A) by penetrating unbroken skin

(B) by means of insect bites

(C) through the mouth in contaminated food

(D) in improperly cooked pork

(E) in improperly cooked fish

36. Which of the following diseases of humans is transmitted by the bite of ticks?

(A) Tularemia

(B) Rocky Mountain spotted fever

(C) Sleeping sickness

(D) Psittacosis

(E) Amebiasis

Questions 37–39

In the diagrams below, water and sugar solutions are separated by cellophane membranes, as indicated. These cellophane membranes are permeable to water molecules and impermeable to sugar molecules. Assume that temperatures are constant and that the cellophane bags are filled equally.

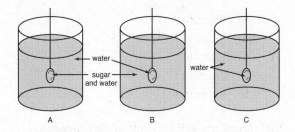

37. In diagram *A*

(A) the bag will shrink as water molecules move from the bag to the outside
(B) the addition of sugar to the water in the container will cause the turgidity of the bag to increase
(C) diffusion does not occur
(D) water molecules diffuse into the bag because there is a greater concentration of water outside than inside the bag
(E) there is a net movement of water molecules out of the cellophane bag because of a concentration difference

38. In diagram *B*

(A) the bag will shrink
(B) the bag will swell
(C) there will be a net movement of water molecules into the bag
(D) there will be a net movement of sugar molecules into the bag
(E) sugar draws water out of the bag

39. In diagram *C*

(A) water will diffuse into the bag causing it to swell
(B) water will diffuse out of the bag causing it to shrink
(C) there will be no change in the size of the bag
(D) osmosis occurs in the system
(E) the addition of glass marbles to the container will cause the bag to shrink

40. An organism which obtains energy from the oxidation of inorganic substances is

(A) chemosynthetic
(B) photosynthetic
(C) parasitic
(D) saprophytic
(E) holozoic

41. In a typical lake, the important producers are

(A) commensals
(B) zooplankton
(C) nekton
(D) phytoplankton
(E) benthos

42. Photosynthesis

(A) results in a decrease in dry weight
(B) requires the energy provided by respiration
(C) produces carbon dioxide and water
(D) results in an increase in dry weight
(E) uses oxygen and glucose as raw materials

43. The failure of one or more pairs of chromosomes to separate during meiosis is called

(A) polyploidy
(B) deletion
(C) translocation
(D) nondisjunction
(E) aneuploidy

44. Xylem is the principal constituent of a plant product called

(A) wood
(B) bark
(C) latex
(D) pith
(E) resin

45. One side effect that may be produced by the antigen-antibody reaction of the body is

(A) an allergic reaction
(B) dehydration
(C) convulsions
(D) infection
(E) pain

46. The body responds to an invasion of viruses by producing

(A) antibodies
(B) vaccine
(C) antibiotics
(D) antigens
(E) immune serum

47. The active substance which appears in a virus-infected cell and which prevents infection by a second virus is called

(A) autolysis
(B) interferon
(C) lysozyme
(D) bacteriophage
(E) rickettsias

48. Which of the following gases binds most tightly to hemoglobin?

(A) Oxygen
(B) Carbon dioxide
(C) Carbon monoxide
(D) Nitrogen
(E) Ozone

49. The Rh factor is produced due to

(A) a hormonal reaction
(B) an antigen-antibody reaction
(C) a form of anemia
(D) phagocytosis
(E) a vitamin deficiency

50. Which of the following vitamins is important for proper vision?

(A) Vitamin A
(B) Vitamin B
(C) Vitamin C
(D) Vitamin E
(E) Vitamin K

51. Roughage is important in the human diet because it

(A) contains vitamins
(B) speeds up digestion
(C) stimulates the walls of the large intestine
(D) slows digestion
(E) stimulates the production of antibodies

52. "Animal starch," a nutrient stored in various types of animal cells, is more properly known as

(A) angstrom
(B) antigen
(C) myosin
(D) glycogen
(E) actin

53. When the thyroid gland produces insufficient amounts of thyroxine,

(A) tetany occurs
(B) the basal metabolism rate increases
(C) irregularities in sodium metabolism develop
(D) acromegaly develops
(E) the basal metabolism rate decreases

54. Among the contributions of the ancient Greek scholars

    (A) was the law of independent assortment

    (B) was the concept of biogenesis

    (C) was the concept of recapitulation

    (D) were elements of the theory that living organisms have evolved

    (E) was the preformation theory

55. The two scientists most responsible for determining the structure, and thus the mechanism of duplication, of DNA were

    (A) Pauling and Crick

    (B) Morgan and Franklin

    (C) Watson and Pauling

    (D) Watson and Crick

    (E) Franklin and Pauling

56. Paul Ehrlich is best known for his discoveries in

    (A) immunization

    (B) attenuation

    (C) chemotherapy

    (D) antibiosis

    (E) phytopathology

57. The first person to show that blood circulates through the body was

    (A) Galen

    (B) Vesalius

    (C) Paracelsus

    (D) Harvey

    (E) Pasteur

58. In general, short food chains are more efficient than long food chains because in short food chains

    (A) there can be no carnivores

    (B) there is more energy produced in each stage

    (C) there are fewer producers

    (D) there is less energy loss

    (E) there are more producers

59. A population displaying a great number of homologous structures is considered to be

    (A) an order

    (B) a class

    (C) a family

    (D) a genus

    (E) a species

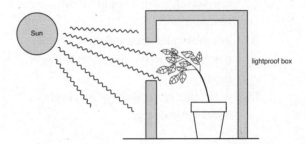

60. Under the conditions of uneven lighting imposed upon the plant in the diagram above, the plant bends toward the light because

    (A) the plant needs more light in order to carry on photosynthesis

    (B) the plant grows away from darkness

    (C) this is a growth response caused by the unequal distribution of growth-promoting substances in the plant stem

    (D) the plant is attracted to light

    (E) this is a growth response in an attempt to overcome the growth repressing effects of darkness

61. After two half-lives of radioactive decay, what percentage of the original number of atoms would remain unchanged?

    (A) 12.5%

    (B) 25%

    (C) 37.5%

    (D) 50%

    (E) 75%

62. The kinetic-molecular theory explains the difference between solids, liquids, and gases. One of the postulates of this theory is that

(A) molecules are in constant motion and move in straight lines

(B) molecules of a gas have great attraction for each other

(C) the kinetic energy of gas molecules is inversely proportional to the temperature

(D) gas molecules are extremely large in comparison to the distances between them

(E) when two molecules collide, both always lose energy

63. The basic energy-producing reaction in the sun is the conversion of

(A) mass to energy due to pressure

(B) helium to hydrogen

(C) fuels to heat

(D) heavy elements into lighter elements

(E) hydrogen to helium

64. A term to describe the solar system when the earth is presumably in the center is

(A) rotation

(B) parallax

(C) geocentric

(D) heliocentric

(E) ecliptic

65. The Milky Way galaxy is best described as

(A) a spherical grouping of about fifty million stars spread over approximately 2,000 light-years

(B) the solar system together with its moons and asteroids

(C) a disk-shaped grouping of billions of stars which spreads over approximately 100,000 light-years

(D) a galactic system comprising all the constellations

(E) a spherical grouping of over a billion stars

66. Forms of an atom with the same number of protons but different numbers of neutrons are known

(A) cations

(B) anions

(C) moles

(D) isotopes

(E) allotropes

67. When an astronomer detects a shift toward the red end of the spectrum, which of the following may he correctly infer?

(A) The chemical composition of a star has changed.

(B) He has discovered a new star.

(C) A star is stationary.

(D) The star he is observing is moving closer.

(E) The star he is observing is moving away.

68. One example of geological crosscutting is

   (A) a fault
   (B) an oxbow
   (C) a moraine
   (D) a floodplain
   (E) a stalagmite

69. Fossilized resin from ancient coniferous trees is called

   (A) amber
   (B) basalt
   (C) pumice
   (D) dolomite
   (E) halite

70. One outstanding and distinguishing feature of sedimentary rocks is

   (A) their complete lack of fossils
   (B) that they are formed exclusively of precipitates
   (C) that they are formed exclusively of crystals
   (D) the presence of different layers
   (E) that they are formed by the cooling of magma

71. The form of radiation with the greatest penetrating power is

   (A) alpha particles
   (B) beta particles
   (C) fission
   (D) fusion
   (E) gamma rays

72. As a result of nuclear fission

   (A) there is an increase in mass
   (B) light atomic nuclei fuse
   (C) X-rays are emitted
   (D) much energy is consumed
   (E) larger nuclei split into smaller ones

73. Color aberrations encountered when using lenses are corrected by

   (A) use of convex lenses
   (B) use of concave lenses
   (C) use of achromatic lenses
   (D) reducing the field or the aperture
   (E) proper focusing

74. When an object is immersed in a liquid

   (A) it displaces its own weight
   (B) it displaces a volume equal to its weight
   (C) it displaces a weight equal to its volume
   (D) it is buoyed up by a volume of liquid
   (E) it displaces its own volume of liquid

75. The energy transfer mechanism by which energy from the sun reaches the earth is

   (A) conduction
   (B) radiation
   (C) convection
   (D) vaporization
   (E) diffusion

Questions 76 and 77 are based on the following table, which summarizes the parts of the earth's crust as well as some basic information about those parts:

Layer	Thickness (km)	Composition	Temperature (°C)	Density (g/cm³)
Continental crust	30–60	Granitic silicate rock	20–600	2.8
Oceanic crust	5–8	Basaltic silicate rock	20–1,300	3.3
Mantle	2,800	Solid silicate	100–3,000	5.0
Outer core	2,150	Liquid iron-nickel	3,000–6,500	12
Inner core	1,230	Solid iron-nickel	7,000	12

76. About how far is it from the surface of the earth to its center?

(A) 62 km
(B) 620 km
(C) 6,200 km
(D) 62,000 km
(E) 620,000 km

77. What is the general relationship between the depth of a layer of the earth and its density?

(A) the greater the depth, the greater the density
(B) the greater the depth, the lower the density
(C) as the depth increases, the density increases and then decreases
(D) as the depth increases, the density decreases and then increases
(E) there is no pattern that relates these two factors

—————————

78. For every known subatomic particle, there is believed to exist

(A) an isotope
(B) an ionized equivalent
(C) an antiparticle
(D) coherent radiation
(E) a thermoelectric effect

79. What name is applied to an atom that carries a negative electric charge?

(A) catalyst
(B) electron
(C) anion
(D) isotope
(E) cation

80. The continual change in the plane in which a Foucault pendulum swings is evidence that

(A) the earth rotates
(B) the moon revolves around the earth
(C) the earth revolves around the sun
(D) the sun is the center of the solar system
(E) the earth is round

81. When a glass rod is rubbed with a silk cloth

(A) the glass rod gains protons and becomes negatively charged
(B) the glass rod gains protons and becomes positively charged
(C) the glass rod remains neutral
(D) the glass rod loses electrons and becomes negatively charged
(E) the glass rod loses electrons and becomes positively charged

82. The First Law of Thermodynamics states that

(A) energy can be created but not destroyed
(B) energy cannot be created but can be destroyed
(C) energy cannot be created or destroyed
(D) the amount of entropy increases during chemical reactions
(E) the amount of entropy stays constant during chemical reactions

83. Which of the following would increase the rate of a chemical reaction between gas molecules?

(A) increasing the temperature and increasing the pressure
(B) increasing the temperature and decreasing the pressure
(C) decreasing the temperature and increasing the pressure
(D) decreasing the temperature and decreasing the pressure
(E) increasing the temperature only

84. Work is accomplished when

(A) direction is imposed upon a moving object
(B) energy output equals energy input
(C) a machine operates without expending energy
(D) force is exerted upon an object, causing it to move
(E) a weight is held stationary at a certain height

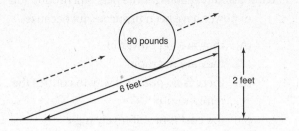

85. In the diagram above, how much effort is required to push the 90-pound barrel up the inclined plane?

(A) 45 pounds effort
(B) 30 pounds effort
(C) 15 pounds effort
(D) 10 pounds effort
(E) 5 pounds effort

86. Avogadro's number, the number of molecules in one mole of a substance, is

(A) 186,000
(B) 22.4
(C) 100
(D) 6.02×10^{23}
(E) 9.8

87. Compared to the earth, the sun is

(A) much larger and of greater density
(B) much larger and of lesser density
(C) much smaller and of greater density
(D) much smaller and of lesser density
(E) about the same size and density

88. Newton's First Law states that an object will maintain its motion unless acted upon by an unbalanced force. This is also known as the concept of

(A) acceleration
(B) action-reaction
(C) momentum conservation
(D) friction
(E) inertia

89. Fusion reactions for the peaceful production of power have been unsuccessful because

    (A) they are too powerful
    (B) they are too rapid
    (C) there is no practical way to control the temperature
    (D) the cost is prohibitively high
    (E) radioactive electricity is too dangerous

90. Laser-generated light

    (A) is polarized
    (B) is chaotic
    (C) is coherent
    (D) is disordered
    (E) has waves of different frequencies

91. Kinetic theory with respect to gases is based primarily on

    (A) the motion of particles
    (B) the attraction of molecules for each other
    (C) the ionization of gas molecules
    (D) sublimation
    (E) vaporization

92. High-altitude satellites will someday fall to earth because of

    (A) drag caused by cosmic radiation
    (B) drag caused by infrared radiation
    (C) centrifugal force
    (D) centrifugal force and the moon's gravity
    (E) drag caused by air and particles

93. An acidic solution would have

    (A) a pH < 7 and more hydrogen ions than hydroxide ions
    (B) a pH < 7 and more hydroxide ions than hydrogen ions
    (C) a pH > 7 and more hydrogen ions than hydroxide ions
    (D) a pH > 7 and more hydroxide ions than hydrogen ions
    (E) a pH = 7 and more hydrogen ions than hydroxide ions

94. Compared to earth, an object on the moon would have

    (A) the same mass and a greater weight
    (B) the same mass and a smaller weight
    (C) a greater mass and the same weight
    (D) a greater mass and a greater weight
    (E) a smaller mass and a smaller weight

95. The thermodynamic measure of disorder is called

    (A) entropy
    (B) spontaneity
    (C) momentum
    (D) redundancy
    (E) valence

96. Through a microscope, minute particles are observed to be in an almost constant state of random movement, a phenomenon called

    (A) surface tension
    (B) capillarity
    (C) osmosis
    (D) diffusion
    (E) Brownian motion

97. Igneous rocks include which of the following?

   (A) Sandstone
   (B) Limestone
   (C) Diamond
   (D) Obsidian
   (E) Shale

98. The atomic number of an element refers to

   (A) the total number of electrons and protons it possesses
   (B) the number of neutrons in the atomic nucleus
   (C) the number of protons in the atomic nucleus
   (D) its sequential number in the atomic scale
   (E) the total number of neutrons, electrons, and protons it possesses

99. Which type of mixture will not settle out but will scatter a beam of light (exhibit the Tyndall Effect)?

   (A) a solution
   (B) a suspension
   (C) a heterogeneous mixture
   (D) an aerosol
   (E) a colloid

100. The family of elements on that periodic table that includes chlorine, fluorine, and bromine is

   (A) the noble gases
   (B) the alkali metals
   (C) the transition metals
   (D) the halogens
   (E) the metalloids

101. When iron rusts

   (A) iron atoms are reduced and gain electrons
   (B) iron atoms are reduced and lose electrons
   (C) iron atoms are oxidized and gain electrons
   (D) iron atoms are oxidized and lose electrons
   (E) iron atoms react to form iron molecules

102. The change in state of matter from a solid directly to a gas is called

   (A) melting
   (B) freezing
   (C) boiling
   (D) sublimation
   (E) vaporization

103. In any given process

   (A) energy may be created
   (B) energy may be destroyed
   (C) energy may neither be created nor destroyed
   (D) the energies of the reactants and products are variable
   (E) energy and work are totally unrelated

104. In accordance with Einstein's theory of relativity, as a body gains speed

   (A) its mass decreases proportionately
   (B) its mass increases proportionately
   (C) only electrons in the outer shells of its atoms are affected
   (D) mass and energy are not related
   (E) only energy is lost

105. What kind of bonding would be found in a substance that is hard, brittle, and dissolved in water to produce a solution that conducts electricity

(A) ionic
(B) polar covalent
(C) nonpolar covalent
(D) molecular
(E) van der Waals

106. Carbon-12 and Carbon-14 are examples of

(A) allotropes
(B) isotopes
(C) carbon dating
(D) anions
(E) radioactivity

107. Gamma radiation is frequently used successfully to treat tumors and cancer tissue because

(A) such tissues are immune to radiation
(B) such tissues are more sensitive to radiation than are healthy tissues
(C) it acts faster than surgery without the risks of surgery
(D) the induced rate of radioactive decay is indicative of the extent of cure
(E) gamma radiation is low-energy radiation

108. Heat is a form of energy caused by

(A) the exchange of electrons between atoms
(B) the conversion of matter to energy
(C) the motion of molecules
(D) the conversion of energy to matter
(E) its absorption from the environment

109. By mixing all of the colors of the visible spectrum of light we produce

(A) infrared light
(B) black light
(C) purple light
(D) green light
(E) white light

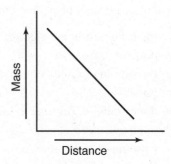

110. Which two factors affect the gravitational force on an object?

(A) charge and distance
(B) charge and mass
(C) mass and friction
(D) mass and distance
(E) friction and distance

111. The change of certain substances from solid to gaseous states without passing through the liquid state is called

(A) sublimation
(B) fusion
(C) convergence
(D) thermal coefficient
(E) reciprocation

Questions 112 and 113

Humidity is a measure of water-holding capacity of the atmosphere and may be expressed in terms of the number of grams of water vapor held per cubic meter of air.

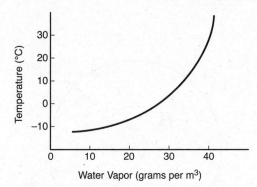

112. According to the illustration above, one may conclude that

   (A) humidity increases at lower temperatures
   (B) humidity decreases at lower temperatures
   (C) temperature does not affect humidity
   (D) higher temperatures decrease humidity
   (E) humidity is directly proportional to temperature

113. From the illustration above, one may also conclude that

   (A) if the humidity increases the temperature will rise
   (B) if the humidity decreases the temperature will rise
   (C) humidity increases uniformly as temperature increases
   (D) saturated air cannot retain its water if the temperature is lowered
   (E) saturated air can hold additional water if the temperature is lowered

114. Although ahead of his time, Roger Bacon contributed to science by stating that intuition or reason is insufficient to justify scientific theory and that, to give certainty to science, there must be

   (A) research
   (B) data
   (C) facts
   (D) observation
   (E) experimentation

115. Electromagnetic waves of extremely high frequency are called

   (A) photons
   (B) matter waves
   (C) gamma rays
   (D) X-rays
   (E) beta rays

DIRECTIONS: Each group of questions below consists of five lettered choices followed by a list of numbered phrases or sentences. For each numbered phrase or sentence select the one choice that is most closely related to it. Each choice may be used once, more than once, or not at all in each group.

Questions 116–118

(A) Distillation
(B) Evaporation
(C) Radiolysis
(D) Polymerization
(E) Transmutation

116. Nuclear reactions that change one element into another

117. The radioactive disintegration of radium to radon

118. The joining of small molecules into larger molecules

Questions 119–120

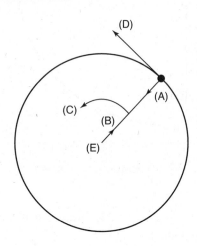

The diagram above represents the circular path of a moving weight tied to the end of a string. The five lettered choices are indicated on the diagram.

119. The velocity of the weight

120. The centripetal force on the moving weight

If there is still time remaining, you may review your answers.

ANSWER KEY
Trial Test

NATURAL SCIENCES

1.	B	31.	E	61.	B	91.	A
2.	D	32.	C	62.	A	92.	E
3.	C	33.	B	63.	E	93.	A
4.	D	34.	B	64.	C	94.	B
5.	A	35.	A	65.	C	95.	A
6.	D	36.	B	66.	D	96.	E
7.	D	37.	D	67.	E	97.	D
8.	D	38.	A	68.	A	98.	C
9.	E	39.	C	69.	A	99.	E
10.	B	40.	A	70.	D	100.	D
11.	D	41.	D	71.	E	101.	D
12.	B	42.	D	72.	E	102.	D
13.	D	43.	D	73.	C	103.	C
14.	D	44.	A	74.	E	104.	B
15.	A	45.	A	75.	B	105.	A
16.	E	46.	A	76.	C	106.	B
17.	C	47.	B	77.	A	107.	B
18.	A	48.	C	78.	C	108.	C
19.	B	49.	B	79.	C	109.	E
20.	C	50.	A	80.	A	110.	D
21.	B	51.	C	81.	E	111.	A
22.	E	52.	D	82.	C	112.	B
23.	B	53.	E	83.	A	113.	D
24.	C	54.	D	84.	D	114.	E
25.	A	55.	D	85.	B	115.	C
26.	E	56.	C	86.	D	116.	E
27.	B	57.	D	87.	B	117.	E
28.	B	58.	D	88.	E	118.	D
29.	D	59.	E	89.	C	119.	D
30.	C	60.	C	90.	C	120.	A

SCORING CHART

After you have scored your Trial Examination, enter the results in the chart below, then transfer your score to the Progress Chart on page 12. As you complete the Sample Examinations later in this part of the book, you should be able to achieve increasingly higher scores.

Total Test	Number Right	Number Wrong	Number Omitted
120			

ANSWER EXPLANATIONS

1. **(B)** Protozoans include some 30,000 single-celled organisms, some of which cause malaria, some types of dysentery, and African sleeping sickness.

2. **(D)** Mitochondria are the sites where energy is transferred from molecules of carbohydrate to those of ATP.

3. **(C)** Pasteur proved that life arises from life and that spontaneous generation is not possible.

4. **(D)** Ribosomes are found scattered in the cytoplasm of living cells and in association with the endoplasmic reticulum. They are composed of ribonucleic acid and protein and function in the synthesis of proteins such as enzymes.

5. **(A)** If a cell is placed in a highly concentrated solution (a hypertonic solution), water will migrate out of the cell in an attempt to equalize the concentrations inside and outside the cell.

6. **(D)** Basic food production for most of the biological world is accomplished by photosynthetic producers such as plants or algae.

7. **(D)** Photosynthesis is an energy-storing biochemical reaction in which the radiant energy of sunlight is stored in simple sugars in the form of chemical bonds. During its light reactions, water is split into hydrogen and oxygen.

8. **(D)** Root hair cells are hairlike extensions of the epidermal cells of most kinds of plant roots. These provide greatly increased surfaces for water absorption.

9. **(E)** A photosynthetic organism possesses chlorophyll and, in the presence of radiant energy, synthesizes glucose from carbon dioxide and water and stores energy.

10. **(B)** Tropisms are plant responses to external stimuli. Phototropism is a response to light, geotropism is a response to gravity, and thigmotropism is a response to touch.

11. **(D)** Hydroponics is the growing of plants in a liquid or moist environment (without soil) to which essential mineral nutrients are added.

12. **(B)** Most plants survive and grow best in soils of slightly acid to neutral soils (pH 5.8–7.0).

13. **(D)** Fermentation is a metabolic process in which sugars (carbohydrates) are converted to acids, alcohols, or common gases such as carbon dioxide.

14. **(D)** In plants, diploid spore-mother cells undergo meiosis to produce haploid spores.

15. **(A)** Analogous structures are similar due to a common function, such as the wings of a bird and the wings of an insect. Homologous structures are those that share common ancestry in evolutionary history, such as the wing of a bat and the arm of a monkey.

16. **(E)** A person with O negative blood will reject all blood types except O negative, but because he lacks antigens to A, B, or Rh positive, can donate blood to anyone (universal donor).

17. **(C)** Carotene is a precursor of vitamin A.

18. **(A)** The semicircular canals are innervated by the auditory nerve and are associated with the inner ear and function to keep the body aware of its position with respect to gravity and motion.

19. **(B)** Thyroxin controls the rate of metabolism by controlling the cellular respiration of food.

20. **(C)** The sympathetic nervous system responds to perceived emotional situations such as anger or fear. One body response to anger or fear is accelerated heartbeat.

21. **(B)** The corpus luteum secretes progesterone, which regulates the menstrual cycle and prepares the body for pregnancy.

22. **(E)** Mitosis is both a quantitative and qualitative division of the nucleus of a cell which results in precise and equal distribution of chromatin and, therefore, DNA to each daughter cell.

23. **(B)** Deoxyribonucleic acid (DNA) is the only substance transmitted qualitatively and quantitatively from one generation to the next.

24. **(C)** Mutations are alterations in DNA that can be passed on to the next generation. They are the source of variation from one generation to another. Those mutations that make an individual better able to adapt to the environment may be passed on to future generations so that the individual will be better able to survive and reproduce.

25. **(A)** It was once believed that in sperm were preformed miniature humans that grew to become adults. One of these perfectly preformed humans was known as a homunculus.

26. **(E)** The data indicate that, at the time of permanent wilting, soil moisture is fairly constant, no matter what species of plant is concerned.

27. **(B)** The arctic tundra is treeless and the home of caribou and numerous lichen. It is also the summer breeding ground for numerous migratory birds.

28. **(B)** Phytoplankton are plant species located primarily at the upper levels of the ocean. At deeper levels there would not be enough sunlight to enable them to survive.

29. **(D)** The abyssal zones of the oceans are the deepest ocean trenches.

30. **(C)** The balance between any predator-prey group is delicate; an increase in the population of the prey is typically followed by an increase in the population of the predator, and vice versa.

31. **(E)** Commensalism is a relationship between two species in which one benefits from the other without harming it or giving benefit to it.

32. **(C)** The Cenozoic Era is the last of the great periods of geologic time and is characterized by the advent of mammals and seed plants.

33. **(B)** Pulmonary veins return oxygenated blood from the lungs to the left atrium of the heart.

34. **(B)** Coronary arteries branch from the aorta and carry blood to the heart muscle.

35. **(A)** Hookworm larvae on the ground penetrate unbroken skin, commonly the feet of barefoot children in warm climates.

36. **(B)** Rocky Mountain spotted fever is caused by a rickettsia transmitted to humans through the bite of a tick.

37. **(D)** Sugar molecules inside the bag lower the concentration of water molecules in comparison to the water outside. Therefore, water molecules diffuse into the bag.

38. **(A)** The bag, containing only water, has a higher concentration of water molecules than the surrounding water, which also contains sugar molecules. Water will, therefore, diffuse out of the bag and the bag will shrink.

39. **(C)** A state of equilibrium exists and there will be no net diffusion of water either into or out of the bag.

40. **(A)** Some bacteria, such as iron and sulfur using bacteria, obtain energy through the oxidation of iron and sulfur compounds respectively.

41. **(D)** Phytoplankton are photosynthetic organisms and because they are so numerous, they are important producers.

42. **(D)** Photosynthesis produces the carbohydrate glucose and therefore increases the dry weight of the plant.

43. **(D)** The failure of homologous chromosomes to separate in the anaphase of the first meiotic division, or the failure of the sister chromatids of a chromosome to separate in the anaphase of the second meiotic division, is called nondisjunction.

44. **(A)** Wood is the tree tissue inside the vascular cambium and is a term synonymous with xylem.

45. **(A)** A single injection of a foreign protein into the body may hypersensitize an individual so that future exposure to the same protein results in an allergic reaction.

46. **(A)** A virus invading the body is an antigen. The body's immune system responds by producing antibodies.

47. **(B)** Interferon is produced by body cells into which the foreign nucleic acid of a virus has entered. It renders uninfected cells immune to other viruses.

48. **(C)** While both carbon dioxide and oxygen bind to and release from hemoglobin, carbon monoxide binds very tightly and releases with difficulty. This is the reason carbon monoxide inhalation is so often fatal.

49. **(B)** Rh-negative individuals develop antibodies to the Rh antigen, and these destroy Rh-positive cells.

50. **(A)** Vitamin A, or retinol, is essential for the formation of pigments needed for vision. Vitamin C prevents scurvy, and Vitamin K aids in the proper formation of blood clots. Vitamin E is an important antioxidant, and the B vitamins are essential for proper metabolism.

51. **(C)** Roughage, such as whole-grain cereals, is important to the diet because it stimulates the large intestine.

52. **(D)** In humans and other animals, excess glucose is converted into a starch called glycogen, which is stored in muscles and in the liver, where it is readily available.

53. **(E)** Thyroxine deficiency in humans leads to cretinism in early childhood and to a lowered metabolic rate in adults.

54. **(D)** Anaximander, a Greek philosopher (611–547 B.C.), proposed an explanation of evolution based upon observation and reasoning.

55. **(D)** Watson and Crick determined the double helix structure of DNA.

56. **(C)** Ehrlich studied the effects of chemicals upon body tissues and discovered salvarsan, a chemical used to treat syphilis. He was the first to use a systematic approach to treat chemotherapeutic investigations.

57. **(D)** William Harvey demonstrated in the 1620s that blood circulates through the body.

58. **(D)** At each level in a food chain there is a loss of useful energy. For this reason, shorter food chains with fewer energy transfers are more efficient.

59. **(E)** One definition identifies a species on the basis of its number of shared homologous structures.

60. **(C)** Uneven light is responsible for the unequal distribution of growth-promoting substances in the stem, thus causing uneven stem elongation.

61. **(B)** The half-life of a radioactive substance is the length of time necessary for 50% of its atoms to decay. After two half-lives of radioactive decay, 25% of the original atoms would remain unchanged.

62. **(A)** The kinetic-molecular theory holds that matter is composed of molecules that are in constant motion, move in straight lines, and collide.

63. **(E)** Hydrogen atoms in the sun undergo fusion. Four atoms of hydrogen fuse to form one atom of helium with a minute quantity of mass left over. This mass is converted into energy.

64. **(C)** *Geocentric* describes a concept pertaining to the solar system that supposes that the earth is the center of the system.

65. **(C)** The Milky Way is a large spiral galaxy shaped like a disk and is approximately 5,000 light-years thick and 100,000 light-years in diameter.

66. **(D)** Isotopes are forms of an atom with the same number of protons (atomic number) but different numbers of neutrons, and thus also different mass numbers.

67. **(E)** A shift toward the red end of the spectrum means that the light wavelengths are increasing and indicates that the star being viewed is moving away from the viewer.

68. **(A)** A fault is a fracture of the earth's crust accompanied by a shift of one side with respect to the other.

69. **(A)** Amber is fossilized resin.

70. **(D)** Probably the most distinguishing feature of sedimentary rock is the fact that it has a layered structure.

71. **(E)** Alpha particles have the lowest penetrating power, beta an intermediate amount, and gamma rays the greatest.

72. **(E)** Fission is the "splitting" of larger atoms into smaller ones.

73. **(C)** Color or chromatic aberration is the failure of the different colors contained in white light to meet in a common point, called the focal point, after they pass through a convex lens. It may be reduced by use of an achromatic lens.

74. **(E)** A submerged object displaces its own volume.

75. **(B)** Since there is no matter in outer space, energy can be transferred only via radiation. Both conduction and convection require physical contact between molecules for heat transfer to take place.

76. **(C)** Adding up all the depths of the layers gives the distance to the center of the earth, about 6,200 km. Note that the exact distance is not required; only the order of magnitude is necessary.

77. **(A)** A look at the last column shows that as the layers go in toward the center of the earth, the density increases.

78. **(C)** In many situations, such as pair annihiliation, a particle and its antiparticle interact and disappear. An example of an antiparticle is the positron, a particle identical to the electron, except that it has the opposite charge.

79. **(C)** Anions are negatively charged ions. Cations are positively charged.

80. **(A)** A Foucault pendulum is so constructed that it always swings in the same plane. The rotation of the earth makes the pendulum appear to change the plane in which it swings.

81. **(E)** Static electricity can be produced by rubbing a glass rod with a piece of silk, during which the silk takes up electrons to become negatively charged. The glass rod gives up electrons to become positively charged.

82. **(C)** The First Law of Thermodynamics is a statement of the law of conservation of energy, which states that energy is neither created nor destroyed.

83. **(A)** The rates of chemical reactions depend upon collisions. Greater temperatures mean molecules move faster and collide more often, and greater pressures also increase collision rates.

84. **(D)** Work is defined as the force exerted upon an object multiplied by the distance the object is moved.

85. **(B)** The ratio of the height of the inclined plane to its hypotenuse determines the effort required to move the barrel up the inclined plane.

86. **(D)** Avogadro's number, the number of molecules in a mole of a substance, is 6.02×10^{23}.

87. **(B)** The sun is very much larger than the earth and being made primarily of gases (as opposed to the earth, which is solid) is of much lower density.

88. **(E)** Newton's First Law of Motion summarizes the principle of inertia, which states that an object's motion will be unchanged unless it is altered by a force or forces that act upon it.

89. **(C)** Nuclear fusion promises unlimited supplies of energy with much less environmental danger than from fission reactions. However, to date, no useful fusion reactor has been designed.

90. **(C)** Laser-generated light is coherent, ordered, and nonchaotic, and each wave has the same frequency, phase, and direction.

91. **(A)** The current kinetic-molecular theory is a concept based on studies of the motion of molecules.

92. **(E)** All earth satellites will eventually fall back to earth because of drag which is caused by air molecules (even though sparse) and particulate matter in space.

93. **(A)** An acidic solution has a greater concentration of hydrogen ions (H^+) than hydroxide ions (OH^-) and a pH less than 7.0.

94. **(B)** The mass of an object does not change with location, but an object on the moon has less weight because the moon is smaller than the earth and exerts less gravitational attraction.

95. **(A)** Entropy is the thermodynamic measure of disorder and always increases during any spontaneous process.

96. **(E)** Brownian movement is the result of molecular activity. Under the microscope, visible particles appear to be in a state of erratic motion because they are continually being bombarded (bumped) from all sides by molecules in motion.

97. **(D)** Igneous rocks are formed from cooling magma and lava. Obsidian is a glassy rock found where lava has cooled. Shale, limestone, and sandstone are sedimentary rocks, while diamond is a metamorphic rock, being formed from the action of heat and pressure.

98. **(C)** The number of protons in an atomic nucleus is the atomic number.

99. **(E)** Colloids are mixtures that have particles small enough that they do not settle out but large enough to scatter a beam of light. A suspension has larger particles and settles out, whereas a true solution has smaller particles that do not scatter a beam of light.

100. **(D)** The halogens include group 17 (or VIIA) on the periodic table.

101. **(D)** Iron atoms are oxidized by oxygen, and in the process they lose electrons.

102. **(D)** A physical change from a solid to a gas without a liquid as an intermediate is known as sublimation.

103. **(C)** The First Law of Thermodynamics states that energy may be neither created nor destroyed.

104. **(B)** Mass and velocity are proportional; as speed approaches the velocity of light, mass approaches infinity.

105. **(A)** Ionic compounds tend to be hard and brittle, dissolve in water, and when dissolved produce ions that conduct an electric current.

106. **(B)** Carbon-12 and Carbon-14 both are carbon atoms, but with different mass numbers (due to a different number of neutrons). This makes them isotopes of each other.

107. **(B)** Tumor cells, which grow rapidly, are more sensitive to radiation generally than are healthy cells. Therefore, radiation therapy is often a successful tumor therapy.

108. **(C)** Heat is a form of energy existing in matter resulting from the motion of its molecules. There is no molecular motion at absolute zero.

109. **(E)** Visible light is white and includes wavelengths from red to violet with orange, yellow, green, and blue in between.

110. **(D)** Gravitation attraction depends on the mass of the objects involved (the greater the mass, the greater the attraction) and distance (the greater the distance, the weaker the attraction).

111. **(A)** The direct change from the solid state to the gaseous state is called sublimation. An example is the sublimation of ice or snow when air flows over it at below freezing temperatures.

112. **(B)** ⎱ The ability of the air to hold moisture in vapor form is inversely proportional
113. **(D)** ⎰ to the temperature.

114. **(E)** Roger Bacon is credited with the introduction of the experimental method of science.

115. **(C)** Gamma rays are high frequency, high energy, and short wavelength electromagnetic radiation.

116. **(E)** Transmutation, in the historic sense, is the conversion of base metals to gold or silver; in modern physics, it is the transformation of one element into another by one or more nuclear reactions.

117. **(E)** Radioactive decay of certain elements accounts for one form of transmutation, which was unknown before its discovery by Becquerel.

118. **(D)** Polymerization is the joining of small molecules to produce larger molecules using heat, pressure, and selected catalysts.

119. **(D)** ⎱ The weight tied to the end of the string tends to move in a straight line but is held in circular orbit by the string. Centripetal force acts in the direction toward the
120. **(A)** ⎰ axis or center.

Background and Practice Questions

16

DESCRIPTION OF THE NATURAL SCIENCES EXAMINATION

The CLEP Examination in Natural Sciences measures your general knowledge and your ability to use principles and ideas in the biological and physical sciences. It covers material that is generally taught in a college course for nonscience majors. The exam is given in two parts, each consisting of approximately 60 questions and each requiring 45 minutes to complete. See the following chart for approximate percentages of examination items:

Natural Sciences Exam

	Content and Item Types	Time/Number of Questions
50%	**Biological Science**	120 questions
	10% Origin and evolution of life, classification of organisms	90 minutes
	10% Cell organization, cell division, chemical nature of the gene, bioenergetics, biosynthesis	
	20% structure, functions, and development in organisms; patterns of heredity	
	10% Concepts of population biology with emphasis on ecology	
50%	**Physical Science**	
	7% Atomic and nuclear structure and properties, elementary particles, nuclear reactions	
	10% Chemical elements, compounds and reactions; molecular structure and bonding	
	12% Heat, thermodynamics, and states of matter; classical mechanics, relativity	
	4% Electricity and magnetism, waves, light, and sound	
	7% The universe: galaxies, stars, the solar system	
	10% The earth: atmosphere, hydrosphere, structure, properties, surface features, geological processes, history	

The questions on this exam include aspects of natural science that may not have been covered in courses you have taken in school. Your ability to answer these questions will depend on the extent to which you have maintained a general interest in these subjects and kept current by reading science articles and science-based materials in magazines, newspapers, books, and other materials written for the nonscientist.

THE KINDS OF QUESTIONS THAT APPEAR ON THE EXAMINATION

There are two important aspects of the examination questions: (1) the knowledge and abilities they test for, and (2) the formats in which they are presented.

Some questions require knowledge of basic scientific concepts, facts, and principles; others require application of knowledge; and a third group requires interpretation and understanding of data presented in various forms (graphs, diagrams, tables, lists). The following questions provide examples of each type of question.

Knowledge of Concepts, Facts, and Principles

DIRECTIONS: Each of the questions or incomplete statements below is followed by five suggested answers or completions. Select the one that is best in each case.

1. A plant tissue whose cells disintegrate, causing leaves to separate from their stems, is called

    (A) the annulus
    (B) a bud scar
    (C) the collenchyma
    (D) the abscission layer
    (E) the cambium

2. When a glowing wood splint introduced into a tube of gas subsequently bursts into flame, what gas is in the tube?

    (A) Nitrogen
    (B) Chlorine
    (C) Oxygen
    (D) Helium
    (E) Carbon dioxide

Ability to Apply Knowledge

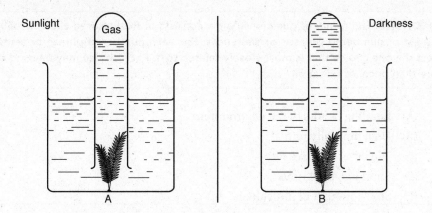

In the diagrams above, aquatic photosynthetic plants are placed under inverted test tubes which are filled with water. Except for light, all environmental and genetic factors are constant and the same for each.

3. After exposing plant A to several hours of sunlight, while plant B is maintained in darkness, it may correctly be concluded that, with respect to gas production,

   (A) plant A carried on photosynthesis
   (B) plant A carried on both photosynthesis and respiration
   (C) darkness inhibits respiration
   (D) sunlight is necessary for gas production
   (E) sunlight inhibits respiration

Ability to Interpret and Understand Data

(A) Limiting factors of the environment
(B) High mortality rate
(C) High reproductive rate
(D) Short length of time
(E) Small number of individuals

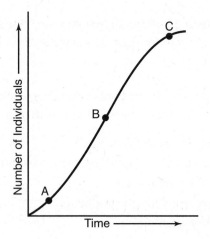

4. A condition limiting the growth rate at position A on the curve

5. A condition limiting the growth rate at position B on the curve

6. A condition limiting the growth rate at position C on the curve

What Formats Are Used

Most questions are in interrogative or sentence-completion form, and require you to select the correct answer from five choices that follow the question. In the preceding group, questions 1–3 are in this format.

A second type lists the answer choices first, and then gives a list of numbered phrases or sentences. You are required to select, for each phrase or sentence, the answer choice that best fits it. Questions 4–6 above, based on a graph, are in this category.

Notice that the directions for the two formats differ.

Answers and Explanations for Sample Questions

1. **(D)** The abscission layer is a layer of plant cells that disintegrates, causing leaves and other structures to separate from the plant.

2. **(C)** A standard laboratory test for oxygen production is that a glowing wood splint bursts into flame in the presence of oxygen.

3. **(D)** Plants A and B are exposed to identical conditions except for sunlight/darkness. There is no evidence that photosynthesis or respiration is occurring. An unidentified gas produced by A is the only observable outcome of this experiment.

4. **(E)** The graph represents a standard growth (sigmoid) curve. Over a period of time a
5. **(C)** small number of individuals existing under normal conditions will increase in
6. **(A)** number while food, space, etc., are ample, but, as the numbers of individuals increase, competition for food, space, etc., increases and the accumulation of metabolic wastes at the same time slows growth.

PRACTICE QUESTIONS ON NATURAL SCIENCES

Biology

DIRECTIONS: Each of the questions or incomplete statements below is followed by five suggested answers or completions. Select the one that is best in each case.

1. At the tissue level of organization

   (A) cells retain their separate functional identity
   (B) dissimilar cells are associated to conduct a variety of functions
   (C) cells are completely independent
   (D) similar cells are associated in the performance of a particular function
   (E) there is no cellular specialization

2. A cell's metabolic requirements are proportional to its volume. Its ability to meet these requirements and to exchange substances with its environment is

   (A) dependent on its activity
   (B) inversely proportional to its surface area
   (C) dependent on its environment
   (D) a function of both its activity and its environment
   (E) proportional to its surface area

3. Cellular metabolism is controlled by organic catalysts called

   (A) hormones
   (B) vitamins
   (C) auxin
   (D) phlogistons
   (E) enzymes

4. An organism which utilizes radiant energy in food synthesis is

   (A) holozoic
   (B) parasitic
   (C) chemosynthetic
   (D) saprophytic
   (E) photosynthetic

5. The typical consumers in an ecosystem are

   (A) saprophytic
   (B) photosynthetic
   (C) parasitic
   (D) chemosynthetic
   (E) holozoic

Questions 6 and 7

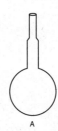
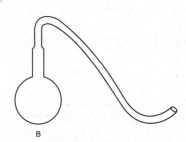

A   B

Pasteur placed a nutrient broth in each of two flasks similar to those illustrated above. Both flasks were open to air, but flask B was open only through its curved neck. The broth in each flask was boiled initially to kill the contained organisms, and then the flasks were left standing. Living organisms soon reappeared in flask A but no life appeared in flask B.

6. Since flask B remained free of life indefinitely, it can be concluded that

(A) life does not arise spontaneously from the nutrient broth
(B) flask A permits microorganisms to enter readily
(C) the curved neck of flask B apparently prevents microorganisms from entering the flask
(D) all of the above
(E) none of the above

7. The evidence generated by this experiment supports

(A) Koch's postulates
(B) The Hardy-Weinberg Law
(C) the Germ Theory of disease
(D) Virchow's theory of biogenesis
(E) the Cell Theory

8. In the "dark reactions" of photosynthesis

(A) chemical energy is changed to radiant energy
(B) organic synthesis occurs
(C) carbon dioxide is absorbed
(D) radiant energy is released
(E) radiant energy is changed to chemical energy

9. Photosynthesis

(A) produces oxygen and inorganic compounds
(B) produces carbon dioxide and water
(C) produces carbon dioxide and organic compounds
(D) produces oxygen and organic compounds
(E) produces oxygen and water

10. A process which results, in part, in the production of carbon dioxide and water is

(A) respiration
(B) photosynthesis
(C) secretion
(D) osmosis
(E) phosphorylation

11. An orientation growth movement by plants in response to an external stimulus is a

(A) tropism
(B) synergism
(C) polymorphism
(D) cyclosis
(E) taxis

12. The tendency of the roots of a plant to grow down is known as

(A) phototropism
(B) photosynthesis
(C) geotropism
(D) geoattraction
(E) gravitropism

13. Which of the following is an organic compound found in the cell walls of hard wood?

(A) Lignin
(B) Suberin
(C) Pectin
(D) Cutin
(E) Resin

14. When you eat a celery "stalk," you are eating

(A) root tissue
(B) stem tissue
(C) leaf tissue
(D) fruit
(E) seed

15. Water loss by plants is known as

   (A) evaporation
   (B) transpiration
   (C) stomata
   (D) condensation
   (E) chloroplasticity

16. If a species has more than one pair of chromosomes, during meiosis recombination of genes may occur as a result of the reassortment of non-homologous chromosomes and by

   (A) mutation
   (B) fertilization
   (C) polyploidy
   (D) nondisjunction
   (E) crossing-over

17. In plants, selected cells of the haploid, gamete-producing generation

   (A) become or produce spores
   (B) undergo meiosis
   (C) undergo cleavage
   (D) become or produce eggs or sperm
   (E) are polyploid

18. Structures which are similar because of anatomy and development are said to be

   (A) analogous
   (B) dioecious
   (C) monoecious
   (D) homologous
   (E) homosporous

19. The Rh factor assumes serious proportions when

   (A) an Rh-negative mother carries an Rh-positive fetus in a first pregnancy
   (B) an Rh-negative mother carries an Rh-negative fetus in a second pregnancy
   (C) an Rh-positive mother carries an Rh-negative fetus
   (D) an Rh-positive mother carries an Rh-positive fetus
   (E) an Rh-negative mother carries an Rh-positive fetus in a second pregnancy

20. Carotene functions in maintaining

   (A) night vision
   (B) normal blood clotting
   (C) normal nerves
   (D) fertility
   (E) normal tooth and bone development

21. A change in the sequence of nucleotides in DNA is called

   (A) duplication
   (B) transition
   (C) mutation
   (D) transcription
   (E) induction

22. Impairment of the spinal accessory nerves would affect

   (A) muscles of the shoulder
   (B) facial muscles
   (C) the parotid gland
   (D) swallowing
   (E) muscles of the tongue

23. Teeth are innervated by the

    (A) oculomotor nerve
    (B) facial nerve
    (C) vagus nerve
    (D) trochlear nerve
    (E) trigeminal nerve

24. Stimulation by the parasympathetic nervous system would result in

    (A) weaker heartbeat
    (B) erection of hair
    (C) dilated pupils
    (D) higher blood pressure
    (E) increased sweat secretion

25. Pathologic conditions caused by defects in hormonal action are called

    (A) atrophy
    (B) pheromones
    (C) infectious diseases
    (D) deficiency diseases
    (E) functional diseases

26. Oxytocin

    (A) stimulates basal metabolism
    (B) regulates calcium metabolism
    (C) constricts blood vessels
    (D) regulates phosphorus metabolism
    (E) stimulates lactation

27. All of the following may occur during synapsis in meiosis *except*:

    (A) crossing-over
    (B) transduction
    (C) inversion
    (D) translocation
    (E) duplication

28. The appearance of variations in a population may be attributed to either genetic change or

    (A) genetic drift
    (B) changed environmental factors
    (C) nonrandom mating
    (D) parthenogenesis
    (E) adaptive radiation

29. Which one of the following is *not* a type of RNA?

    (A) Template RNA
    (B) Ribosomal RNA
    (C) Messenger RNA
    (D) Gametic RNA
    (E) Transfer RNA

30. The concept that all eggs have existed since the creation of the world is entailed in the beliefs of

    (A) pangenesists
    (B) animaculists
    (C) epigenesists
    (D) ovists
    (E) parthenogenesists

31. The ovary of a flower matures into

    (A) a seed
    (B) an embryo
    (C) a fruit
    (D) the endosperm
    (E) the receptacle

32. You would expect to observe moose and spruce trees in the

    (A) alpine tundra
    (B) coniferous forest
    (C) tropical rain forest
    (D) grasslands
    (E) deciduous forest

33. Nekton includes marine organisms which

    (A) exist only in darkness
    (B) swim by their own propulsion
    (C) exist to a depth of 5,000 feet
    (D) exist in the deepest ocean trenches
    (E) float on the surface

34. A student of cytogenetics would be concerned with

    (A) convergent evolution
    (B) the cellular basis of inheritance
    (C) prenatal development
    (D) the genetic changes in populations
    (E) parallel evolution

35. A paleontologist is a biologist concerned primarily with studying

    (A) birds
    (B) snakes
    (C) rocks
    (D) insects
    (E) fossils

36. An interrelationship between two organisms in which one receives all of the benefits at the expense of the other is called

    (A) parasitism
    (B) commensalism
    (C) mutualism
    (D) symbiosis
    (E) saprophytism

37. In the human circulatory system, leakage of blood back into the heart is prevented by the

    (A) tricuspid valve
    (B) aortic valve
    (C) ventricular valves
    (D) semilunar valves
    (E) bicuspid valve

38. Blood leaves the human liver through the hepatic vein and returns to the heart through the

    (A) hepatic portal system
    (B) anterior vena cava
    (C) azygous vein
    (D) inferior mesenteric artery
    (E) inferior vena cava

39. Children in developed countries do not need to be immunized against which of the following infectious diseases?

    (A) Tetanus
    (B) Diphtheria
    (C) Measles
    (D) Polio
    (E) Cholera

40. The greatest significance of sexual reproduction is that it

    (A) ensures invariable genetic lines
    (B) permits new combinations of genes
    (C) ensures that traits are never lost
    (D) eliminates the need for meiosis
    (E) stimulates mating

41. A plant heterozygous for a particular gene (Aa) is crossed with a plant that is homozygous recessive for the gene (aa). What is the probability any given offspring will exhibit the dominant trait?

    (A) 1/8
    (B) 1/4
    (C) 1/2
    (D) 3/4
    (E) 7/8

42. In an individual with genotype "AaBb," the probability of producing gametes with dominant genes ("AB") is

    (A) unpredictable
    (B) 1/16
    (C) 1/8
    (D) 1/4
    (E) 1/2

43. A mutation to a gene will be expressed by a protein having an incorrect sequence of

    (A) molecules
    (B) glycolipids
    (C) covalent bonds
    (D) amino acids
    (E) enzymes

44. An ecological niche

    (A) is a micro-habitat
    (B) is really nondistinguishable
    (C) may be occupied by only one species
    (D) may be occupied by any number of species
    (E) may be occupied by only one individual

45. An organism which exhibits bilateral symmetry

    (A) always has a right and left leg
    (B) always has a right side and a left side
    (C) exhibits universal symmetry internally
    (D) could never possess an anterior or posterior end
    (E) would give birth to living young

46. Enzyme reactions typically have an opposite or contrary reaction. The contrary reaction to the enzyme reaction called hydrolysis is called

    (A) condensation
    (B) reduction
    (C) amination
    (D) phosphorylation
    (E) oxidation

47. Which of the following is the correct formula for a carboxylic acid group, such as might be found in amino acids?

    (A) CNH_2
    (B) NH_2
    (C) $COONH_2$
    (D) COH
    (E) COOH

48. When a living cell is placed in a fluid and there is net movement of water molecules out of the cell, the fluid is said to be

    (A) isotonic
    (B) hypotonic
    (C) plasmolyzed
    (D) hypertonic
    (E) hydrolyzed

49. An organism capable of synthesizing its own food is described as

    (A) holozoic
    (B) heterotrophic
    (C) autotrophic
    (D) parasitic
    (E) saprophytic

50. Heterotrophic organisms relying upon decomposing organic materials for nutrition are

    (A) parasitic
    (B) autotrophic
    (C) holozoic
    (D) saprophytic
    (E) chemotrophic

51. In 1772, Joseph Priestley demonstrated that green plants

    (A) carry on photosynthesis
    (B) absorb water from the soil
    (C) give off carbon dioxide
    (D) absorb minerals from the soil
    (E) give off oxygen

52. An enzyme-regulated process in living cells resulting in the transfer of energy to ATP is

    (A) reduction
    (B) assimilation
    (C) osmosis
    (D) absorption
    (E) respiration

53. Cellular organelles called ribosomes are the sites of

(A) enzyme storage
(B) protein synthesis
(C) chromosomal replication
(D) cellular respiration
(E) photosynthesis in plants

54. What is the principal absorbing structure of typical roots?

(A) Root cap
(B) Root hair cell
(C) Endodermis
(D) Hair roots
(E) Xylem

55. The loss of water by transpiration is the result of

(A) capillarity
(B) diffusion
(C) mass movement
(D) cohesive forces
(E) adhesive forces

56. The classification of bacteria is determined chiefly by their

(A) cell membranes and capsules
(B) movements and environments
(C) morphological characteristics
(D) anatomical characteristics
(E) physiological characteristics

57. The union of a sperm and an egg is called

(A) germination
(B) homospory
(C) fertilization
(D) reduction
(E) meiosis

58. The most significant benefit of flowering to humans is

(A) double fertilization
(B) the production of fruit and seeds
(C) pollination
(D) alternation of generations
(E) aesthetic

59. Antigens are foreign proteins which stimulate the production of

(A) fibrin
(B) globulins
(C) cytochrome
(D) antibodies
(E) lymphocytes

60. A deficiency of vitamin D may cause

(A) muscular cramps
(B) stunted growth
(C) xerophthalmia
(D) retardation of bone and tooth formation
(E) paralysis

61. Molecules that often function as enzyme cofactors and are essential to a healthy diet are known as

(A) amino acids
(B) proteins
(C) lipids
(D) vitamins
(E) substrates

62. Scientific research on the human cerebral cortex reveals that

    (A) the parasympathetic system is centered here
    (B) it controls smooth muscle
    (C) it controls endocrine secretions
    (D) it controls subconscious muscle coordination
    (E) specific areas control specific functions

63. The phases of mitosis occur in the following sequence:

    (A) prophase, anaphase, metaphase, telophase, and interphase
    (B) interphase, telophase, prophase, anaphase, and metaphase
    (C) interphase, prophase, metaphase, telophase, and anaphase
    (D) interphase, telophase, prophase, anaphase, and metaphase
    (E) prophase, metaphase, anaphase, telophase, and interphase

64. The constancy of linkage groups may be altered by

    (A) transduction
    (B) crossing-over
    (C) recombination
    (D) synapsis
    (E) assimilation

65. The "dark" reactions of photosynthesis take place in portions of the chloroplast called

    (A) grana
    (B) stomata
    (C) carotene
    (D) chlorophyll
    (E) stroma

66. Cytoplasmic streaming within living cells is called

    (A) translocation
    (B) transpiration
    (C) helicotropism
    (D) helicotaxis
    (E) cyclosis

67. Cellular respiration in mitochondria may

    (A) result in further energy storage
    (B) form ATP, an energy-yielding molecule
    (C) form ADP, an energy-related substance
    (D) release sugar molecules
    (E) release a variety of cellular hormones

68. Fibrinogen is

    (A) a precursor of certain hormones
    (B) formed from fibrin during clotting
    (C) an antibody to specific antigens
    (D) a source of globulin
    (E) a reservoir of antibodies for immune response

69. Systolic pressure is

    (A) the lowest pressure of the blood, between heartbeats
    (B) the result of a leak in a heart valve
    (C) the blood pressure in veins
    (D) the pressure on the blood as the ventricles contract
    (E) the blood pressure in arteries

70. During the infection process of bacteria by viral particles, it has been demonstrated that

    (A) the virus enters the bacterial cell "head first"
    (B) the virus enters the bacterial cell "tail first"
    (C) only the viral protein enters the cell
    (D) only the DNA of the virus enters the cell
    (E) the complete viral particle enters the cell

71. In the prophase of mitosis,

    (A) homologous chromosomes become paired
    (B) the centriole reappears
    (C) chromosomes are doubled and the duplicate chromatids may be observed
    (D) tetrads of chromatids appear
    (E) synapsis takes place

72. Marine organisms which move by drifting are referred to as

    (A) plankton
    (B) neritic
    (C) littoral
    (D) sessile
    (E) nekton

73. Genes, which control inheritance, are composed of the chemical

    (A) adenosine triphosphate (ATP)
    (B) ribonucleic acid (RNA)
    (C) adenosine diphosphate (ADP)
    (D) deoxyribonucleic acid (DNA)
    (E) acetylcholine

74. Nephrons

    (A) are functional units of the pancreas
    (B) are functional units of the liver
    (C) are functional units of the spleen
    (D) are functional units of the thyroid gland
    (E) are functional units of the kidney

Questions 75 and 76

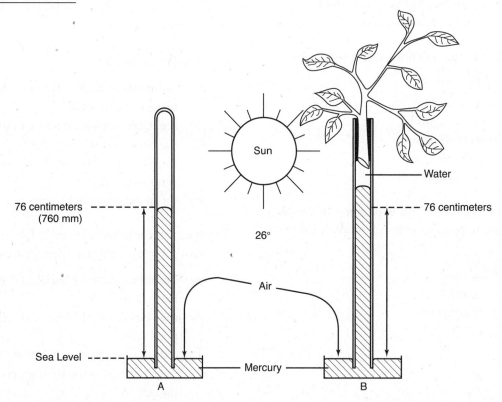

In the diagrams shown above, figure A illustrates a simple mercury barometer, a column of mercury in a sealed glass tube, the open end of which is immersed in a container of mercury which is exposed to atmospheric pressure at sea level. Figure B illustrates a living plant stem, with leaves, sealed in water in the upper end of the glass tubing, which is likewise filled with mercury.

75. What causes the mercury in figure A to rise to a height of 76 centimeters?

   (A) Adhesive forces
   (B) Cohesive forces
   (C) Sunlight heating the mercury, which expands
   (D) Atmospheric pressure on the mercury in the dish
   (E) The vacuum above the mercury in the glass tube

76. The mercury in figure B rises above 76 centimeters because

   (A) the plant stem absorbs mercury, pulling the mercury up the tube
   (B) plants grow better at sea level
   (C) of external and internal forces, including transpirational pull
   (D) the top of the glass tube is not sealed, thus destroying the vacuum
   (E) atmospheric pressure is highest at sea level

---

77. The existence of monotremes, the egg-laying mammals, suggests that

   (A) birds and mammals exhibit parallel evolution
   (B) mammals evolved before birds
   (C) mammals acquired the ability to nurse before any of them substituted live birth for egg-laying
   (D) the environment is more favorable to egg-laying
   (E) birds and mammals have little in common

78. Experiments using radioactive carbon as a tracer have demonstrated that all living cells

   (A) require radiant energy
   (B) are dependent upon photosynthesis
   (C) carry out chemosynthesis
   (D) are able to assimilate carbon compounds
   (E) produce organic substances and release oxygen

79. Etiolation in plants is the result of

   (A) synergism
   (B) insufficient light
   (C) photoperiodism
   (D) parthenocarpy
   (E) taxis

80. Eutrophication of a lake may occur

   (A) when essential nutrients are insufficient
   (B) as a result of too many fish
   (C) during prolonged high temperatures
   (D) when there is insufficient phosphorus
   (E) when there is excess phosphorus

81. Gene frequencies in a population are sometimes modified or changed by factors of little significance or bearing on genetics. What is the genetic effect of such changes called?

   (A) Cultural effect
   (B) Parallelism
   (C) Morphogenesis
   (D) Radiation
   (E) Random genetic drift

82. That each organism develops from the undifferentiated material of the fertilized egg is the premise of

(A) pangenesis
(B) regeneration
(C) special creation
(D) fertilization
(E) epigenesis

83. An undesirable result of the widespread use of antibiotics to cure bacterial diseases is

(A) the advent of entirely new bacterial diseases
(B) that the antibiotics may cause mutations of the pathogens
(C) the development of antigenicity
(D) the development of resistant strains by pathogens
(E) loss of virulence by some pathogens

84. The adrenocorticotropic hormone is one of seven produced by the anterior lobe of the pituitary gland. Its primary function is to

(A) stimulate the pancreas to release insulin
(B) stimulate the thyroid to release thyroxin
(C) stimulate the adrenal cortex to secrete the hormone cortisone
(D) stimulate the ovaries to release estrogens
(E) stimulate skeletal growth

85. When one species cannot survive without the benefits received from another species, the relationship is called

(A) coordination
(B) mutualism
(C) neutralism
(D) aggregation
(E) commensalism

86. Which of the following elements is found in proteins but not in nucleic acids or carbohydrates?

(A) carbon
(B) nitrogen
(C) phosphorous
(D) sulfur
(E) oxygen

87. The movement of ions into a living cell against a concentration gradient with the expenditure of energy is called

(A) active transport
(B) osmosis
(C) plasmolysis
(D) phagocytosis
(E) pinocytosis

88. Those viruses which attack and parasitize bacteria are called

(A) interferon
(B) bacteriozymes
(C) rickettsias
(D) lysozymes
(E) bacteriophages

89. When no oxygen is available to cells, they may produce ATP by

(A) glycolysis
(B) anaerobic respiration
(C) use of the TCA cycle
(D) cytochrome interaction
(E) the citric acid cycle

90. Niacin functions in maintaining

(A) normal bone formation
(B) normal nerve functioning
(C) normal blood clotting
(D) normal cellular oxidations
(E) night vision

91. By the conversion of ATP to ADP, cells

    (A) produce amino acids to make proteins
    (B) obtain energy for cellular activities
    (C) synthesize fats
    (D) dissociate to form various ions
    (E) store energy in complex carbohydrates

92. In the farsighted eye,

    (A) light rays converge in front of the retina
    (B) the cornea is defective
    (C) light rays converge in the fovea
    (D) vision is not blurred
    (E) light rays converge behind the retina

93. According to the Watson and Crick model of DNA, the bases are paired as follows:

    (A) adenine-thymine and cytosine-guanine
    (B) adenine-uracil and cytosine-guanine
    (C) adenine-cytosine and guanine-thymine
    (D) adenine-guanine and cytosine-thymine
    (E) adenine-thymine and guanine-uracil

94. Which of the following plants does not produce multicellular embryos?

    (A) Clover
    (B) Elodea
    (C) Tree ferns
    (D) Club mosses
    (E) Spirogyra

95. Which of the genotypes for hemophilia illustrated below would inherit the disease? The gene for hemophilia is recessive.

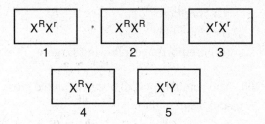

    (A) 1, 3, and 5
    (B) 2 and 4
    (C) 4 and 5
    (D) 3 and 5
    (E) 1, 2, and 4

96. Which of the following types of molecules yield the greatest amount of energy per gram when oxidized?

    (A) Carbohydrates
    (B) Proteins
    (C) Vitamins
    (D) Glycoproteins
    (E) Lipids

97. Isolation of a population over a long period of time produces

    (A) adaptive radiation
    (B) hybridization
    (C) inbreeding
    (D) interspecific competition
    (E) parallel evolution

98. As a result of photosynthesis

    (A) CO_2 is stored in carbohydrates
    (B) light energy is converted into stored chemical energy
    (C) entropy is neutralized
    (D) energy is released
    (E) ATP is energized

99. A deficiency of folic acid could result in

    (A) a type of anemia
    (B) sterility
    (C) beriberi
    (D) gray hair
    (E) hemorrhage following surgery

100. You would expect to observe buffalo grass and bison in the

    (A) desert
    (B) tropical rain forest
    (C) deciduous forest
    (D) arctic tundra
    (E) grasslands

101. For the biologist, mutations are

    (A) the primary source of variability that permits evolution to occur
    (B) seldom inherited complications of inheritance patterns
    (C) predictable but impossible to create
    (D) nonstable variations of inheritance patterns
    (E) are noninherited genetic aberrations

102. Bacterial genes for resistance to antibiotics are readily shared and are carried on bacterial structures called

    (A) plasmids
    (B) spores
    (C) cell membranes
    (D) ribosomes
    (E) plastids

103. One of the reasons that Mendel was successful when others before him failed was that

    (A) he studied the inheritance of single contrasting characters
    (B) he understood mutations
    (C) he was able to verify his results by making chromosome studies
    (D) he concerned himself with genes, not with how they expressed themselves
    (E) he was lucky

104. A cellular activity that results in a decrease in dry weight is

    (A) osmosis
    (B) photosynthesis
    (C) diffusion
    (D) respiration
    (E) reduction

105. Pavlov's experiment with dogs involved varying patterns of food presentation and bell-ringing, which, in turn, resulted in a shift of the stimulus causing the dog's salivation. This is a type of reaction called

    (A) imprinting
    (B) proprioception
    (C) conditioned reflex
    (D) visual accommodation
    (E) intelligent behavior

106. Conversion of molecular nitrogen to ammonia or nitrate is carried out only by

    (A) certain bacteria and photosynthesis
    (B) bacteria and fungi
    (C) earthworms and soil bacteria
    (D) lightning, certain bacteria, and blue-green algae
    (E) lightning, decomposition, and fungi

Questions 107–108

The following list represents factors that affect the growth, reactions, distribution, and reproduction of living organisms:

   (A) Genetic
   (B) Climatic
   (C) Edaphic
   (D) Biotic
   (E) Fire

107. The factor(s) involved in high soil alkalinity

108. The factor(s) involved in competition between garden beans and weeds

Questions 109–111

   (A) Adenosine triphosphate
   (B) Deoxyribonucleic acid
   (C) Disaccharide
   (D) Nucleotide
   (E) Phospholipid

109. A chemical compound found in chromosomes that stores hereditary information

110. The immediate source of energy for cellular activities

111. Energy-rich molecules formed in the mitochondrion

Answer Explanations

1. **(D)** By definition, a tissue is a group of similar cells specialized to perform a particular function or functions.

2. **(E)** Cells exchange substances with their environments through their surface membranes. The ratio of cell surface to cell volume has a direct effect on cellular metabolism and size.

3. **(E)** Enzymes are proteins produced by living cells. Enzymes control cellular metabolism.

4. **(E)** Photosynthesis is the biochemical process which occurs in living cells containing chlorophyll; it occurs only when radiant energy is present and results in the production of the basic food glucose.

5. **(E)** Typical holozoic organisms obtain nourishment by ingesting (eating) their food.

6. **(D)** Flask A permits microorganisms to enter readily and the material broth supports their existence and growth. Flask B severely restricts or prevents the entrance of microorganisms and, due to the lack of microorganismsin its broth, one must conclude that microorganisms do not arise spontaneously.

7. **(D)** Biogenesis is the concept that life arises only from preexisting life, a proposal first suggested by Virchow.

8. **(B)** The dark reactions of photosynthesis include the reduction of CO_2 and its combination into 3-and-6-carbon sugars. This is followed by a series of reactions in which the sugar ribulose is replaced.

9. **(D)** $6CO_2 + 6H_2O + \text{Radiant Energy} \rightarrow C_6H_{12}O_6 + 6O_2$

10. **(A)** $C_6H_{12}O_6 + 6O_2 \rightarrow 6CO_2 + 6H_2O + \text{energy (respiration)}$

11. **(A)** Tropisms are growth responses of plants to environmental stimuli such as light, water, gravity, and touch.

12. **(C)** A tropism is an attraction of a plant to some external stimulus. The attraction toward the earth is known as geotropism. Attraction to light (as in the sun) is known as phototropism.

13. **(A)** Hard woods contain fibers (a type of cell) in addition to tracheids. The cell walls of fibers contain lignin, which resists decay and gives strength.

14. **(C)** Typically, celery has a short, cushiony stem to which the "stalks" are attached. Celery has a compound leaf, i.e., a leaf consists of a petiole, or "stem," and leaflets.

15. **(B)** The loss of water from the leaves of plants is known as transpiration. Water and gases are exchanged through openings known as stomata.

16. **(E)** The two activities responsible for gene recombination in individuals with more than one pair of chromosomes are crossing-over and the reassortment of nonhomologous chromosomes.

17. **(D)** The typical plant life cycle is an "alternation of generations," i.e., the alternation of a diploid, spore-producing generation with a haploid, gamete-producing generation.

Following meiosis, haploid spores give rise to the gametophyte generation; haploid gametes, produced by the gametophyte, fuse (fertilization) to produce the zygote, which develops into the diploid sporophyte generation.

18. **(D)** Homologous structures have similarities of structure, embryonic development, and relationships.

19. **(E)** An Rh-negative mother carrying an Rh-positive fetus in a first pregnancy develops antibodies to the Rh antigen, which, in turn, destroy the Rh positive red blood cells of the fetus in a second pregnancy.

20. **(A)** Carotenes are a group of orange to red pigments found in the chromoplastids of certain plant cells. The pigments are converted to vitamin A.

21. **(C)** Any change of the nucleotide sequences in DNA is called a mutation, and the activity that causes it is also called a mutation.

22. **(A)** Spinal nerves typically innervate muscles and organs of the body, while cranial nerves innervate muscles and organs associated with the head.

23. **(E)** Nerve innervations are specific, i.e., the trigeminal nerve innervates the teeth; the optic nerve innervates the eye.

24. **(A)** The sympathetic nervous system typically responds to situations involving anger, fear, etc., with bodily response that provides greater courage, strength, etc. The parasympathetic nervous system tends to counter these by reducing blood pressure, decreasing heart rate, etc.

25. **(E)** Disease may be caused by invading organisms and their products, such as diphtheria or poliomylitis; by deficiencies of minerals and vitamins, such as scurvy or rickets; or by defects in hormonal production and secretion such as goiter. The latter are called functional diseases.

26. **(E)** Endocrine secretions—hormones—are specific in action. Oxytoxin stimulates lactation, or the release of milk.

27. **(B)** Crossing-over, inversion, translocation, and duplication are events which frequently happen to chromatin materials during meiosis.

28. **(B)** The total development of any individual is determined by its genetic makeup as affected by its environment. Changes in genetic makeup through new gene combinations or by mutation, and/or by changed environmental factors are the only causes of variation in a population.

29. **(D)** No type of RNA is designated "gametic RNA." The RNA of gametes is not so designated.

30. **(D)** Ovists contend that miniature organisms were contained in eggs and that all eggs were created together and have existed since the beginning of the world.

31. **(C)** By definition, a fruit is the matured ovary of a flower.

32. **(B)** The coniferous forest biome, the taiga, is dominated by conifers, especially spruce trees. It is populated by bears, rodents, birds, and moose.

33. **(B)** Nekton includes large fishes, giant squids, and whales which swim in direct relation to their food supply and independent of wave or current actions.

34. **(B)** Cytogenetics is that branch or division of cytology which emphasizes the behavior of the genetic apparatus, or chromosomes of the cell.

35. **(E)** Paleontology is concerned with a study of life of past geological time periods as revealed by fossil remains.

36. **(A)** A parasite derives its food from the living tissue and at the expense of other organisms.

37. **(D)** Semilunar valves are found at the entrance of both the pulmonary artery and the aorta.

38. **(E)** The hepatic vein empties into the inferior vena cava, which returns blood to the heart.

39. **(E)** Cholera is not a disease of the developed world, so immunizations against it are not necessary. Cholera primarily arises from impure drinking water, especially water contaminated by sewage.

40. **(B)** Sexual reproduction is the only reproductive measure which permits new combinations of genes, thus establishing the basis for evolution and adaptation to a constantly changing environment.

41. **(C)** If a plant that is Aa is crossed with a plant that is aa, the offspring will be 50% Aa (exhibiting the dominant trait) and 50% aa (exhibiting the recessive trait).

42. **(D)** The chance of an AB segregation of genes following meiosis in an individual with an "AaBb" genotype is one in four.

43. **(D)** Gene mutations cause incorrect amino acid sequences, because each codon of nucleic acid bases indicates a specific amino acid.

44. **(C)** In biotic communities, most populations can be assigned to one of several roles such as a food producer, a first-order consumer, a parasite, a scavenger, etc. Each role is recognized as a niche and only one species occupies a particular and specific niche in a community.

45. **(B)** Animals with bilateral symmetry have right and left sides, a front and back, and are usually active movers.

46. **(A)** Properties of enzymes include inactivation by heat, sensitivity to changes in acidity, limitation (usually) to one substrate, and specificity in regard to the type of reaction carried out. In addition, there is always a contrary reaction. The contrary reaction to oxidation is reduction, and the contrary reaction to hydrolysis is condensation.

47. **(E)** The carboxylic acid functional group is COOH.

48. **(D)** A hypertonic solution is one with a higher osmotic pressure than the reference (in this case, the living cell) solution.

49. **(C)** An autotrophic organism is able to manufacture its own food, usually by photosynthesis.

50. **(D)** A saprophytic organism derives its food from nonliving organic matter.

51. **(E)** Priestley discovered the opposing natures of photosynthesis and respiration. Respiration uses oxygen and releases carbon dioxide, while photosynthesis uses carbon dioxide and releases oxygen.

52. **(E)** In respiration the energy of foodstuffs is converted through a series of enzyme-regulated reactions into ATP, adenosine triphosphate, the principal energy storage molecule.

53. **(B)** Ribosomes are RNA-containing organelles that are the sites of the synthesis of proteins.

54. **(B)** Root hair cells increase the absorbing surface area of roots.

55. **(B)** Transpiration is the evaporation of water from the aerial part of plants. Evaporation is the result of the molecular activity called diffusion.

56. **(E)** There are over 2,000 species of bacteria. Bacteria have few morphological/ anatomical characteristics. Bacteria are distinguished by their growth in selected nutrient media and by such tests as the production of acid, gas, etc.—all of which are physiological traits.

57. **(C)** By definition, fertilization is the union or fusion of an egg and sperm, which results in the formation of a fertilized egg, or zygote.

58. **(B)** Flowering plants produce the cereal grains in addition to numerous fruits and seeds, all of which are essential to the nutrition of humans and other animals.

59. **(D)** An antigen is any substance which, when introduced into one body, causes the body to produce antibodies against it.

60. **(D)** The physiological function of vitamin D is the regulation of calcium and phosphorus metabolism, hence, bone and tooth formation.

61. **(D)** Vitamins are chemicals needed in small amounts, primarily because they serve as enzyme cofactors.

62. **(E)** Billions of nerve cell bodies make up the cerebral cortex. By various means (i.e., disease, surgery, electrical stimulation), it has been shown that specific regions of the cerebral cortex control specific functions such as hearing, movement, balance, memory, etc.

63. **(E)** Mitosis is a process consisting of recognized phases which occur in the order prophase, metaphase, anaphase, telophase, and interphase.

64. **(B)** A linkage group consists of a series of inherited traits which are inherited as a "package" because they are in a linear arrangement along a single chromatid. Crossing-over, the exchange of segments between the chromatids of a tetrad, may disrupt this inheritance package.

65. **(E)** The dark reactions of photosynthesis use the energy of ATP, which is formed in the light, for their essential processes, all of which take place in the clear stroma, which surround the grana of the chloroplast.

66. **(E)** A streaming movement of the cytoplasm (cyclosis) within a cell during periods of photosynthesis apparently presents the contained chloroplastids of each cell to maximum light exposure in sequence.

67. **(B)** Enzymes that control respiration are generally found in the mitochondria and, under suitable conditions, the oxidation of pyruvic acid to carbon dioxide and water with the production of ATP molecules can be demonstrated.

68. **(B)** Under the influence of the enzyme thrombin, fibrinogen is converted into fibrin, which gradually forms a mesh in which blood cells become embedded, thus forming a clot.

69. **(D)** Systole is that phase of the heart's action in which blood is forced out of the ventricles.

70. **(D)** Research shows that when a virus is grown in a medium containing radioactive phosphorus-32, the phosphorus is assimilated by the virus and becomes part of the viral DNA. Additional research, using a culture medium containing radioactive sulfur-35, demonstrates that sulfur becomes part of the viral protein but not the DNA. Subsequent studies reveal that only the phosphorus-32 DNA enters bacterial cells while sulfur-35 viral protein does not.

71. **(C)** The prophase is recognized as the phase of mitosis in which the chromatids may be observed in the doubled chromosomes.

72. **(A)** Plankton is the myriad of small, microscopic, free-floating aquatic organisms found at or near the surface and subject to tides and currents.

73. **(D)** The genetic material must be able to contain a code and to copy itself exactly. Deoxyribonucleic acid, often abbreviated DNA, has this capability. In addition, it meets the requirements of being able to mutate and undergo crossing-over.

74. **(E)** Nephrons are the functional units of the kidneys that, while secreting quantities of fluid, reabsorb blood sugar and amino acids as well as urea, various ions, and a large amount of water.

75. **(D)** Atmospheric pressure on the surface of the mercury in the sealed tube pushes the mercury to a height of 760 millimeters. This is the basis of the common mercury barometer.

76. **(C)** Atmospheric pressure on the surface of the mercury and the effects of transpirational pull—the evaporation of water from the stem and leaves of the plant—work together in raising the level of the mercury in figure B above 760 millimeters of mercury.

77. **(C)** Monotremes, the most primitive group of mammals, constitute the lowest evolutionary animal group that nurses its young.

78. **(D)** Carbon is an element basic to all organic compounds and is essential to the synthesis of carbohydrates, fats, and proteins.

79. **(B)** Insufficient light stimulates stem elongation, which, when carried to extremes, is known as etiolation.

80. **(E)** Eutrophication occurs when chemical fertilizers containing phosphorus and nitrogen wash into a lake, causing photoplankton and bottom vegetation to reach high productivity. This tremendous growth blocks out light, causing deeper plants to die while certain decomposers use all the oxygen, thus suffocating the fish.

81. **(E)** Random genetic drift is one of the ways by which changes in gene frequency are explained when mutation and natural selection do not account for evolution.

82. **(E)** According to epigenesis, the individual arises from the undifferentiated material of the egg.

83. **(D)** The widespread use of antibiotics to cure bacterial diseases commonly results in the development of resistance and resistant strains of pathogenic organisms. The use of certain chemicals in controlling insects and other biological pests also results in their development of resistance.

84. **(C)** In response to various sources of stress, the adrenocorticotropic hormone (ACTH) is one of seven hormones produced by the anterior lobe of the pituitary gland. It stimulates the adrenal cortex to release cortisone, which, in turn, causes the stomach to develop ulcerations, shrinks the lymph nodes, increases blood pressure, and lowers the white blood cell count.

85. **(B)** The distinguishing factor of mutualism is that at least one of the species cannot survive without the other.

86. **(D)** Both proteins and nucleic acids contain nitrogen. Nucleic acids contain phosphorous but not sulfur, whereas proteins contain sulfur but not phosphorous.

87. **(A)** The transport of ions against a concentration gradient in the direction opposite to that which would occur in osmosis or by diffusion is active transport. The cell expends energy to accomplish this.

88. **(E)** Bacteriophages are viruses that attack and invade bacterial cells converting bacterial DNA to viral DNA.

89. **(B)** Fermentation takes place in yeasts and other cells in the absence of free oxygen, and a similar type of reaction takes place in muscle cells. This process produces lactic acid from which the energy-bearing ATP molecule is formed.

90. **(B)** Niacin is usually thought of as the vitamin that prevents pellagra. Persons consuming insufficient niacin may also develop disorders of the digestive system, skin, and the nervous system.

91. **(B)** In the cellular process that converts ATP to ADP, energy is released for use in cellular activities.

92. **(E)** In the farsighted eye, the misshapen lens focuses the image behind the retina.

93. **(A)** In the complex DNA molecule, the bases adenine and thymine are always paired, as are cytosine and guanine.

94. **(E)** Algae (spirogyra), slime molds, and fungi are the plant groups that do not produce multicellular embryos. All other plants, including mosses and liverworts, and all vascular plants, including club mosses, ferns, gymnosperms, and flowering plants, produce multicellular embryos.

95. **(D)** In human sex-linked inheritance, females, with two X chromosomes, are the "carriers" of the recessive gene for such sex-linked traits as the disease hemophilia. The male Y chromosome lacks a gene for the trait in question. When a male inherits an X chromo-

some with the recessive gene (X^r), the recessive gene is expressed because no normal gene is present to prevent it.

96. **(E)** Proteins and carbohydrates yield about 4 cal of energy per gram, whereas fats, or lipids, produce about 9 calories per gram.

97. **(A)** Under conditions of isolation, exemplified by Darwin's finches, the production of a number of diverse species from a single ancestral one is referred to as adaptive radiation.

98. **(B)** Photosynthesis results in the conversion of radiant, or light, energy into chemical energy and its storage in the glucose molecule.

99. **(A)** Folic acid is important for normal bone marrow function and a deficiency could result in certain types of anemia.

100. **(E)** Native perennial grasses of the grasslands (prairies) of North America include the so-called buffalo grass, and the predominant animal is the bison.

101. **(A)** Mutations are the primary source of variability that permits evolution to occur. Mutations are recognized today as the source of the accumulated changes described by Darwin in the *Origin of Species*.

102. **(A)** Bacterial genes for resistance to antibiotics are carried on bacterial structures called plasmids. These, in turn, are readily shared or exchanged between different species of bacteria.

103. **(A)** Prior to Mendel, most students of inheritance attempted to study inheritance patterns involving all or groups of supposedly inheritable traits. The usual result was confusion and chaos.

104. **(D)** Respiration is a biochemical process that releases energy and carbon dioxide. Dry weight is lost during respiration because organic compounds are used up.

105. **(C)** In response to a given stimulus, animals, including man, produce a certain response. If a second stimulus is presented simultaneously with the first, the initial response after multiple repetitions will be transferred to the second stimulus and the response will occur even in the absence of the first stimulus. This is called a conditioned reflex.

106. **(D)** Under natural conditions only lightning, certain bacteria, and blue-green algae are able to "fix" nitrogen.

107. **(C)** ⎫ In their environment, all living things are affected by and respond to various
108. **(D)** ⎭ combinations of genetic, climatic, edaphic (soil factors), biotic (living organisms), and fire stimuli.

109. **(B)** Deoxyribonucleic acid, DNA, is found in chromosomes and stores hereditary information in coded form.

110. **(A)** ⎫ In the mitochondria, during cellular respiration, energy is transformed from
111. **(A)** ⎭ carbohydrate molecules to energy-rich adenosine triphosphate (ATP) for use throughout the cell.

Astronomy

1. Retrograde motion is the

   (A) apparent backward motion of a planet
   (B) apparent backward motion of the moon
   (C) seasonal movement between the vernal equinox and the autumnal equinox
   (D) reciprocal movement of the earth's axis
   (E) retreat of a meteorite

2. Which of the following statements about the motion of the moon is correct?

   (A) The moon revolves around the earth about once every 365 days, and the same side of the moon always faces the earth.
   (B) The moon revolves around the earth about once every 30 days, and the same side of the moon always faces the earth.
   (C) The moon revolves around the earth about once every 24 hours, and the same side of the moon always faces the earth.
   (D) The moon revolves around the earth about once every 365 days, and the moon rotates so that different sides of the moon face the earth at different times in the lunar cycle.
   (E) The moon revolves around the earth about once every 30 days, and the moon rotates so that different sides of the moon face the earth at different times in the lunar cycle.

3. To say that the solar system is heliocentric means that

   (A) the earth is the center of the solar system
   (B) the sun is the center of the solar system
   (C) the sun is highest in the sky
   (D) the sun is lowest in the sky
   (E) the center reflects the perimeter

4. A star that increases to a maximum brightness and does not return to its original condition is known as a

   (A) nova
   (B) supernova
   (C) giant
   (D) supergiant
   (E) binary star

5. During a solar eclipse

   (A) the earth's shadow is cast on the moon
   (B) the moon's shadow is cast on the earth
   (C) the earth's shadow falls on the sun
   (D) the earth moves between the sun and moon
   (E) the sun moves between the earth and moon

6. An early Egyptian achievement, based on a knowledge of astronomy, was the

   (A) recording of eclipses
   (B) recording of earthquakes
   (C) invention of time
   (D) development of a 365-day calendar
   (E) development of a decimal system

7. Radio waves of broadcasting frequency are reflected by

   (A) ozone in the stratosphere
   (B) an ionized layer of the troposphere
   (C) a nonionized layer of the troposphere
   (D) the exosphere
   (E) the ionosphere

8. An eclipse of the moon

   (A) occurs when the earth passes into the shadow of the moon
   (B) occurs when the moon passes between the sun and the earth
   (C) occurs every eight years
   (D) can occur only during a new moon
   (E) can occur only during a full moon

9. The Hawaiian Islands are just east of the international dateline, and Wake Island is west. When it is July 4 at Pearl Harbor, what is the date at Wake Island?

   (A) July 2
   (B) July 3
   (C) July 4
   (D) July 5
   (E) July 6

10. The laws of which scientist describes the paths of the planets in their orbits around the sun?

    (A) Brahe
    (B) Newton
    (C) Copernicus
    (D) Kepler
    (E) Ptolemy

11. At the time of the summer solstice in the Northern Hemisphere,

    (A) the sun's rays are tangent to the poles
    (B) the sun's rays are perpendicular to the equator
    (C) days and nights are equal over the entire earth
    (D) the sun is directly overhead at the Tropic of Cancer
    (E) the sun is directly overhead at the Tropic of Capricorn

12. Small celestial bodies whose orbits generally lie between Mars and Jupiter are called

    (A) comets
    (B) meteoroids
    (C) asteroids
    (D) planets
    (E) micrometeorites

13. One piece of evidence for the earth's rotation is

    (A) the solar eclipse
    (B) the lunar eclipse
    (C) the changing phases of the moon
    (D) the tilt of the earth's axis
    (E) the circulation of air as reported on weather maps

14. According to Isaac Newton, a combination of the earth's forward motion and "falling" motion, caused by the sun's gravitational force, defines

    (A) the earth's declination
    (B) parallax
    (C) its perturbation
    (D) perihelion
    (E) the earth's orbit

Answer Explanations

1. **(A)** Occasionally planets appear to become stationary and then to drift westward for a short time; then the planet resumes its normal eastward motion. This is known as retrograde motion.

2. **(C)** The moon revolves around the earth about once a month, and the same side of the moon always faces the earth.

3. **(B)** By definition: having the sun as a center.

4. **(B)** A supernova is a star that has collapsed under intense gravitation and then exploded.

5. **(B)** When the moon lies directly between the earth and the sun we witness a solar eclipse.

6. **(D)** The Egyptians were the first to develop a 365-day calendar.

7. **(E)** A layer of the atmosphere characterized by electrical properties and the presence of ionized particles is called the ionosphere. Radio waves from the earth travel upward to these ionized layers and are reflected back to earth.

8. **(E)** In an eclipse, both the sun and the center of the earth lie in the ecliptic plane and so must the moon lie in the ecliptic plane for, if it is too far from the ecliptic plane, it cannot pass into the shadow of the earth to cause a lunar eclipse. When lying in the ecliptic plane, the moon is, by its location, in the "full moon" phase.

9. **(D)** The International Date Line is designated ± 12 hours based on Greenwich time. Points east and west of this line differ in time by 24 hours.

10. **(D)** While all the scientists mentioned made major contributions to astronomy, it was Kepler who described mathematically the elliptical paths of the planets around the sun.

11. **(D)** On June 21, the sun is as far north as it will go and is directly over the Tropic of Cancer, 23° 27′ north of the equator. This date and this position of the sun mark the summer solstice.

12. **(C)** Asteroids include thousands of small planets between Mars and Jupiter with diameters of a fraction of a mole to almost 500 miles.

13. **(E)** Winds are deflected to the right of their paths in the Northern Hemisphere and to the left of their paths in the Southern Hemisphere, deviations which are the result of the earth's rotation. This deviation is called the Coriolis effect. The circulation of air as indicated on weather maps, is, therefore, a direct effect of the earth's rotation.

14. **(E)** Using his laws of motion, Isaac Newton demonstrated that the earth's orbit depends on its forward motion and its "falling" motion.

Earth Science

DIRECTIONS: Each of the questions or incomplete statements below is followed by five suggested answers or completions. Select the one that is best in each case.

1. A contemporary source of support for the theory of the spheroidal shape of the earth is

    (A) the Foucault pendulum
    (B) photographs taken by astronauts
    (C) computer data
    (D) Coriolis forces
    (E) parallax of stars

2. A crystalline calcite column hanging from a cave ceiling is called a

    (A) stalagmite
    (B) anthracite
    (C) dolomite
    (D) alabaster
    (E) stalactite

3. Which planet has the shortest orbit time of all the planets in our solar system?

    (A) Mercury
    (B) Venus
    (C) Mars
    (D) Jupiter
    (E) Saturn

4. Rocks that are formed by heat or pressure altering another rock type are known as

    (A) igneous rocks
    (B) sedimentary rocks
    (C) metamorphic rocks
    (D) inclusion rocks
    (E) extrusion rocks

5. A degrading of rock by a combination of mechanical and chemical forces is

    (A) weathering
    (B) crosscutting
    (C) lamination
    (D) intrusion
    (E) intumescence

6. A surface separating young rocks from older ones is

    (A) a moraine
    (B) a bench
    (C) a stack
    (D) an unconformity
    (E) a disjunction

7. An earthquake that follows a larger earthquake and originates at or near the same focus is called

    (A) the epicenter
    (B) surface wave
    (C) an aftershock
    (D) seismogram
    (E) reflected wave

8. A dark-brown residue formed by the partial decomposition of plants that grow in marshes and other wet places is called

    (A) coal
    (B) dolomite
    (C) peat
    (D) chert
    (E) coquins

9. Perihelion means

   (A) that the earth is at its summer solstice
   (B) the point in the earth's orbit most distant from the sun
   (C) the point in the earth's orbit nearest to the sun
   (D) that the earth is crossing the Tropic of Cancer
   (E) that the earth is crossing the Tropic of Capricorn

10. Rocks formed by solidification of molten material are called

   (A) sedimentary
   (B) igneous
   (C) fossiliferous
   (D) metamorphic
   (E) monomineralic

11. The gradual domelike buildup of calcite mounds or columns on the floors of caves results in formations called

   (A) stalactites
   (B) diamonds
   (C) gypsum
   (D) dolomite
   (E) stalagmites

12. A fracture line of the earth's crust where one portion has shifted vertically in reference to the other is called

   (A) a fault
   (B) a P wave
   (C) an L wave
   (D) an S wave
   (E) a tremor

13. The condition in which warm air overlying cooler air functions to prevent the upward movement of air is called

   (A) temperature profile
   (B) temperature inversion
   (C) fog
   (D) negative feedback
   (E) heat island

Answer Explanations

1. **(B)** Photographs taken from outer space show the earth to be a sphere.

2. **(E)** Crystalline calcite columns called stalactites are formed over long periods of time by dripping water.

3. **(A)** The planet closest to the sun, Mercury, has the shortest orbital period (about 88 days).

4. **(C)** Metamorphic rocks are formed by the action of heat and/or pressure on igneous or sedimentary rocks.

5. **(A)** Mechanical weathering is the breaking of rock into smaller pieces, each retaining the characteristics of the original material. Chemical weathering results when chemical actions alter the rock by either the removal or addition of elements.

6. **(D)** Breaks in the rock record are called unconformities. One easily recognized unconformity consists of tilted or folded sedimentary rocks that are overlaid by other, more flat-lying rock strata.

7. **(C)** Aftershocks are earthquakes of less severity that usually follow the primary earthquake.

8. **(C)** As a layer of sphagnum (peat moss) grows over water, older growth is pressed deeper in the water and into darkness where it dies. Initial decay products contain much tannin and this slows down bacterial decay. This becomes the peat of commerce.

9. **(C)** On or about January 3 each year the earth is about 92 million miles from the sun, and is closer than at any other time of the year. This is called perihelion.

10. **(B)** Rock formed by the cooling of magma is known as igneous rock.

11. **(E)** The calcite mounds built up on cave floors are called stalagmites.

12. **(A)** When portions of the earth's crust fracture as a result of earthquakes, these fracture lines are called faults.

13. **(B)** When air is very stable, there is little or no verticle mixing and, therefore, little dilution. Warm air overlying cooler air prevents upward air movement, which results in the atmospheric pollutants being trapped below. This condition is called a temperature inversion.

Physics

1. During the process called nuclear fission,

    (A) alpha particles are emitted
    (B) light atomic nuclei fuse
    (C) there is an increase in mass
    (D) radioactive fragments are often formed
    (E) much energy is consumed

2. Chromatic aberration may be eliminated by the use of

    (A) a convex lens
    (B) a concave lens
    (C) monochromatic light
    (D) proper focusing
    (E) a wider lens

3. When a musical note is raised one half step in pitch, it is called

    (A) tremolo
    (B) syncopation
    (C) sharp
    (D) flat
    (E) overtone

4. Pressure in a liquid

    (A) is inversely proportional to depth
    (B) decreases with depth
    (C) is variable at all points at the same level
    (D) is the same at different points at different levels
    (E) is the same at all points at the same level

5. A device in which chemical energy is converted into electrical energy is the

    (A) induction coil
    (B) rectifier
    (C) vacuum tube
    (D) amplifier
    (E) fuel cell

6. The condition created when two wires are connected through such a low resistance that current flow is excessive is called

    (A) a short circuit
    (B) induction
    (C) rectification
    (D) a circuit breaker
    (E) transition

7. Electronics is a field of applied science concerned with

    (A) the flow of electrons along a wire
    (B) the flow of electrons through gases or through a vacuum
    (C) the flow of electrons in liquids
    (D) amplitude modulation
    (E) frequency modulation

8. A prism separates white light because

    (A) parallel rays are reflected
    (B) parallel rays are focused
    (C) the angle of incidence equals the angle of reflection
    (D) the different frequencies are refracted differently
    (E) light rays are absorbed

9. The speed of sound in air is approximately how many miles per hour?

(A) 330
(B) 440
(C) 550
(D) 660
(E) 770

10. A shift in the wavelength of light or sound, when the source of the light or sound is moving relative to an observer, is known as the

(A) Bernoullian effect
(B) Compton effect
(C) Doppler effect
(D) Edison effect
(E) Coriolis effect

11. In scientific terminology, the prefix associated with the exponential expression 10^3 is

(A) centi
(B) kilo
(C) nano
(D) milli
(E) pico

12. Magnetic fields produced by an alternating current carried in a wire

(A) are indefinite and variable
(B) cannot exist in a vacuum
(C) cannot be demonstrated
(D) can be explained by Gilbert's Theory
(E) cannot penetrate nonmagnetic materials

13. In reference to electrical circuitry, the ohm represents

(A) the unit of current
(B) a force between two electric fields
(C) the difference of potential
(D) the flow of coulombs
(E) the unit of resistance

14. Work requires that

(A) direction be changed
(B) a force be exerted over a distance
(C) a definite rate be maintained
(D) the rate of motion increase
(E) the rate of motion decrease

15. In using a lever,

(A) force is gained when the force arm is longer than the weight arm
(B) force is gained when the force arm is shorter than the weight arm
(C) force is gained when the force arm and the weight arm are equal
(D) distance is gained when the force arm is longer than the weight arm
(E) distance is gained when the fulcrum is central

16. Attics should have provision for ventilation so that hot summer air may be removed by

(A) conduction
(B) expansion
(C) convection
(D) entropy
(E) radiation

17. Many runners participate in 5K, or 5 kilometer road races. About how many miles is this?

    (A) 0.3
    (B) 0.6
    (C) 3.0
    (D) 6.0
    (E) 9.0

18. Every object remains in its state of rest or in its state of uniform motion unless

    (A) its velocity changes
    (B) its acceleration varies
    (C) internal forces change
    (D) internal forces remain constant
    (E) unbalanced external forces change that state

19. According to Newton's third law of motion,

    (A) force is proportional to mass times acceleration
    (B) momentum equals mass times velocity
    (C) the weight of a body is equal to the gravitational attraction exerted upon it by the earth
    (D) the weight of a body is equal to the gravitational attraction exerted upon it by the sun
    (E) to every action, there is an equal and opposite reaction

Questions 20–22

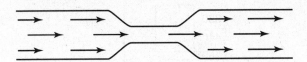

20. A fluid moving through a constriction, as illustrated above, speeds up and at the same time

    (A) its temperature also increases
    (B) its temperature decreases
    (C) its molecules begin to cling together
    (D) the pressure of the fluid within the constriction decreases
    (E) the pressure of the fluid within the constriction increases

21. The phenomenon illustrated is known as

    (A) the Doppler effect
    (B) Borelli's constant
    (C) Bernoulli's principle
    (D) the Mach effect
    (E) Pascal's law

22. One application of the phenomenon illustrated is in the

    (A) calculation of barometric pressure
    (B) verification of translational motion
    (C) design of airplane wings
    (D) determination of wave frequency
    (E) design of internal guidance systems

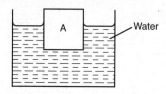

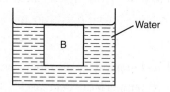

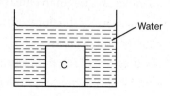

In the figures illustrated above, cubes A, B, and C, which have equal dimensions, are shown in containers of water.

23. With respect to the relative densities of the cubes, it may be concluded that

(A) cube C has the greatest density
(B) cube C sinks because its density is equal to the density of water
(C) cube A has the greatest density
(D) cube B has the greatest density
(E) water has less buoyant force than cube A or B

24. Cube C sinks to the bottom because

(A) cube C has a very low density
(B) the weight of the displaced water is greater than the weight of cube C
(C) cube C displaces too much water
(D) the weight of the displaced water is equal to the weight of cube C
(E) the weight of the displaced water is less than the weight of cube C

25. The phenomenon illustrated in these figures is best summarized or explained by

(A) Faraday's postulates
(B) Boyle's law
(C) Dalton's theory
(D) Archimedes' principle
(E) Kepler's laws

_____

26. The energy exerted by a moving bowling ball as it strikes the pins is

(A) rolling energy
(B) mass energy
(C) kinetic energy
(D) potential energy
(E) transferred energy

27. If a container of perfume is unstoppered in a closed room where there are no air currents or air circulation, we soon smell perfume because of the process called

(A) osmosis
(B) diffusion
(C) transpiration
(D) capillarity
(E) surface tension

28. When electricity flows through a wire wound in the form of a coil, the coil functions as

(A) a generator
(B) a resistor
(C) an electromagnet
(D) an electrostatic generator
(E) an electroscope

29. When the nucleus of a radium atom emits an alpha particle,

(A) only its atomic number changes
(B) only its mass changes
(C) neither its mass nor atomic number changes
(D) both its mass and atomic number change
(E) it becomes uranium

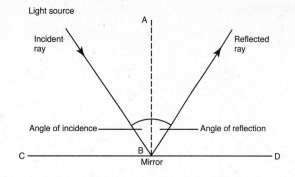

The diagram above illustrates the reflection of a ray of light from a mirror. The imaginary line *AB* is perpendicular to line *CD*.

30. The nature of a reflected ray of light is such that

(A) the angle of incidence is greater than the angle of reflection
(B) the angle of reflection always equals the angle of incidence
(C) the angle of reflection is greater than the angle of incidence
(D) the angle of reflection varies and changes
(E) the sum of the angle of incidence and the angle of reflection is a right angle

31. A vibrating string on a musical instrument will produce a low pitch if it is

(A) short, stretched, and of small diameter
(B) long, stretched, and of small diameter
(C) long, loose, and of small diameter
(D) long, loose, and of large diameter
(E) short, stretched, and of large diameter

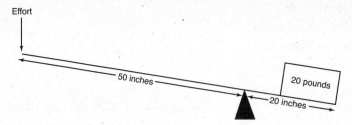

32. The force required to lift the 20-pound load in the illustration above is

    (A) 2 pounds
    (B) 8 pounds
    (C) 10 pounds
    (D) 20 pounds
    (E) 40 pounds

33. What is the mechanical advantage of the lever illustrated above?

    (A) 1
    (B) 2.5
    (C) 5
    (D) 7.5
    (E) 10

34. In the transmission of electric power, alternating current is used because

    (A) its voltage is readily transformed
    (B) it is cheaper
    (C) it is readily grounded
    (D) it is ready to use in household appliances
    (E) it has greater resistance

35. Ultraviolet radiation can cause a metal to emit electrons, a process called

    (A) ionization
    (B) facsimile transmission
    (C) electron transformation
    (D) the Compton effect
    (E) the photoelectric effect

36. Materials which transmit no light are referred to as

    (A) luminous
    (B) opaque
    (C) transparent
    (D) lucid
    (E) translucent

37. Concave lenses cause light rays to diverge by

    (A) reflection
    (B) absorption
    (C) diffraction
    (D) dispersion
    (E) diffusion

38. The acoustical engineer is chiefly concerned with

    (A) amplitude
    (B) frequencies
    (C) loudness
    (D) reverberations
    (E) wavelength

39. When a bullet is fired upward vertically, it gains in

    (A) momentum
    (B) speed
    (C) kinetic energy
    (D) potential energy
    (E) inertia

40. Work is the

   (A) direction of movement
   (B) distance of movement
   (C) rate of movement
   (D) product of the rate of movement multiplied by the distance moved
   (E) product of the force on an object multiplied by the distance it moves

41. A rubber rod is rubbed with fur, and the rod acquires a negative charge. What is the best explanation for this?

   (A) The rod has gained electrons from the fur.
   (B) The rod has lost electrons from the fur.
   (C) The rod has gained protons from the fur.
   (D) The rod has lost protons from the fur.
   (E) The rod has gained neutrons from the fur.

42. Transformers

   (A) are coils of wire carrying electric current
   (B) change the voltage of alternating current
   (C) have the capacity to store electric charges
   (D) change the voltage of direct current
   (E) are used to break circuits

43. According to Boyle's Law, when the temperature is constant, the volume of a given quantity of gas is inversely proportional to the

   (A) viscosity
   (B) temperature
   (C) density
   (D) surface tension
   (E) pressure

44. Roger Bacon contributed the

   (A) heliocentric theory
   (B) idea of the rotation of the earth
   (C) experimental approach to science
   (D) concept of buoyancy and density
   (E) idea of the sphericity of the earth

45. The Coriolis force, a significant influence on the movement of ocean waters, is caused by

   (A) the upwelling of cold water
   (B) the gyre
   (C) tidal currents
   (D) the earth's rotation
   (E) tsunamis

46. The inward force that is necessary to keep an object in circular motion is called

   (A) centrifugal force
   (B) inertia
   (C) centripetal force
   (D) net force
   (E) weightlessness

47. When an object exhibits inertia it

   (A) resists changes in its motion
   (B) resists friction and slowing down
   (C) responds directly to friction forces
   (D) exhibits velocity in a specified direction
   (E) possesses direction and magnitude

48. Which of the following is the fuel used in a modern nuclear power plant?

   (A) Hydrogen-2
   (B) Hydrogen-3
   (C) Uranium-235
   (D) Uranium-238
   (E) Plutonium-241

49. The phenomenon called interference is produced when

(A) light waves are bent
(B) light waves are parallel
(C) two or more waves of the same frequency are superimposed
(D) the velocities of sound in air are identical
(E) the frequencies of wave vibrations are equal

50. Which of the following molecules contains a double bond?

(A) H—C≡C—H

(B)
```
        H
        |
   H — C — O — H
        |
        H
```

(C)
```
        F
        |
   F — C — F
        |
        F
```

(D)
```
        H       H
        |       |
   H — C — O — C — H
        |       |
        H       H
```

(E)
```
   H         H
    \       /
     C = C
    /       \
   H         H
```

51. At the higher altitudes, the existence of a satellite is limited because of drag caused by

(A) cosmic rays from the sun
(B) air and other particles in space
(C) infrared radiation from the sun
(D) centrifugal force
(E) both cosmic rays and centrifugal force

52. According to Einstein's theory of relativity, as the speed of a spaceship approaches the speed of light,

(A) metabolism and mass increase
(B) metabolism and mass decrease
(C) metabolism and mass remain constant
(D) aging, relative to earth, would slow down
(E) aging, relative to earth, would speed up

53. How much work is done in lifting a 10 kg box to a height of 2 meters?

(A) 20 Joules
(B) 40 Joules
(C) 100 Joules
(D) 200 Joules
(E) 400 Joules

54. When a gas is compressed by pressure and the temperature is held constant,

(A) its component molecules are compressed
(B) space between its molecules decreases
(C) its volume increases
(D) its molecules speed up
(E) its molecules slow down

55. The natural tendency of molecules and/or energy to go from a more ordered to a less ordered state is known as

(A) osmosis
(B) diffusion
(C) conservation of energy
(D) entropy
(E) passive transport

56. The velocity of an object is a description of

(A) distance and time
(B) its acceleration
(C) its resistance to inertia
(D) its mass and weight
(E) its speed and direction

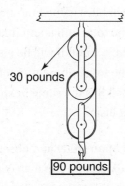

30 pounds

90 pounds

57. What is the mechanical advantage of the block and tackle illustrated above?

(A) 1
(B) 2
(C) 3
(D) 6
(E) 9

58. The conversion of alternating current to direct current is called

(A) amplification
(B) modulation
(C) transistorization
(D) induction
(E) rectification

59. That property of matter which tends to maintain any motionless body at rest is called

(A) friction
(B) mass
(C) inertia
(D) force
(E) velocity

60. Electric current in which the direction of flow is reversed at regular intervals is called

(A) effective current
(B) alternating current
(C) direct current
(D) induced current
(E) universal current

61. In connection with nuclear reactions, that mass which is just sufficient to make the reaction self-sustaining is called

(A) a fusion mass
(B) a fission mass
(C) a critical mass
(D) a supercritical mass
(E) a subcritical mass

62. Echoes are

(A) decibels
(B) reflected sound waves
(C) interference
(D) reinforcement
(E) diffracted sound waves

63. The correct units for work and energy in the SI system of measurement are

(A) work = newtons and energy = calories
(B) work = newtons and energy = joules
(C) work = joules and energy = newtons
(D) work = joules and energy = joules
(E) work = watts and energy = joules

Questions 64–67

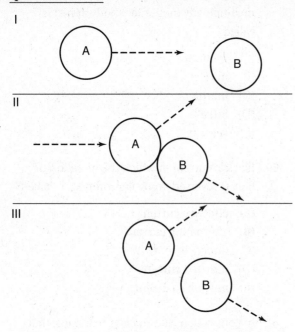

I

II

III

The three diagrams above illustrate a sequence in which ball A is moving toward stationary ball B in diagram I; strikes ball B in diagram II; and both balls are moving after ball A strikes ball B in diagram III.

64. In diagram I, the moving ball (ball A)

(A) has a momentum equal to that of ball B
(B) accelerates in direct proportion to its mass
(C) accelerates in indirect proportion to its mass
(D) has zero momentum
(E) has a momentum equal to its mass times its velocity

65. When ball A collides with ball B (diagram II)

(A) ball A's momentum will increase
(B) ball A will retain its initial velocity
(C) ball A's momentum will remain constant
(D) ball A will slow down
(E) the force of the collision represents a gain in momentum

66. After the collision of ball A with ball B (diagram III)

(A) both ball A and ball B will be moving
(B) ball A will have slowed down and changed direction
(C) ball A will have lost momentum; ball B will have gained momentum
(D) the total initial and final velocities of balls A and B will be equal
(E) the total momentum of ball A and ball B is the same before and after the collision

67. Based upon study and observation of the three diagrams, one may conclude that, in accord with Newton's Second Law,

(A) momentum decreases mass
(B) momentum increases mass
(C) velocity is constant
(D) a force is necessary for acceleration
(E) energy is gained following the collision

68. One of the following is not an acceptable statement with respect to magnetic fields:

(A) They require the presence of matter.
(B) Lines of force are changeable.
(C) They can penetrate glass and wood.
(D) They can penetrate thin sheets of copper.
(E) They may exist in a vacuum.

69. Which of the following is a unit used to express a measure of luminous intensity?

(A) volt
(B) roentgen
(C) erg
(D) candela
(E) luminous flux

70. Which of the following is not an example of luminescence?

(A) Electroluminescence
(B) Fluorescence
(C) Phosphorescence
(D) Bioluminescence
(E) Incandescence

71. When white light is directed through a glass prism a spectrum is formed due to which process?

(A) absorption
(B) dispersion
(C) reflection
(D) refraction
(E) diffusion

Questions 72 and 73 refer to the following diagram, which illustrates the basic characteristics of waves.

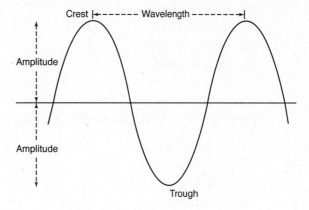

72. Amplitude may be thought of as

(A) an interaction between two different waves
(B) the number of crests passing a given point per second
(C) the distance between two adjacent crests
(D) a complete cycle, from crest to trough
(E) one-half of the vertical distance between crests and troughs

73. Interference is

(A) the simultaneous arrival of two different waves at a single point in space
(B) the combining of two different waves at some point in space
(C) the interaction of two or more waves
(D) "in phase" if two interacting waves are of the same frequency and shape and if they meet crest to crest and trough to trough
(E) all of the above

74. The total of the number of neutrons and protons in the atomic nucleus is called the

(A) atomic number
(B) atomic valence
(C) mass number
(D) nucleic number
(E) ionic number

75. The ratio of the weight of a given mineral to the weight of an equal volume of water is its

(A) molecular weight
(B) specific gravity
(C) specific density
(D) specific weight
(E) atomic weight

76. Pressures exerted by the water over a submerged object such as a submarine

(A) are equal to the area divided by the force
(B) are dependent upon direction
(C) are not affected by rate of flow
(D) are lower nearest the bottom
(E) are equal to the weight of a column of water above it

77. The Kelvin scale is an absolute scale since its zero point, absolute zero, is

(A) the freezing point of water
(B) the temperature at which water reaches its greatest density
(C) the coldest possible temperature
(D) the same temperature as outer space
(E) the temperature of liquid nitrogen

DIRECTIONS: The group of questions below consists of five lettered choices followed by a list of numbered phrases or sentences. For each numbered phrase or sentence select the one choice that is most closely related to it. Each choice may be used once, more than once, or not at all.

Questions 78–80

(A) Alpha particle
(B) Beta particle
(C) Electron
(D) Neutron
(E) Isotope

78. A negatively charge particle emitted from the nucleus during radioactive decay

79. A form of an atom with the same atomic number but a different mass number

80. A subatomic particle located in the nucleus of the atom

Answer Explanations

1. **(D)** When an atom undergoes fission, it splits into two smaller atoms called fission fragments, and these are usually radioactive.

2. **(C)** Chromatic aberration is the failure of different colors (wavelengths) of light to meet at the focal point after passing through a convex lens. This can be corrected by combining two or more lenses to ensure that the various colors of light meet at the focal point. The use of monochromatic light (light of one or a few nearly similar wavelengths) also eliminates the condition.

3. **(C)** In music, sharps are notes that are raised one half step in pitch.

4. **(E)** Pressure is exerted equally in all directions at a given level.

5. **(E)** In a fuel cell, gaseous hydrocarbons are the oxidizable material, and air supplies oxygen.

6. **(A)** A "short" is an electrical circuit with a very low resistance.

7. **(B)** Electronics is that branch of physics that studies the emission behavior and effects of electrons in vacuums and in gases.

8. **(D)** When white light passes through a prism it is broken up into an array of colors called a spectrum. The shortest rays of light bend the most and are the violet end of the spectrum. The longest rays bend the least and are the red end of the spectrum. All other colors fall in between, i.e., orange, yellow, green, and blue.

9. **(E)** The speed of sound in air is about 340 m/s at room temperature. This is the equivalent of 770 m/s (also known as Mach 1).

10. **(C)** When the source of a light wave or a sound wave is moving relative to the observer, a change in the observed frequency of light or sound occurs and this change or shift is called the Doppler effect.

11. **(B)** The decimal equivalent to the exponential expression 10^3 is 1,000. The prefix KILO means 1,000.

12. **(A)** When an alternating current is carried in a wire, a changing magnetic field is produced which, in turn, generates a varying electric field.

13. **(E)** The ohm is the unit of electrical resistance in a given circuit.

14. **(B)** Work is performed when an effort or a force causes a body to move.

15. **(A)** A lever is in balance when the effort and load are in balance, i.e., effort $\times$ length of force arm = load $\times$ length of weight arm. If other factors remain constant, increasing the length of the force arm gives a gain in force.

16. **(C)** Convection currents transfer heat energy in air by a circulatory motion due to variation in density and the forces of gravity.

17. **(C)** One kilometer is just over 0.6 miles, so a 5 kilometer race is about 3 miles.

18. **(E)** Inertia is that property of every object that causes it to remain at rest, or, if in motion, to remain at a constant velocity unless made to change by external forces.

19. **(E)** Whenever something is lifted, pulled, or pushed, it pushes down or resists in return.

20. **(D)** The pressure of a moving fluid (including gases) changes with and is inversely proportional to its speed of motion.

21. **(C)** According to Bernoulli's principle, when a fluid flows through a constriction, it speeds up and its pressure, therefore, decreases.

22. **(C)** An airplane wing is so shaped that air molecules moving over the top surface have farther to travel and, in so doing, they must speed up. This creates a lower air pressure on the top of the wing and the result is lift.

23. **(A)** ⎫ All matter consists of atoms. The density of a substance depends on the masses of
24. **(E)** ⎭ its atoms and the closeness in which its atoms are packed. A given object, when placed in water, displaces a volume of water equal to its weight.

25. **(D)** According to Archimedes' Principle, a floating object displaces an amount of water equal to its own weight.

26. **(C)** Kinetic energy is the energy possessed by a moving object.

27. **(B)** All molecules, except when at absolute zero temperature, tend to remain in constant motion and to spread out throughout all space available to them. This is diffusion.

28. **(C)** The magnetic field around any long straight wire is circular when an electric current passes through the wire. If an electric current is passed through a coil of wire, the strength of the magnetic field is equal to the number of coils of wire and the amount of current in the coil.

29. **(D)** Radium emits charged helium atoms called alpha particles, and these are very heavy. This results in a loss of mass. Radium ($_{88}$Ra) has an atomic number of 88, the 88 representing 88 protons or alpha particles. Since helium is $_2$He and comes from the radium atom, the loss of two from the radium to the helium means that the atom is now $_{86}$R, which is another element—radon.

30. **(B)** When a ray of light strikes an object at a specific angle and is reflected, it bounces off the reflecting surface at the same angle at which it approached.

31. **(D)** Small-diametered musical strings produce a high pitch if stretched tightly and large diametered strings produce a low pitch if strung loosely.

32. **(B)** Effort multiplied by the length of the effort arm equals the load multiplied by the length of the load arm.

33. **(B)** Mechanical advantage is calculated either by dividing the load by the effort or by dividing the length of the effort arm by the length of the load arm.

34. **(A)** Electric power transmission is normally transmitted efficiently at higher voltages. Alternating current is easier to transmit and its voltage is readily transformed.

35. **(E)** The outermost electrons of certain metals are not held strongly by the nucleus. Light of certain frequencies can dislodge surface electrons and this movement of electrons constitutes an electric current, which is called the photoelectric effect.

36. **(B)** Opaque substances do not permit light penetration.

37. **(C)** Parallel rays of light passing through a concave lens bend outward or spread apart and this is called diffraction.

38. **(D)** Reverberations are sound echoes which distort vocal and musical sounds.

39. **(D)** Potential energy is the energy possessed by a body because of its position. A bullet fired into the air has potential energy because it will fall back to earth due to gravity.

40. **(E)** Work is determined by multiplying the force on an object by the distance it is moved.

41. **(A)** Static charge is obtained via the loss or gain of electrons, which are negatively charged subatomic particles. An object that takes on a negative charge would have an excess of electrons. Protons are held tightly in the nucleus and are not gained or lost.

42. **(B)** Transformers are used to increase or decrease the voltage of alternating current.

43. **(E)** At a constant temperature, the volume of a gas is inversely proportional to the pressure.

44. **(C)** Roger Bacon advocated observation and experimentation as sources of scientific information.

45. **(D)** Many factors affect the earth's surface water currents. The most significant factor is the Coriolis force that is caused by the earth's rotation and that deflects currents to the right of their path in the Northern Hemisphere and to the left in the Southern Hemisphere.

46. **(C)** Centripetal force is the inward force that holds an object, such as a satel-lite, in circular motion in its orbit.

47. **(A)** Inertia is the tendency of a body in motion to remain in motion or the tendency of a body at rest to remain at rest.

48. **(C)** The modern nuclear power plant makes use of the energy released during the fission of the Uranium-235 isotope.

49. **(C)** When sound waves of the same frequency reach a single point simultaneously they combine in a process called interference.

50. **(E)** The double chemical bond occurs when two electron pairs are shared by bonded atoms.

51. **(B)** Any body anywhere in space is subject to drag caused by the air molecules and other particles found throughout space.

52. **(D)** Speed and time as measured by an observer on a rocket traveling at a speed near the speed of light are different from the speed and time measured by an observer on earth. To the space traveler, light from earth is catching up to the spaceship at one speed; to the observer on earth, light is catching up to the spaceship at a different speed. Both observers are correct.

53. **(D)** The amount of work done if lifting an object is the weight of the object (10 kg) times gravity (about 10 m/s^2) times the height (2 m) = 200 Joules

54. **(B)** In a sense, the same number of molecules occupies less space when a gas is compressed and the temperature is held constant.

55. **(D)** Entropy is the natural tendency of processes to go from a more to a less ordered state.

56. **(E)** Velocity is linear motion in a specific direction.

57. **(C)** Mechanical advantage, in a pulley system, is determined by the number of ropes that support the weight.

58. **(E)** A rectifier is a device used to convert alternating current to direct current.

59. **(C)** The property of any object that keeps it at rest or at a constant velocity unless it is forced to change by external forces is called inertia.

60. **(B)** In alternating current, the direction of current flow is reversed at regular intervals.

61. **(C)** In a nuclear reaction, the minimum mass required to support a self-sustaining chain reaction is called the critical mass.

62. **(B)** Echoes are reflected sound waves.

63. **(D)** Both work and energy are measured in Joules in the SI system. Calories are a measure of work and energy in the English system, and Newtons are units of force, not work.

64. **(E)** The momentum of any moving body is the product of its mass times its velocity.

65. **(D)** ⎫ When two bodies collide, total momentum after the collision equals total
66. **(E)** ⎬ momentum before the collision. Speed and direction may change because the original momentum is redistributed during the collision.

67. **(D)** The acceleration of a body is directly proportional to the force acting on it and inversely proportional to its mass.

68. **(A)** Magnetic fields exist in vacuums and can also penetrate most kinds of matter.

69. **(D)** The power of a light source is called its luminous intensity. A unit of luminous intensity is the candela.

70. **(E)** Incandescence is the emission of radiation by a hot body which makes the body visible.

71. **(D)** When a ray of light moves from one medium to another, such as air through glass, the ray bends. This is refraction. The different wavelengths of white light are, therefore, separated into the visible spectrum since each has its own refractive index.

72. **(E)** Amplitude is measured from a zero point and is one-half the vertical distance between the crest of a wave and its trough.

73. **(E)** Interference is the combining of two different waves which meet at a point in space. If they meet crest to crest, trough to trough, they are in phase. If they combine out of phase, they cancel out. If waves of different frequencies combine, they reinforce each other part of the time and cancel each other part of the time.

74. **(C)** The total of the number of neutrons and protons in the atomic nucleus equals the mass number.

75. **(B)** The number, which represents the ratio of the weight of a given mineral to the weight of an equal volume of water, is its specific gravity.

76. **(E)** Pressures in fluids increase with depth and are higher as depth increases due to the effects of gravity and the weight of the column of water above an object at any given depth.

77. **(C)** The Kelvin scale is an absolute scale because its zero is the coldest possible temperature, absolute zero.

78. **(B)** Beta particles are negatively charged electrons emitted during radioactive decay. The process involves the conversion of a proton to a neutron and an electron, which is ejected from the nucleus at high speed.

79. **(E)** Isotopes are forms of atoms with different numbers of neutrons, and thus the same atomic number but a different mass number.

80. **(D)** The two subatomic particles located in the nucleus of the atom are the proton and the neutron. Electrons are located in the energy levels outside the nucleus.

Chemistry

> **DIRECTIONS:** Each of the questions or incomplete statements below is followed by five suggested answers or completions. Select the one that is best in each case.

1. A radioactive sample of an isotope has a half-life of 20 days. What fraction of the sample will remain after 80 days?

   (A) 1/2
   (B) 1/4
   (C) 1/8
   (D) 1/16
   (E) 1/32

2. In a process called electrolysis,

   (A) there is an interaction between electric currents and magnets
   (B) the motions of electrons in magnetic fields are studied
   (C) chemical compounds are synthesized
   (D) chemical compounds are decomposed by means of electric current
   (E) ionizing radiation may be measured

3. A 200 ml of a gas at a pressure of 100 kPa (1 atmosphere) is compressed to 50 ml. What happens to the pressure of the gas in the container, assuming the temperature does not change?

   (A) The pressure decreases to 25 kPa.
   (B) The pressure decreases to 50 kPa.
   (C) The pressure increases to 150 kPa.
   (D) The pressure increases to 200 kPa.
   (E) The pressure increases to 400 kPa.

4. Elements included in the alkali metal family are unique in that they

   (A) are all dense metals
   (B) have varying combining qualities
   (C) are highly reactive
   (D) form negative ions
   (E) have two valence electrons

Questions 5 and 6

$$H \cdot + \cdot H \rightarrow H : H$$

5. The two joined hydrogen atoms shown above illustrate

   (A) surface tension
   (B) ionization
   (C) mass number
   (D) hydrogen bonding
   (E) covalent bonding

6. In the hydrogen molecule, H_2, illustrated

   (A) each atom shares its electron with the other atom
   (B) two hydrogen isotopes are attracted to each other
   (C) positively charged electrons neutralize each other
   (D) the atomic number of each of its hydrogen atoms is four
   (E) hydrogen molecules are held together by surface tension

7. Proteins are long chain organic polymers made of smaller units or building blocks known as

   (A) peptides
   (B) amino acids
   (C) nucleotides
   (D) monosaccharides
   (E) esters

8. The reaction of sodium and chlorine to produce sodium chloride is shown below. What type of reaction is this?

$$2 \, Na_{(s)} + Cl_{2(g)} \rightarrow 2 \, NaCl_{(s)}$$

(A) Decomposition
(B) Combustion
(C) Metathesis
(D) Single displacement
(E) Synthesis

9. Which ion is responsible for the acidic properties of chemicals such as hydrochloric acid?

(A) Oxide
(B) Peroxide
(C) Hydroxide
(D) Hydrogen
(E) litmus

10. Forms of an atom with the same number of protons but a different number of neutrons are known as

(A) allotropes
(B) isotopes
(C) polymers
(D) buffers
(E) isomers

11. Which of the following should give you the least concern?

(A) Carcinogens in soft drinks
(B) Strontium 90 in dairy products
(C) DDT in fresh vegetables
(D) Riboflavin and niacin in bread
(E) Herbicidal residues in vegetables

12. Atoms having the same atomic number but having different mass numbers

(A) have the same number of protons and neutrons
(B) have the same number of electrons and neutrons
(C) are called isotopes
(D) are artificially made by man and do not occur naturally
(E) cannot be made artificially and occur naturally only

13. A solution can be exemplified by

(A) a scattering of fine particles in water
(B) a dispersion of sugar molecules in water
(C) a dispersion of particles which are larger than molecules but too small to be microscopic
(D) a dispersion in which the suspended particles eventually settle out
(E) the immiscibility of the dispersed substances

14. The process shown below, which occurs when an ionic compound such as sodium bromide is dissolved in water, is known as

$$NaCl_{(s)} \rightarrow Na^{+1}_{(aq)} + Cl^{-1}_{(aq)}$$

(A) aquification
(B) saturation
(C) solvation
(D) dissociation
(E) decomposition

15. The energy liberated or consumed in exothermic and endothermic chemical processes is primarily that of

(A) vaporization
(B) compression
(C) chemical bonds
(D) catalysts
(E) enzymes

16. In general, the rate of chemical reactions is related to

    (A) the temperature and concentration of the reacting substances
    (B) the exothermic quotient
    (C) the endothermic quotient
    (D) the availability of ions
    (E) the availability of cations

17. A substance consisting of two or more ingredients which are not in chemical combination is called

    (A) a substance
    (B) a mixture
    (C) a molecule
    (D) an oxide
    (E) a compound

18. The atoms of nonmetals tend to gain electrons, resulting in the creation of negatively charged atoms called

    (A) cations
    (B) acid-base pairs
    (C) Bronsted-Lowry ions
    (D) anions
    (E) reduced ions

19. What best accounts for the similarities in the properties of elements in the same family (such as sodium and potassium)?

    (A) They have the same number of protons.
    (B) They have the same number of neutrons.
    (C) They have the same number of electrons.
    (D) They have the same number of valence electrons.
    (E) They have the same number of isotopes.

20. Mass number represents

    (A) atomic mass expressed in grams
    (B) the number of atoms in one gram atomic mass
    (C) atomic mass
    (D) the sum of the protons and neutrons in an atom
    (E) atomic number

21. The chemical reaction:

$$C_6H_{12}O_6 + 6O_2 \rightarrow 6CO_2 + 6H_2O$$

represents both the oxidation of glucose when it is burned in a flame and the oxidation of glucose when it is utilized within a living cell. The oxidation reaction in either example involves the

    (A) gain of electrons by atoms being reduced
    (B) loss of electrons by the atoms being oxidized
    (C) gain of electrons by the oxidizing agent
    (D) loss of electrons by the reducing agent
    (E) all of the above

Questions 22 and 23

According to Boyle's law, the pressure and volume of a confined gas are inversely proportional. As a consequence, the product of the pressure and the volume of a gas are constant at a given temperature, i.e., $PV =$ constant.

22. If the pressure of a volume of a gas is halved

    (A) its volume is halved
    (B) its volume is doubled
    (C) its volume remains constant
    (D) its volume decreases according to a geometric progression
    (E) its volume increases according to a geometric progression

23. Which of the following illustrates the pressure-volume relationship for a gas?

(P = pressure and V = volume)

(A)

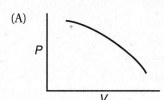

(B)

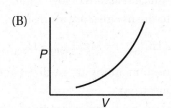

(C)

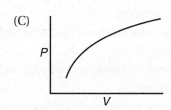

(D)

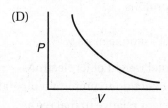

(E)

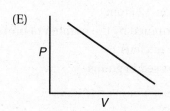

24. Which of the following is a characteristic property of the noble gases?

(A) They are highly reactive.

(B) They are chemically nonreactive.

(C) They react readily with metals but not nonmetals.

(D) They exist as diatomic molecules, such as He_2 and Ar_2.

(E) They are highly flammable.

25. Substances with identical chemical formulas but with different physical and chemical properties are called

(A) ethers

(B) ions

(C) polymers

(D) esters

(E) isomers

26. Which chemical element is found in all proteins?

(A) Sulfur

(B) Potassium

(C) Phosphorus

(D) Manganese

(E) Nitrogen

27. The atomic number of an element means

(A) the number of electrons in its nucleus

(B) the number of neutrons in its nucleus

(C) the sum of its electrons and neutrons

(D) the number of protons in its nucleus

(E) the number of protons in its orbits

28. In the chemical reaction

$$2\ C_6H_{12}O_6 \rightarrow C_{12}H_{22}O_{11} + H_2O$$

a disaccharide sugar is formed. This kind of reaction is called

(A) condensation

(B) the dark reaction

(C) oxidation

(D) the light reaction

(E) reduction

29. When the disaccharide sugar in the equation above undergoes digestion

(A) water and CO_2 are the end products

(B) energy is stored

(C) water is consumed

(D) water is the end product

(E) condensation occurs

30. The family of nonmetallic chemical elements known as the halogens includes

    (A) silicon
    (B) fluorine
    (C) nitrogen
    (D) oxygen
    (E) lithium

31. The chemistry of plastics could well be called the chemistry of

    (A) synergy
    (B) the halogen family
    (C) detergents
    (D) polymers
    (E) biodegradability

32. The smallest existing particle of any chemically pure compound is the

    (A) electron
    (B) proton
    (C) nucleus
    (D) ion
    (E) molecule

33. The changing of one atom into another is called

    (A) ionization
    (B) radiography
    (C) nuclear fusion
    (D) transmutation
    (E) transduction

34. In the process called respiration, which occurs in all living cells, carbon atoms gain oxygen and glucose is

    (A) dissolved
    (B) oxidized
    (C) reduced
    (D) precipitated
    (E) catalyzed

35. In the chemical reaction below, what happens to the magnesium atoms?

    $$Mg_{(s)} + 2\,HCl_{(aq)} \rightarrow MgCl_{2(aq)} + H_{2(g)}$$

    (A) Magnesium atoms are oxidized and lose electrons.
    (B) Magnesium atoms are oxidized and gain electrons.
    (C) Magnesium atoms are reduced and lose electrons.
    (D) Magnesium atoms are reduced and gain electrons.
    (E) Magnesium atoms are oxidized and lose protons.

36. An element's atomic mass is

    (A) the total weight of its electrons
    (B) dependent upon uniform temperatures
    (C) its weight relative to that of the carbon-12 atom
    (D) determined by the number of protons in its nucleus
    (E) expressed in grams

Answer Explanations

1. **(D)** If one half-life is 20 days, then 80 days is four half-lives; so the amount of material will be the original amount divided in half four times, or 1/16 of the original amount.

2. **(D)** In electrolysis, an electric current is passed through a liquid causing a chemical reaction. In industry, sodium may be produced (purified) by the electrolysis of liquid sodium chloride.

3. **(E)** According to Boyle's Law, the pressure and volume of a gas are inversely related (move in opposite directions); so if the volume is reduced by a factor of 4, the pressure is increased by a factor of 4.

4. **(C)** Alkali metals are very reactive, readily giving up one electron to form ions.

5. **(E)** } A covalent bond occurs when two atoms share a pair of electrons.
6. **(A)** }

7. **(B)** Proteins are chains of amino acids, connected via peptide bonds.

8. **(E)** The reaction shows two elements combining to make a single product, a process known as a synthesis (or combination) reaction.

9. **(D)** Acidic properties are the result of hydrogen ions, whereas basic properties result from hydroxide ions.

10. **(B)** Isotopes are forms of an atom with the same number of protons (atomic number) but different numbers of neutrons, yielding different mass numbers.

11. **(D)** Riboflavin and niacin are vitamins; all of the other substances listed are hazardous to health.

12. **(C)** Atoms of any element that differ in the number of neutrons in their nucleus are different in mass and are called isotopes.

13. **(B)** Homogenous mixtures have the same composition at the microscopic level throughout. When the dispersed particles are on a molecular scale the mixture is referred to as a solution.

14. **(D)** The process shows an ionic solid dissociating into its ions when placed in water.

15. **(C)** Energy transformations in chemical reactions are concerned with the energy of chemical bonds. Energy loss may be due to the formation of chemical bonds, or energy may be added to break the chemical bonds.

16. **(A)** The rates of chemical reactions are controlled by only a few factors, the most common being the concentrations of the reactants, the temperature, the nature of the reactants, and catalysts.

17. **(B)** A mixture is any portion of matter consisting of two or more substances which can be separated from each other by physical means, i.e., without reacting to form new substances.

18. **(D)** An ion is an atom or a group of atoms functioning as a unit and carrying an electrical charge. Those with positive charges are called cations, those with negative charges anions.

19. **(D)** The chemical properties of the elements result from their valence (or highest energy level) electrons.

20. **(D)** Mass number is the total number of neutrons and protons in the atom's nucleus.

21. **(E)** In oxidation-reduction reactions a transfer of electrons is involved. Atoms that gain electrons are reduced and atoms that lose electrons are oxidized. The atoms giving up electrons are called reducing agents and the atoms receiving electrons are called oxidizing agents.

22. **(B)** ⎫ According to Boyle's law, the pressure and the volume of a confined gas are inversely
23. **(D)** ⎭ proportional.

24. **(B)** The noble gases are characterized by being chemically inert (nonreactive).

25. **(E)** Isomers are chemical compounds that have the same number of atoms of the same elements, but differ in structural arrangements and properties.

26. **(E)** Nitrogen is found in all amino acids and, hence, in all proteins.

27. **(D)** The atomic number of an element is the number of protons in its nucleus.

28. **(A)** Disaccharides form by the joining of two monosaccharide units in a condensation reaction in which a molecule of water is split out.

29. **(C)** Disaccharides can react with water in the presence of a catalyst to form monosaccharides. This is digestion and a water-consuming reaction.

30. **(B)** Halogens include fluorine, chlorine, bromine, etc.

31. **(D)** Polymers are molecules composed of two or more small and repeated units that are chemically bonded together. They may be linear, branched, or three-dimensional. Plastic materials are polymers.

32. **(E)** The molecule cannot be further broken down without destroying it and changing its characteristics.

33. **(D)** The concept that atoms (elements) may be changed from one to another is called transmutation.

34. **(B)** When any elements or compounds combine with oxygen they are said to be oxidized. This involves the loss of hydrogen, the loss of electrons.

35. **(A)** In the reaction shown, the magnesium goes from an element with an oxidation number of 0 to an ionic form with an oxidation number of +2. This increase in oxidation number is caused by a loss of electrons and is known as oxidation. The opposite process of gaining electrons results in a decrease in oxidation number and is known as reduction.

36. **(C)** An atom's mass is a characteristic of a particular element and the atoms of each element have their own specific atomic mass. Carbon-12 has been assigned an atomic mass of 12; the atoms of all the other elements are assigned atomic masses relative to the atomic mass of the isotope of carbon.

History of Science

1. The scientist who first developed an atomic theory based on experimental evidence was

   (A) J.J. Thomson
   (B) Ernest Rutherford
   (C) Democritus
   (D) John Dalton
   (E) Aristotle

2. That living organisms have evolved was first theorized by

   (A) Lamarck
   (B) ancient Greek philosophers
   (C) Darwin and Wallace
   (D) Romans in the first century B.C.
   (E) the geologist Charles Lyell

3. A famous anatomist during the Renaissance was

   (A) Linnaeus
   (B) Michelangelo
   (C) Pliny
   (D) Bacon
   (E) Galen

4. A Roman naturalist, literary man, and government worker who composed an encyclopedia called "Historia Naturalis" ("Natural History") was

   (A) Lucretius
   (B) Galen
   (C) Celsus
   (D) Pliny the Elder
   (E) Dioecorides

5. A pupil of Thales, one of the earliest Greek scholars to be concerned with human evolution, and one who believed in transmutations as a cause of diversity was

   (A) Anaximander
   (B) Galen
   (C) Heraclitus
   (D) Pliny
   (E) Empedocles

6. A stimulus which influenced the thinking of both Darwin and Wallace was

   (A) Lyell's *Principles of Geology*
   (B) Malthus' writing on population
   (C) Lucretius' poem "De Rerum Natura"
   (D) Lamarck's *Philosophie Zoologique*
   (E) the writings of Aristotle

7. The ancient Greek scholar who became the "father of medicine" was

   (A) Aristotle
   (B) Theophrastus
   (C) Alemaeon
   (D) Hippocrates
   (E) Empedocles

8. The 365-day calendar was first proposed by

   (A) Pythagoras
   (B) Archimedes
   (C) the Babylonians
   (D) the Egyptians
   (E) the Greeks

9. The field of immunization had its beginning with the work of

   (A) Lister
   (B) Jenner
   (C) Koch
   (D) Pasteur
   (E) Ehrlich

10. According to Ptolemy,

    (A) the sun is the center of the solar system
    (B) the earth is round, with a circumference of 24,000 miles
    (C) the universe is infinite
    (D) the earth is a flat, floating disc
    (E) the earth is the center of the solar system

11. The first person to prove experimentally that atoms were made of smaller particles was

    (A) J.J. Thomson
    (B) Ernest Rutherford
    (C) Antoine Lavoisier
    (D) John Dalton
    (E) Robert Millikan

12. A highly significant contribution of Isaac Newton was his

    (A) heliocentric theory
    (B) universal law of gravitation
    (C) concept of the atom
    (D) photon theory of light energy
    (E) phlogiston theory

13. Who was the earliest Greek scholar to hold that the entire universe is subject to natural law?

    (A) Aristotle
    (B) Thales
    (C) Anaximander
    (D) Theophrastus
    (E) Empedocles

14. The recording of eclipses was first undertaken by the

    (A) Babylonians
    (B) Egyptians
    (C) Greeks
    (D) Chinese
    (E) Romans

15. Sterile and antiseptic surgical procedures were introduced by

    (A) Fleming
    (B) Semmelweis
    (C) Banting
    (D) Lister
    (E) Gorgas

16. The first to show that a connection exists between electricity and magnetism was

    (A) Henri Becquerel
    (B) Michael Faraday
    (C) Guglielmo Marconi
    (D) Benjamin Franklin
    (E) Han Christian Oersted

17. An early Greek physician whose writings considered medical ethics was

    (A) Galen
    (B) Hippocrates
    (C) Anaximander
    (D) Aristotle
    (E) Theophrastus

18. The Greek scholar who was the first to relate fossils to living plants and animals was

    (A) Anaximander
    (B) Theophrastus
    (C) Empedocles
    (D) Xenophanes
    (E) Aristotle

Answer Explanations

1. **(D)** Although Democritus was the first person to come up with the idea of the atom, it was John Dalton who first developed a theory summarizing what was known of atoms based on experimental evidence.

2. **(B)** The early Greek philosophers Anaximander and Xenophanes formulated ideas concerning the origins of life and evolution.

3. **(B)** Michelangelo made dissections of human internal structures so as to represent the features accurately and in proper relation to each other. His statues give evidence of his knowledge of human anatomy.

4. **(D)** Pliny the Elder (A.D. 23–79) compiled a comprehensive encyclopedia called "Natural History."

5. **(A)** Anaximander proposed that humans evolved.

6. **(B)** Malthus' writing on population presented the theme that humans multiply more rapidly than does food supply, thereby creating conditions for the competition for existence.

7. **(D)** The "Hippocratic Oath" honors Hippocrates as the "father of medicine."

8. **(D)** The Egyptians first proposed the 365-day calendar.

9. **(B)** Jenner was not the first to use vaccinations, but he developed the practicality and usefulness of the procedure.

10. **(E)** Ptolemy developed a model of the universe that accounted for the movements of the planets in circular orbits around a motionless earth.

11. **(A)** J.J. Thomson discovered the electron in his experiments with cathode ray tubes. He showed that electrons were negatively charged basic particles of all matter.

12. **(B)** Newton was the first person to recognize gravity as a universal force relative to both "the falling apple" and the orbits of the planets.

13. **(B)** Thales supported both the concept of rational inquiry into nature and the school of thought that presumed that the entire universe is controlled by natural law.

14. **(A)** Earliest written records, found in Babylonia and Mesopotamia, describe eclipses and other astronomical events inscribed in the clay and stone tablets of the time.

15. **(D)** Prior to Lister, most surgical procedures were complicated by infection. Lister devised methods of sterilizing the operating room and its equipment by spraying carbolic acid over the hands of the surgeons and the immediate surroundings while the surgery was in progress.

16. **(E)** Oersted was first to demonstate the connection between electricity and magnetism and was the first to propose the principle on which the electric motor is based.

17. **(B)** Hippocrates is called the "father of medicine." His professional writings, entitled "The Law," "The Physician," and "Oath," describe the contemporary attributes and ethics of Greek medicine and of the physicians who practiced it.

18. **(D)** Xenophanes was the first Greek scholar to compare fossils to living organisms.

ANSWER SHEET
Sample Examination 1

NATURAL SCIENCES

1. Ⓐ Ⓑ Ⓒ Ⓓ Ⓔ	31. Ⓐ Ⓑ Ⓒ Ⓓ Ⓔ	61. Ⓐ Ⓑ Ⓒ Ⓓ Ⓔ	91. Ⓐ Ⓑ Ⓒ Ⓓ Ⓔ
2. Ⓐ Ⓑ Ⓒ Ⓓ Ⓔ	32. Ⓐ Ⓑ Ⓒ Ⓓ Ⓔ	62. Ⓐ Ⓑ Ⓒ Ⓓ Ⓔ	92. Ⓐ Ⓑ Ⓒ Ⓓ Ⓔ
3. Ⓐ Ⓑ Ⓒ Ⓓ Ⓔ	33. Ⓐ Ⓑ Ⓒ Ⓓ Ⓔ	63. Ⓐ Ⓑ Ⓒ Ⓓ Ⓔ	93. Ⓐ Ⓑ Ⓒ Ⓓ Ⓔ
4. Ⓐ Ⓑ Ⓒ Ⓓ Ⓔ	34. Ⓐ Ⓑ Ⓒ Ⓓ Ⓔ	64. Ⓐ Ⓑ Ⓒ Ⓓ Ⓔ	94. Ⓐ Ⓑ Ⓒ Ⓓ Ⓔ
5. Ⓐ Ⓑ Ⓒ Ⓓ Ⓔ	35. Ⓐ Ⓑ Ⓒ Ⓓ Ⓔ	65. Ⓐ Ⓑ Ⓒ Ⓓ Ⓔ	95. Ⓐ Ⓑ Ⓒ Ⓓ Ⓔ
6. Ⓐ Ⓑ Ⓒ Ⓓ Ⓔ	36. Ⓐ Ⓑ Ⓒ Ⓓ Ⓔ	66. Ⓐ Ⓑ Ⓒ Ⓓ Ⓔ	96. Ⓐ Ⓑ Ⓒ Ⓓ Ⓔ
7. Ⓐ Ⓑ Ⓒ Ⓓ Ⓔ	37. Ⓐ Ⓑ Ⓒ Ⓓ Ⓔ	67. Ⓐ Ⓑ Ⓒ Ⓓ Ⓔ	97. Ⓐ Ⓑ Ⓒ Ⓓ Ⓔ
8. Ⓐ Ⓑ Ⓒ Ⓓ Ⓔ	38. Ⓐ Ⓑ Ⓒ Ⓓ Ⓔ	68. Ⓐ Ⓑ Ⓒ Ⓓ Ⓔ	98. Ⓐ Ⓑ Ⓒ Ⓓ Ⓔ
9. Ⓐ Ⓑ Ⓒ Ⓓ Ⓔ	39. Ⓐ Ⓑ Ⓒ Ⓓ Ⓔ	69. Ⓐ Ⓑ Ⓒ Ⓓ Ⓔ	99. Ⓐ Ⓑ Ⓒ Ⓓ Ⓔ
10. Ⓐ Ⓑ Ⓒ Ⓓ Ⓔ	40. Ⓐ Ⓑ Ⓒ Ⓓ Ⓔ	70. Ⓐ Ⓑ Ⓒ Ⓓ Ⓔ	100. Ⓐ Ⓑ Ⓒ Ⓓ Ⓔ
11. Ⓐ Ⓑ Ⓒ Ⓓ Ⓔ	41. Ⓐ Ⓑ Ⓒ Ⓓ Ⓔ	71. Ⓐ Ⓑ Ⓒ Ⓓ Ⓔ	101. Ⓐ Ⓑ Ⓒ Ⓓ Ⓔ
12. Ⓐ Ⓑ Ⓒ Ⓓ Ⓔ	42. Ⓐ Ⓑ Ⓒ Ⓓ Ⓔ	72. Ⓐ Ⓑ Ⓒ Ⓓ Ⓔ	102. Ⓐ Ⓑ Ⓒ Ⓓ Ⓔ
13. Ⓐ Ⓑ Ⓒ Ⓓ Ⓔ	43. Ⓐ Ⓑ Ⓒ Ⓓ Ⓔ	73. Ⓐ Ⓑ Ⓒ Ⓓ Ⓔ	103. Ⓐ Ⓑ Ⓒ Ⓓ Ⓔ
14. Ⓐ Ⓑ Ⓒ Ⓓ Ⓔ	44. Ⓐ Ⓑ Ⓒ Ⓓ Ⓔ	74. Ⓐ Ⓑ Ⓒ Ⓓ Ⓔ	104. Ⓐ Ⓑ Ⓒ Ⓓ Ⓔ
15. Ⓐ Ⓑ Ⓒ Ⓓ Ⓔ	45. Ⓐ Ⓑ Ⓒ Ⓓ Ⓔ	75. Ⓐ Ⓑ Ⓒ Ⓓ Ⓔ	105. Ⓐ Ⓑ Ⓒ Ⓓ Ⓔ
16. Ⓐ Ⓑ Ⓒ Ⓓ Ⓔ	46. Ⓐ Ⓑ Ⓒ Ⓓ Ⓔ	76. Ⓐ Ⓑ Ⓒ Ⓓ Ⓔ	106. Ⓐ Ⓑ Ⓒ Ⓓ Ⓔ
17. Ⓐ Ⓑ Ⓒ Ⓓ Ⓔ	47. Ⓐ Ⓑ Ⓒ Ⓓ Ⓔ	77. Ⓐ Ⓑ Ⓒ Ⓓ Ⓔ	107. Ⓐ Ⓑ Ⓒ Ⓓ Ⓔ
18. Ⓐ Ⓑ Ⓒ Ⓓ Ⓔ	48. Ⓐ Ⓑ Ⓒ Ⓓ Ⓔ	78. Ⓐ Ⓑ Ⓒ Ⓓ Ⓔ	108. Ⓐ Ⓑ Ⓒ Ⓓ Ⓔ
19. Ⓐ Ⓑ Ⓒ Ⓓ Ⓔ	49. Ⓐ Ⓑ Ⓒ Ⓓ Ⓔ	79. Ⓐ Ⓑ Ⓒ Ⓓ Ⓔ	109. Ⓐ Ⓑ Ⓒ Ⓓ Ⓔ
20. Ⓐ Ⓑ Ⓒ Ⓓ Ⓔ	50. Ⓐ Ⓑ Ⓒ Ⓓ Ⓔ	80. Ⓐ Ⓑ Ⓒ Ⓓ Ⓔ	110. Ⓐ Ⓑ Ⓒ Ⓓ Ⓔ
21. Ⓐ Ⓑ Ⓒ Ⓓ Ⓔ	51. Ⓐ Ⓑ Ⓒ Ⓓ Ⓔ	81. Ⓐ Ⓑ Ⓒ Ⓓ Ⓔ	111. Ⓐ Ⓑ Ⓒ Ⓓ Ⓔ
22. Ⓐ Ⓑ Ⓒ Ⓓ Ⓔ	52. Ⓐ Ⓑ Ⓒ Ⓓ Ⓔ	82. Ⓐ Ⓑ Ⓒ Ⓓ Ⓔ	112. Ⓐ Ⓑ Ⓒ Ⓓ Ⓔ
23. Ⓐ Ⓑ Ⓒ Ⓓ Ⓔ	53. Ⓐ Ⓑ Ⓒ Ⓓ Ⓔ	83. Ⓐ Ⓑ Ⓒ Ⓓ Ⓔ	113. Ⓐ Ⓑ Ⓒ Ⓓ Ⓔ
24. Ⓐ Ⓑ Ⓒ Ⓓ Ⓔ	54. Ⓐ Ⓑ Ⓒ Ⓓ Ⓔ	84. Ⓐ Ⓑ Ⓒ Ⓓ Ⓔ	114. Ⓐ Ⓑ Ⓒ Ⓓ Ⓔ
25. Ⓐ Ⓑ Ⓒ Ⓓ Ⓔ	55. Ⓐ Ⓑ Ⓒ Ⓓ Ⓔ	85. Ⓐ Ⓑ Ⓒ Ⓓ Ⓔ	115. Ⓐ Ⓑ Ⓒ Ⓓ Ⓔ
26. Ⓐ Ⓑ Ⓒ Ⓓ Ⓔ	56. Ⓐ Ⓑ Ⓒ Ⓓ Ⓔ	86. Ⓐ Ⓑ Ⓒ Ⓓ Ⓔ	116. Ⓐ Ⓑ Ⓒ Ⓓ Ⓔ
27. Ⓐ Ⓑ Ⓒ Ⓓ Ⓔ	57. Ⓐ Ⓑ Ⓒ Ⓓ Ⓔ	87. Ⓐ Ⓑ Ⓒ Ⓓ Ⓔ	117. Ⓐ Ⓑ Ⓒ Ⓓ Ⓔ
28. Ⓐ Ⓑ Ⓒ Ⓓ Ⓔ	58. Ⓐ Ⓑ Ⓒ Ⓓ Ⓔ	88. Ⓐ Ⓑ Ⓒ Ⓓ Ⓔ	118. Ⓐ Ⓑ Ⓒ Ⓓ Ⓔ
29. Ⓐ Ⓑ Ⓒ Ⓓ Ⓔ	59. Ⓐ Ⓑ Ⓒ Ⓓ Ⓔ	89. Ⓐ Ⓑ Ⓒ Ⓓ Ⓔ	119. Ⓐ Ⓑ Ⓒ Ⓓ Ⓔ
30. Ⓐ Ⓑ Ⓒ Ⓓ Ⓔ	60. Ⓐ Ⓑ Ⓒ Ⓓ Ⓔ	90. Ⓐ Ⓑ Ⓒ Ⓓ Ⓔ	120. Ⓐ Ⓑ Ⓒ Ⓓ Ⓔ

Sample Natural Sciences Examinations

17

This chapter has two sample CLEP natural sciences examinations. Each examination is followed by an answer key, scoring chart, and answer explanations.

SAMPLE NATURAL SCIENCES EXAMINATION 1

Number of Questions: 120

TIME LIMIT: 90 MINUTES

DIRECTIONS: Each of the questions or incomplete statements below is followed by five suggested answers or completions. Select the one that is best in each case.

1. The smallest and least complex unit of living matter is the

   (A) electron
   (B) atom
   (C) organelle
   (D) cell
   (E) molecule

2. Homologous structures, such as the anterior pairs of appendages of vertebrates, are modified for various functions such as flying, swimming, etc. This is called

   (A) mutations
   (B) parallel evolution
   (C) convergent evolution
   (D) adaptive radiation
   (E) metamorphosis

3. If a living cell is placed in a hypertonic solution, the cell will

   (A) experience a net migration of water molecules inward, and cell turgidity will increase.
   (B) experience a net migration of water molecules inward, and cell turgidity will decrease.
   (C) experience a net migration of water molecules outward, and cell turgidity will increase.
   (D) experience a net migration of water molecules outward, and cell turgidity will decrease.
   (E) experience no net migration of water molecules, and cell turgidity will be unchanged.

4. Which one of the following factors does *not* influence enzyme activity?

   (A) Temperature
   (B) pH
   (C) Humidity
   (D) Inhibitors
   (E) Concentration

5. Heterotrophs

   (A) utilize radiant energy
   (B) cannot synthesize organic materials from inorganic substances
   (C) are food synthesizers
   (D) oxidize inorganic materials
   (E) synthesize organic materials from inorganic substances

6. The process by which living cell membranes use energy to move ions and molecules into and out of cells, when this cannot be explained by diffusion, is called

   (A) osmosis
   (B) transpiration
   (C) absorption
   (D) imbibition
   (E) active transport

7. A deficiency of vitamin K can potentially lead to

   (A) scurvy
   (B) pellagra
   (C) clotting disorders
   (D) night blindness
   (E) anemia

8. Cellular respiration

   (A) stores energy
   (B) uses oxygen and organic compounds as raw materials
   (C) increases dry weight
   (D) occurs only in the presence of radiant energy
   (E) uses carbon dioxide and water as raw materials

9. The movement of genes from one part of a population to another as a result of migration and interbreeding is called

   (A) genetic drift
   (B) gene flow
   (C) natural selection
   (D) directional selection
   (E) nonrandom mating

10. Plants grown in the dark become

   (A) plasmolyzed
   (B) asphyxiated
   (C) synergistic
   (D) etiolated
   (E) parthenocarpic

11. In plants, water is normally conducted upward by a tissue called the

   (A) phloem
   (B) cortex
   (C) cuticle
   (D) pith
   (E) xylem

12. A condition of the human body in which the chemical and physical internal environment is favorable for cellular activities is

   (A) osmotic equilibrium
   (B) chemostasis
   (C) analogous balance
   (D) homeostasis
   (E) neural equilibrium

13. Primitive plants having neither vascular tissues nor multicellular embryos are called

   (A) bryophytes
   (B) thallophytes
   (C) pteridophytes
   (D) spermatophytes
   (E) xerophytes

14. Plants basic in many food chains are

    (A) fungi
    (B) bryophytes
    (C) gymnosperms
    (D) pteridophytes
    (E) algae

15. The first step in the formation of a blood clot is the disintegration of platelets and the release of

    (A) thrombin
    (B) fibrinogen
    (C) fibrin
    (D) thromboplastin
    (E) prothrombin

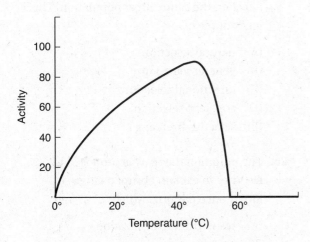

The illustration above represents enzyme activity as a function of temperature.

16. One may conclude, on the basis of the above illustration, that enzymatic activity

    (A) is greatest at 60°C
    (B) is stopped by temperatures above 60°C
    (C) is not affected by temperature
    (D) is independent of temperature
    (E) is greatest at 20°C

17. A child with type O blood cannot have parents with which of the following blood type combinations?

    (A) Both parents type A
    (B) Both parents type B
    (C) Both parents type O
    (D) One parent type AB and one parent type O
    (E) One parent type A and one parent type B

18. A common enteric bacterium, *Escherichia coli*, is used as a standard to identify water contaminated by sewage, is often identified as the pathogen causing food-borne diseases, and

    (A) is the organism used in a citric acid fermentation
    (B) is the organism used in preparing rabies vaccine
    (C) is the organism of choice for cleaning up toxic wastes
    (D) is one of the organisms suitable for and subjected to genetic engineering techiques
    (E) is the recognized pathogen responsible for vascular wilting diseases of vegetables

19. Nerve impulses from sensory receptors are conducted to the central nervous system

    (A) through the ventral root ganglion
    (B) along a motor neuron
    (C) through the dorsal root ganglion
    (D) through a Doric valve
    (E) across a synapse between connector and motor neurons

20. The transmission of genetic information from one generation to the next requires

    (A) replication of DNA molecules
    (B) replication of RNA molecules
    (C) replication of messenger RNA molecules
    (D) replication of all forms of nucleic acid
    (E) replication of the protein portion of nucleoproteins

21. Transpiration benefits plants by

    (A) assisting in the upward translocation of dissolved minerals
    (B) assisting in the upward translocation of organic substances
    (C) assisting in the downward translocation of organic substances
    (D) helping the plant to retain heat
    (E) maintaining a constant root pressure

22. What is the expected hereditary result of matings involving the interaction of multiple, incompletely dominant genes?

    (A) Inbreeding
    (B) Blending of the involved traits
    (C) Hybridization
    (D) Segregation
    (E) Independent assortment

23. In the prophase of the first meiotic division,

    (A) dyads of chromatids appear following synapsis
    (B) cell plate formation is initiated
    (C) the centriole reappears
    (D) the chromosome number is haploid
    (E) tetrads of chromatids appear following synapsis

24. Floods and fires repeatedly destroyed all life on earth, but acts of special creation repopulated the earth: this doctrine was called

    (A) catastrophism
    (B) adaptation
    (C) uniformitarianism
    (D) natural selection
    (E) Lamarckianism

25. A farmer sprays his crop with a new insecticide that annihilates all but a few of the target population of insects. He continues to use the insecticide and several years later notices the population is back in full force, but the insecticide has little to no effect on the same target population. This is an example of

    (A) natural selection
    (B) genetic selection
    (C) directional selection
    (D) constant selection
    (E) selective breeding

26. The mutation theory was proposed by De Vries to explain abrupt changes in inheritance patterns which

    (A) result from hybridization
    (B) breed true
    (C) do not breed true in subsequent generations
    (D) are environmentally induced
    (E) are based on mitotic errors

27. Antiseptic surgery was first performed by

    (A) Louis Pasteur
    (B) John Tyndall
    (C) Lazaro Spallanzani
    (D) John Needham
    (E) Joseph Lister

28. Changes that occur within the gene pools of populations, such as the increasing incidence of antibiotic resistance in bacteria is

(A) genetic drift
(B) microevolution
(C) macroevolution
(D) anagenesis
(E) biogenesis

29. Which of the following is a polar molecule?

(A) Methane, CH_4
(B) Carbon dioxide, CO_2
(C) Water, H_2O
(D) Chlorine, Cl_2
(E) Carbon tetrachloride, CCl_4

30. The basic physiological reaction of vision is

(A) physical
(B) chemical
(C) analgesic
(D) ketogenic
(E) electrical

31. Marine organisms found between the limits of high and low tide exist in the

(A) neritic zone
(B) abyssal zone
(C) zone of perpetual darkness
(D) bathyal zone
(E) littoral zone

32. Most of the photosynthesis in the oceans is carried out by

(A) green algae
(B) blue-green algae
(C) brown algae
(D) red algae
(E) diatoms

33. When corresponding structures of different species are based on similarities in function only, they are said to be

(A) homologous
(B) divergent
(C) parallel
(D) convergent
(E) analogous

34. An interrelationship between organisms in which one organism benefits at the expense of the other is known as

(A) commensalism
(B) mutualism
(C) parasitism
(D) symbiosis
(E) synergism

35. The time period described as the age of reptiles is the

(A) Ordovician period
(B) Proterozoic Era
(C) Mesozoic Era
(D) Cenozoic Era
(E) Miocene epoch

36. In the digestive system of humans, the stomach-produced enzyme rennin splits the

(A) ester bond of fats
(B) phosphate esters of DNA
(C) peptide bonds of trypsinogen
(D) phosphate esters of RNA
(E) peptide bonds in casein

37. Rodent control is necessary to prevent outbreaks of the following bacterial disease:

(A) psitticosis
(B) amebiasis
(C) plague
(D) typhoid fever
(E) polio

38. If a couple has three sons, what is the probability that the fourth child will be a daughter?

   (A) 1/16
   (B) 1/8
   (C) 1/4
   (D) 1/2
   (E) 3/4

39. In a cross between a mother who is homozygous recessive for gene "r" and a heterozygous father for the gene, the genotypes of the offspring will be

   (A) ½ RR, ½ Rr
   (B) ½ RR, ¼ Rr, ¼ rr
   (C) ¼ RR, ¼ Rr, ½ rr
   (D) ½ Rr, ½ rr
   (E) ¼ RR, ½ Rr, ¼ rr

40. The frequency of crossing-over between two linked genes is

   (A) controlled by sex chromosomes
   (B) controlled by the law of independent assortment
   (C) controlled by the Hardy-Weinberg Law
   (D) inversely proportional to the distance separating them
   (E) directly proportional to the distance separating them

41. An antigen stimulates the production of

   (A) blood groups
   (B) platelets
   (C) toxins
   (D) an antibody
   (E) Rh

42. Addition of detergents containing phosphates can disturb aquatic ecosystems because the phosphates

   (A) kill bacteria
   (B) poison fish
   (C) stimulate algae growth
   (D) fertilize crop plants
   (E) form deposits in rock

Questions 43–46

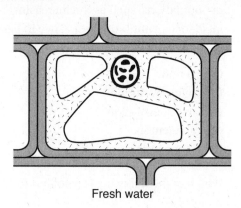

Fresh water

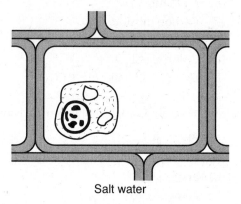

Salt water

The plant cells diagrammed above are located in fresh water and in salt water, respectively, as indicated.

43. Water has moved out of the cell in salt water by a process called

   (A) diffusion
   (B) imbibition
   (C) capillarity
   (D) adhesion
   (E) plasmolysis

44. The cell in fresh water is "plump" with water, a condition referred to as

   (A) rigid
   (B) plasmolyzed
   (C) saturated
   (D) hydrolyzed
   (E) turgid

45. The condition of the cell in the salt water is a result of

(A) the flow of water out of the cell
(B) a net movement of water out of the cell
(C) salt pulling the water out of the cell
(D) the forces of imbibition
(E) the force called cohesion

46. In the case of the cell in fresh water

(A) nothing is able to move into the cell
(B) adhesive forces hold water in the vacuoles
(C) the vacuoles continue to lose and to take in water by diffusion
(D) the cell walls are impermeable to water
(E) the cell walls are impermeable to salt

────────────────────

47. The figure below shows a food chain. Assume that there are 1,000 units of energy available at the level of the grasses. How much energy will be available by the time the coyote consumes its prey?

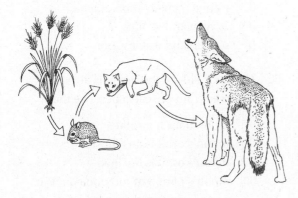

(A) 999 units
(B) 900 units
(C) 90 units
(D) 9 units
(E) 1 unit

48. Stems increase in diameter mainly because of cell division by the

(A) cork cambium
(B) endodermis
(C) medullary rays
(D) cortex
(E) vascular cambium

49. The evaporation of water from the aerial surfaces of plants is called

(A) translocation
(B) hydrotropism
(C) hydroponics
(D) aquaculture
(E) transpiration

50. Which hormone is responsible for the "fight or flight" mechanism in humans?

(A) Thyroxin
(B) Melatonin
(C) Adrenaline
(D) Insulin
(E) Calcitonin

51. The primary significance of mitosis is the fact that

(A) it is quantitative
(B) the chromosome number is increased
(C) it results in the production of either eggs or sperm
(D) the chromosome number is reduced
(E) it is qualitative

52. The area in the retina of the human eye lacking both rods and cones is called the

(A) alveolus
(B) fundibulum
(C) fovea
(D) blind spot
(E) cornea

53. During the initial stages of blood clot formation, blood platelets require

    (A) calcium ions
    (B) the antihemophilic factor
    (C) thrombin
    (D) prothrombin
    (E) cytochrome

54. Which molecule is primarily responsible for the metabolism of glucose in the human body?

    (A) Adenosine triphosphate (ATP)
    (B) Lactase
    (C) Insulin
    (D) Glucagon
    (E) Amylase

DIRECTIONS: Each group of questions below consists of five lettered choices followed by a list of numbered phrases or sentences. For each numbered phrase or sentence select the one choice that is most closely related to it. Each choice may be used once, more than once, or not at all in each group.

Questions 55–57

    (A) Cuvier
    (B) Darwin
    (C) Lamarck
    (D) Lyell
    (E) Tyson

55. Proposed the doctrine of catastrophism

56. Suggested that the events in the geologic history of the earth were the product of the same natural forces that are active today

57. Proposed the doctrine of uniformitarianism

Questions 58–60

    (A) Cambrian period
    (B) Devonian period
    (C) Jurassic period
    (D) Carboniferous period
    (E) Tertiary period

58. A period of psilopsids, lycopsids, and seed ferns

59. The period of modern mammals and herbacious angiosperms

60. The age of the great coal swamps

DIRECTIONS: Each of the questions or incomplete statements below is followed by five suggested answers or completions. Select the one that is best in each case.

61. The two gases that make up the majority of the earth's atmosphere are

    (A) oxygen and carbon dioxide
    (B) oxygen and nitrogen
    (C) nitrogen and carbon dioxide
    (D) oxygen and ozone
    (E) oxygen and water vapor

62. The same side of the moon is always observed from the earth because the

    (A) moon does not rotate
    (B) moon's orbit is an ellipse
    (C) moon's orbit is inclined
    (D) moon's period of rotation equals its period of revolution
    (E) moon's period of rotation is greater than its period of revolution

63. The point in a space vehicle or satellite's path that is farthest from earth is known as

    (A) apogee
    (B) perigee
    (C) terminal velocity
    (D) reentry point
    (E) gravitational inertia

64. There are always two calendar days in effect except

(A) during the summer solstice
(B) the instant it is noon at Greenwich, England
(C) the instant it is noon at longitude 180°
(D) on February 29
(E) the instant of crossing the International Date Line

65. Low offshore sand ridges that parallel coastlines are called

(A) baymouth bars
(B) spits
(C) barrier islands
(D) tombolos
(E) drifts

66. The theory that landmasses move over the surface of the globe is called

(A) catastrophism
(B) plate tectonics
(C) sedimentation
(D) fossilization
(E) discontinuity

67. A chemical that contains water as a part of its crystal structure is

(A) a dessicant
(B) a hydrate
(C) not flammable
(D) an ionic substance
(E) a covalent molecule

68. Chemical elements that follow uranium in the periodic chart and that have an atomic number higher than uranium (92) are called

(A) transuranium elements
(B) isotopes
(C) transmutation elements
(D) nucleons
(E) curies

69. Electrons in atoms emit light energy when they

(A) absorb energy from an outside source
(B) emit energy, return to the ground state and then give off that energy
(C) absorb energy, enter an excited state and then give off that energy
(D) emit a gamma ray
(E) absorb a neutron and become energized

70. Which of the following compounds has ionic bonds?

(A) Hydrochloric acid, HCl
(B) Carbon monoxide, CO
(C) Carbon dioxide, CO_2
(D) Calcium chloride, $CaCl_2$
(E) Methane, CH_4

71. Electron microscopes provide a greater magnification than light microscopes because

(A) there is a laser effect
(B) electrons travel faster than photons
(C) their magnifications are greater
(D) electrons have longer wavelengths than visible light
(E) electrons have shorter wavelengths than visible light

72. Which of the following is a major advantage of using aluminum for beverage containers?

(A) It requires very little energy to turn aluminum ore into aluminum metal.
(B) It takes less energy to manufacture aluminum than it does to manufacture steel.
(C) Unlike other metals, aluminum can be recycled.
(D) Obtaining aluminum via recycling is relatively inexpensive.
(E) There is abundant aluminum in the earth's crust.

73. If one were to observe a variety of samples of quartz, the property that would vary mostly would be

(A) streak
(B) density
(C) specific gravity
(D) color
(E) cleavage type

74. How are rocks, ores, and minerals related to each other?

(A) Ores are highly concentrated forms of valuable rocks.
(B) Ores are rocks that contain valuable minerals.
(C) Rocks are made of minerals, which exist as crystals.
(D) Rocks are combinations of minerals, while ores are a single mineral.
(E) Ores are combinations of minerals and rocks.

75. Which of the following is an organic compound?

(A) Calcium carbonate, $CaCO_3$
(B) Nitric acid, HNO_3
(C) Ethanol, CH_3CH_2OH
(D) Calcium iodide, CaI_2
(E) Magnesium oxide, MgO

76. Which of the following is not an acceptable statement with respect to magnetic fields?

(A) Lines of force are unchanging.
(B) They do not require the presence of matter.
(C) They can penetrate wood.
(D) They may exist in a vacuum.
(E) They can penetrate glass.

77. The unit of measurement of electric current is the

(A) ohm
(B) volt
(C) ampere
(D) coulomb
(E) watt

78. What are the two major metals obtained from the earth's crust, in terms of quantity?

(A) Lead and silicon
(B) Gold and magnesium
(C) Copper and calcium
(D) Iron and aluminum
(E) Iron and silicon

79. Which of the following cannot be emitted from the nucleus of an atom during radioactive decay?

(A) An alpha particle
(B) A beta particle
(C) A gamma ray
(D) A neutron
(E) A carbon atom

80. The tendency of systems to move to states of greater disorder is known as

(A) free energy
(B) thermodynamics
(C) heat capacity
(D) conservation of energy
(E) entropy

81. The faint outer atmosphere of the sun is known as the

(A) photosphere
(B) chromosphere
(C) corona
(D) sunspot layer
(E) spicule

82. The sun and most stars have which two elements as their main components?

(A) Hydrogen and carbon
(B) Iron and lithium
(C) Helium and lithium
(D) Hydrogen and helium
(E) Helium and iron

83. In order to apply a force to one object, one must be able to

(A) exert a force on the object
(B) use centrifugal force
(C) use centripetal force
(D) overcome gravity
(E) maintain a constant velocity

84. Energy is defined as the

(A) rate of doing work
(B) rate of supply of energy
(C) capacity to accelerate
(D) capacity to resist acceleration
(E) capacity to do work

85. A fundamental particle of negative charge is

(A) a proton
(B) an electron
(C) a neutron
(D) a meson
(E) a quark

86. In reference to light or sound waves, the Doppler effect occurs when

(A) the source and the receiver are in motion relative to one another
(B) waves are of unequal length
(C) waves are parallel
(D) the source and the receiver are stationary
(E) the source and the receiver are at different temperatures

87. A self-sustaining reaction in which the first atoms to react trigger more reactions is called

(A) a photochemical reaction
(B) a chain reaction
(C) an accelerator reaction
(D) an electrical reaction
(E) a biophysical reaction

88. The statement below that correctly describes the relationship between a gas and its pressure, volume, and temperature is

(A) pressure and volume are related directly
(B) pressure and temperature are related inversely
(C) pressure and volume are related inversely
(D) temperature and volume are related inversely
(E) pressure and number of moles are related inversely

89. The source of short, consistently timed radio bursts from neutron stars is known as a

(A) pulsar
(B) nebula
(C) quasar
(D) Red dwarf
(E) parsec

90. For every force there is a force of reaction which is

(A) equal and parallel
(B) unequal and transverse
(C) equal and transverse
(D) equal and opposite
(E) unequal and opposite

91. Electricity produced by a nuclear power plant

    (A) has higher voltage
    (B) has lower voltage
    (C) is radioactive
    (D) is the same as any other electricity
    (E) is direct current only

92. The temperature at which all molecular motion would theoretically cease is

    (A) 0°C
    (B) 273°C
    (C) 0°F
    (D) 273 K
    (E) 0 K

93. Dalton's atomic theory included all of the following statements except

    (A) All matter is made of indivisible particles known as atoms.
    (B) Atoms of an element can have several isotopes, which differ in mass number.
    (C) Atoms combine in definite ratios in compounds.
    (D) Atoms may combine physically as in mixtures or chemically as in compounds.
    (E) Atoms do not change identity when they undergo a chemical reaction.

94. The efficiency of machines is always reduced by

    (A) temperature
    (B) sublimation
    (C) momentum
    (D) friction
    (E) refraction

95. The valence or charge of an element from the halogen family (group VIIA or 17 on the periodic table), such as chlorine is

    (A) +1
    (B) −1
    (C) +7
    (D) −7
    (E) 0

96. The family of elements on the periodic table characterized by their chemical inertness is the

    (A) alkali metals
    (B) halogens
    (C) noble gases
    (D) metalloids
    (E) alkaline earth elements

97. Substances that increase the rate of chemical reactions are called

    (A) ions
    (B) isotopes
    (C) catalysts
    (D) neutralizers
    (E) bases

98. Of the four known forces in the universe, the strong force

    (A) is a force of repulsion
    (B) holds the particles inside the atomic nucleus together
    (C) causes the sun to shine
    (D) holds atoms and molecules together
    (E) produces radioactivity

99. Separation of the components in liquid solution by distillation is dependent upon

    (A) varying solubilities
    (B) heat of solidification
    (C) adsorption
    (D) differences in volatility
    (E) absorption

100. The products of the reaction of an acid and a base are

    (A) an anhydride and water
    (B) a salt and an anhydride
    (C) two ionic salts
    (D) a salt and water
    (E) water and hydrogen gas

101. Chemical formulas enable us to determine the kind and number of atoms in a compound, each element's percentage, and

(A) the number and kinds of isotopes
(B) its physical properties
(C) its nuclear reactions
(D) its half-life
(E) its molar mass

102. Thermosetting plastics polymerize irreversibly under conditions of

(A) freezing
(B) bonding
(C) volitilization
(D) heat or pressure
(E) crystallization

103. By A.D. 1000, when western Europe was beginning to emerge from the Dark Ages, intellectual development was hindered because

(A) most Arabic and Greek knowledge had been lost
(B) scientists hesitated to experiment
(C) alchemy was supreme
(D) there were formal centers of learning
(E) the Christian Church advocated Aristotle's logic

104. The emission of a beta particle from a radioisotope would lead to which changes in the atomic number and mass number?

(A) The atomic number increases by 1, and the mass number remains unchanged.
(B) The atomic number remains unchanged, and the mass number increases by 1.
(C) The atomic number remains unchanged, and the mass number decreases by 1.
(D) The atomic number decreases by 1, and the mass number increases by 1.
(E) The atomic number decreases by 1, and the mass number remains unchanged.

105. Which of the following statements about isotopes is true?

(A) Isotopes have the same atomic number but different mass numbers.
(B) Isotopes have the same mass number but different atomic numbers.
(C) Isotopes have different atomic numbers and different mass numbers.
(D) Isotopes are different molecular forms of an element.
(E) Isotopes emit radiation.

106. Lines that run parallel to the equator of a planet and are identified as being north or south of the equatorial line are known as

(A) equatorials
(B) lines of latitude
(C) lines of longitude
(D) Greenwich mean time lines
(E) meridian lines

107. In referring to wave phenomena, the term wavelength means

(A) the bending of the direction of wave motion
(B) the interaction of waves arriving simultaneously at the same point
(C) the distance between crests
(D) one-half of the distance in height between a crest and a trough
(E) the number of crests passing a point in a given time

108. The height of transverse sound waves is expressed as

(A) frequency
(B) wavelength
(C) rarefaction
(D) modulation
(E) amplitude

109. Einstein showed that, although energy and matter can be converted into each other,

(A) there is more energy than matter

(B) there is more matter than energy

(C) the total amount of energy and matter remains constant in the universe

(D) the total amount of energy and matter in the universe is unstable

(E) the conversion of matter to energy requires the input of energy, which is lost

110. In medicine, the X-rays that enable physicians to photograph the skeleton make use of

(A) radioactive rays

(B) electron beams

(C) kinetic energy

(D) very-high-frequency electromagnetic waves

(E) Brownian movement

111. Electron emission by certain heated metals is

(A) the photoelectric effect

(B) electromagnetic induction

(C) commutation

(D) the thermionic effect

(E) transformation

112. When dissolved in water, inorganic bases produce which of these ions in greatest concentrations

(A) sulfate ions

(B) various ions

(C) hydrogen ions

(D) nitrate ions

(E) hydroxide ions

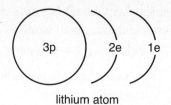

lithium atom

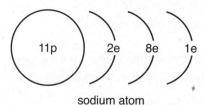

sodium atom

113. The diagrams above show the lithium and sodium atoms. The chemical and physical properties of lithium and sodium are similar because

(A) both possess an uneven number of protons

(B) each has a single electron in its outermost energy level

(C) both possess an uneven number of electrons

(D) both have the same atomic number

(E) both are heavy metals

114. Christian theology and Aristotelian philosophy were reconciled in *Summa Theologica*, written by

(A) Francis Bacon

(B) Albertus Magnus

(C) Roger Bacon

(D) Thomas Aquinas

(E) Pope Paul III

115. If the corner of a cube of sugar is placed in contact with iodine solution, the entire cube quickly becomes the color of iodine due to

(A) capillarity

(B) surface tension

(C) kinetic energy

(D) potential energy

(E) convection

116. Transfer of heat energy in solids occurs via which mechanism?

(A) Radiation
(B) Convection
(C) Cohesion
(D) Capillary action
(E) Conduction

117. According to the concept of the conservation of mass, when two or more elements react chemically,

(A) the sum of their masses equals the mass of the compound formed
(B) the sum of their masses is less than the mass of the compound formed
(C) the sum of their masses is greater than the mass of the compound formed
(D) atoms may be created, modified, or destroyed
(E) atoms may be changed from one kind to another

118. The process by which substances are separated by utilization of differences in the degree to which they are absorbed to the surface of any inert material is

(A) fractional distillation
(B) chromatography
(C) filtration
(D) neutralization
(E) isomerism

119. The maintenance of acid-base balance is accomplished by chemical substances called

(A) ionizers
(B) polarizers
(C) buffers
(D) neutralizers
(E) catalysts

120. The chemical equation

$$Mg_{(s)} + 2HCl_{(aq)} \rightarrow MgCl_{2(aq)} + H_{2(g)}$$

shows which type of reaction taking place?

(A) Combustion
(B) Redox
(C) Neutralization
(D) Single displacement
(E) Double replacement

STOP

If there is still time remaining, you may review your answers.

ANSWER KEY
Sample Examination 1

NATURAL SCIENCES

1.	D	31.	E	61.	B	91.	D
2.	D	32.	E	62.	D	92.	E
3.	D	33.	E	63.	A	93.	B
4.	C	34.	C	64.	B	94.	D
5.	B	35.	C	65.	C	95.	B
6.	E	36.	E	66.	B	96.	C
7.	C	37.	C	67.	B	97.	C
8.	B	38.	D	68.	A	98.	B
9.	B	39.	D	69.	C	99.	D
10.	D	40.	E	70.	D	100.	D
11.	E	41.	D	71.	E	101.	E
12.	D	42.	C	72.	D	102.	D
13.	B	43.	A	73.	A	103.	E
14.	E	44.	E	74.	D	104.	A
15.	D	45.	B	75.	C	105.	A
16.	B	46.	C	76.	A	106.	B
17.	D	47.	E	77.	C	107.	C
18.	D	48.	E	78.	D	108.	E
19.	C	49.	E	79.	E	109.	C
20.	A	50.	C	80.	E	110.	D
21.	A	51.	E	81.	C	111.	D
22.	B	52.	D	82.	D	112.	E
23.	E	53.	B	83.	A	113.	B
24.	A	54.	C	84.	E	114.	D
25.	C	55.	A	85.	B	115.	A
26.	B	56.	D	86.	A	116.	E
27.	E	57.	D	87.	B	117.	A
28.	B	58.	B	88.	C	118.	B
29.	C	59.	E	89.	A	119.	C
30.	B	60.	D	90.	D	120.	D

SCORING CHART

After you have scored your Sample Examination 1, enter the results in the chart below; then transfer your score to the Progress Chart on page 12.

Total Test	Number Right	Number Wrong	Number Omitted
120			

ANSWER EXPLANATIONS

1. **(D)** Of the choices given, the cell is the smallest and least complex unit of living matter. (If one accepts viruses as units of living matter, then these are smaller and less complex.)

2. **(D)** Homologous structures have a basic structural plan that becomes modified or specialized in various directions to meet different modes of life. This is adaptive radiation.

3. **(D)** If a living cell is placed in a hypertonic solution, then water will migrate out of the cell in an attempt to create an equal solution concentration. This will make the cell turgor decrease.

4. **(C)** Humidity has no effect on enzyme activity. Most enzymes are highly sensitive to pH and temperature.

5. **(B)** Heterotrophic organisms require organic compounds as food.

6. **(E)** Active transport occurs when cell membranes expend energy to transport ions and molecules in and out of cells at rates or directions that cannot be explained solely by the factors that affect diffusion.

7. **(C)** Vitamin K is essential for proper blood clotting. A deficiency of Vitamin C leads to scurvy.

8. **(B)** Cellular respiration combines oxygen and organic compounds to release energy, carbon dioxide, and water.

9. **(B)** Gene flow is defined as the movement of genes from one population to another by way of interbreeding of individuals in the two populations.

10. **(D)** The absence of light stimulates stem elongation in plants and results in the failure of chlorophyll synthesis. This is etiolation.

11. **(E)** In plants, xylem functions mainly in the upward movement of water and dissolved minerals and in the support and strengthening of stems. Phloem is the vascular tissue that transports sugars and metabolic products from the leaves downward.

12. **(D)** Homeostasis is the chemical and physical control over the internal conditions of the body which maintains an environment favorable for carrying out cellular activities.

13. **(B)** Thallophytes, or thallus plants, lack xylem and phloem, the conducting tissues, and they also do not develop multicellular embryos.

14. **(E)** Under normal favorable conditions in the seas and in freshwater lakes and streams, algae are so prolific that they constitute the basic food in many established food chains.

15. **(D)** In blood clotting, in the presence of the antihemophilic factor, blood platelets stick to torn tissue and release thromboplastin and serotonin.

16. **(B)** As indicated on the graph, at temperatures approaching 60°C, enzyme activity stops.

17. **(D)** In order for parents to have a child with type O blood, each parent must have the ability to contribute an allele for that type of blood. A parent with type AB blood can contribute an allele for only A or B, which means a type O child is an impossibility.

18. **(D)** The common enteric bacterium, *Escherichia coli*, has been found suitable for selected genetic-engineering activities, including genetic alteration for the production of human-type insulin.

19. **(C)** All nerve impulses from sensory receptors are conducted to the central nervous system through a dorsal root ganglion.

20. **(A)** The genetic information of an organism is stored in its DNA molecules, coded according to the sequence of bases along the DNA chain. For the transmission of genetic information to occur, there must be exact duplication of the DNA molecules.

21. **(A)** Transpiration is the evaporation of water from the aerial parts of plants. It has the beneficial effect of transporting dissolved minerals upward from the roots to the stem and leaves.

22. **(B)** The hereditary result of matings involving multiple, incompletely dominant genes is blending of the traits in question. For example, in matings of a wheat homozygous for red grains ($X_1X_1X_2X_2$) with a wheat homozygous for white kernels ($x_1x_1x_2x_2$), the following combinations of genes for color of the grains can be expected: *XXXX*, *XXXx*, *XXxx*, *Xxxx*, and *XXXX* with varying grain colors from dark red to white as the result.

23. **(E)** During the first meiotic division, chromosome reduction has not yet occurred. Hence, the chromatids of any pair of chromosomes are still in groups of four, or tetrads.

24. **(A)** According to *catastrophism* sudden and violent events changed the earth's surface and destroyed all life, and subsequent acts of special creation repopulated the earth.

25. **(C)** Directional selection is defined as selection that changes the frequency of an allele in a constant direction, either toward or away from fixation for that allele.

26. **(B)** Mutations are abrupt and unexpected changes in inheritance patterns that breed true.

27. **(E)** Joseph Lister initiated the era of antiseptic surgery when he began spraying the surgical scene with carbolic acid.

28. **(B)** Microevolution is evolution resulting from small specific genetic changes that can lead to a new subspecies.

29. **(C)** Water molecules, with two lone pairs of electrons on the central oxygen atoms, are polar. The polar nature of a water molecule is responsible for the ability of water to form

hydrogen bonds, allowing ice to float, and water to have a high boiling point and heat capacity.

30. **(B)** The basic type of reaction in respect to vision or sight is chemical. The chemical reactions occur in the cells of the retina.

31. **(E)** The littoral zone exists from the high tide level to the area 200 meters deep.

32. **(E)** Often called the "grass of the sea," diatoms carry out most of the photosynthesis that takes place in the oceans and are the principal source of food of the animals that inhabit them.

33. **(E)** The key to analogous structures is the word *function*. The wing of a bird and the wing of a bee are similar in only one category: function. Structurally, they are unrelated.

34. **(C)** In parasitism, the parasite benefits at the expense of the host. In mutualism, both benefit. In commensalism, one benefits, and the other has little benefit or harm.

35. **(C)** The giant reptiles flourished in the geologic time period called the Mesozoic Era.

36. **(E)** Rennin is a digestive enzyme secreted by the stomach which is partially responsible for casein digestion.

37. **(C)** Plague still exists in certain parts of the world and, since it is associated with rodents and their fleas, rodent control is a necessary control measure.

38. **(D)** In each instance of sex determination in humans, the probability that any one individual will be male or female is one-half at the time of conception.

39. **(D)** The cross between Rr and rr will give 50% Rr and 50% rr.

40. **(E)** Since the probability of crossing-over between two linked genes on a pair of chromosomes is directly proportional to the distance separating them, crossing-over frequencies are greatest in widely separated genes.

41. **(D)** An antigen is any substance that, when introduced into the body, causes the body to produce antibodies.

42. **(C)** Phosphates stimulate the growth of algae, which often form a layer thick enough on the surface of a lake or pond to dramatically reduce oxygen exchange into the water.

43. **(A)** Diffusion in this instance is the movement of water molecules from an area of high concentration of water molecules to or toward an area of low or lower concentration of water molecules.

44. **(E)** Turgid or turgor pressure is a positive pressure developed within living plant cells, and therefore in stems and leaves, as a result of internal water pressure.

45. **(B)** The cell in the salt water has lost water by diffusion, the net movement of water molecules out of the cell.

46. **(C)** Diffusion is the movement of water molecules as a result of their molecular activity. In the case of the cell in fresh water, as in the case of the cell in salt water also, water molecules move freely into and out of the cell.

47. **(E)** At each trophic level, only about 10% of the energy from the previous level is available.

48. **(E)** Cell division by the vascular cambium produces xylem internally and phloem externally, thus adding to the diameter of the stem.

49. **(E)** Water which moistens the cell walls of leaf mesophyll cells evaporates since these cell walls are exposed to the internal gaseous atmosphere of the leaf. This water loss is called transpiration.

50. **(C)** The hormone adrenaline, or epinephrine, is responsible for the "fight or flight" mechanism in mammals.

51. **(E)** Mitosis is a qualitative distribution of chromatin to each of two different daughter cells. Its primary significance is that each daughter cell receives identical chromatin materials.

52. **(D)** The point where the optic nerve enters the eyeball has neither rods nor cones and, therefore, has no sight capability. It is called the blind spot.

53. **(B)** The antihemophilic factor causes blood platelets to swell into spherical masses and these tend to prevent the loss of other blood components.

54. **(C)** The hormone insulin is primarily responsible for the metabolism of glucose in mammals. Amylase and lactase are enzymes and not hormones.

55. **(A)** Cuvier suggested that there must have been many floods (catastrophes) that killed most of the organisms living at the time, followed by repeated special creations to repopulate the earth. This idea is called catastrophism.

56. **(D)** ⎫ Lyell opposed catastrophism and special creation. He stated that events
57. **(D)** ⎭ in the geological history of the earth were the products of the same natural forces active today, i.e., erosion, sedimentation, etc. This doctrine is called uniformitarianism.

58. **(B)** The Devonian period was the beginning of true land plants with stomata, vascular tissues, and multicellular embryos.

59. **(E)** During the Tertiary, early modern mammals assumed dominance, together with the flowering (seed) plants.

60. **(D)** During the Carboniferous, giant ferns, clubmosses, and horsetails grew in widespread low and swampy regions of the earth. These later formed layers of dead vegetation which did not decompose. This plant material became coal.

61. **(B)** The atmosphere of earth is made of 78% nitrogen, 21% oxygen, about 1% argon, and less than 1% other gases.

62. **(D)** The periods of rotation and revolution of the moon are the same, $27\frac{1}{3}$ days. Because of this, the same "face" of the moon is always turned toward the earth.

63. **(A)** A satellite's greatest distance from earth while in orbit is known as apogee, and the closest point is known as perigee.

64. **(B)** When it is noon at Greenwich, England, it is 12:00 P.M./00:00 A.M. at the International Date Line. At this instant, only one calendar day is in effect, worldwide.

65. **(C)** Barrier islands are low sand ridges that lie offshore along moderately sloping coastlines.

66. **(B)** Plate tectonics is the concept that continents drift in relation to one another on the earth's surface.

67. **(B)** Hydrates are ionic compounds with water molecules as part of their crystal structures.

68. **(A)** Transuranium elements have atomic numbers above 92, are synthetic radioactive elements, and do not exist naturally.

69. **(C)** An electron that has gained a quantum of energy will have a higher energy level, or exist in an excited state. When this energy is released and the electron returns to the ground state, the energy is emitted as a form of electromagnetic radiation.

70. **(D)** Ionic bonds are formed between metals and nonmetals. Metals are found on the left side of the periodic table, and nonmetals on the right.

71. **(E)** The wavelength of electrons is very short and, therefore, permits a higher degree of resolution than with a light microscope.

72. **(D)** While obtaining pure aluminum metal from its ore (bauxite) is relatively expensive in terms of energy, recycling aluminum is quite inexpensive compared to recycling other metals.

73. **(A)** Samples of quart are all silicon dioxide, SiO_2, and thus have the same density, hardness, and cleavage type. Differences in the streak test results of types of quartz are the result of metal ion impurities in the crystal structure.

74. **(D)** The term *ore* refers to a specific mineral that contains a metal of commercial value (aluminum oxide or bauxite is an ore of aluminum). Rocks are physical combinations of minerals.

75. **(C)** Organic compounds are carbon based but do not include carbonates or bicarbonates.

76. **(A)** Magnetic fields vary according to their sources, the positions of their sources, and the intensities of their sources.

77. **(C)** Electrical current is measured in amperes, one ampere being equal to one coulomb of charge past a point in one second.

78. **(D)** The two most widely obtained minerals from the earth's crust are iron and aluminum. These are not the two most valuable, but they are the most widely mined.

79. **(E)** Radioactive decay can involve the emission of an alpha particle (a helium nucleus), a beta particle (an electron), a gamma ray (high energy electromagnetic energy), or a neutron, but not a larger atom.

80. **(E)** The tendency of systems to move toward a state of greatest disorder is known as entropy.

81. **(C)** The outer atmosphere of the sun is known as the corona. The photosphere and chromosphere lie beneath the corona but above the surface of the sun.

82. **(D)** The sun and most stars create energy via the fusion of hydrogen into helium, and these two elements make up the vast majority of stars.

83. **(A)** For every force in one direction, there is an equal force in the opposite direction. To move an object in one direction, a stationary base or anchor is required to overcome the force directed in the opposite direction.

84. **(E)** By definition, energy is the capacity to do work.

85. **(B)** By definition, an electron is a fundamental particle of negative electricity.

86. **(A)** The Doppler effect is the apparent change in the pitch of sounds produced by moving objects when an observer is stationary or moving at a different speed than the producer of the sound.

87. **(B)** In a chain nuclear reaction, neutrons strike other atoms, which, in turn, release neutrons, which strike additional atoms. When a chain reaction can be sustained, the number or amount of fissionable material is described as a critical mass.

88. **(C)** Pressure and volume are inversely related: as the pressure on a gas increases, its volume decreases. This concept is known as Boyle's Law. Pressure and temperature are directly related (Gay-Lussac's Law), while volume and temperature are also directly related (Charles's Law).

89. **(A)** Pulsars are periodic radio wave bursts from neutron stars.

90. **(D)** For every force in one direction, there is an equal force in the opposite direction.

91. **(D)** The nature of electricity is not affected by the source of its production— hydro-electric power plants, nuclear power plants, or plants that burn fossil fuels.

92. **(E)** Absolute zero is equal to 0 Kelvin or –273°C. At this temperature, all molecular motion would cease.

93. **(B)** Dalton could not have known about isotopes of atoms, as no subatomic particles had yet been discovered. He thought that all atoms of an element were identical.

94. **(D)** Friction is a force that opposes motion when two objects in contact with each other attempt to move relative to each other. Friction uses energy and, therefore, reduces mechanical efficiency.

95. **(B)** Elements in group 17, the halogen family, are one electron short of an octet, or eight valence electrons. This means they tend to gain one electron to form a –1 ion.

96. **(C)** The noble gases, with their complete valence energy levels, are chemically inert.

97. **(C)** A catalyst is a substance that initiates or speeds up a chemical reaction without being permanently altered.

98. **(B)** The *strong force* holds the particles inside the atomic nucleus together. The *gravitational force* holds objects to the ground. The *electromagnetic force* holds atoms and molecules together and holds electrons to the atomic nucleus. The *weak force* permits some atomic nuclei to break down, producing radioactivity and causing the sun to shine.

99. **(D)** Distillation is a process of boiling a liquid and condensing its vapor. Two or more liquids will usually have different boiling points so they may be separated by first boiling off the vapor of one liquid and condensing it and then boiling off the vapor of the second liquid and condensing it.

100. **(D)** An acid and a base react to produce a salt and water. This type of process is known as a neutralization reaction.

101. **(E)** A chemical formula is a description, using chemical symbols, of the ratio of atoms in a chemical compound. If the weight ratio and the atomic mass of the elements of a compound are known, the molecular weight of the compound can be calculated.

102. **(D)** The family of plastics referred to as "thermosetting" consists of substances that polymerize irreversibly under heat or pressure, forming a hard mass.

103. **(E)** Albertus Magnus and Saint Thomas Aquinas endeavored to harmonize the teachings of Aristotle with church doctrine. Roger Bacon, in opposition, demonstrated the values of observation and experimentation and argued against the age-old scholastic method of education.

104. **(A)** A beta particle has a charge of –1 and a mass of essentially 0. This means that emission of a beta particle from a nucleus will increase the atomic number by 1 and have no effect on the mass number.

105. **(A)** Isotopes are forms of an atom with the same atomic number but different mass numbers. This is due to a different number of neutrons, but the same number of protons. Different molecular forms of an element, such as O_2 and O_3, are known as allotropes.

106. **(B)** Lines of latitude run parallel to the equator and are identified as being north or south of that imaginary line. Lines of longitude run perpendicular to latitude lines and are identified as being east or west of the prime meridian, located in Greenwich, England.

107. **(C)** Wavelength is the measure of distance between two adjacent crests.

108. **(E)** Amplitude of a sound vibration is one-half of the vertical distance between the crest and the trough.

109. **(C)** Energy and matter can be neither created nor destroyed, but energy and matter can be converted into one another, the total amount in the universe remaining constant.

110. **(D)** X-rays, discovered in 1895 by W.C. Roentgen, are very-high-frequency electromagnetic waves that enable one to photograph the skeleton. X-rays also have numerous other uses in science and industry.

111. **(D)** When certain metals are heated, they emit electrons, a phenomenon called the thermionic effect.

112. **(E)** A base is a substance which produces hydroxyl ions (OH^-) when dissolved in water.

113. **(B)** In general, the chemical and physical properties of lithium and sodium are similar because the higher energy level of each atom contains a single electron.

114. **(D)** Thomas Aquinas taught that there is no conflict between faith and reason.

115. **(A)** The force of adhesion between a solid and a liquid based on the relative attraction of the molecules of the liquid in each other and for the solid is called capillarity.

116. **(E)** Heat transfer in solids takes place by conduction, involving direct contact of molecules.

117. **(A)** The law of conservation of mass holds that there is no detectable gain or loss of mass in or as a result of chemical change.

118. **(B)** Various substances may be separated by using the degree to which they are absorbed onto an inert material. If the inert material is paper, the process is called paper chromatography.

119. **(C)** A buffer is any substance capable of neutralizing acids and bases to maintain a given hydrogen ion concentration.

120. **(D)** A single displacement reaction involves the reaction of an element and a compound to form a different element and a different compound.

ANSWER SHEET
Sample Examination 2

NATURAL SCIENCES

1. Ⓐ Ⓑ Ⓒ Ⓓ Ⓔ	31. Ⓐ Ⓑ Ⓒ Ⓓ Ⓔ	61. Ⓐ Ⓑ Ⓒ Ⓓ Ⓔ	91. Ⓐ Ⓑ Ⓒ Ⓓ Ⓔ
2. Ⓐ Ⓑ Ⓒ Ⓓ Ⓔ	32. Ⓐ Ⓑ Ⓒ Ⓓ Ⓔ	62. Ⓐ Ⓑ Ⓒ Ⓓ Ⓔ	92. Ⓐ Ⓑ Ⓒ Ⓓ Ⓔ
3. Ⓐ Ⓑ Ⓒ Ⓓ Ⓔ	33. Ⓐ Ⓑ Ⓒ Ⓓ Ⓔ	63. Ⓐ Ⓑ Ⓒ Ⓓ Ⓔ	93. Ⓐ Ⓑ Ⓒ Ⓓ Ⓔ
4. Ⓐ Ⓑ Ⓒ Ⓓ Ⓔ	34. Ⓐ Ⓑ Ⓒ Ⓓ Ⓔ	64. Ⓐ Ⓑ Ⓒ Ⓓ Ⓔ	94. Ⓐ Ⓑ Ⓒ Ⓓ Ⓔ
5. Ⓐ Ⓑ Ⓒ Ⓓ Ⓔ	35. Ⓐ Ⓑ Ⓒ Ⓓ Ⓔ	65. Ⓐ Ⓑ Ⓒ Ⓓ Ⓔ	95. Ⓐ Ⓑ Ⓒ Ⓓ Ⓔ
6. Ⓐ Ⓑ Ⓒ Ⓓ Ⓔ	36. Ⓐ Ⓑ Ⓒ Ⓓ Ⓔ	66. Ⓐ Ⓑ Ⓒ Ⓓ Ⓔ	96. Ⓐ Ⓑ Ⓒ Ⓓ Ⓔ
7. Ⓐ Ⓑ Ⓒ Ⓓ Ⓔ	37. Ⓐ Ⓑ Ⓒ Ⓓ Ⓔ	67. Ⓐ Ⓑ Ⓒ Ⓓ Ⓔ	97. Ⓐ Ⓑ Ⓒ Ⓓ Ⓔ
8. Ⓐ Ⓑ Ⓒ Ⓓ Ⓔ	38. Ⓐ Ⓑ Ⓒ Ⓓ Ⓔ	68. Ⓐ Ⓑ Ⓒ Ⓓ Ⓔ	98. Ⓐ Ⓑ Ⓒ Ⓓ Ⓔ
9. Ⓐ Ⓑ Ⓒ Ⓓ Ⓔ	39. Ⓐ Ⓑ Ⓒ Ⓓ Ⓔ	69. Ⓐ Ⓑ Ⓒ Ⓓ Ⓔ	99. Ⓐ Ⓑ Ⓒ Ⓓ Ⓔ
10. Ⓐ Ⓑ Ⓒ Ⓓ Ⓔ	40. Ⓐ Ⓑ Ⓒ Ⓓ Ⓔ	70. Ⓐ Ⓑ Ⓒ Ⓓ Ⓔ	100. Ⓐ Ⓑ Ⓒ Ⓓ Ⓔ
11. Ⓐ Ⓑ Ⓒ Ⓓ Ⓔ	41. Ⓐ Ⓑ Ⓒ Ⓓ Ⓔ	71. Ⓐ Ⓑ Ⓒ Ⓓ Ⓔ	101. Ⓐ Ⓑ Ⓒ Ⓓ Ⓔ
12. Ⓐ Ⓑ Ⓒ Ⓓ Ⓔ	42. Ⓐ Ⓑ Ⓒ Ⓓ Ⓔ	72. Ⓐ Ⓑ Ⓒ Ⓓ Ⓔ	102. Ⓐ Ⓑ Ⓒ Ⓓ Ⓔ
13. Ⓐ Ⓑ Ⓒ Ⓓ Ⓔ	43. Ⓐ Ⓑ Ⓒ Ⓓ Ⓔ	73. Ⓐ Ⓑ Ⓒ Ⓓ Ⓔ	103. Ⓐ Ⓑ Ⓒ Ⓓ Ⓔ
14. Ⓐ Ⓑ Ⓒ Ⓓ Ⓔ	44. Ⓐ Ⓑ Ⓒ Ⓓ Ⓔ	74. Ⓐ Ⓑ Ⓒ Ⓓ Ⓔ	104. Ⓐ Ⓑ Ⓒ Ⓓ Ⓔ
15. Ⓐ Ⓑ Ⓒ Ⓓ Ⓔ	45. Ⓐ Ⓑ Ⓒ Ⓓ Ⓔ	75. Ⓐ Ⓑ Ⓒ Ⓓ Ⓔ	105. Ⓐ Ⓑ Ⓒ Ⓓ Ⓔ
16. Ⓐ Ⓑ Ⓒ Ⓓ Ⓔ	46. Ⓐ Ⓑ Ⓒ Ⓓ Ⓔ	76. Ⓐ Ⓑ Ⓒ Ⓓ Ⓔ	106. Ⓐ Ⓑ Ⓒ Ⓓ Ⓔ
17. Ⓐ Ⓑ Ⓒ Ⓓ Ⓔ	47. Ⓐ Ⓑ Ⓒ Ⓓ Ⓔ	77. Ⓐ Ⓑ Ⓒ Ⓓ Ⓔ	107. Ⓐ Ⓑ Ⓒ Ⓓ Ⓔ
18. Ⓐ Ⓑ Ⓒ Ⓓ Ⓔ	48. Ⓐ Ⓑ Ⓒ Ⓓ Ⓔ	78. Ⓐ Ⓑ Ⓒ Ⓓ Ⓔ	108. Ⓐ Ⓑ Ⓒ Ⓓ Ⓔ
19. Ⓐ Ⓑ Ⓒ Ⓓ Ⓔ	49. Ⓐ Ⓑ Ⓒ Ⓓ Ⓔ	79. Ⓐ Ⓑ Ⓒ Ⓓ Ⓔ	109. Ⓐ Ⓑ Ⓒ Ⓓ Ⓔ
20. Ⓐ Ⓑ Ⓒ Ⓓ Ⓔ	50. Ⓐ Ⓑ Ⓒ Ⓓ Ⓔ	80. Ⓐ Ⓑ Ⓒ Ⓓ Ⓔ	110. Ⓐ Ⓑ Ⓒ Ⓓ Ⓔ
21. Ⓐ Ⓑ Ⓒ Ⓓ Ⓔ	51. Ⓐ Ⓑ Ⓒ Ⓓ Ⓔ	81. Ⓐ Ⓑ Ⓒ Ⓓ Ⓔ	111. Ⓐ Ⓑ Ⓒ Ⓓ Ⓔ
22. Ⓐ Ⓑ Ⓒ Ⓓ Ⓔ	52. Ⓐ Ⓑ Ⓒ Ⓓ Ⓔ	82. Ⓐ Ⓑ Ⓒ Ⓓ Ⓔ	112. Ⓐ Ⓑ Ⓒ Ⓓ Ⓔ
23. Ⓐ Ⓑ Ⓒ Ⓓ Ⓔ	53. Ⓐ Ⓑ Ⓒ Ⓓ Ⓔ	83. Ⓐ Ⓑ Ⓒ Ⓓ Ⓔ	113. Ⓐ Ⓑ Ⓒ Ⓓ Ⓔ
24. Ⓐ Ⓑ Ⓒ Ⓓ Ⓔ	54. Ⓐ Ⓑ Ⓒ Ⓓ Ⓔ	84. Ⓐ Ⓑ Ⓒ Ⓓ Ⓔ	114. Ⓐ Ⓑ Ⓒ Ⓓ Ⓔ
25. Ⓐ Ⓑ Ⓒ Ⓓ Ⓔ	55. Ⓐ Ⓑ Ⓒ Ⓓ Ⓔ	85. Ⓐ Ⓑ Ⓒ Ⓓ Ⓔ	115. Ⓐ Ⓑ Ⓒ Ⓓ Ⓔ
26. Ⓐ Ⓑ Ⓒ Ⓓ Ⓔ	56. Ⓐ Ⓑ Ⓒ Ⓓ Ⓔ	86. Ⓐ Ⓑ Ⓒ Ⓓ Ⓔ	116. Ⓐ Ⓑ Ⓒ Ⓓ Ⓔ
27. Ⓐ Ⓑ Ⓒ Ⓓ Ⓔ	57. Ⓐ Ⓑ Ⓒ Ⓓ Ⓔ	87. Ⓐ Ⓑ Ⓒ Ⓓ Ⓔ	117. Ⓐ Ⓑ Ⓒ Ⓓ Ⓔ
28. Ⓐ Ⓑ Ⓒ Ⓓ Ⓔ	58. Ⓐ Ⓑ Ⓒ Ⓓ Ⓔ	88. Ⓐ Ⓑ Ⓒ Ⓓ Ⓔ	118. Ⓐ Ⓑ Ⓒ Ⓓ Ⓔ
29. Ⓐ Ⓑ Ⓒ Ⓓ Ⓔ	59. Ⓐ Ⓑ Ⓒ Ⓓ Ⓔ	89. Ⓐ Ⓑ Ⓒ Ⓓ Ⓔ	119. Ⓐ Ⓑ Ⓒ Ⓓ Ⓔ
30. Ⓐ Ⓑ Ⓒ Ⓓ Ⓔ	60. Ⓐ Ⓑ Ⓒ Ⓓ Ⓔ	90. Ⓐ Ⓑ Ⓒ Ⓓ Ⓔ	120. Ⓐ Ⓑ Ⓒ Ⓓ Ⓔ

SAMPLE NATURAL SCIENCES EXAMINATION 2

Number of Questions: 120

TIME LIMIT: 90 MINUTES

> **DIRECTIONS:** Each of the questions or incomplete statements below is followed by five suggested answers or completions. Select the one that is best in each case.

1. The term most appropriate to the passage of molecules across cellular membranes is

   (A) selective permeability
   (B) porosity
   (C) mass movement
   (D) capillarity
   (E) imbibition

2. According to the principle of biogenesis,

   (A) organic evolution is a reality
   (B) life comes from preexisting life
   (C) life arose from minerals
   (D) life arose as the result of special creation
   (E) life arises directly from nonliving matter

3. Both inductive and deductive reasoning may be involved in formulating a scientific hypothesis. An example of inductive reasoning is

   (A) the assumption that a particular genetic pattern would result from the mating of two specific parental types
   (B) the consideration of the numbers of different kinds of individuals that resulted from a genetic mating
   (C) the generalization that the inheritance patterns in plants are identical to those in animals
   (D) the prediction of genetic patterns based on reasoning alone
   (E) the presumption of genetic ratios that might result from an experimental mating

4. When a living cell is placed in a hypertonic fluid, there will be

   (A) a net movement of water molecules into the cell
   (B) no net movement of water molecules into or out of the cell
   (C) an increase in cell turgidity
   (D) an increase in Brownian movement
   (E) a net movement of water molecules out of the cell

5. When an organism is incapable of synthesizing its food from inorganic materials, it is described as

   (A) chemosynthetic
   (B) autotrophic
   (C) autophobic
   (D) heterotrophic
   (E) photosynthetic

6. Which of the following chemicals is responsible for the ability of plants to convert light energy into plant material?

   (A) Carotene
   (B) Chlorophyll
   (C) Anthocyanins
   (D) Stomata
   (E) Hemoglobin

7. As a result of the process called cellular respiration,

   (A) dry weight increases
   (B) oxygen and organic compounds are produced
   (C) water and carbon dioxide are consumed
   (D) dry weight decreases
   (E) water and organic compounds are produced

8. An energy-releasing process occurring continuously in all living cells is

   (A) respiration
   (B) osmosis
   (C) catalysis
   (D) diffusion
   (E) photosynthesis

9. Which of the following are plant hormones?

   (A) Calcitonin and insulin
   (B) Auxin and adrenaline
   (C) Gibberelin and prostaglandin
   (D) Auxin and gibberelin
   (E) Auxin and calcitonin

10. The total amount of organic matter in a population is referred to as

   (A) alluvium
   (B) humus
   (C) laterite
   (D) schist
   (E) biomass

11. In plants one of the functions of the xylem is to

   (A) manufacture organic substances from carbon dioxide and water
   (B) reduce transpiration
   (C) increase stem diameter by continued cell division
   (D) conduct water upward
   (E) conduct food substances

12. A grain of wheat is

   (A) a fruit
   (B) a seed
   (C) an epicotyl
   (D) a cotyledon
   (E) a hypocotyl

13. Water loss from plants by transpiration is decreased by

   (A) rainfall
   (B) increased air circulation
   (C) increased temperature
   (D) increased humidity
   (E) decreased humidity

14. Variation in a population may arise due to

   (A) mutation
   (B) independent assortment
   (C) changes in chromosome structure
   (D) changes in the chromosome number
   (E) all of the above

15. In plants, fertilization

   (A) gives rise to the gametophyte
   (B) precedes spore formation
   (C) precedes gamete formation
   (D) restores the diploid condition
   (E) may take place between two spores

16. What is the function of genes?

   (A) To produce mutations
   (B) To produce DNA
   (C) To produce transfer RNA
   (D) To produce all cellular components
   (E) To direct cells to produce specific proteins

17. Within the cytoplasm of living cells, the structures that "read" the genetic code, thereby directing the production of specific enzymes, are the

   (A) ribosomes
   (B) lysosomes
   (C) Golgi complex
   (D) macrosomes
   (E) mitochondria

18. Recombinant DNA research

   (A) permits the creation of entirely new species
   (B) permits the reassortment of genes between different species
   (C) utilizes X-ray techniques
   (D) produces predictable results in every case
   (E) is of no concern to environmental stability

19. Which of the following may be a problem associated with recombinant DNA research and the release of resulting strains of microorganisms into the environment?

   (A) The ultimate cost of development and production
   (B) The extremely limited target areas
   (C) The fact that expectations, at best, are meager
   (D) The fact that all current techniques are uncontrollable
   (E) The difficulty of tracing and recalling such released organisms

20. Nerve impulses along motor nerves leave the central nervous system

   (A) along a dorsal root axon
   (B) along a ventral root axon
   (C) after passing through a dorsal root ganglion
   (D) along a connector dendrite
   (E) along dendrites of sensory neurons

21. The capability of focusing both eyes on the same object is

   (A) stigmatism
   (B) binocular vision
   (C) glaucoma
   (D) hypermetropia
   (E) myopia

22. The hormone that regulates calcium metabolism in humans is

   (A) thyroxin
   (B) insulin
   (C) prolactin
   (D) parathormone
   (E) melatonin

23. The mutual exchange of chromosome fragments, which is called crossing-over, occurs during

   (A) interphase
   (B) fertilization
   (C) telophase
   (D) synapsis
   (E) cytoplasmic reorganization

24. The theory proposing the inheritance of acquired characteristics was proposed by

   (A) Alfred R. Wallace
   (B) Charles Darwin
   (C) Jean Baptiste de Lamarck
   (D) Sir Charles Lyell
   (E) Thomas Hunt Morgan

25. The mutation theory was eventually shown to strengthen Darwin's theory of natural selection because it provided

   (A) an explanation for genetic coding
   (B) for cytoplasmic inheritance
   (C) an explanation for pangenesis
   (D) a source of inheritable variations
   (E) the bridge between biometrics and the Mendelean ratios

26. Which of the following diseases has been eradicated from the earth?

   (A) Polio
   (B) Measles
   (C) Mumps
   (D) Smallpox
   (E) Yellow fever

27. The first to use the word *cell* after studying plant tissue with his microscope was

(A) Brown
(B) Leonardo da Vinci
(C) Hooke
(D) Grew
(E) Schleiden and Schwann

28. The primary characteristic of the disease acquired immune deficiency syndrome (AIDS) is that

(A) it causes a parasitic infection of the digestive tract
(B) it stimulates the development of several types of cancer
(C) it causes a defect in a person's natural immunity against disease
(D) there is no infectious agent
(E) it causes damage to brain tissues

29. The scientist responsible for proving that blood circulates through the body was

(A) Pasteur
(B) Paracelsus
(C) Harvey
(D) Galen
(E) Hippocrates

30. You would expect to encounter numerous epiphytes and a variety of arboreal mammals in

(A) a tropical rain forest
(B) a deciduous forest
(C) a coniferous forest
(D) an alpine tundra
(E) a taiga

31. Marine organisms found on the continental shelf live in the

(A) zone of perpetual darkness
(B) neritic zone
(C) littoral zone
(D) abyssal zone
(E) bathyal zone

32. A diet completely free of cholesterol would include

(A) a balance of all food types, including lean meat
(B) fruits and dairy products
(C) foods of plant origin only
(D) whole grains and dairy products
(E) vegetables and lean meat

33. Homologous structures are indicative of

(A) common ancestry
(B) convergence
(C) parallel evolution
(D) divergence
(E) similar function

34. An organism which obtains its food from nonliving organic materials is called a

(A) symbiont
(B) saprophyte
(C) commensal
(D) parasite
(E) buffer

35. The time period described as the age of glaciers is called the

(A) Eocene epoch
(B) Late Mesozoic
(C) Triassic period
(D) Early Mesozoic
(E) Pleistocene epoch

36. Repeated pruning of a row of shrubs commonly results in a dense growth of the shrub branches. The fact that the same shrubs, if not pruned, develop longer main stems with fewer branches is attributed to the action of auxin and is called

(A) phototropism
(B) thigmotropism
(C) disbudding
(D) apical dominance
(E) parthonocarpy

37. Goiter is caused by a lack of which element in the diet?

   (A) Iron
   (B) Calcium
   (C) Magnesium
   (D) Iodine
   (E) Copper

38. The process of rapidly heating foods to kill bacteria is known as

   (A) sterilization
   (B) homogenization
   (C) pasteurization
   (D) immunization
   (E) inoculation

39. The mating between a homozygous recessive male for trait "A" and a heterozygous female for the same trait would give which genotypes in the offspring?

   (A) 1/2 AA 1/2 Aa
   (B) 1/2 Aa 1/4 AA 1/4 aa
   (C) 1/2 Aa 1/2 aa
   (D) 1/4 AA 1/2 Aa 1/4 aa
   (E) 1/2 aa 1/4 Aa 1/4 AA

40. An enzyme catalyzes the reaction of a specific molecule known as a(an)

   (A) product
   (B) intermediate
   (C) transition state
   (D) substrate
   (E) activated complex

41. In a single-celled organism such as the amoeba, pinocytic vesicles function by

   (A) bringing some solid particles into the cell
   (B) discharging needlelike barbs containing poison
   (C) propelling the organism
   (D) reacting to environmental stimuli
   (E) excreting waste substances from the cell

42. Amino acid analysis of proteins has been advanced by

   (A) mass spectroscopy
   (B) better understanding of anabolic reactions
   (C) chromatography and electrophoresis
   (D) production and study of autoradiographs
   (E) DNA sequencing methods

43. Saprophytes

   (A) utilize radiant energy
   (B) rely upon the absorption of nutrients from decomposing organic materials
   (C) eat, digest, and assimilate food materials
   (D) oxidize inorganic materials
   (E) exist at the expense of living organisms

44. A main trigger for synthesis of Vitamin D by epithelial cells is

   (A) intake of calcium
   (B) intake of iron
   (C) exposure to calcitonin
   (D) exposure to sunlight
   (E) exposure to heat

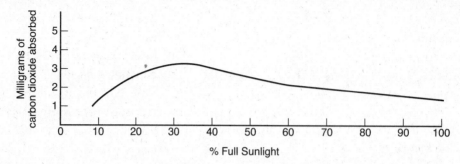

The graph represents the relationship between the rate of photosynthesis (expressed as milligrams of carbon dioxide absorbed per 0.5 square meter of leaf area per hour) and light intensity (expressed as percentages of full sunlight) for woodland ferns.

45. Under the conditions noted above, one may conclude that

(A) ferns use the most sunlight at 100% full sunlight
(B) photosynthesis decreases dry weight
(C) optimum light intensity for ferns is 30–40% full sunlight
(D) photosynthesis increases dry weight
(E) equal increases in light intensity throughout the range of 0–100% of full sunlight bring about equal increases in the rate of photosynthesis for ferns

46. One may also infer that

(A) ferns prefer shade
(B) absorbed carbon dioxide increases to 4 or more milligrams in ferns when exposed to greater than 100% full sunlight
(C) fern leaves are inefficient when it comes to photosynthesis
(D) ferns use more carbon dioxide at 10–50% full sunlight than at 60–100% full sunlight
(E) ferns would grow best in 100% full sunlight

47. Which of the following best describes a nerve impulse?

(A) The transmission of coded signals along a nerve fiber
(B) A wave of depolarization passing along a nerve fiber
(C) A flow of electrons along a nerve fiber
(D) A chemical reaction
(E) A wave of contraction passing along the myelin sheath

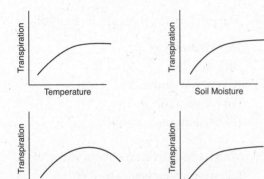

48. The graphs above illustrate the approximate rates of water loss by the aerial parts of plants (transpiration) under varying environmental conditions. On the basis of the information conveyed by the graphs, one may correctly infer that

(A) air velocity is the principal factor affecting transpiration
(B) transpiration is affected by multiple factors
(C) genetic factors exert the primary control over transpiration
(D) the oxygen concentration in soil moisture has no effect on transpiration
(E) plants having high concentrations of anthocyanins have high transpiration rates

49. When the dorsal root of a reflex arc is cut,

(A) stimulation of the distal end causes no reaction
(B) stimulation of the distal end causes a normal reaction
(C) the reflex reaction will occur normally
(D) the sensory stimulus will travel along the ventral root
(E) new nerve pathways will develop immediately

50. The main control of hormonal regulation in the body is performed by the

(A) pituitary gland
(B) adrenal glands
(C) pancreas
(D) thyroid gland
(E) parathyroid glands

51. An example of a sex-linked disease is

(A) multiple sclerosis
(B) hemophilia
(C) Down syndrome
(D) cystic fibrosis
(E) diabetes

52. The inherited variations commonly referred to in treatises on natural selection and evolution, are, in reality,

(A) merely chance variations
(B) induced by the environment
(C) special creations
(D) mutations
(E) acquired characteristics

53. Deoxyribonucleic acid consists of simple sugars, phosphate units, and four specific nitrogenous bases:

(A) cytosine, guanine, thymine, and uracil
(B) adenine, guanine, thymine, and uracil
(C) adenine, cytosine, guanine, and thymine
(D) adenine, cytosine, thymine, and uracil
(E) adenine, cytosine, guanine, and uracil

54. The best dietary sources of polyunsaturated fats include

(A) oils of plant origin
(B) fats of animal origin
(C) milk, cream, cheese, and butter
(D) hydrogenated vegetable oils
(E) trans fats

55. A Renaissance artist renowned for his knowledge of human musculature was

(A) Albertus Magnus
(B) Galen
(C) Michelangelo
(D) Vesalius
(E) De Chauliac

56. The ancient Greek scholar who devoted much study to and wrote much about plant reproduction and seed development, and who is referred to as the "father of botany" is

(A) Aristotle
(B) Empedocles
(C) Thales
(D) Anaximander
(E) Theophrastus

57. Salts of the heavy metals, such as lead or mercury, when taken into the body, accumulate in the marrow of long bones and interfere with

(A) coagulation of the blood
(B) formation of thrombin from prothrombin
(C) formation of erythrocytes
(D) maturation of phagocytes
(E) release of calcium from platelets

58. The primary function of root hair cells is

(A) anchorage
(B) storage
(C) photosynthesis
(D) absorption
(E) synergism

59. With respect to dietary fibers, which of the following statements is correct?

(A) A high-fiber diet is high in carbohydrates.
(B) Oat bran may lower cholesterol.
(C) A high-fiber diet may cause colon cancer.
(D) Dry beans and peas are low in dietary fiber.
(E) A high-fiber diet is usually a high-calorie diet.

60. When environmental conditions become unfavorable, certain species of bacteria

(A) develop flagella
(B) become aerobic
(C) form spores
(D) become anaerobic
(E) develop capsules

61. When certain types of atmospheric particles act as nuclei on which water condensation occurs, these fog-forming nuclei are called

    (A) hydrologic nuclei
    (B) condensation nuclei
    (C) hydroscopic nuclei
    (D) hygroscopic nuclei
    (E) aquifers

62. The earth's orbit around the sun is most like

    (A) a parabola
    (B) a circle
    (C) an ellipse
    (D) a hyperbola
    (E) a spiral

63. One significant scientific contribution of the Babylonians was the

    (A) Pythagorean theorem
    (B) combining of mathematics with experimental theory
    (C) recording of eclipses
    (D) science of alchemy
    (E) principle of Archimedes

64. The laws of conservation of mass were verified experimentally by

    (A) Priestly
    (B) Democritus
    (C) Dalton
    (D) Rutherford
    (E) Lavoisier

65. A star that suddenly increases in brightness and then slowly fades is known as a

    (A) supernova
    (B) nova
    (C) giant star
    (D) visual binary
    (E) white dwarf

66. A mixture that does not settle out upon standing and that displays the Tyndall Effect is a

    (A) solution
    (B) suspension
    (C) colloid
    (D) precipitate
    (E) filtrate

67. Deposits of glacial till forming various ridge patterns are called

    (A) bergschrunds
    (B) moraines
    (C) uplifts
    (D) displacements
    (E) sediments

68. An offshore ridge formed by coral is called

    (A) a fjord
    (B) continental shelf
    (C) sediment
    (D) a barrier reef
    (E) an upwelling

69. The smallest particles possessing the properties of elements are

    (A) neutrons
    (B) isotopes
    (C) protons
    (D) atoms
    (E) electrons

70. Throughout the universe, the force that holds atoms and molecules together is called the

    (A) weak force
    (B) nuclear force
    (C) strong force
    (D) electromagnetic force
    (E) fifth force

71. The measure of the disorder of a system is known as

(A) chaos
(B) enthalpy
(C) entropy
(D) randomness
(E) nonequilibrium condition

72. Color is primarily the property of those wavelengths of light which are

(A) absorbed
(B) reflected
(C) produced
(D) attracted
(E) adsorbed

73. Why is gravity the dominant force throughout the universe?

(A) The electromagnetic force only holds atoms and molecules together.
(B) The hypothetical "fifth force" is a repulsive force.
(C) The weak force allows some atomic nuclei to break down.
(D) The strong force is vastly stronger than the gravitational force.
(E) Both the strong force and the weak force have very short ranges.

74. Which of the following changes when an object accelerates?

(A) Speed only
(B) Direction only
(C) Both speed and direction
(D) The object's weight, but not its mass
(E) The forces acting on the object

75. An object is traveling at 20 m/s. Five seconds later it is moving at 60 m/s. The acceleration of the object is

(A) 0.6 m/s^2
(B) 4.0 m/s^2
(C) 8.0 m/s^2
(D) 12.0 m/s^2
(E) 10.0 m/s^2

76. A solution into which more solute can be dissolved is said to be

(A) unsaturated
(B) saturated
(C) supersaturated
(D) diluted
(E) concentrated

77. Which of the following statements describing cathode rays is *not* correct?

(A) They are bent by electric fields but not by magnetic fields.
(B) They cast shadows.
(C) They travel in straight lines.
(D) They are bent by both electric and magnetic fields.
(E) They consist of electrons.

78. Radio waves and light waves differ with respect to

(A) amplitude
(B) wavelength
(C) visibility
(D) velocities
(E) diffraction

79. Chemical bonds in which a pair of electrons are shared unevenly between two atoms are called

(A) hydrogen bonds
(B) ionic bonds
(C) nonpolar covalent bonds
(D) polar covalent bonds
(E) London dispersion forces

80. In electricity, the unit of resistance is the

(A) ohm
(B) watt
(C) volt
(D) ampere
(E) coulomb

81. Which of the following accounts for the high boiling point of water?

    (A) its high molecular weight (molar mass)
    (B) the ability of water molecules to attract to many surfaces
    (C) the ability of water molecules to form hydrogen bonds
    (D) the ability of water molecules to evaporate easily
    (E) the ability of water molecules to dissolve many other substances

82. Simple machines such as levers enable humans to

    (A) gain both force and distance
    (B) gain both mechanical advantage and speed
    (C) decrease the force arm and increase the weight arm without increasing force
    (D) eliminate friction
    (E) trade force for distance, or vice versa

83. Heat transfer is accomplished by conduction, radiation, and

    (A) vaporization
    (B) convection
    (C) expansion
    (D) entropy
    (E) insulation

84. Quantum mechanics is concerned with the

    (A) change in velocity of electrons
    (B) likely location of electrons in atoms
    (C) transmission of heat energy through gases and liquids
    (D) deflection of air flow caused by the earth's rotation
    (E) tendencies of materials to fail as a result of repeated stress

85. A property of matter which tends to make it resist any change in motion is called

    (A) gravity
    (B) force
    (C) mass
    (D) acceleration
    (E) inertia

86. Any physical system is said to possess energy if it

    (A) has the capacity to do work
    (B) has mass
    (C) is at absolute zero
    (D) resists acceleration
    (E) resists gravity

87. A fundamental particle with a positive charge found in the nuclei of all atoms is

    (A) an ion
    (B) a meson
    (C) a proton
    (D) an electron
    (E) a neutron

88. Approximately what percentage of the potential energy of fossil fuels such as coal is actually delivered to homes and businesses as useful energy?

    (A) 95%
    (B) 75%
    (C) 65%
    (D) 35%
    (E) 25%

89. In a nuclear chain reaction, the process continues due to the emission of which particles from the decaying nuclei?

    (A) Protons
    (B) Electrons
    (C) Gamma rays
    (D) Photons
    (E) Neutrons

90. To say that a football player weighs 220 pounds means that

(A) his body is attracted by the sun with a force equal to 220 pounds
(B) his body is attracted by the sun and the moon with a combined force equal to 220 pounds
(C) his body is attracted by the earth with a force equal to 220 pounds
(D) he has a negative mass equal to 220 pounds
(E) he has a positive mass equal to 220 pounds

91. Water held behind a dam represents what kind of energy?

(A) Kinetic
(B) Potential
(C) Mass
(D) Conserved
(E) Transformed

92. Which of the following is not currently used as a source of electrical power generation?

(A) Fission energy
(B) Fusion energy
(C) Hydroelectric energy
(D) Tidal motion
(E) Geothermal energy

93. In the process called evaporation, the faster molecules of a liquid are able to escape the attractive forces of their slower neighboring molecules. This results in

(A) an increase in temperature
(B) a decrease in temperature
(C) adhesion
(D) cohesion
(E) friction

94. Specific gravity is a measure of the relative density of a liquid compared to

(A) water
(B) air
(C) ice
(D) mercury
(E) oxygen

95. Which are the products of the reaction between an acid, such as HCl, and a base, such as NaOH?

(A) Hydrogen gas and water
(B) Oxygen gas and a salt
(C) Water and a salt
(D) A salt and hydrogen gas
(E) Water and oxygen gas

96. Which element is located in the noble gas family?

(A) Oxygen
(B) Sodium
(C) Chlorine
(D) Chromium
(E) Neon

97. When exposed to light, chlorophyll fluoresces. This effect is the

(A) return of electrons to the chlorophyll molecule
(B) reflection of light by the chlorophyll molecule
(C) beginning of glucose synthesis
(D) absorption of light at one wavelength and the emission of light energy at a different wavelength
(E) shifting of electrons to the innermost orbits of the chlorophyll atoms

98. One class of organic compounds constitutes the building blocks of proteins and is characterized by possessing

   (A) a carboxyl group only
   (B) an NH_2 group in addition to a carboxyl group
   (C) hydrocarbons
   (D) an alkyl group
   (E) esters

99. Which of the following is an example of a chemical change?

   (A) Wax melting
   (B) Wood burning
   (C) Tearing a piece of paper
   (D) Attracting iron to a magnet
   (E) Dissolving sugar in water

100. In chemical equations, the total mass of the reactants

   (A) equals the total mass of the products
   (B) is less than the total mass of the products
   (C) is greater than the total mass of the products
   (D) is not relative to the total mass of the products
   (E) is determined by the atomic number of the reactant

101. The majority of freshwater usage in the world today is for which purpose?

   (A) Drinking and washing by people
   (B) Agricultural uses
   (C) Cooling factories and power plants
   (D) Hydroelectric power
   (E) Recreational uses

102. Scholasticism represents a philosophical attempt during the Middle Ages to harmonize Roman Catholic beliefs and

   (A) the astronomical works of Copernicus
   (B) the anatomical and physiological works of Vesalius
   (C) Galileo's "behavior of moving objects"
   (D) the works and teachings of Aristotle
   (E) early Byzantine and Moslem sciences

103. Which of the following is not a major air pollutant today?

   (A) Carbon monoxide (CO)
   (B) Ozone (O_3)
   (C) Unburned hydrocarbons
   (D) Nitrogen oxides (NO_x)
   (E) Carbon dioxide (CO_2)

104. The process of an atom gaining electrons is known as

   (A) neutralization
   (B) oxidation
   (C) reduction
   (D) decomposition
   (E) synthesis

105. An alpha particle is best described as

   (A) an electron
   (B) a photon
   (C) a quantum of light energy
   (D) a hydrogen nucleus
   (E) a helium nucleus

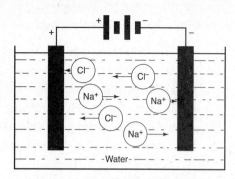

106. After study of the illustration above, one may conclude that

   (A) water molecules are attracted by the electrodes
   (B) sodium ions are attracted to the positive electrode
   (C) sodium chloride dissociates when placed in water
   (D) chlorine ions are attracted to the negative electrode
   (E) current flow causes an increase in water temperature

107. One may also conclude that

   (A) the solution will not conduct current
   (B) only sodium ions conduct current
   (C) only chlorine ions conduct current
   (D) the closed circuit illustrated results in neutrality
   (E) when ions are present they are attracted to electrodes having opposite electrical charges

108. Certain metals and alloys, such as nichrome wire, are used in electrical heating devices (toasters, for example) because of their

   (A) low melting point
   (B) high specific resistance
   (C) great current flow
   (D) capacity to discharge electrons
   (E) capacity to modify electrons

109. A unique feature of lasers is

   (A) the abrupt spreading of their beam of light
   (B) their production of coherent radiation
   (C) the Peltier effect
   (D) the Seebeck effect
   (E) the very narrow beam of light produced

110. Compared to visible light, infrared light has

   (A) a longer wavelength and more energy
   (B) a longer wavelength and less energy
   (C) a shorter wavelength and more energy
   (D) a shorter wavelength and less energy
   (E) the same wavelength and the same energy

111. When an electric current is passed through electrodes immersed in an electrolyte, ions of the electrolyte

   (A) precipitate
   (B) dissociate
   (C) crystallize
   (D) combine
   (E) neutralize

112. According to the law of reflection,

    (A) the angle of incidence is equal to the angle of reflection

    (B) the angle of incidence is less than the angle of reflection

    (C) the angle of incidence is greater than the angle of reflection

    (D) the angle of incidence equals the angle of reflection squared

    (E) the angle of reflection equals the angle of incidence squared

113. Which of the following is considered a greenhouse gas that has been increasing in amounts due to human activity?

    (A) carbon dioxide
    (B) water vapor
    (C) ozone
    (D) sulfur dioxide
    (E) carbon monoxide

114. A coil of wire carrying an electric current behaves as

    (A) a stator
    (B) a commutator
    (C) a transistor
    (D) a bar magnet
    (E) a capacitor

DIRECTIONS: Each group of questions below consists of five lettered choices followed by a list of numbered phrases or sentences. For each numbered phrase or sentence select the one choice that is most closely related to it. Each choice may be used once, more than once, or not at all in each group.

Questions 115–117

    (A) Binary stars
    (B) Black holes
    (C) Dwarfs
    (D) Supernovas
    (E) Variable stars

115. Stars which fluctuate in brightness

116. Stars attracted by their mutual gravitations

117. Stars which increase in brightness multifold

Questions 118–120

    (A) Avogadro's law
    (B) Boyle's law
    (C) Kinetic-molecular theory
    (D) First law of thermodynamics
    (E) Uncertainty principle

118. States that energy may be neither created nor destroyed

119. Is based on the concept that we cannot know both the position and the momentum of an electron at the same time

120. Assumes that gases consist of independently moving molecules

If there is still time remaining, you may review your answers.

ANSWER KEY
Sample Examination 2

NATURAL SCIENCES

1.	A	31.	B	61.	B	91.	B
2.	B	32.	C	62.	C	92.	B
3.	B	33.	A	63.	C	93.	B
4.	E	34.	B	64.	E	94.	A
5.	D	35.	E	65.	B	95.	C
6.	B	36.	D	66.	C	96.	E
7.	D	37.	D	67.	B	97.	D
8.	A	38.	C	68.	D	98.	B
9.	D	39.	A	69.	D	99.	B
10.	E	40.	D	70.	D	100.	A
11.	D	41.	A	71.	C	101.	B
12.	A	42.	C	72.	B	102.	D
13.	D	43.	B	73.	E	103.	E
14.	E	44.	D	74.	C	104.	C
15.	D	45.	C	75.	C	105.	E
16.	E	46.	D	76.	A	106.	C
17.	A	47.	B	77.	A	107.	E
18.	B	48.	B	78.	B	108.	B
19.	E	49.	A	79.	D	109.	E
20.	B	50.	A	80.	A	110.	B
21.	B	51.	B	81.	C	111.	B
22.	D	52.	D	82.	E	112.	A
23.	D	53.	C	83.	B	113.	E
24.	C	54.	A	84.	B	114.	D
25.	D	55.	C	85.	E	115.	E
26.	C	56.	E	86.	A	116.	A
27.	C	57.	C	87.	C	117.	D
28.	C	58.	D	88.	E	118.	D
29.	C	59.	B	89.	E	119.	E
30.	A	60.	C	90.	C	120.	C

SCORING CHART

After you have scored your Sample Examination 2, enter the results in the chart below; then transfer your score to the Progress Chart on page 12.

Total Test	Number Right	Number Wrong	Number Omitted
120			

ANSWER EXPLANATIONS

1. **(A)** Cellular membranes are selectively permeable since they permit different kinds of molecules to pass at varying rates or not at all and this permeability may constantly change.

2. **(B)** According to biogenesis, all life comes from preexisting life.

3. **(B)** Inductive reasoning is reasoning from a part or parts to a whole, or from particulars to general. Deductive reasoning is the derivation of a conclusion by reasoning alone.

4. **(E)** A hypertonic solution has a higher osmotic pressure than the protoplasm of the cell in question and, therefore, water will diffuse out of the cell with a consequent decrease in turgor pressure.

5. **(D)** Autotrophic organisms have the ability to synthesize their food from inorganic materials; heterotrophic organisms lack this ability.

6. **(B)** The green pigment chlorophyll absorbs energy from the sun, and that energy is used to carry out the chemical reactions by which plants produce sugars and starches.

7. **(D)** In cellular respiration organic substances are broken down to release their stored energy. This results in a decrease in dry weight.

8. **(A)** All living cells carry on cellular respiration, which is a process that provides energy for the cell's use.

9. **(D)** Both auxin and gibberelin are plant hormones. Calcitonin, adrenaline, and insulin are human hormones.

10. **(E)** The total weight of protoplasm in a community is referred to as biomass.

11. **(D)** Xylem is the principal water-conducting tissue in vascular plants.

12. **(A)** A fruit is the matured ovary of a flower. A grain of wheat is a matured ovary of the wheat plant.

13. **(D)** Any factor that affects the evaporation of water from an open container will have a similar effect on transpiration by plants. Transpiration is defined as the evaporation of water from the aerial parts of plants.

14. **(E)** Variation may occur in a population as a result of any chromosomal change affecting its DNA, chromosome number, or structure; the position of genes; or independent assortment during meiosis.

15. **(D)** The fusion of two haploid (N) gametes in plants restores the diploid ($2N$) chromosome number.

16. **(E)** Genes direct cells to produce specific enzymes, all of which are proteins, and these act as the cellular "machines" that control or determine cellular traits.

17. **(A)** All cellullar proteins, including enzymes, are produced by ribosomes, which are composed of RNA and proteins and which follow the instructions received from the DNA code of the nucleus.

18. **(B)** Techniques utilized in the field of recombinant DNA research permit the transfer or reassortment of genes between different species. However, its results are not readily predictable, may affect food chains, and may upset the delicate environment.

19. **(E)** Gene-splicing produces new kinds of individuals within species. The interactions of these new kinds of organisms with the environment are not only unpredictable, but also potentially hazardous if something "goes wrong."

20. **(B)** Motor nerve impulses leave the central nervous system along ventral root axons, while sensory impulses move toward the central nervous system along dorsal roots.

21. **(B)** The human visual system is binocular and stereoscopic, i.e., the images of the two eyes fit together to produce roundness and depth.

22. **(D)** Parathormone, released by the parathyroid glands, controls the metabolism of calcium in the human body. Calcium plays a role in nerve signaling, muscle contraction, and bone and teeth formation and maintenance.

23. **(D)** Synapsis is the pairing of the chromosomes during the prophase and metaphase of the first meiotic division. Since each chromosome consists of two daughter chromatids during this period, a tetrad of four chromatids exists and crossing-over occurs often.

24. **(C)** Lamarck proposed the theory of the inheritance of acquired characteristics, frequently referred to as the theory of "use and disuse."

25. **(D)** The mutation theory proposed by de Vries strengthened Darwin's theory of natural selection because it provided a good explanation for the source of inheritable variations, something Darwin was not able to do.

26. **(C)** Smallpox as a disease has been eradicated from the face of the earth. The other diseases are rare in North America but much more common elsewhere.

27. **(C)** Robert Hooke was the first to use the term *cell* in describing the microscopic units that comprise the tissues and organs of multicellular plants and animals.

28. **(C)** Although AIDS is a very complex disease distinguished by various symptoms, it is primarily characterized by causing major defects in an individual's immunity to disease.

29. **(C)** William Harvey discovered both arteries and veins, and predicted that smaller blood vessels, which we know are called capillaries, would also exist. He described the circulation of blood in the body.

30. **(A)** In the tropical rain forest with its excessive rains, the ground level environment is poor. Therefore, many forms of plants and animals are tree dwellers.

31. **(B)** The neritic environment is identified as a region of shallow water adjoining the seacoast and above the continental shelf.

32. **(C)** Cholesterol is not found in foods of plant origin.

33. **(A)** Homologous structures are similar from the standpoint of structure, embryonic development, and relationship and thus indicate common ancestry.

34. **(B)** A saprophyte is a heterotrophic plant that obtains its nourishment from nonliving organic matter.

35. **(E)** In the Pleistocene epoch climates cooled dramatically and there were two glacial periods during which the ice advanced twice.

36. **(D)** Auxin (plant hormone) is produced primarily by terminal buds, and among its induced responses are stem elongation and lateral bud inhibition. Removal of terminal buds by pruning permits lateral buds to grow into branches.

37. **(D)** Goiter, visible clinically as a grossly enlarged thyroid gland, is caused by a lack of iodine in the diet. The addition of small amounts of iodine to salt has largely eliminated this disease. Seafood also contains iodine.

38. **(C)** Pasteurization, or the heating of food to kill bacteria, was developed by Louis Pasteur.

39. **(A)** The offspring of AA mated with Aa will give 1/2 AA and 1/2 Aa.

40. **(D)** Enzymes act upon substrates. Each enzyme exhibits a great deal of specificity for a single substrate (or small number of similar substrates).

41. **(A)** Solid food particles such as bacterial cells may be brought into the cell by pinocytosis and released into the cytoplasm as a food vacuole.

42. **(C)** Chromatography permits the separation of amino acids and relies upon the different solubilities of amino acids and on their differential absorption on paper.

43. **(B)** Saprophytes are heterotrophic plants which obtain their nourishment from nonliving organic matter.

44. **(D)** The synthesis of Vitamin D by epithelial cells is triggered primarily by exposure to sunlight.

45. **(C)** ⎫ Study of the graph indicates that optimum light intensity for the ferns is
46. **(D)** ⎭ 30–40%, since this represents the light intensity at which there is greatest absorption of CO_2. Similarly, ferns use more CO_2 at 10–50% of full sunlight than at 60–100%. On the basis of the information given, no other conclusions are valid.

47. **(B)** The resting nerve fiber is polarized, having its outside positively charged and its inside negatively charged. A stimulus causes a wave of depolarization to pass along the fiber, from which it recovers in about 0.001 second.

48. **(B)** Transpiration is the loss of water from the aerial parts of plants; its rate is affected by several environmental factors, including solar radiation, humidity, air movement, soil moisture, and temperature.

49. **(A)** Sensory nerve impulses travel to the spinal cord along the dorsal root of a reflex arc. When the dorsal root has been cut, no sensory nerve impulse may travel to the spinal cord.

50. **(A)** The master hormonal gland is the pituitary gland, located at the base of the brain.

51. **(B)** Hemophilia is a sex-linked disease and is far more prevalent in males. Down Syndrome is caused by having three copies of chromosome 21, rather than the normal two copies. Cystic fibrosis is an autosomal recessive disease.

52. **(D)** Mutations are the source of the inherited variations and support the theory of evolution by providing the variations needed for natural selection.

53. **(C)** The specific nitrogenous bases of deoxyribonucleic acid are the amino acids adenine, cytosine, guanine, and thymine.

54. **(A)** Polyunsaturated fats are found in largest proportions in plant fats such as sunflower, corn, and soybean oils and in selected fish.

55. **(C)** Michelangelo Buonarroti was a great student of human anatomy who performed many of his own dissections. Evidence of his vast knowledge of anatomy is found in his paintings and sculptures.

56. **(E)** Theophrastus' writings on plants have been preserved and represent the extent of the Greeks' knowledge of science. His greatest work was "Historia Plantarum."

57. **(C)** Erythrocytes are formed in the marrow of long bones. Injury to bone marrow, caused by the deposition of heavy metals, interferes with erythrocyte production.

58. **(D)** Root hair cells increase the absorbing surface of roots and are the principal water-absorbing structures of typical land plant roots.

59. **(B)** Oat bran has a high proportion of soluble fiber, and it is soluble fiber that lowers cholesterol.

60. **(C)** Spore formation is a response of certain bacteria to an environment which becomes unfavorable. Bacterial spores have thick, resistant spore walls and the living bacterial cell within is in a state of suspended animation. When conditions become favorable, the bacterial cell converts back to its active way of life.

61. **(B)** When the atmosphere is saturated with water vapor, minute bits of particulate matter known as condensation nuclei serve as surfaces for the condensation of water vapor.

62. **(C)** Kepler's greatest discovery was the fact that planetary orbits, including that of the earth, are ellipses.

63. **(C)** Ancient civilizations, including the Babylonians, relied on astrology in predicting the future. Astrological events are tied to the behavior of the sun, moon, and planets. It is, therefore, not surprising that early Babylonian writings included references to eclipses.

64. **(E)** Lavoisier showed that mass is conserved in a chemical or physical change.

65. **(B)** Stars that fluctuate in brightness are called variables. In one type, the eruptive variable, a sudden brightening occurs; this is called a nova.

66. **(C)** Solutions do not settle out over time due to the small size of their particles. They do not show the Tyndall Effect. Suspensions, due to the larger size of their particles, will settle out over time and do show the Tyndall Effect. Colloids, with intermediate sized particles, exhibit the Tyndall Effect, but do not settle out over time.

67. **(B)** Glaciers cause the erosion, transportation, and deposition of mineral matter, and this mass of rock debris deposited as residual matter is referred to as a moraine.

68. **(D)** A barrier reef is a long, narrow coral embankment lying offshore.

69. **(D)** Atoms are the smallest units of elements that can exist and that possess all the properties of the specific elements.

70. **(D)** The electromagnetic force is the force that holds atoms and molecules together.

71. **(C)** Entropy is the physical quantity that describes the amount of disorder in a chemical or physical system.

72. **(B)** Those wavelengths of the total visible spectrum which are reflected are blended and perceived by the eye as color.

73. **(E)** The strong force and the weak force have very short ranges and are felt only inside the atomic nucleus. The electromagnetic force acts only to hold atoms and molecules together. Gravity, however, is felt throughout the universe.

74. **(C)** Velocity is comprised of both speed and direction. Unbalanced force causes a change in velocity.

75. **(C)** Acceleration is the change in velocity divided by the time involved. The velocity went from 20 m/s to 60 m/s for a change in velocity of 40 m/s. That took 5 seconds for an acceleration of $(40 \text{ m/s})/5 \text{ s} = 8 \text{ m/s}^2$.

76. **(A)** An unsaturated solution can have more solute dissolved in it. Diluted and concentrated are terms that describe the amounts of solute dissolved, not whether more can be dissolved.

77. **(A)** Characteristics of cathode rays include traveling in straight lines, casting shadows, consisting of electrons, and being bent by both electric and magnetic fields.

78. **(B)** Radio waves and light waves are different parts of the electromagnetic spectrum differing primarily in that they have different wavelengths.

79. **(D)** Chemical bonds in which electrons are shared are known as covalent bonds. Uneven sharing results in polar covalent bonds, while even sharing results in nonpolar covalent bonds. Ionic bonds involve the transfer (gain and loss) of electrons between atoms.

80. **(A)** The ohm is the unit of electrical resistance in a material.

81. **(C)** Water's high boiling point (as well as its ability to "bead up" and its high heat capacity) is the result of its formation of hydrogen bonds, or weak attraction between water molecules.

82. **(E)** A lever is a machine which can be used to gain force or distance, since the length of the force arm multiplied by the force used equals the length of the weight arm multiplied by the weight.

83. **(B)** Heat energy is transferred within a medium by conduction, radiation, and convection.

84. **(B)** Quantum theory identifies the smallest units of energy, the quantum, and quantum mechanics explains their behavior inside the atom.

85. **(E)** Inertia is the tendency of a body at rest to remain at rest or the tendency of a body in motion to remain in motion.

86. **(A)** Energy may be defined as the capacity to perform work.

87. **(C)** Protons are one of the fundamental types of particles found in the nuclei of all atoms. Protons have positive charges.

88. **(E)** Only about 1/4 of the energy stored in fossil fuels is actually delivered to its end point. Most useful energy is lost during transmission and generation of the electricity.

89. **(E)** Nuclear chain reactions are both initiated and maintained by the absorption of a neutron by a nucleus. The process continues because the splitting of the nucleus can also emit more neutrons, allowing a self-sustaining process.

90. **(C)** Weight is defined as the force of gravity upon an object.

91. **(B)** Potential energy is that energy possessed by an object because of its position.

92. **(B)** While it has great potential, no functioning fusion plants exist today. This is largely because of our inability to generate and maintain the high temperatures the process requires.

93. **(B)** The heat of vaporization is the heat energy absorbed by the molecules of an evaporating liquid. The result is cooling or a decrease in temperature.

94. **(A)** The specific gravity of a liquid is the ratio of the density of the liquid to the density of water where both densities are obtained in air at the same temperature.

95. **(C)** The general reaction for an acid and a base is acid + base $\rightarrow$ salt plus water. Acids tend to react with metals to produce hydrogen gas.

96. **(E)** The noble gases include the inert elements in group 18 (VIIIA) on the periodic table. Group 17 (VIIA) is known as the halogens, and includes fluorine and chlorine.

97. **(D)** Fluorescence is the emission of light of one wavelength by a substance subsequent to the absorption of radiant energy of a different wavelength. Subsequent to the absorption of radiant energy by chlorophyll, electrons of some of its atoms may move to outer electron orbits, resulting in the excited state of these moved electrons. When these moved electrons return to their normal orbits, light of a different wavelength is emitted.

98. **(B)** Proteins are polymers consisting of long chains of amino acids, each unit of which is built from an amino group and a carboxyl group.

99. **(B)** In a chemical change, the chemical identity of the products differs from that of the starting materials. In other words, new substances are formed.

100. **(A)** In any chemical reaction, the total molecular mass of the reactants always equals the total molecular mass of the products.

101. **(B)** Over 70% of the freshwater used in the world today is used for agricultural purposes.

102. **(D)** Scholasticism was a philosophical movement during the Middle Ages attempting to combine the teachings of Aristotle and St. Augustine with fixed religious dogma.

103. **(E)** While we hear a great deal about carbon dioxide as a greenhouse gas it is not considered a major air pollutant as the others are.

104. **(C)** The gaining of an electron is known as reduction, and the losing of an electron is known as oxidation.

105. **(E)** An alpha particle has two protons and two neutrons, but no electrons, making it have a mass of 4 amu and a charge of +2. It is the nucleus of a helium atom.

106. **(C)** Dissociation is the breaking up of a chemical substance into its ionic constituents. In this instance NaCl dissociates to form Na^+ ions and Cl^- ions when placed in water.

107. **(E)** Ionic behavior responds to the concept that like (electrical) charges repel each other and unlike charges attract each other.

108. **(B)** Metals possessing high specific resistance to the conduction of electric current heat up since it takes more energy to push current through wires having high resistance and this energy is converted to heat.

109. **(E)** A laser is a device that can focus a beam of light to concentrate a great amount of electromagnetic energy on a very small area.

110. **(B)** Infrared light is less energetic than visible light and has a longer wavelength. For all parts of the electromagnetic spectrum, the longer the wavelength, the smaller the frequency and the lower the energy. Ultraviolet light has a shorter wavelength than visible light, along with a higher frequency and a greater energy.

111. **(B)** Molecules of an electrolyte dissociate when it conducts an electric current and simultaneously the newly formed ions migrate with anions moving toward the anode and cations moving toward the cathode.

112. **(A)** When electromagnetic waves strike a surface, they are said to be reflected, and careful measurements will reveal that the angle of incidence is equal to the angle of reflection.

113. **(E)** While both water and carbon dioxide are considered greenhouse gases, there is no evidence that human activity has increased the amount of water vapor in the atmosphere.

114. **(D)** The magnetic field generated in a coil of wire when an electric current passes through it behaves in a manner similar to a bar magnet.

115. **(E)** Stars that fluctuate in brightness are known as variable stars.

116. **(A)** Stars which move about each other and which are attracted by their mutual gravitation are called binary stars.

117. **(D)** When a star increases its brightness several million times it is called a supernova.

118. **(D)** According to the first law of thermodynamics, energy may be transformed from one type to another, but may be neither created nor destroyed.

119. **(E)** An electron is displaced by the energy transmitted to it by the photon that strikes it. The electron will then be in a different location. Thus, the energy and the original position of the electron remain unknown, a phenomenon called the uncertainty principle.

120. **(C)** A theory concerning the nature of gases that assumes that gases consist of independently moving molecules is named the kinetic-molecular theory.

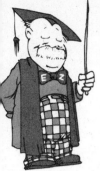
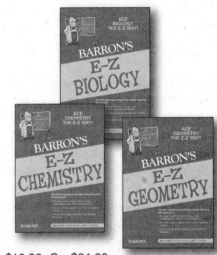
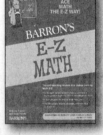
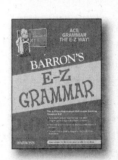
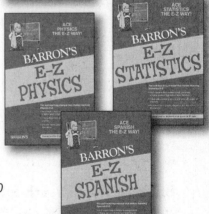
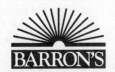

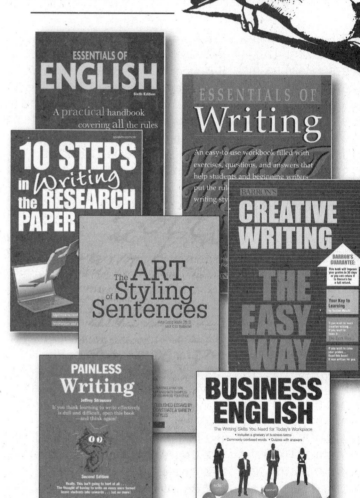
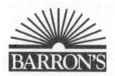

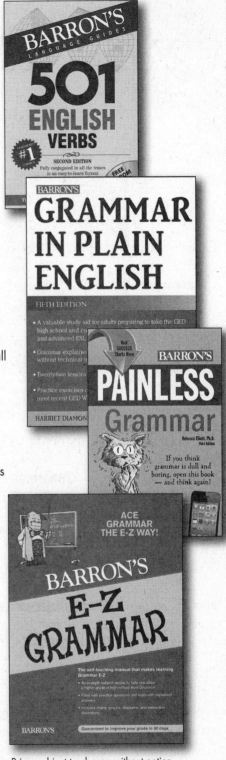
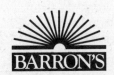

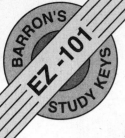

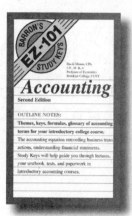
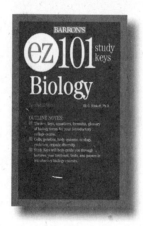
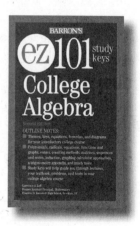